MEDICINE SCIENCES AND BIOENGINEERING

PROCEEDINGS OF THE 2014 INTERNATIONAL CONFERENCE ON MEDICINE SCIENCES AND BIOENGINEERING (ICMSB 2014), KUNMING, YUNNAN, CHINA, 16–17 AUGUST 2014

Medicine Sciences and Bioengineering

Editor

Mings Wang
Central China Normal University, China

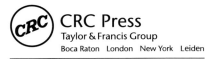

CRC Press
Taylor & Francis Group
Boca Raton   London   New York   Leiden

CRC Press is an imprint of the
Taylor & Francis Group, an **informa** business

A BALKEMA BOOK

CRC Press/Balkema is an imprint of the Taylor & Francis Group, an informa business

© 2015 Taylor & Francis Group, London, UK

Typeset by diacriTech, Chennai, India

Published by: CRC Press/Balkema
       P.O. Box 11320, 2301 EH Leiden, The Netherlands
       e-mail: Pub.NL@taylorandfrancis.com
       www.crcpress.com – www.taylorandfrancis.com

ISBN: 978-1-138-02684-1 (Hardback)
ISBN: 978-1-315-73451-4 (eBook PDF)

Table of contents

Preface   xv

Committees   xvii

Section 1: Medicine

Numerical simulation of performance for axial flow maglev blood pump   3
Z.-Q. Wang, H.-C. Wu, P. Chen, Z.-Y. Zhang & Y.-W. Ren

Design and analysis of maglev-hydrodynamic supporting for centrifugal blood pumps   7
H.-C. Wu, P. Chen, Z.-Y. Zhang & Y.-W. Ren

Anti-cancer research on *Melodinus sp.* (Apocynaceae Juss.)   13
Y. Lu, T. Bradshaw, B. Hazra, S.P. Voravuthikunchai, T. Srichan, M. Qazzaz, S. Debnath,
T.J. Khoo & C. Wiart

Behavioral research on elderly sports fitness activities   19
Y.-Q. He

Research and development of multilayer array modulation collimator for precise
radiotherapy   25
L. Lin & H.-L. Zhang

The estimations for the multifactorial interaction between factors and confidence intervals   31
X.-D. Wang & J. Tian

The protection of amyloid precursor protein 17 peptide on diabetic encephalopathy   39
D. Zhang & H. Meng

The effect of different concentrations of rocuronium bromide used for anesthesia induction on
introperative recurrent laryngeal nerve monitoring of the patients with thyroid operation   45
P. Chen, Y.-H. Pan & F. Liang

Application and prospect of process control in the modern production of Chinese
materia medical   51
M.-S. Miao, L. Guo, S. Tian, P.-F. Li & L.-L. Jiang

The wireless control system for high frequency portable X-ray machine based on MCU   57
X. Tan, Q.-C. Liu & B.-F. Xu

Bisimulation-based consistency checking on syndrome Tan-Yu-Bi-Zu in rheumatoid
arthritis between textbook and clinical practice   63
G. Zheng, L.-R. Wang, H.-H. Shi, R. Li, M. Jiang & A.-P. Lu

Farrerol improves the blood pressure, plasma biochemical indices and aortic media
thickness in spontaneously hypertensive rats   69
X.-J. Qin, X.-M. Hou, T.-G. Liang & Q.-S. Li

Application of neck elastic tourniquet in thyroid surgery   75
Y.-M. Li, W.-J. Sun & S. Yan

To explore the famous TCM doctor Wang Xing-Kuan's rule of prescriptions for
coronary heart disease on the basis of association rule — 79
H.-W. Gong, Y. Wen, J.-Y. Li, H.-Y. Qu, X. Du, L. Jiang, J.-F. Yan & J.-R. Fan

Apprehending big data of TCM from the perspective of the complexity of the symptoms — 85
H.-W. Gong, J.-H. Lu, H. Chen, Y. Wen, W.-C. Liu, X. You & J.-F. Yan

A method to measure the trans-lamina cribrosa pressure difference in rabbits — 89
*F. Zhao, C. Wang, Z. Wei, Z.-H. Liu, B.-Q. Xu, D.-Y. Yang, K.-G. Liu, N.-L. Wang &
Y.-B. Fan*

miRNAs and targets that underlie glomerular development — 93
X. Wu, Y.-F. Ding, J.-Y. Zhao, G. Guo, Y.-Q. Li, T.-B. Li, J.-L. Wang & S.-Y. Cui

Performance research of a single cell as a microreactor by microchip electrophoresis
with laser-induced fluorescence — 99
C.-T. Liang, Y. Sun, Y.-Q. Rong, S.-M. Wang & S.-W. Liang

Linear correlation analysis method of normality test for medical statistical data — 105
M. Lei & J. Zuo

A comparative study on the application of three-dimensional ultrasound to breast
intraductal lesion — 109
S.-N. Liu, G. Sun & Y.-X. Liu

Roles of different ionic currents in the automaticity of central and peripheral
sinoatrial node — 115
H. Zhang, X. Zheng, W. Zhao, D. Zhao & X. Huang

Effect of using six sigma in improving service efficiency in endoscopy departments — 121
H.-L. Ku & C.-L. Lee

Research progress in induced liver cancer model of rats — 125
*D.-F. Cao, Y. Sun, L. Wang, D.-K. Wang, Q. Wu, Y. Li, G.-Q. Huang, J.-H. Zhao,
W.-Y. Hou & Y. Jiang*

The study of gray matter lesions in multiple sclerosis via proton magnetic resonance
spectroscopy — 129
J. Ma & Z.-H. Wang

The optimization of scan parameters on head and neck in children by somatom
definition flash — 133
J. Ma, J. Ma, Y. Wang, X.-M. Mu & F.-L. Kong

Development of thoracic impedance detection system based on embedded — 137
X.-Y. Yan, T. Chen, S.-M. Gao & Y.-L. Song

Altered functional connectivity of the entorhinal cortex in mild cognitive impairment — 143
Y.-Q. Zhang, Y. Liu, C.-S. Yu & T.-Z. Jiang

Sedative and hypnotic effects of *Schisandra* polysaccharides — 149
C.-M. Wang, W.-J. Sun, H. Li, J.-H. Sun, H. Jia, J.-G. Chen & X.-T. Fan

Three polymorphisms in Programmed Cell Death 1 Ligand (PD-L1) gene are not
associated with Aplastic Anemia (AA) in Chinese Han populations — 155
*Z.-J. Ming, Y.-G. Jiang, M. Miao, W.-P. Wang, Y. Zhang, X.-G. Zhang &
Y.-H. Qiu*

Quantitative relationship between mental fatigue and sustained attention: A CPT study — 161
Y.-X. Lv, Y. Xiao & Q.-X. Zhou

vi

Standardized development of the thyroid operation anesthesia under neuromuscular
electric monitoring   167
P. Chen, Y.-H. Pan, J. Zhao & Y.-D. Han

The effect of different concentrations of vecuronium bromide used for anesthesia induction on
intraoperative recurrent laryngeal nerve monitoring of the patients with thyroid operation   173
P. Chen, Y.-H. Pan & F. Liang

Study on the determination of anticancer drug nedaplatin in a spectrophotometer   177
J. Peng, J. He, Q.-K. Wang & S.-P. Pu

Species and plant morphology, biological characteristics of Banlangen (*Radix isatidis*)
in China   181
G. Chen, S.-P. Wang, X. Huang, J. Hong, M.-H. Ge, L.-H. Zhang & L. Du

Expression changes of Hes1 of PC12 cells after OGD   187
J.-T. He, L. Yan, J.-Q. Wang, Y. Cui, Z.-S. Li, J. Mang, Y.-K. Shao & Z.-X. Xu

Cell immunophenotypic assays more accurately diagnose and classify the different
subtypes of acute leukemia   193
Q. Chi, Y.-Z. Lun & Z.-G. Yu

Conditioned medium mediated immune protection in In Vitro model of endogenous
neurotoxin N-methyl-salsolinol in an astrocyte dependent manner   199
F.-L. Wang, X.-H. Wang, F. Zeng, H. Qing & Y.-L. Deng

Analyzing couplet medicines in Ma Xiang's treatment of chronic gastritis:
Chinese prescription based on association rules   203
W.-X. Zhang, H.-H. Zhang, X.-S. Liang, L. Bian, Z.-Z. Li & Y.-F. Gu

Comprehensive rehabilitation treatment and nursing after a surgical repair of hand
tendon injuries   207
J.-H. Wang & Z.-Y. Guo

An evaluation of the safety and time-saving by the fully automatic ampoule
opening device   211
J.-H. Wang, X.-L. Li, L. Zhong & C.-P. Song

Zeta potential of different size of urinary crystallites in lithogenc patients and
healthy subjects   215
Y.-B. Li, X.-L. Wen & J.-M. Ouyang

Individualized nursing intervention in patients with chronic hepatitis C antiviral
treatment adherence   221
X.-L. Cheng, Y.-C. Cao, C.-J. Liu & Y.-F. Sun

Unexpected difficult intubation inspired by asymptomatic lingual thyroid   227
Y.-D. Han, K. Li & P. Chen

Development and validation of bioactive components of *Xiao xianggou* (*Ficus*)   231
H.-Q. Lv, X.-Z. Chen, Z.-J. Xie & C.-P. Wen

Active constituents' determination in *Schisandra chinensis* by HPLC and evaluation
of the uncertainty   237
J.Y.-X. Qin, X. Ye, C. Yan & D.-S. Gao

Reconstruction of central aortic pressure using continuous peripheral arterial blood
pressure at two separate sites on lower arms   243
C. Ma, J. Liu, P.-D. Zhang & X.-P. Yang

Experimental study on reduction of Aβ by berberine in serum and brain of diabetic rats 249
Y. Zhou, Y. Tan, L. Li, D.-X. Wang & Y. Zhao

Metabonomic characterization of aging rats by means of RRLC-Q-TOF-MS-based techniques 253
J.-H. Sun, C.-M. Wang, H. Jia, H.-X. Sun, C.-Y. Zhang, J.-G. Chen & H. Li

Precision analysis of the Nintendo Balance Board for assessment of wheelchair stability 259
X.-Z. Jiang, L.-L. Yang & C. Zhang

Blood lipid components in functional tradeoffs and risk of coronary heart disease due to type 2 diabetes mellitus 265
Q. Guo, R. Gong, G.-H. Xia, L.-M. Tian, S.-H. Zhou, L.-Y. Zhang & H.-Q. Niu

Application of problem-based learning in the clinical practice teaching of neurology 273
W. Sun & J.-L. Liu

Neuroprotective effects of Breviscapine against oxidative-stress-induced cell death in PC12 cells: Involvement of Nrf2/HO-1 pathway 277
G.-L. Jin, H.-L. Qin, H.-B. He, F. Cheng, D.-C. Gong, B. Xu, L.-L. Jia, W. Xi, H.-W. Wang & X.-F. Xing

Oxidative stress injury caused by 1800-MHz electromagnetic radiation 283
H. Liu, M.-L. Wang, R.-G. Zhong, X.-M. Ma, Q.-L. Liu, Y. Li, F. Xie & Q.-X. Hou

Clinical analysis of Baoxinbao film for elderly patients with unstable angina pectoris 289
L.-J. Guo

A preliminary study of high pressure CO_2 on the crystal transformation of heat-sensitive drugs 293
D.-D. Hu, S.-Z. Zhang, Q. Wang, H. Zhang & W.-Q. Wang

Effect of external use of fresh aloe juice on the scald model of rats 299
M.-S. Miao & L. Guo

A detection method of lung cancer—characteristic expired gases based on a cross-responsive sensor array 305
J.-C. Lei, C.-J. Hou, D.-Q. Huo, X.-G. Luo, M. Yang, Y.-J. Li & M.-Z. Bao

Detection of follicle stimulating hormone expressed in CHO cell 311
R.-M. Hua, L. Jiang & B. Zeng

The protective potential of fasudil hydrochloride in liver injury induced by intestinal ischemia reperfusion in rats 317
X. Hu, X.-F. Tian, Z. Fan, L. Chu, Y. Li, L. Lv, D.-Y. Gao & J.-H. Yao

Simulation and prediction of the material foundation of Rhubarb based on molecular docking 323
Y.-Y. Rong, L. Lu, Y.-X. Tian, J.-X. Lin, Q.-X. Guan, S.-W. Liang, L. Zhao & S.-M. Wang

Analysis of effect of Pueraria lobata flavone in the cerebral ischemia-reperfusion rats using ^{1}H-NMR-based metabonomics 331
C.-W. Wu, Q.-X. Guan, S.-M. Wang, F. Yang, L. Zhao, L. Lu & Y.-Y. Rong

Solid-phase synthesis of octapeptide GHGKHKNK 341
X. Han, M.-C. Zhang, S. Jiang, L.-P. An, G.-Y. Xv, G.-H. Wang & P.-G. Du

The anti-inflammatory activity of a natural occurring coumarin: Murracarpin 347
W.-M. Shi, H.-Q. Liu, L.-F. Li & L.-H. Wu

Complete structural assignment of a new natural product from the roots of Raphanus Sativus L.
F. Wang, H. Chen, Y.-B. Wang & S.-M. Wang
353

Pharmacokinetic analysis of five rhubarb aglycones in rat plasma after oral administration and the influence of borneol on their pharmacokinetics
F. Wang, Q.-X. Guan, L. Lu, L. Zhao, X.-S. Guo, S.-W. Liang & S.-M. Wang
357

Section 2: Bioinformatics and Biomedical Engineering

Study actuality of immune optimization algorithm
Y. Miao, H.-M. Yang, W.-L. Shi, L.-Y. Zhang & Y.-N. Cao
367

Zinc oxide nanorod biosensor for detection of Alpha Feto Protein in blood serum
A. Manoharan & S.S. Ang
373

Region-Of-Interest tomography with noisy projection data
R. Ye & Y. Tang
379

Gene biclustering based on Independent Component Analysis and Non-negative Matrix Factorization
L.-Q. Zhao, S.-J. Wan, Z.-G. Zhang, H. Jiang, X.-R. Jia & Y.-H. Zhou
385

A recognition method based on the curvature feature for identifying dental anatomical reference points from 3D digital models
A. Lv, B.-W. He, J. Yao & D. Tong
391

Bioinformatics analyses for the Mycobacterium *tuberculosis* secreted proteins prediction
L. Wang, Z. Jin & Z. Sun
397

Analyzing method of exercise intensity based on wavelet frequency band energy quotient
X.-F. Cheng, H. Yang & W. Jiang
403

Neuroprotective effects against ischemia injury derived from Smad7-modulated ActA/Smads pathway activation
Y.-K. Shao, Z.-H. Xu, Y.-M. Wang, Y.-T. Wang, J.-Q. Wang, C.-L. Mei, J. Mang & J.-T. He
409

Structure of clustering based on inquiry of TCM data storage management system in wireless sensor network
J.-Q. Liang & J.-C. He
415

A simple enzyme glucose biosensor based on Ag doped Fe_3O_4 nanoparticles
Y.-Y. Li, J. Han, P. Wang, K. Li & Y.-H. Dong
421

Design and implementation of a cursor control system based on steady-state visual evoked potential
X. Zou, Q.-G. Wei & Z.-W. Lu
427

Design of a tonometer pressing force measuring device
J.-H. Zhao, Y.-J. Wang, J. Zhang & J.-G. Ma
435

From "unusual sequences" to human diseases
F.-J. Huang & Z.-Z. Wu
443

Modeling of virtual spine based on multi-body dynamics
F. Pan, Z. Gao, C. Ding, J.-Z. Wang & J.-H. Wang
449

Image registration based on weighted residual complexity using local entropy
J. Zhang, M.-H. Zhang, W. Yang & Z.-T. Lu
455

Preparation of modified TiO_2 nanorods and research of light photocatalytic activity
M.-J. Li, X.-Y. Cui, Y.-K. Yin, S.-Z. Rong, X.-D. Jin, Q.-H. Wu & Y.-H. Hao
461

Gradient projection method on Electrical Impedance Tomography   465
D.-Y. Jiang, H. Xu, Z. Zhou & N. Li

Multidimensional multigranularity data mining for health-care service management   469
J. K. Chiang & C.-C. Chu

Packed fiber solid-phase extraction of monoamine neurotransmitters in human plasma
using composite nanofibers composed of polyvinyl pyrrolidone and polystyrene as
sorbent prior to HPLC-fluorescence detection   505
X.-X. Wu, K.-W. Shen, J.-J. Deng, Y. Wang, L. Ma & X.-J. Kang

Exploring the treatment laws of Sinomenium Acutum through text mining   481
N. Ge, G. Zheng, A.-R. Qi, D. Yang, S.-D. Yang, W.-J. Wang & S.-M. Li

Biomechanical research on treatment of fracture of femoral shaft   489
X.-Y. Wang & J.-H. Zhou

Locating robot capsule looped by magnet ring   495
W.-A. Yang, Y. Li, C. Hu & F.-Q. Qin

Establishment of an innovative personnel training platform by virtue of the laboratory
built by central and local government together   501
H. Li, W.-J. Sun, C.-M. Wang, J.-H. Sun, H. Jia, H.-X. Sun, C.-Y. Zhang, X.-T. Fan &
J.-G. Chen

Extraction, isolation, purification and structure of a new polysaccharide from
Hypomesus olidus   505
X.-Y. Guan & X.-J. Liu

Practice and reflection in the diagnostic bilingual teaching   513
X.-X. Du, W.-J. Sun & C.-M. Wang

Exploration of pharmacy graduation design quality assurance system   517
J.-H. Sun, G.-H. Wang & G.-Y. Xu

Practice and reflection on the integration and optimization of general surgery
teaching course system   521
S. Jing, W.-J. Sun & W.-H. Jiang

Antibacterial property of silver nanoparticles with block copolymer shells   525
X.-L. Li, B.-G. Dai, H.-X. Zhang, R. Wang, S.-L. Yuan & X. Li

Effect of chiral N-isobutyryl-cysteine on PC12 cells response   529
J. Mang, J.-Q. Wang, H.-Y. Lui, J.-T. He, Y.-K. Shao & Z.-X. Xu

Induction of Programmed Cell Death through mitochondria-dependent pathways
in Tamba black soybean (Glycine max)   533
J.-J. Li, L. Zhang, J.-J. Zhang, P. Wang, L.-M. Chen & H.-J. Nian

Considering geometric transformations in noninvasive ultrasonic measurement of
arterial elasticity   539
L.-L. Niu, M. Qian, L. Meng, Y. Xiao, X.-W. Huang & H.-R. Zheng

The improved mosaic algorithm for spine medical image based on the SUFR   543
H.-M. Liu, J.-H. Zhang & J.-H. Gong

Interaction of IVIG and camptothecin   551
Y.-C. Liu, X.-X. Wei, X.-Y. Xu, X.-J. Yao, R.-X. Lei, X.-D. Zheng & J.-N. Liu

Reduction of dopamine increases methylglyoxal-induced mitochondrial dysfunction in SH-SY5Y cells 559
B.-J. Xie, F.-K. Lin, K. Ullah, L. Peng, H. Qing & Y.-L. Deng

A sensitive determination of 1-acetyl-6,7-dihydroxyl-1,2,3,4-tetrahydroisoquinoline (ADTIQ) in rat substantia nigra by Multiple Reaction Monitoring (MRM) 565
B.-J. Xie, H.-Y. Wu, K. Ullah, L. Peng, H. Qing & Y.-L. Deng

Effect of unitary, binary and ternary carboxylates on crystal phase selection in the process of calcium oxalate crystallization 571
Y.-B. Li, Q.-Z. Gan & J.-M. Ouyang

On-chip microbubble destruction by surface acoustic waves 577
L. Meng, F.-Y. Cai, F. Li, L.-L. Niu & H.-R. Zheng

Assessing Cerebral Auto-regulation using Least angle regression 581
X.-C. Wu, J. Liu, P.-D. Zhang & X.-P. Yang

Importance of bioinformatics in modernization of Traditional Chinese Medicine 587
Y. Bai, Z.-Y. Xin, G.-H. Cui, C.-H. Sui, W.-L. Li, S.-F. Dong, L.-Q. Han, W.-X. Zhao & G.-Y. Xu

Application of case-based learning model in the clinical practice of orthopedic graduates 591
W.-H. Jiang & W. Sun

The effect of 1800 MHz electromagnetic radiation on telomerase expression in NIH/3T3 cells 595
Y. Li, M.-L. Wang, Q.-L. Liu, Q.-X. Hou & H. Liu

A reliable method for cloud data storage security 599
F. Yang & Y.-T. Rao

Thinking on strengthening university library health information service model innovation in the age of big data 603
J.-Y. Lu, J.-Z. Zhou, H.-L. Ruan & G.-C. Luo

Application of synthetic index method in the evaluation of rational drug use in primary health institutions 607
S. Wang & G. Gao

Study on near infrared spectroscopy to detect cerebral blood oxygen parameter in computing task 613
C.-J. Guo

Differences in medical education teaching between China and Japan 619
S. Jing, W.-J. Sun, J.-G. Chen & H. Li

Improvement of medical students' cultivation in international exchange 623
X.-D. Qiu, W.-J. Sun, W.-Y. Zhao, X.-X. Du & S.-W. Zhao

Optimization for fundus molecular imaging 627
Y.-H. Liu, P. Zhang, D.-M. Xie, T.-C. Wang & Z.-X. Xie

BDNF of the hippocampal CA3 relates to the spatial memory in rats exposed to music 633
Y.-S. Xing, Y. Xia & D.-Z. Yao

Section 3: Ecology, Environment and Chemistry

Differential microbial community complexity levels between different locations in the GuJingGong pits 641
K.-Q. Li, H.-M. Zhang, A.-J. Li, H.-K. He, Q.-W. Zhou & Z.-Z. Zhang

Effect of ultrasonic pretreatment on the oil removal of ASP flooding produced water 647
F.-J. Xia

Antibiotics-resistant profiles of airborne *enterococcus faecalis* in an enclosed-type Chicken shed 653
Z.-M. Miao, S. Li, Y.-J. Tang & R.-M. Wang

GC-MS fingerprint of *Acanthopanax brachypus* in China 657
H.-B. Hu, X.-D. Zheng, H.-S. Hu & Y. Wu

Research and practice of diversified pharmaceutical talent training model 663
H.-Q. Wang & P.-G. Du

Antioxidant study of the polysaccharides from *Cordyceps militaris*, natural quercetin and N-acetylneuraminic acid 667
S.-D. Guo

Stability and antimicrobial activity of microencapsulated clove oil 671
Q.-L. Xu, Y.-G. Xing, D. Cao, D.-F. Zhang, Z.-M. Che, W.-F. Han, Y. Meng, H.-B. Lin & L. Jiang

Research on the test of gas emission control method of vehicular pyrolysis furnace for medical waste 677
L.-H. Wu, J.-S. Han & Z. Wang

Study for problems and solutions of the paperless electronic prescription 683
A.-N. Li & S.-L. Hu

Detection of genetically modified herbicide tolerant soybeans using multiplex-nested PCR 687
Y.-W. Qiu, M.-H. Zhang, Y. Liu, Z. Zhen, A.-X. Wang, X.-J. Gao & Y.-B. Yu

Research on the effect of attracting insects about the composite LED lamppost 693
W.-B. Qiu & S.-Y. Lin

Changes of functional connectivity patterns of V1 with eyes open and closed 697
J.-J. Wang & T.-Z. Jiang

Production of L-lactic acid by *Escherichia coli* JH12 using rice straw hydrolysate as carbon source 701
Y. Liu, X. Zhao, J.-J. Gu, J.-H. Wang, S.-D. Zhou & W. Gao

Study on the multiple wavelength HPLC integration fingerprint of active fractions from a purified sample of Naodesheng 705
B. Liu, Z.-C. Li, C. Chen, S.-M. Wang & S.-W. Liang

Kinetics study of glutathione peroxidase 4 mutant using H_2O_2 as oxidizing substrate 713
X. Guo, Z.-L. Fan, Y. Yu, Y.-L. Zhang, S. Wang, C. Ma, J.-Y. Wei, J. Song, R.-Q. Xing, D.-L. Liu & H.-W. Song

Study on the job satisfaction of public health staff 719
W.-J. Zhong, W.-D. Yang & B. Li

Study on extracts constituents of *nux prinsepiae uniflorae* 723
Y. Wu, X.-D. Zheng, H.-B. Hu & J.-Y. Zhao

Optimization of fermentation conditions for bacteriocin production by *Lactobacillus plantarum* 727
L.-X. Jie, H. Liu, T. Han, H.-X. Zhang & Y.-H. Xie

Study on characteristic of apple pectins of pH-modification and heat-modification 733
J. Dou, Y.-R. Guo, J. Li, L. Liu & H. Deng

Study on kinetics of sludge reduction in domestic wastewater with nitrogen
removal filler 737
L.-H. Gao, J.-M. Liu, H.-Z. Wang, J.-J. Wang, L. Shi & Y.-L. Shen

Effect of steam blanching on drying characteristics of Jin Yin Hua, the flower bud of
Lonicera japonica Thunb. 743
Z.-H. Liu, X.-S. Wen, G.-D. Wei & Y.-Q. Zhang

Optimization of oligonucleotide pools amplification for SELEX 749
C.-X. Zhang, X.-F. Lv, X.-H. Wang, H. Qing & Y.-L. Deng

Antioxidant responses of two *in vitro* shoots of snow lotus (*Saussurea involucrata*
Kar.et Kir.) to salt stress 753
Y. Ou, L. Zhao, J. Sun, X.-C. Zhao & J. Ye

Research progress on chemical compositions of *Hymenocallis littoralis* 759
Y.-B. Ji, Y.-B. Liang, N. Chen, D. Zhao, D.-X. Song, C.-R. Xu & X.-M. Cao

A study on the influence of living habits on indoor air quality 763
W.-H. Wang, J. Xu & J.-S. Liang

Separation of polysaccharide from wolfberry fruit and determination by infrared
spectroscopy based on nonlinear modeling 769
H. Zhang, Z.-T. Xu & H.-S. Zhao

Transformation of trichothecene acetyldeoxynivalenol to deoxynivalenol by bacterial
acetyltransferase 775
W. Wang, S.S.M. Soliman, X.-Z. Li, H.-H. Zhu, L. Yang, Y.-L. Yin & T. Zhou

Binuclear lanthanide complexes derived from aroylhydrazines with
8-hydroxyquinoline-2-carboxaldehyde and a series of DNA intercalators 783
R.-X. Lei, D.-P. Ma, X.-W. Zhang, Y.-C. Liu, X.-D. Zheng, J.-N. Liu & Z.-Y. Yang

Analysis of two pairs of grape early-ripening bud sports varieties based on iPBS markers 793
D.-L. Guo & X.-Y. Zhang

Antimicrobial characters of bacteriocin produced by *Streptococcus lactis* S5-3 799
J.-C. Zhang, H. Liu, Y.-H. Xie & H-X. Zhang

Quality characteristics of WCA and PCA during cold storage 805
Y.-Y. Li, Y.-R. Guo, G. Bai, J. Dou & H. Deng

Ionic liquids improve the biotransformation of isoeugenol to vanillin by *Bacillus
fusiformis* CGMCC1347 811
L.-Q. Zhao, R.-X. Chen, Y.-L. Chen, J.-M. Fang, W.-B. Chen & J.-F. Wang

New method for producing diosgenin 817
X. Li, L.-P. Wang, C.-L. Shi & B. Zhang

Sulfate-reducing bacteria anaerobic metabolism carbon source test of Huainan coal 821
C. Qi, X.-G. Ge, S. Liu, G.-X. Zhao, L. Yang & Y.-K. Ye

Optimization of PCR-SSCP analysis conditions on the analysis of microbial
communities of the strong-flavor Chinese liquor fermentation 829
X.-X. Chen & L. Yuan

Author index 837

Medicine Sciences and Bioengineering – Wang (Ed.)
© *2015 Taylor & Francis Group, London, ISBN: 978-1-138-02684-1*

Preface

The 2014 International Conference on Medicine Sciences and Bioengineering (ICMSB2014) was held in Kunming, Yunnan, China on August 16-17, 2014. ICMSB2014 was aimed at researchers, engineers, industry professionals and academics, who were broadly welcomed to present their latest research results, academic developments or theory practice. Topics of interest include but are not limited to Medicine, Bioinformatics, and Biomedical Engineering. It was a great pleasure to see the delegates exchanging ideas and establishing sound relationships at the conference.

All the accepted papers are now published as a conference proceeding volume by CRC Press / Balkema (Taylor & Francis Group). The review process has been extremely strict and was operated by a peer-review group made up of 2-3 experts in the related fields. The acceptance of full drafts was approved according to a combination of various standards including originality, structure, novelty, expression, etc. All this hard work led to a rich and profound conference program consisting of oral presentations and poster exhibitions. We sincerely hope that ICMSB2014 will not merely serve as a platform for academic communication, but also as an opportunity for international business cooperation and mutual benefit.

The final conference program comprised 151 papers divided into 3 sessions. Thanks to the great endeavor of all the TPC members, the review process ran smoothly and properly, thus each and every paper was reviewed before the review deadline.

Heartfelt thanks are also extended to all the volunteers and staff, without whose long hours' hard work, the conference would not have been such an obvious success. Last but not least, we would also like to express our sincere gratitude to all the participants, speakers, authors, and presenters for their constant support and valued contributions to the conference.

ICMSB2014 Organizing Committee

Medicine Sciences and Bioengineering – Wang (Ed.)
© 2015 Taylor & Francis Group, London, ISBN: 978-1-138-02684-1

Committees

Technical Program Committee

General Chair

Professor Cuie Wen
Professor of Surface Engineering
Faculty of Science, Engineering and Technology
School of Engineering
Industrial Research Institute Swinburne
Swinburne University of Technology
Hawthorn, VIC, Australia

Yuncang Li, *Institute for Frontier Materials, Deakin University, Australia*
E.G. Rajan, *Pentagram Research Centre Pvt Ltd, India*
V.K. Bairagi, *University of Pune, India*
Jubaraj Bikash Baruah, *Indian Institute of Technology Guwahati, India*
Shihua Zhang, *Academy of Mathematics and Systems Science, Chinese Academy of Science, China*
N. Dinesh Kumar, *Vignan Institute of Technology & Science, JNTU Hyderabad, India*
C.T. Kavitha, *Sree Sastha Institute of Engineering and Technology, Affiliated to Anna University, India*
Chen De-yu, *Nantong University, China*
Rachad M. Shoucri, *Royal Military College of Canada, Canada*
Bing-Huei Chen, *College of Human Ecology, Fu Jen Catholic University, Taiwan*
Shu-Yen Wan, *Chang Gung University, Taiwan*
Ahmad Yusairi Bani Hashim, *Universiti Teknikal Malaysia Melaka, Malaysia*
Po-Hsun Cheng, *National Kaohsiung Normal University, Taiwan*
Selcuk Comlekci, *Süleyman Demirel University, Turkey*
J.M. Garcia-Aznar, *Universidad de Zaragoza, Spain*
Elena Zaitseva, *University of Zilina, Slovakia*
Burhan Ergen, *Firat University, Turkey*
Erlong Yu, *Anhui University of Engineering Science & Technology, China*
Jincheng Zhang, *Light Engineering Institute of Zhengzhou, China*
Ryohei Yoneyama, *University of Kitakyushu, Japan*
Tingting Gu, *Finance and Economics Institute of the Inner Mongol, China*
Wenxin Bai, *He'nan University of Technology, China*
Norma J. Richmond, *University of North Texas, USA*
Takeshi Taniguchi, *Ryukoku University, Japan*
Warren Murphy, *Southampton Solent University, UK*
Dawei Miao, *University of Xiangtan, China*
Linjiang Jiang, *Yang'en University, China*
Yanhua Zhu, *Technical College of Zhuzhou, China*
Zhe Wei, *Western Anhui University, China*

Yazheng Zhou, *Guangxi Technical College, China*
Yongqin Sun, *University of Science and Technology of Hebei, China*
Wu Huang, *Five City University, China*
Zhaoquan Li, *Hainan Medical College, China*
Jinqiu Song, *Hebei University of Technology, China*
Lan Liu, *Fujian Normal University, China*

Medicine

Medicine Sciences and Bioengineering – Wang (Ed.)
© *2015 Taylor & Francis Group, London, ISBN: 978-1-138-02684-1*

Numerical simulation of performance for axial flow maglev blood pump

Zhi-qiang Wang, Hua-chun Wu*, Pu Chen, Zheng-yuan Zhang & Yong-wu Ren
School of Mechanical and Electrical Engineering, Wuhan University of Technology, Wuhan, Hubei Province, China

ABSTRACT: To solve the existing problems of mechanical bearings used for blood pumps such as friction and wear, which lead to short life and heating and cause thrombosis and hemolysis, a hybrid maglev supporting structure that consists of radial permanent magnetic bearing and axial hybrid magnetic bearing for axial flow maglev blood pump was designed. Performance analysis of radial permanent magnetic bearing by using the three-dimensional software ANSYS has been studied. Moreover, computational fluid dynamics analysis was performed to quantify the hydro-dynamics of an axial flow maglev blood pump. The hybrid magnetic bearing structures of an axial flow blood pump were designed. Simulation results show that permanent magnetic bearing could ensure the rotor was suspended at the radial position. The pressure performance curve demonstrates the ability of an axial flow maglev blood pump to deliver adequate flow rates with desired increases in pressure. This result provides an important basis for structure design and hemolysis issue improvement of an axial flow maglev blood pump.

1 INTRODUCTION

A blood pump is an important part of any ventricular assist device. At present, the blood pump used in clinical practice is a mechanical pump, which has more advantages such as simple structure, small size, and high reliability (Qu Zheng et al., 2008). But the existing problem of mechanical bearings such as friction and wear will lead to short life and heating and cause thrombosis and hemolysis (Boyang Su & Zengsheng Chen, 2013). Magnetic bearings with no mechanical contacting have been used in the rotor supporting of blood pumps as a means to extend pump life by eliminating material wear, decreasing heat generation, and minimizing both red blood cell damage and formation of blood clots. The blood cells can flow freely through the blood pump without being exposed to stresses induced by mechanical bearings. As a subset of artificial blood pumps, maglev axial blood pumps have recently gained tremendous interest due to absence of friction, low heat generation, no need for lubrication, quiet operation, and fast and stable rotation by active control.

Many kinds of blood pumps have been proposed for a long time. Fan Hui-min presented a new implantable axial flow blood pump. A mathematical model was established to simulate flow across the blood pump (Fan Hui-min, 2009). Guan Yong employed an axial flow maglev blood pump that was suspended by two radial permanent magnetic bearings (PMBs) and one axial active magnetic bearing. The blood pump rotor was stably suspended in five degrees of freedom. However, the regions between inducer and impeller and impeller and diffuser were prone to blood stagnation, resulting in thrombus (Guan Yong, 2011). Cheng Shanbao designed a hybrid magnetic bearing (HMB) for a magnetically levitated blood pump, and radial active control and axial pas-sive control could be implemented by the HMB (Cheng Shanbo, 2011). Based on the principle of simple structure, lightweight, and low power consumption, a hybrid maglev supporting structure

---

*Corresponding author: whc@whut.edu.cn

consisting of radial PMB and axial HMB for axial flow maglev blood pump was developed. The method could simplify the blood pump structure and the control system, which facilitates the blood pump implanted in the human body.

2 STRUCTURE OF AXIAL FLOW MAGLEV BLOOD PUMP

The axial flow maglev blood pump is shown in Figure 1. Hybrid maglev supporting structures consist of radial PMB and axial HMB. Each PMB is composed of inner and outer rings; the inner rings were mounted on the rotor body within the impeller hub, and the outer rings were mounted on the runner shell of the blood pump. The radial position of the impeller rotor was controlled by the PMB, and the axial position of the rotor was controlled by the HMB. HMB is a magnetic bearing system formed by active magnetic bearing and a permanent magnet assembly. The method combines the good dynamic performance of active magnetic bearing with the high-density, small-for-size, and non-power-consuming characteristics of PMB.

The fluid structure of a blood pump consists of an inducer region to reduce the tangential flow components and thus avoid flowing prerotation into the pump. The impeller is to impart fluid kinetic energy to the fluid. The diffuser is to provide an adequate pressure head, increase the hydraulic efficiency, and reduce the exit velocity of blood.

In order to improve the performance of the axial flow maglev blood pump, we have optimized the structure design. The three-dimensional structure of the axial flow maglev blood pump is shown in Figure 2.

3 RESULTS AND DISCUSSION

3.1 Levitation performance of radial permanent magnetic bearing

The radial bearing has two pairs of permanent magnet rings (Zhong Wending & Xia Pingchou, 2000). The magnet pairs were placed at the two ends of the motor. Radial bearing capacity curves and axial bearing capacity curves with different displacements are shown in Figure 3.

Figure 3 reveals that no radial force is produced when there is no radial displacement. When the rotor of PMB has a radial displacement, a repulsive force is developed to push the rotor back

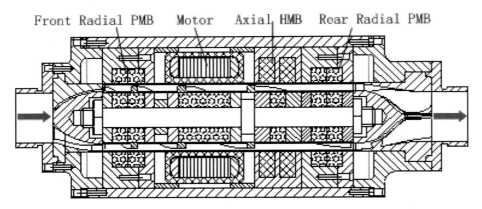

Figure 1.   Schematic of axial flow maglev blood pump

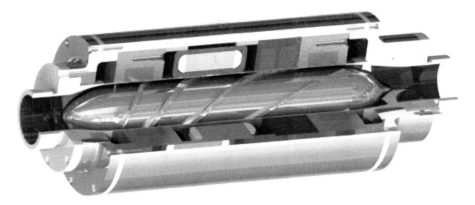

Figure 2.　Three-dimensional structure of axial flow maglev blood pump

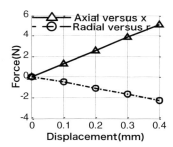

Figure 3.　Force curves with different displacements

to the center. The radial force is approximately proportional to the biased position from the center, and the radial stiffness of the radial magnetic bearings is approximately −5.5 N/mm. In addition, it can be seen that no axial force is produced when there is no axial displacement. When the rotor of PMB has an axial displacement, a repulsive force is developed to push the rotor to deviate the center position. The axial force is approximately proportional to the axial displacement. Figure 3 also indicates that the bearing is radially stable and axially unstable.

3.2　Hydrodynamic performance

Figure 4 illustrates the relationship between static pressure rise and flow rate at each rotational speed of the axial flow maglev blood pump. The numerical simulation condition was the steady state for a specific flow rate and rotational speed. The pressure rise of the axial flow maglev blood pump was determined for flow rates of 3–6 L/min over the rotational speed of 10000–14000 r/min with the standard k-ε turbulence model. When the rotor of the blood pump is maintained at a given rotational speed, the static pressure head across the blood pump decreases with the increase in flow rate due to flow losses. At the equal flow rate, the static pressure across the blood pump will rise in tandem with the increasing of rotational speed. The pressure performance curve demonstrates the ability of the axial flow maglev blood pump to deliver adequate flow rate with desired pressure increases.

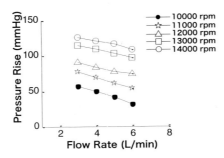

Figure 4.   Pressure rise–flow rate curves

4   SUMMARY

A hybrid maglev supporting structure with radial PMB and axial HMB for the axial flow maglev blood pump was designed. Simulation results show that radial PMB could ensure that the rotor was suspended at the radial position. The pressure performance curve demonstrates the ability of the axial flow maglev blood pump to deliver adequate flow rate with desired pressure increases. However, the performance of HMB should be studied in the future using the three-dimensional analysis software ANSYS and experiments. The entire supporting structure needs to further optimize the design layout to reduce the coupling between electromagnetic bearing and PMB. The rotation characteristics of the rotor need to be verified by further experiments.

ACKNOWLEDGMENTS

The project was supported by the National Natural Science Foundation of China (grant number 51275371), the Fundamental Research Funds for the Central Universities (WUT: 2014-IV-103 and 2014-zy-059).

REFERENCES

Boyang Su & Leok Poh Chua. (2013) Numerical studies of an axial flow blood pump with different diffuser designs. *Journal of Mechanics in Medicine and biology*, [Online] 13 (3), 1350029-1—1350029-16. Available from: doi: 10.1142/S0219519413500292 [Accessed 24th December 2012].

Cheng Shanbo & Mark W. (2011) Optimization of a hybrid magnetic bearing for a magnetically levitated blood pump via 3-DFEA. *Mechatronics*. [Online] 21(2), 1163–1169. Available from: www.elsevier.com/locate/mechatronics [Accessed 1st September 2011].

Fan Hui-min & Hong Fang-wen. (2009) Design of implantable axial-flow blood pump and numerical studies on its performance. *Journal of Hydrodynamics,* [Online] 21(4), 445–452. Available from: doi: 10.1016/S1001-6058(08)60170-5 [Accessed August 2009].

Guan Yong & Li Hongwei. (2011) System design of magnetic bearing system in an axial-flow artificial blood pump. *Journal of Shandong University (Engineering Science)*, 41(1), 151–155.

Katharine H. Fraser & Tao Zhang. (2012) A quantitative comparison of mechanical blood damage parameters in rotary ventricular assist devices: shear stress, exposure time and hemolysis index. *Journal of biomechanical engineering*, [Online] 134(5), 081002-1–081002-11. Available from: http://biomechanical.asmedigitalcollection.asme.org/ on 06/21/2013 Terms of Use: http://asme.org/terms [Accessed August 2008].

Qu Zheng. (2008) *Mechanical Circulatory Support of Modern Treatment of Heart Failure*. Beijing, Science and Technology Literature Publishing House.

Xia Pingchou. (2000) *Permanent Magnetic Actuator*. Beijing. Beijing University of Technology Press.

Zhong Wending. (2000) *Ferromagnetic*. Beijing. Sciences Publishing House.

Zengsheng Chen & Zhaohui Yao. (2013) Hemolysis analysis of axial blood pumps with various structure impellers. *Journal of Mechanics in Medicine and Biology*, [Online] 13(4), 1350054-1–1350054-15. Available from: doi: 10.1142/S0219519413500541 [Accessed 7th May 2013].

Medicine Sciences and Bioengineering – Wang (Ed.)
© 2015 Taylor & Francis Group, London, ISBN: 978-1-138-02684-1

Design and analysis of maglev-hydrodynamic supporting for centrifugal blood pumps

Hua-chun Wu*, Pu Chen, Zheng-yuan Zhang & Yong-wu Ren

School of Mechanical and Electrical Engineering, Wuhan University of Technology, Wuhan, Hubei Province, China

ABSTRACT: Problems of active magnetic bearings used for centrifugal blood pumps exist, such as large size and high power consumption. This paper presents a maglev-hydrodynamic supporting structure for centrifugal blood pumps, which uses both Permanent Magnetic Bearings (PMBs) and hydrodynamic bearings to suspend the impeller. The structure parameters and suspension characteristics of PMBs are analyzed and discussed. The research results show that the axial displacement of the two permanent magnets has an influence on bearing capacity and bearing stiffness of the radial permanent bearing. Using multiple pairs of permanent magnets can improve bearing capacity and bearing stiffness of permanent bearings. When the whole height of the magnetic body is a constant, the single permanent magnet height value is equivalent to the radial thickness value between internal and external permanent magnets, and bearing capacity and bearing stiffness of the radial permanent bearings are the largest.

1   INTRODUCTION

Heart failure treatments generally include heart transplantation, ventricular mechanical assistance, artificial organs' substitution, and so on. Although heart transplantation is a relatively mature technology, there is a serious shortage of donated hearts, which ultimately restricts the technology's applications. Therefore, for supporting the blood circulation of heart failure patients, various kinds of blood pumps have been developed and used at the clinical stage.

These can win over plenty of time for the patients who are awaiting the donor heart. So, blood pumps have been a significant means of saving those patients.

Currently, blood pumps have been developed to the third generation (QU Zheng, 2008, and Hoshi H, 2006). The most important feature of the third generation is that noncontact bearings are applied. When the pump operates, the impeller is suspended and has no physical contact with the pump casing, which can solve the problem of service life, blood damage, etc. Depending on the levitation principle, the third-generation blood pump can be categorized into three types: (i) maglev blood pump, (ii) hydrodynamic suspended blood pump, and (iii) maglev-hydrodynamic suspended blood pump. Although hydrodynamic bearings do not need to provide additional energy and control strategy for the suspension and have low power consumption, high reliability, strong shock resistance, etc., because of their complete dependence on the hydraulic suspension, their gaps are smaller, which results in high shear and hemolysis, and they have difficulty in eliminating thrombosis on account of the smaller gap that is not easily completely flushed; besides, the stability of the hydrodynamic bearing also needs to be further studied (RUAN Xiaodong, 2010). The maglev blood pump is suspended by magnetic force, according to Earnshaw's theory (Earnshaw, 1842), and the impeller cannot be suspended steadily only by permanent magnets. In order to maintain the stability of the system, at least one direction of the motion is supported by active magnetic bearings to restrict the degree of freedom. Therefore, all maglev blood pumps at present

---

*Corresponding author: whc@whut.edu.cn

have an active control system, including sensor, controller, electromagnet, etc. Inevitably, a series of problems arises, i.e., large dimensions, high heat generation, and power consumption, which restricts the development of the maglev blood pump.

For the above problems, hydrodynamic suspension is introduced on the basis of the structure of the maglev to balance the force generated by active magnetic bearings. So, a maglev-hydrodynamic centrifugal blood pump was designed, and we studied the maglev supporting properties through the analysis of three-dimensional static magnetic field coupling.

2 MATERIALS AND METHODS

2.1 Maglev-hydrodynamic supporting for centrifugal blood pump

The maglev-hydrodynamic suspension centrifugal blood pump relies on the motor to drive the impeller to rotate, so the mechanical energy of the motor is transmitted to the blood. Radial PMBs are applied to support the impeller in the radial direction of the blood pump, as a result of the interaction between the axial dynamic pressure generated by the unique structure of the impeller during operation of the pump and the axial force generated by the axial displacement of radial permanent magnetic bearing; the impeller is supported in the axial direction of the blood pump, and the structure is shown in Figure 1.

When the maglev-hydrodynamic suspension centrifugal blood pump operates, blood is brought into the hydrodynamic wedge plane, impeller is separated from the pump casing by the pressure of the liquid film, and hydrodynamic force is generated. When the hydrodynamic force and the axial maglev force keep balance, the impeller will stay in balance in the axial direction. Radial permanent magnet bearings keep the impeller in balance in the radial direction, so the impeller is suspended steadily in the pump cavity; the structure of the centrifugal blood pump is shown in Figure 2.

However, because the liquid pressure of the flow path is uneven, the impeller experiences radial hydraulic eccentric force, which results in a certain offset in the radial direction. If the bearing capacity and stiffness of the radial bearing are small, the impeller has difficulty in resisting the disturbance of blood, so it will lose stability. In order to solve the problem, multipairs permanent magnets are applied to improve the bearing capacity and stiffness of permanent bearings.

2.2 Structure of permanent magnetic bearings for centrifugal blood pumps

Radial PMBs are generally composed of a pair of high-powered magnetic rings that are arranged repulsively, using the magnetic field or the magnetic flux density generated by permanent magnetic rings in the air gap so that the rotor is suspended stably and ensuring that two magnetic rings are not in contact when revolving, thereby reducing motive friction; the structure is shown in Figure 3(a).

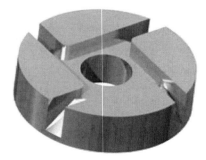

Figure 1:   Impeller structure

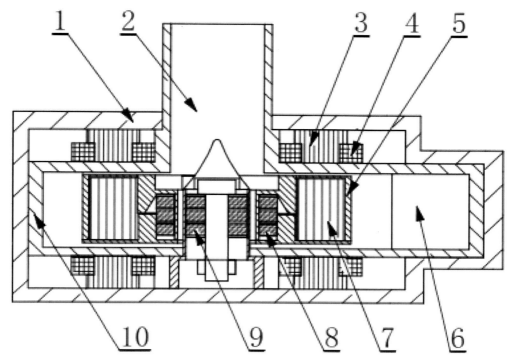

Figure 2:　Blood pump structure

Note: Figure 2 includes pump casing 1, inlet 2, electromagnet 3, coil 4, impeller 5, outlet 6, motor magnetic steel 7, dynamic magnetic ring 8, static magnetic ring 9, and pump cavity 10.

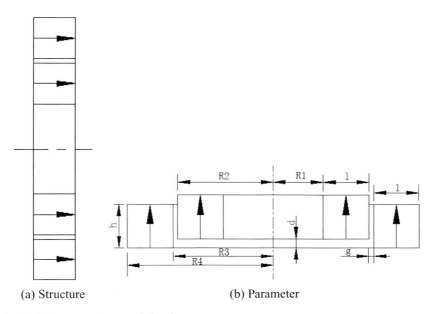

(a) Structure　　　　　　　(b) Parameter

Figure 3:　Radial permanent magnetic bearing

Compared with active magnetic bearings, the permanent magnetic bearing has advantages such as simple structure, low cost, zero response time, etc. Furthermore, an axial displacement exists between two magnetic rings of the permanent magnetic bearing (Figure 3(b)), generated the axial force to make the impeller rotor suspend to the top pump casing. When the pump operates, blood is brought into the hydrodynamic wedge plane and the pressure of the liquid film pushes the impeller away from the top pump casing; as the hydrodynamic force and the axial maglev force keep balance, the impeller stays in balance in the axial direction. The magnetic rings made of high-powered permanent magnetic materials, such as the rare earth elements rubidium, iron, and boron, are magnetized axially.

When the magnetized directions of the two magnetic rings are parallel, using the equivalent magnetic charge method, the universal computational formula of the axial force of bearing is obtained as follows (SUN Lijun, 2005):

$$F_Z = -\frac{J^2 P}{8\pi\mu_0}[2\Phi(d) - \Phi(d+h) - \Phi(d-h)] \tag{1}$$

Where

$$l = R_2 - R_1 = R_4 - R_3 \tag{2}$$

$$P = 2\pi(R_2 + g/2) \tag{3}$$

$$\Phi(x) = (2l+g)\arctan\frac{2l+g}{x} - 2(l+g)\arctan\frac{l+g}{x} +$$
$$g\arctan\frac{g}{x} - \frac{x}{2}[\ln((2l+g)^2 + x^2) - 2\ln(l+g)^2 +$$
$$\ln(g^2 + x^2)] \tag{4}$$

The radial stiffness of bearing is as follows (CAO Guangzhong, 2007):

$$K_r = -\frac{dF_r}{dr} = -\frac{J^2 P}{8\pi\mu_0}[2f(d) - f(d+h) - f(d-h)] \tag{5}$$

Where $f(x)$ is as follows:

$$f(x) = \ln\frac{[(2l+g^2) + x^2](g^2 + x^2)}{[(l+g)^2 + x^2]} \tag{6}$$

Where J represents the magnetized intensity of dynamic and static magnetic rings, P represents the average circumference of dynamic and static magnetic rings, μ_0 represents the vacuum permeability, h represents the magnet thickness, l represents the radial thickness of dynamic and static magnetic rings, g represents the unilateral air gap of dynamic and static magnetic rings, and d represents the axial displacement.

The equations (1) and (5) show that the force F_z is zero when the axial displacement d is zero; at the same time, the radial stiffness K_r becomes maximum and F_z increases as the value of d increases. Under certain conditions, the radial stiffness K_r can be effectively improved by increasing P, h, and l and reducing g and d. Further optimization analysis shows that the values of the optimal design dimension of the magnet thickness h and the radial thickness l of bearing are equivalent.

For a pair of permanent magnets, the bearing capacity of permanent magnetic bearing is quite limited, so usually using multipairs permanent magnets can practically improve bearing capacity and bearing stiffness of PMB. This paper adopts the radial permanent magnetic bearing of repulsion that is magnetized and superposed axially.

3 PERMANENT MAGNETIC BEARINGS' PROPERTIES OF CENTRIFUGAL BLOOD PUMP

The properties of PMB include bearing capacity and stiffness, which are the most important performance index of PMB. The suspension properties of permanent magnetic bearing are interrelated to their material characteristics and the structural configuration. The structural configuration mainly refers to the geometrical dimensions and the relative position of the static and dynamic magnetic rings.

ANSYS software is employed to analyze the support properties of radial PMBs. In order to resolve the limit of dimension for blood pumps, the pair count of magnetic rings is changed; but the total height of magnets is kept constant, which can improve the suspension properties of PMBs. Figure 4 shows the relationship curve of axial displacement and axial force of radial PMBs consisting of one, two, and three pairs of permanent magnet rings. When the axial displacement is 0.5 mm, the axial force of a PMB consisting of one pair of magnetic rings is 2.2 N, that of two pairs is 4.2 N, and that of three pairs is 2.4 N. Obviously, the performance of two pairs is optimized.

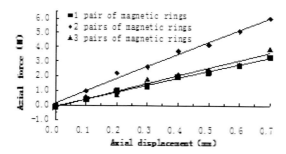

Figure 4:   Relation of force and displacement in the axial direction

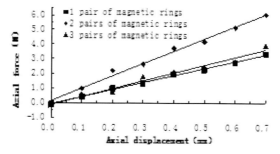

Figure 5:   Relation of force and displacement in the radial direction

Note: Figure 5 shows the relationship curve of the radial force and radial stiffness of radial PMB consisting of 1, 2, and 3 pairs of permanent magnetic rings changing with radial displacement. It can be observed that the radial stiffness of 1 pair of magnetic rings is 2.4 N/mm, that of 2 pairs is 4.7 N/mm, and that of 3 pairs is 3.5 N/mm.

4 SUMMARY

This paper proposes a centrifugal blood pump with a permanent magnetic bearing and hydrodynamic bearings and introduces hydrodynamic suspension and the maglev structure. One permanent magnet is embedded in the impeller hub, and the other is fixed in the center shaft of the pump. It is the interaction between the two permanent magnets that provides the magnetic force to suspend the impeller. As a result of balanced forces acting in the dynamic pressure generated by the operation of impeller and axial force generated by the axial displacement of radial permanent magnetic bearing, the impeller is effectively dynamically suspended between the upper and lower casings of the pump housing during the operation of the pump. Using ANSYS software enables magnetic levitation properties. The conclusions are as follows:

1. The axial displacement of the two permanent magnets has an influence on bearing capacity and bearing stiffness of the radial permanent bearing.
2. Using multipairs permanent magnets can improve bearing capacity and bearing stiffness of PMBs. When the magnetic body height is a constant, the single permanent magnet height value is equivalent to the radial thickness value between internal and external permanent magnets and the bearing capacity and bearing stiffness of the radial permanent bearings are the largest.

ACKNOWLEDGMENTS

The project was supported by National Natural Science Foundation of China with grant number 51275371 and the Fundamental Research Funds for the Central Universities (WUT: 2014-IV-103).

REFERENCES

CAO Guangzhong, WAN Guojun. (2007) Design on the Structure of Multi-pairs Magnetic Rings for Radial Permanent Magnetic Bearing. In: YU Suyuan. (eds.) *Magnetic Bearing Research Progress and the Second Session of China Electromagnetic Bearing Symposium: The second academic conference of Chinese electromagnetic bearing*, EUROCK 2007, 22–24 August 2007, Nanjing, China. pp. 71–77.

Earnshaw S. (1842) On the Nature of Molecular Forces Which Regulated the Constitution of the Aluminiferous Ether. *Trans Camb Phil Soc*, 7: 97–112.

Hoshi H, Shinshi T, Takatani S. (2006) Third-generation Blood Pumps with Mechanical Noncontact Magnetic Bearings. *Journal of Artificial Organs*, 30(5): 324–338.

QU Zheng. (2008) *Mechanical Circulatory Support of Modern Treatment of Heart Failure*. Beijing, Science and Technology Literature Publishing House.

RUAN Xiaodong, LIN Zhe, ZOU Jun, etc. (2010) Study on hydraulic suspension of artificial blood pump. *Set of fluid power transmission and control of the sixth session of national fluid power transmission and control of academic conference papers Chinese Mechanical Engineering Society: The Sixth Fluid Power Transmission and Control Conference of China*. EUROCK 2010, 11–13 August 2010, Lanzhou, China. pp. 410–413.

SUN Lijun, ZHANG Tao, ZHAO Bing, et al. (2005) Study on the Mathematical Model of Permanent Magnetic Bearings. *Chinese Journal of Mechanical Engineering*, 41(4): 69–74.

Medicine Sciences and Bioengineering – Wang (Ed.)
© *2015 Taylor & Francis Group, London, ISBN: 978-1-138-02684-1*

Anti-cancer research on *Melodinus sp.* (Apocynaceae Juss.)

Y. Lu[*]
School of Pharmacy, Faculty of Science, University of Nottingham, Malaysia Campus, Semenyih, Selongar, Malaysia

T. Bradshaw
Centre for Biomolecular Sciences, University of Nottingham, Nottingham, UK

B. Hazra
Department of Pharmaceutical Technology, Jadavpur University, Calcutta, India

S.P. Voravuthikunchai & T. Srichan
Natural Product Research Center, Prince of Songkla University, Hatyai, Thailand

M. Qazzaz
Centre for Biomolecular Sciences, University of Nottingham, Nottingham, UK

S. Debnath
Department of Pharmaceutical Technology, Jadavpur University, Calcutta, India

T.J. Khoo & C. Wiart
School of Pharmacy, Faculty of Science, University of Nottingham, Malaysia Campus, Semenyih, Selongar, Malaysia

ABSTRACT: *Melodinus sp.* a very rare medicinal plant belonging to the family of Apocynaceae. Six different extracts of *Melodinus sp.* leaves and barks were screened for their *in vitro* antitumor activities, among the extracts, the bark and leaf chloroform extract showed significant antitumor activities, the most susceptible cell line is the human breast cancer cell line MCF-7. Besides, HCT-116 colorectal carcinoma cells lines and HT-29 human colon cancer line also have excellent results.

1 INTRODUCTION

Cancer, a cellular malignancy that results in the loss of normal cell-cycle control, such as unregulated growth and the lack of differentiation, can develop in any tissue of any organ, and at any time (Chang & Kinghorn, 2001). Despite the therapeutic advances made in understanding the processes involved in carcinogenesis, cancer has become one of the most serious medical problems today. The worldwide mortality rate increases annually, with more than seven million deaths occurring per year. For this reason, cancer chemotherapy has become a major focus area of research (Reddy *et al.*, 2003). Natural products offer unmatched chemical diversity with structural complexity and biological potency. "Chemoprevention" is defined as a process to delay or prevent carcinogenesis in humans through the ingestion of dietary or pharmaceutical agents. This also implies the identification of chemical entities (specifically cytotoxic entities) that are effective against a range of cancer cell lines, although less active or non-toxic against the normal (healthy) cell population. The search for such anticancer agents from plant sources started in the 1950s and plant products have proven to be an important source of anticancer drugs (Cragg & Newman, 2005). This directly results from the biological and chemical diversity of nature, which allows for the discovery of

---

[*]Correspondences should be addressed to Lu Yao, emilyly@126.com, khyx2lyo@nottingham.edu.my

completely new chemical classes of compounds. A number of natural products are used as chemoprotective agents against commonly occurring cancers. The present study was undertaken to screen the antitumor potential on Melodinus sp. No such studies have been reported on this species to date.

2 MATERIALS AND METHODS

2.1 *Plant material*

In Apocynaceae Family is a rare medicinal plant which has just been discovered in the Malaysia rain forest. The leaves and barks were extracted by hexane, chloroform and ethanol, respectively, and got six crude extracts.

2.2 *Chemicals and reagents*

Dimethyl sulfoxide (R&M), MTT (3-(4,5-dimethylthazol-2-yl)-2,5-diphenyl tetrazolium bromide) (Life Technologies), fetal bovine serum (cell culture, Sigma), RPMI-1640 medium (cell culture, Sigma), defined keratinocyte-SFM, industrial methylated spirits (IMS), methanol (MeOH) (Life Technologies), phosphate buffered saline (PBS) tablets and PBS(dulbecco's phosphate buffered saline) (Sigma), trypan blue (cell culture, Sigma), Trypsin EDTA (0.05% Trypsin, 0.53 mM EDTA.4Na), trypsin-EDTA 10 × solution (Gibco), Penicillin-Streptomycin (liquid, 100 ml/pk) (Gibco). 96-well TC Plate (mammalian cell culture, Orange Scientific), centrifuge tube (Orange Scientific), TC flask (Orange Scientific), minisart syringe filter (SSI), kit, pipette and tips are all from Dragon Med.

2.3 *Protocol — cell lines and cell culture*

2.3.1 *Preparation of plant samples*
Extracts were prepared as 500 ug/ml top stock solutions, dissolved in DMSO, protected from light for a maximum period of 4 weeks. Serial drug dilutions were prepared in medium immediately prior to each assay.

2.3.2 *The MTT assay*
The remainder of the cells were syringed through a 23G needle to attain a single cell suspension. The cells were counted and seeded at a density of 3×10^3 cells per well in a 96-well plate. The cells were suspended in RPMI tissue culture medium per well.

The outer columns of the plate were filled with medium to prevent evaporation from treatment wells in addition to providing blank readings for the plate reader. Cells were additionally seeded in a time zero (to) plate in the same manner as the experimental treatment plate. The cells were incubated overnight at 37°C in a 5% CO_2 environment to allow for attachment. Cells were then treated with serial dilutions of various concentrations the following day. A volume of 20 µL of each dilution was added to respective treatment wells (total volume 200 µL) to yield final concentrations of 0.1 µg/mL, 0.5 µg/mL, 1 µg/mL, 5 µg/mL, 10 µg/mL, 50 µg/mL, 100 µg/mL, 500µg/mL and 1µg/mL. A separate DMSO control trial was done to ensure that it did not affect any of the results obtained. A to measurement was taken to obtain a measurement of cell viability at the time of treatment. Treated cells were incubated for 72 h at 37°C. After the treatment exposure period, MTT was added to each well and incubated at 37°C for 4 h. After incubation, all wells were carefully aspirated and of DMSO was added to each well to solubilize formazan crystals. The plate was then placed in an orbital plate shaker for 2–3 minutes to aid formazan dissolution before obtaining the absorbance reading at 550–570 nm on microplate readers (Anthos Labtec, Perkin Elmer Envision, Biohit plc).

$$Cell\ viability\,(\%) = \frac{(Absorbance\ of\ the\ treated\ wells)}{(Absorbance\ of\ the\ control\ wells)} \times 100 \qquad (1)$$

2.4 *Statistical analysis*

Concentration–response curves and statistical data were calculated using the Prism software package 6.00 for Windows, (GraphPad Software) and data were reported as mean and SD values obtained from a minimum of three determinations. Non-linear best fit was plotted with SD and 95% confidence interval. Wallac Envision® software was used to analyse MTT and tubulin polymerisation data. Qualitative phytochemical analysis of the crude extract was determined as follows (Jérôme *et al.*, 2009; Arab *et al.*, 1997). To calculate IC_{50}, It would need a series of dose-response data and growth inhibition or % cell viability. The values of y are in the range of 0–100. *Linear Regression*: The simplest estimate of IC_{50} is to plot x-y and fit the data with a straight line (linear regression). IC_{50} value is then estimated using the fitted line, i.e., $Y = a * X + b$, $IC_{50} = (50 - b)/a$. *Log transformation*: Frequently, linear regression is not a good fit to dose-response data. The response-curve fits better to a straight line if the x-axis is logarithm-transformed.

3 RESULTS AND DISCUSSION

3.1 *HT-29 human colon cancer cell line*

A range of extracts were evaluated in MTT assays following a 3-day exposure against a panel of human colon cancer cell lines, HT-29. The best growth inhibition was observed with the chloroform extracts of leaves and barks, GI_{50} values of 99.5 µg/ml and 124.2 µg/ml respectively (Table 2, Figure 1).

3.2 *HCT-116 human colon cancer cell line*

All the plant extracts of *Melodinus sp.* showed anti-cancer effect on the HCT-116 cell line. The most extraordinary result was revealed by the leave hexane and chloroform extract, GI_{50} values of 50.22 µg/ml and 50.84 µg/ml respectively against the human colon cancer cell HCT-116. (Table 3, Figure 2, 3).

3.3 *MCF-7 human breast cancer cell line*

Six crude extracts of *Melodinus sp.* had been observed obvious antitumor activity against MCF-7 human breast cancer cell line. Among all the extracts, leaf hexane and chloroform extracts revealed the most significant antitumor activities with GI_{50} values of 53.93 µg/ml and 63.80 µg/ml respectively (Table 4, Figure 4, 5).

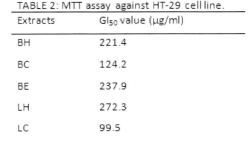

TABLE 2: MTT assay against HT-29 cell line.

Extracts	GI_{50} value (µg/ml)
BH	221.4
BC	124.2
BE	237.9
LH	272.3
LC	99.5
LE	154.6

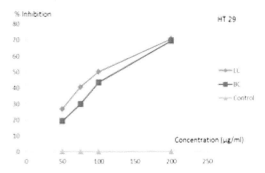

Figure 1:   Effects of extracts on HT-29 cell line growth. LC: leaf chloroform extract, BC: bark chloroform extract. BH: bark hexane extract, BC: bark chloroform, BE: bark ethanol extract, LH: leaf hexane extract, LC: leaf chloroform extract. LE: leaf ethanol extract.

15

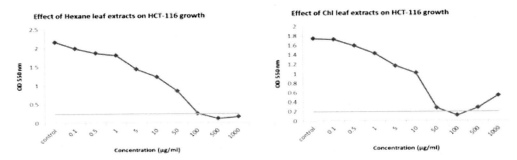

Figure 2 & 3:   Effect of leaf hexane and chloroform extracts on HCT-116 cell line growth.

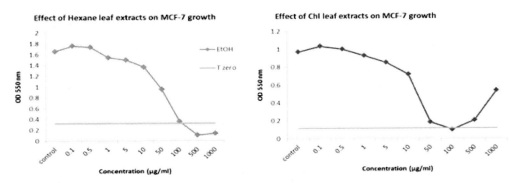

Figure 4 & 5:   Effect of leaf hexane and chloroform extracts on MCF-7 cell line growth.

3.4   *Caco-2 human colon adenocarcinoma cell line*

Extracts were evaluated in MTT assays against a panel of Caco-2 human colon adenocarcinoma cell line. Bark chloroform and leave ethanol extract showed strong antitumor activities with GI50 values of 193.7 µg/ml and 167.1 µg/ml respectively against the human colon cancer cell CaCo-2 (Table 5, Figure 6, 7).

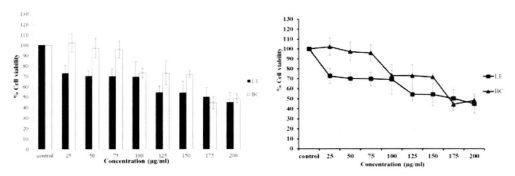

Figure 6 & 7:   Effect of leaf ethanol and bark chloroform extracts on CaCo-2 cell line growth
BC: bark chloroform extract, LE: leaf ethanol extract.

16

Table 3: GI_{50} values against HCT-116.		Table 4: $GI50$ values against MCF-7.		Table 5: GI_{50} values against CaCo-2.	
Extracts	GI_{50} value (μg/ml)	Extracts	GI_{50} value (μg/ml)	Extracts	GI_{50} value (μg/ml)
BH	517.71 ± 22.15	BH	489.14 ± 35.03	BH	>500
BC	66.65 ± 10.31	BC	64.54 ± 21.25	BC	193.7
BE	475.70 ± 37.38	BE	459.62 ± 28.65	BE	>500
LH	50.22 ± 8.23	LH	53.93 ± 9.61	LH	>500
LC	50.84 ± 12.02	LC	63.80 ± 9.86	LC	>500
LE	480.17 ± 24.78	LE	80.42 ± 4.62	LE	167.1

BH: bark hexane extract, BC: bark chloroform extract, BE: bark ethanol extract, LH: leaf hexane extract, LC: leaf chloroform extract, LE: leaf ethanol extract.

4 DISCUSSION

The method used for the MTT (3-(4,5-dimethylazol-2-yl)-2,5-diphenyl tetrazolium bromide) assay was adapted from Mosmann (Mosmann, 1983). The MTT assay is colorimetric in nature and is can be used to assess cell viability from treatment of therapeutic agents or toxic compounds. MTT (yellow) is reduced to a purple formazan in living cells by the activity of cellular enzymes, specifically mitochondrial dehydrogenases, and the intensity of the dye can be quantified by a spectrophotometer. The assay is rapid, economical, and reproducible.

HT-29 cells are human intestinal epithelial cells which produce the secretory component of Immunoglobulin A (IgA), and carcinoembryonic antigen (CEA). Cells are used for tumourigenicity studies. In the present study, six extracts of *Melodinus sp.* leaves and barks were screened for their *in vitro* antitumor activities, among the different extracts tested, the chloroform extracts of leaves and barks revealed significant antitumor activities with GI_{50} values of 99.5 μg/ml and 124.2 μg/ml. The HCT-116 cell line is isolated from a male with colonic carcinoma. These cells are adherent and have a short doubling time of 17.4 hours possess a modal chromosome number of 46. They are also reported to have higher levels of colony formation capability. According to our assay, leave hexane and chloroform extract showed the excellent antitumor activities with GI_{50} values of 50.22 μg/ml and 50.84μg/ml. MCF-7 is an ER+ breast cancer cell line derived from the pleural effusion of a 69-year-old woman who had invasive breast ductal carcinoma in 1970. These cells form tightly cohesive structures thereby illustrating robust cell to cell adhesions and display a luminal epithelial phenotype. In this study, leave hexane and chloroform extract revealed significant antitumor activities with GI_{50} values of 53.93 μg/ml and 63.80 μg/ml. The CaCo-2 cell line is an immortalized line of heterogeneous human epithelial colorectal adenocarcinoma cells. The CaCo-2 cell line is widely used with in vitro assays to predict the absorption rate of candidate drug compounds across the intestinal epithelial cell barrier. The assay requires that drug absorption rates be determined 21 days after CaCo-2 cell seeding to allow for monolayer formation and cell differentiation. CaCo-2 may also refer to a cell monolayer absorption model. Cell-based functional assays, such as the Caco-2 drug transport model for assessing intestinal transport, are extremely valuable for screening lead compounds in drug discovery. Bark chloroform and leave ethanol extract showed significant antitumor activities with GI_{50} values of 193.7 μg/ml and 167.1 μg/ml. It is known that nature is able to produce a wide variety of chemical entities of novel structure. Many of the new and novel compounds isolated from natural sources might otherwise have never been discovered, especially those of considerable complexity requiring the development of methods for the creation of new ring systems. Natural products appeared to be a promising source for new types of compounds with antitumor activity (Hartwell, 1976).

5 CONCLUSION

Plant substances continue to serve as a wellspring of drugs for the world population and several plant-based drugs are in extensive clinical use (Handa, 2007). Preliminary antitumor screening of six extracts of *Melodinus sp.* showed that the chloroform extract of barks and all the extracts of leaves had promising growth inhibition on the four human cancer cell lines. The results obtained suggest that further isolation studies can be performed on *Melodinus sp.* to identify the active constituents responsible for the antitumor activities.

REFERENCES

Chang, L., Kinghorn AD (2001) *Flavonoids as cancer chemopreventative agents. Bioactive Compounds from Natural Sources, Isolation, Characterisation and Biological Properties* Corrado-Tringali (Ed).

Cragg, G., Newman DJ (2005) Plants as a source of anticancer agents. *Journal of Ethnopharmacology* 100, 72–79.

"Extraction of plant secondary metabolites", in *Natural Products Isolation*, Satyajit D. Sarker and Alexander I. Gray, Eds., pp. 339–342, 2nd edition, 2006.

Handa SS (2007) Status of Medicinal and Aromatic Plants (MAPs) *Utilization Globally Including Issues of Quality Control and Technologies for Large Scale Production of Plant Based Products.* United Nations Industrial Development Organization (UNIDO).

Hartwell J (1976) Types of Anticancer Agents Isolated From Plants. *Cancer Treatment Reports* 60.

Jérôme Rollin, Claire Bléchet, Sandra Régina, Arthur Tenenhaus, Serge Guyétant, Xavier Gidrol. The Intracellular Localization of ID2 Expression Has a Predictive Value in Non Small Cell Lung Cancer. *PLoS ONE*, 4(1): 7, 2009.

M. Kamalinejad, F. Mojab, N. Ghaderi, and H. R. Vahidipour, "Phytochemical screening of some species of Iranian plants", *Iranian Journal of Pharmaceutical Research*, vol. 2, pp. 77–82, 2003.

Mosmann T (1983) Rapid colorimetric assay for cellular growth and survival: application to proliferation and cytotoxicity assays. J Immunol Methods 65:55–63.

Reddy, L., Odhav B. and Bhoola KD (2003) *Natural products for cancer prevention: a globalperspective.* Pharmacology and therapeutics 99: 1–13. (referenced: Denmark-Wahnefried et al., 2001).

S. Arab, E. Russel, W. B. Chapman, B. Rosen, C. A. Lingwood. Expression of the verotoxin receptor glycolipid, globotriaosylceramide, in ovarian hyperplasias. *Oncology Research*, 9(10): 553–563, 1997.

Medicine Sciences and Bioengineering – Wang (Ed.)
© 2015 Taylor & Francis Group, London, ISBN: 978-1-138-02684-1

Behavioral research on elderly sports fitness activities

Yan-qun He*

School of Physical Education of Hunan University of Technology, Zhuzhou, Hunan, China

ABSTRACT: With the progressive development of national fitness activities, sports activities in cities are surging. The wave of awareness on elderly fitness especially demonstrates the wide range of China's fitness campaign. Currently, China's elderly accounts for a large proportion of the population, and the improvement in health conditions means that elderly sports fitness is making a difference. However, with various types of fitness approaches elderly sports fitness is not normative and there is a lack of formal management of administrative departments and regulations. By analyzing behavioral data on elderly fitness, reform orientation of elderly fitness is studied and a new approach is put forward herewith.

1 INTRODUCTION

The key purposes for elderly people to perform physical fitness activities are to train their physical fitness to be in the optimum state, help them enhance their physique, improve immune ability, relax pressure, improve life quality, and change their attitude toward life. In developed countries, importance is attached to the proportion of elderly people and the coverage rate of elderly physical fitness is valued. Furthermore, many good advices are put forward to promote elderly fitness campaigns. However, China is different from these countries in the development background and due to the uneven development states of provinces in economy, geography, culture, and sports there are barriers to promoting physical fitness campaigns for elderly people. Exposed problems not only include the popularizing rate of elderly people but also refer to behavioral problems, moral issues, normative problems, scientific problems, and humanization problems during the process of performing fitness activities (Lin Zhao-Rong, 2003). As a matter of fact, the level and achievement of elderly people's physical fitness according to from mood and time. By observing elderly people's fitness achievements of different time intervals, corresponding strategies can be made to meet their needs in fitness. To increase their professional knowledge and awareness about physical training is the crucial step, which can ensure that they participate in healthy body–building exercises. Behavioristics of elderly people's physical fitness is to differentiate exercise habits of human beings from those of animals, especially to make a distinction between various aspects of humanized exercise behaviors. Behavioral analysis refers to the analysis of human beings' lifestyle and behaviors in human habitats. Relevant rules can be found out through the methods of interview, observation, and statistics. Behavioral research provides new perspectives to analyze effectiveness and rationality of elderly people's physical fitness and improve various facilities for elderly people to exercise.

---

*About the author: He Yanqun (1981–), female; born in Chaling, Hunan; a lecturer in the School of Physical Education of Hunan University of Technology who mainly teaches and studies fitness and health education.

2 SPORTS BEHAVIORAL CHARACTERISTICS OF ELDERLY PEOPLE

2.1 *Behavior choice of elderly people at different age groups*

Elderly fitness campaigns cater to the age group of elderly people, for whom it is quite necessary to have physical exercise. The term elderly people refers to those who are between 65 and 85 years, whereas individuals between 45 and 65 years are middle aged. People's capacity for exercise decreases with age growth. Therefore, it is indispensable to promote orderly physical training with age growth. The rhythm of life changes with lifestyle. People stepping into the aged group will show decline in organs, immune competence, resistibility, and coordination between locomotive organs and the body. In a word, overall physical fitness will show a dramatic decline. Therefore, it is quite necessary to improve the physical fitness of elderly people (Zhou Xin-xin, 2007). Furthermore, elderly people should keep a positive lifestyle and enthusiasm about fitness. A survey on the residents of urban Zhuzhou City indicates that 92.5% of people in urban communities of Zhuzhou like or love sports; people who stand neutral account for 4.5%, and only 3% of them dislike sports. This survey shows a strong awareness among urban Zhuzhou citizens on exercise and fitness, and they value sports as a good way to keep health and prolong life.

2.2 *Psychological features of elderly physical fitness*

Aged people need to invest more energy in keeping healthy, and they pay more attention on life quality and physical training. In psychology, aged people face various pressures from environment and disease. Less concern from society causes loneliness in the elderly. Unbalanced physiological conditions and separation from social needs give them an integrated sense of being "old people." Compared with the middle-aged group and young people, they experience an apparent sense of loneliness and a sense of loss and some even lose confidence in life and themselves (Wang Cun-wen, 2009).

A survey of elderly people in the Tianyuan District of Zhuzhou shows that 94% females but only 6% males agreed to accept investigation; 94% females like sports, compared with 70% males. Only 50% of interviewees were satisfied with the fitness facilities of their neighborhood. As for ages, 50% were between 60 and 70 years and the other 50% were over 70 years. Thus, it can be seen that there is a massive base for regional elderly fitness programs, except that relevant sports facilities are lacking. Therefore, elderly people can make use of their own advantages to enhance physical training and help themselves remove anxiety and unease at old age. Through exercising at centralized sites and taking part in group activities, they can establish friendship and eliminate a sense of loneliness. A survey in Foshan shows that 70% of exercise participants at community sports facility sites are elderly people, compared with 30% middle-aged ones.

3 ANALYSIS ON TYPES OF FITNESS FOR ELDERLY PEOPLE

People at advanced ages (advanced age refers to ages over 80 years) must be cautious when participating in physical fitness as organ functions decline remarkably. Due to muscle atrophy and rarefaction of bones, advanced-aged people cannot stand high-strength sports; such activities are likely to cause damage of bones, joints, and muscles. After exercise, advanced-aged people will take a long time to recover. If overfatigue occurs after exercise, somatic functions will show decline, contrary to the purpose of exercise. It is advisable for advanced-aged people to choose general movements to exercise joints and muscle groups. These movements should be slow and rhythmic, such as walking, jogging, tai chi, qigong, eight trigrams boxing, therapeutic massage, gate ball, sunbaths, air baths, cold baths, etc. When doing fitness exercises, if elderly people feel uncomfortable they should not carry on with the exercise. Instead, they should take a rest to recover. In addition, advanced-aged people had better exercise under medical supervision. They need to do checkups before, during, and after exercise, such as heart rate, blood pressure, and electrocardiogram checks. Exercise intensity or exercise item should be adjusted in accordance with the checkup results (Song Hai-xia, 2010).

A survey on the physical exercise behaviors of elderly people in Zhuzhou presents the following results. Fifty percent of elderly people feel satisfaction about keep-fit through exercising; elderly people who are over 70 years expect that the society should contribute more to the fitness of elderly people, among which 80% consider that the society should enlarge relevant investment. The satisfaction degree about exercise quality of elderly people between 60 and 70 years is only 65%. It is fully illustrated that there is great potential in the field of physical exercise of elderly people, and they need more fitness resources and greater guarantees.

Through analysis, it is found that types of elderly fitness are mainly classified into dynamic exercise and static exercise. Dynamic exercise refers to large amounts of sustained aerobic exercise, such as jogging, which is the favorite sports of most people. and the purpose is to train body harmony and keep athletic ability. Frequent jogging can effectively enhance and improve cardiovascular system, respiratory system, digestive system, and nervous system function so that it inhibits or delays senescence and prolongs life.

Basic requirements for jogging are as follows: keep the body straight slightly leaning forward. The thigh drives the calf. The whole sole of the foot touches down. Arms swing naturally. Both eyes should smoothly inspect ahead, accompanied by rhythmic breathing. The other mode of exercise is static exercise, which is slow and beneficial to the internal function of the body. Such kind of exercises includes qigong and tai chi. Tai chi, with a long history in China, is not only a martial art but also a sport and fitness regime. It was derived from the marksmanship and long-handle modus of blade of ancient cavalrymen. Its fundamental usage is to open, close, and spread, just like playing spear and long-handle broadsword at stilts. Tai chi started from the infinite, which generates two complementary forces; they are further divided into three forces. Three forces generate four aggregates. Four aggregates generate eight trigrams. A special Chinese boxing called tai chi is created in accordance with the principle of yin and yang from the Book of Changes, meridian of traditional Chinese medicine, Daoism, and expiration and inspiration. Tai chi is consistent with the nature of yin and yang, body constitution, and nature laws.

4 BEHAVIORISTIC ANALYSIS OF ELDERLY PHYSICAL FITNESS

4.1 Choice of time range for elderly physical fitness

Elderly people are likely to exercise in the morning or at night. It is investigated that most elderly people like to exercise from 6am to 8am in the morning. They do not like to sleep in late and like to keep early hours. Another large part of elderly people likes to exercise in the evening. Exercise time in these two sections is between 30 minutes and 120 minutes. As elderly people have limited physical strength, they can keep the exercise habit (Zhu Zhuang-zhi, 2004). However, the choice of time range is not rational, because many elderly people cannot maintain abundant physical strength every day, and it is uncertain whether everyday exercise may hurt the body of elderly people.

4.2 Fitness site choice of elderly people

Fitness sites of elderly people focus on lakesides, riversides, and squares of cities. Generally, squares of every city are main sites for elderly people to exercise. But due to shortage of leadership and organization, exercise at squares is scattered, spontaneous, and temporary and far from normative. Currently, elderly people select parks as their new fitness sites, because parks can provide better environment to stretch the body and ease the mind. However, 41% of them are satisfied with these sites, whereas 44.6% express dissatisfaction (Liu Lin-jian, 2004). Investigation shows that elderly people tend to choose afforested free sites with fresh air, and nobody chooses professional fitness centers requiring financial investment. It is desirable for elderly people to change the current status and choose better professional sites for group exercise and amusement.

4.3 Analysis on instructions for maintaining physical fitness of elderly people

A national investigation of elderly people shows that 44% of them receive fitness guidance, whereas 56% have no professional guidance. Reasons may be that professional guidance is not attractive to elderly people and the operation philosophy of professional fitness training centers does not cater to the need of elderly people. Actually, 69% of interviews on elderly people show that those who do not have professional guidance hope to receive guidance from professional institutes and they hope to improve self-training knowledge to self-direct and promote the stability of physical training. Behavior selection in this aspect is already expanding the market demand of physical fitness from elderly people.

4.4 Probability analysis of elderly people gathering together to exercise

Elderly people are likely to do something together. Under the influence of their special age, elderly people like crowded and busy environments, and they prefer to exercise with peers. An investigation shows that 70% of elderly people like to gather with those of similar age to exercise. However, some professional agencies only allow a single application system, which is not flexible and lacks internal impetus. It is not necessary to offer highly specialized guidance to elderly people. What they need is instructive communication and the feeling of being involved in the process of exercising.

5 ANALYSIS OF APPROACHES TO IMPROVE PHYSICAL FITNESS OF ELDERLY PEOPLE

5.1 Intensity and time control of physical fitness of elderly people

In accordance with the Health Net and literature on scientific fitness, it is not advisable for elderly people to exercise in the evening, as strenuous exercise will cause sleep to become unstable. The best exercise in the evening is to take a walk for 30–50 minutes, depending on the individual body organism. As for time control, it is suggested to take dynamic exercise at 6:00 to 8:00 in the morning and take static exercise such as a walk at 7:00 to 8:00 in the evening, which is beneficial to sleep quality and preparation to exercise in the next morning (Yue Jin-ku, 2004).

5.2 Professional exercise sites of elder people

Elderly people should select professional exercise items that can guarantee them rationality and safety. And their exercise should be taken care of by specialized persons. Elderly people may enhance their physical quality to meet the challenge of outdoor sports. Substantial sports need to be based on certain amount of exercise. Otherwise, abrupt substantial training may cause illness. Service stations for the exercise of elderly people should be established in communities of cities so as to promote cultural quality of sports and fitness effectiveness of elderly people through professional service. Thus, physical fitness of elderly people can be developed smoothly.

5.3 Selection of a professional guidance agency for elderly people

Elderly people usually select old-fashioned self-exercise. However, what they need are friends, a warm atmosphere, and friendly concern. Therefore, in addition to professional guidance, friendship should be emphasized. For example, some exercises can be conducted in pairs or with many partners to promote coordination capability. Internal communication and collaborative training can help elderly people to develop a sense of belonging and a sense of tacit understanding and pleasure (Yue Jin-ku, 2005). Meanwhile, social sports instructors with long-term contribution should be rewarded. Professional personnel and students from sports departments should also be advocated to be instructors. Thus, elderly people can have more contact and communication with young people, which is beneficial to physical and mental development.

5.4 Choice of elderly people to exercise together

Elderly people like to gather together to exercise, and this is because old people between 65 and 80 years attach more importance to friendship and unity. They like hilarious surroundings because they need more people to show loving care for them and help them with misery and anxiety. Through observation, it is found that professional agencies can learn from the concept of "Group Purchase" to increase their market competitiveness; they can attract elderly people to join their professional training. Meanwhile, elderly people can enhance physical quality and promote professional training level. Moreover, trade associations for elderly people can be established to help them take group training and increase their enthusiasm to select professional guidance agencies.

6 CONCLUSION

The need and realization of elderly fitness is discussed. Currently, the main concern is how to ensure effect and benefit of elderly fitness programs. As aging tendency of population is becoming more and more remarkable, self-quality of aged people should be enhanced to guarantee low mortality. Through group exercise, elderly people can develop a sense of belonging and establish mutual friendship. Through interaction and communication, collaborative exercise can help them obtain pleasure. In the future, more effort should be invested in physical exercise of elderly people, such as improving the fitness system and regulating unreasonable fitness activities. Professional instructors should provide special skills and knowledge to guide physical exercise of elderly people. Facilities should also be ensured to provide intimate service. Behavior judgments should be made according to time, place, and habit. Preparatory work and behavior judgment will determine the effect of elderly fitness programs. To ensure healthy fitness, it is obliged to make behavior prejudging.

ACKNOWLEDGEMENT

Research fund project: Hunan Scientific Research Projects for Colleges and Universities (Project Number: 11C0417).

REFERENCES

Liu Lin-jian. On Exercise Status Quo of Elderly People in Zhejiang Province [J]. *Journal of Haerbin Physical Education Institute*, 2004, 1(80).
Lin Zhao-Rong. Bodybuilding of Urban Middle and Old Aged People [J]. *Journal of Wuhan Institute of Physical Education*, 2003, 5(45).
Song Hai-xia. On Awareness Training of Exercise Behavior [J]. *Shandong Sports Science & Technology*, 2010, 9(40).
Wang Cun-wen. Exercise Status Quo and Countermeasures of Older Age Groups of Communications in Shanghai [J]. *Science Times*, 2009, 2(78).
Yue Jin-ku. Athletic Behavioristics at Volleyball Court [J]. *Harbin Sport Science and Technology*, 2005, 6(60)
Zhou Xin-xin. Survey of Body-Building Exercises of the Aged Citizen in Hangzhou [J]. *Journal of Zhejiang University of Science and Technology*, 2007, 6(66).
Zhu Zhuang-zhi. On Formation, Change and Countermeasures of Exercise Behavior [J]. *Journal of Wuhan Institute of Physical Education*, 2004, 7(54).
Zhang Shu-hui. Research on Improving Sports Behavior Conscious Training [J]. *Journal of Educational Science of Hunan Normal University*, 2003, 11(44).

Medicine Sciences and Bioengineering – Wang (Ed.)
© 2015 Taylor & Francis Group, London, ISBN: 978-1-138-02684-1

Research and development of multilayer array modulation collimator for precise radiotherapy

Lin Lin & Huai-ling Zhang*
School of Information Engineering, Guangdong Medical College, Dongguan, China

ABSTRACT: On the basis of a planar array modulation collimator, a multilayer array modulation collimator is proposed for intensity-modulated radiotherapy. The target area is constructed by multilayer arrays of rectangle modules, which support more flexible adjustments of dose distribution. The structure and operation principle of the collimator is introduced in detail. The combination of this equipment with standard modern linear accelerators and multileaf collimator will be an ideal method to improve boundary conformity and reduce penumbra and dose leakage. The hardware is also compatible with most commercial Monte Carlo–based treatment planning systems.

1 INTRODUCTION

Radiotherapy is widely applied for the treatment of cancer either as a single modality or in combination with other treatments like surgery or chemotherapy. Because radiation damage is not restricted to tumor cells only but affects normal cells as well, it is important that the dose delivered to healthy tissues is as low as possible to minimize the risk of side effects of the treatment. The wish to improve the precision of radiation therapy has stimulated many efforts to develop conformal therapy techniques for delivering a high dose of irradiation to the target while sparing surrounding normal tissues. For example, one can use a large number of blocks, usually made by lead or tungsten alloy, to absorb radiation beams and optimize the beam weights to improve the conformity of the dose distribution to the tumor. For efficiency, the movement of the lead block should be quick and accurate, which can be fulfilled under the guidance of a computer-based treatment planning system (TPS). Recently, three-dimensional treatment planning tools have extended the possibilities of optimizing treatment plans for a particular patient within reasonable time by a proper, manual selection of the number of radiation fields, and for each particular field the beam direction, energy, weight, and wedge angle can be arranged separately (Kawrakow et al., 2004, p. 2883–2898, Chetty et al., 2007, p. 4818–4853, and Yu, 1995, p. 1435–1449). With the application of all kinds of modulation collimators, the shape of treatment fields could be conformed to the beam's eye view projection of the tumor volume, thereby decreasing the dose delivery to nearby healthy tissues. The modulation collimator is a major component of intensity-modulated radiotherapy (IMRT) technology (Keall et al., 2001, p. 2139–2146, Mock et al., 2004, p. 147–154, and Papiez et al., 2005). Several collimators have been developed for IMRT such as the multileaf collimator (MLC) (Poulsen et al., 2011, p. 312–320), sliding window MLC, tomotherapy multileaf intensity collimator, applicator collimator, baffle plate of radiation field, and rapid arc modulation (Palma et al., 2008, p. 996–1001 and Rebecca et al., 2008, p. 16–25). Taking the MLC for example, the accuracy is restricted by the width of leaf, penumbra, and dose leakage. Further, an improvement in accuracy will inevitably lead to an increase in the number of segments that require more complicated driving equipment. So, it is attractive to develop a new type of modulation collimator with higher accuracy and efficiency (Hunter et al., 2008, p. 2347–2355 and Mu et al., 2008, p. 77–88).

---

*Corresponding author: Huai-ling Zhang: huailing@163.com

In this chapter, a new type of collimator named multilayer array modulation collimator (MAMC), developed on the basis of the planar array modulation collimator (PAMC), is introduced in detail. MAMC has a smaller element field that allows more efficient and accurate intensity-modulated conformal radiation therapy. Moreover, it is also promising to put MAMC together with MLC for improvements in performance such as edge response function.

2   PRINCIPLE OF ARRAY MODULATION COLLIMATOR

2.1   *Planar array modulation collimator*

A PAMC, which has been reported in a previous article, consists of two-layer arrays of shield modules with four sides that are parallel to the ray of radiation source. Radiation beam is shielded by modules to result in a square screen area on the plane of isocenter. The modules of upper layer array are immobilized, whereas those of the lower layer can change status between two positions by electromagnetic drive. At one position, the projections of two modules overlap to form one square screen area, as shown in Fig. 1(a). When the lower module, marked as 3, moves to the other position, its projection will also move to the side to form another screen area, marked as 4, adjacent to that formed by the top module, marked as 2. The radiation field, presented as a blank area and marked as 5, can be constructed by different combinations of blocks of the two-layer array. Radiotherapy needs to be performed twice for one target that is smaller than the maximum radiation field. The collimator will take the line between radiation source and isocenter as the axis and rotate through 90° or 180° after the first radiation with an equal dose of radiation.

2.2   *Multilayer array modulation collimator*

A MAMC is developed on the basis of a PAMC in order to realize multiple stage adjustments of radiation intensity. There may be four to five layers of blocks, which can be driven independently as shown in Fig. 1(b). A matrix of projection is fabricated with the dimension determined by the number of layers and arrows per layer. The precision of modulation is equivalent to that of the tomotherapy multileaf intensity collimator. When dealing with large lesions, the radiation area should move to the part out of the maximum range of collimator by swinging around the ray

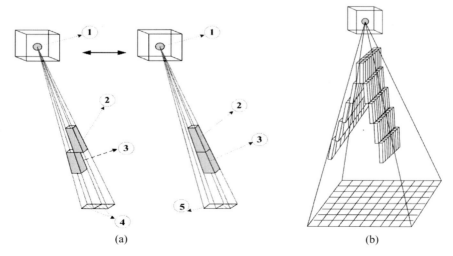

(a)   (b)

Figure 1.   Diagram of arrangement of blocks and the radiation field. (a) Planar array modulation collimator; (b) multilayer array modulation collimator.

source. It is different from the operation of the tomotherapy multileaf intensity collimator, which needs stepping of the therapeutic bed continuously. The radiation dose will not increase for additional illumination because only half of the area is exposed each time, as shown in Fig. 2.

There are two types of arrangements of immobilized modules and projections. One is array distribution, and the other is chessboard distribution, as shown in Fig. 3. In the former, as shown in Fig. 3(a), modules are continuously arranged in one direction and are radially arranged in the vertical direction. For the first radiation, half of the target area is exposed. For the second one, the collimator should rotate through 180° to expose the other half of the target area. For chessboard, shown in Fig. 3(b), modules are radially arranged in both directions and the collimator needs to rotate through 90° to change the radiation field for the second radiation.

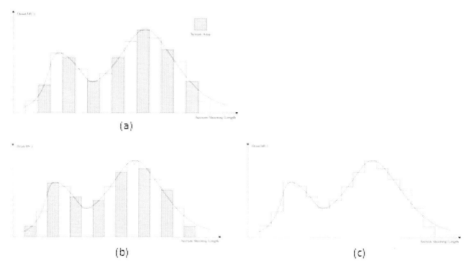

Figure 2. Dose flux along with section shooting length. Parts (a) and (b) represent radiation doses of two statuses before and after rotation. (c) Total dose of two radiations.

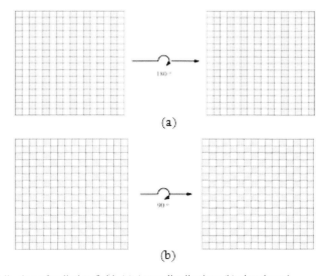

Figure 3. Distribution of radiation field. (a) Array distribution; (b) chessboard.

3 PRECISION AND APPLICATION

We have designed a new method to verify the position of blocks using a two-dimensional ion chamber array (2D array). The edge function of the block was measured, and the accuracy of position was found with 0.2 mm. The error comes from different positions of blocks, which has a nonlinear relationship between movement of blocks and area of projection. The result is a little better than that of common MLC (Venencia & Besa, 2004, p. 37–54).

A special design for image-guided radiation therapy is a multicollimation system in which the ray beam will pass through four-stage collimators including the primary collimator, first collimator, MLC, and PAMC, where MLC acts as the upper collimator of MAMC. The combination of MAMC and MLC can improve the conformity and reduce leakage radiation to the utmost. Fig. 3 illustrates the improvement of boundary conformity where the formation of field boundary is more accurate than in MLC because smaller square elements will fill the leakages of MLC by diving apparatus. MAMC is fit for cooperation with a built-in MLC for body therapy as well as external MLC for head therapy. For head radiation therapy, we have developed a model machine with a total area of 120 mm × 48 mm and an element area of 6 mm × 6 mm. For body therapy, the total area was expanded to 80 mm × 200 mm with an element area of 10 mm × 10 mm. By MLC the ratio of leakage area to projection area is 13.9%, whereas the value is 17.6% for MAMC. However, it will decrease to 11.1% with the combination of the two collimators.

The penumbra characteristic of the collimator was evaluated in the Elekta Synergy linear accelerator (6 MeV). For body treatment, the beam profile is set to 200 mm × 200 mm with the element filled to 10 mm × 10 mm. The edge response function was measured by a 2D array ion chamber (IBA, MatriXX), as shown in Fig. 4. The detectors were put in a water box with a depth of $z = 5$ cm with repeatability better than 1%. MAMC is capable of the task of modulation independently with a similar performance to MLC. The combination of MAMC and MLC will reduce the penumbra obviously from Fig. 5. In Fig. 5, penumbra of three collimators is presented for different field sizes. The measurement sequence came from independent software, and the TPS came from Varian (Eclipse 8.7).

4 SUMMARY

A new collimator called MAMC has been implemented for accurate modulation radiotherapy, which supports more flexible movement compared with its form type PAMC. The accuracy of the current implementation is limited by the dimension of square elements in planar array. This

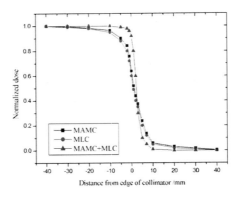

Figure 4. Edge response function of MLC, MAMC, and combination structure.

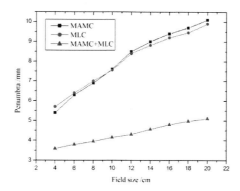

Figure 5. Penumbra of MLC, MAMC, and combination structure at z = 5 cm.

equipment can be assembled to standard modern linear accelerators and MLCs. It has been veri-fied that the conformity can be improved by 2.8%. Reduction of penumbra and lowering of dose leakage are also promising characteristics of this design. We have finished research and devel-opment of the hardware system, and the prototype is in the test state as well. Additional studies are needed to evaluate MAMC for different kinds of anatomic sites and to clinically evaluate the outcomes. In order to avoid duplicate illuminations, we have also developed another type of array modulation collimator that has multiple layers, which will be introduced later.

ACKNOWLEDGMENTS

The authors acknowledge the support given by the Science and Technological Program for Dongguan's Higher Education, Science and Research, and Health Care Institutions (2012108102001).

REFERENCES

C. D. Venencia & P. Besa (2004) Commissioning and quality assurance for intensity modulated radiotherapy with dynamic multileaf collimator: Experience of the Pontificia Universidad Católica de Chile. *Journal of Applied Clinical Medical Physics*, 5(3), 37–54.

C. X. Yu (1995) Intensity-modulated arc therapy with dynamic multileaf collimation: An alternative to tomo-therapy. *Physics in Medicine and Biology*, 40(9), 1435–1449.

D. Palma, E. Vollans & K. James (2008) Volumetric modulated arc therapy for delivery of prostate radiotherapy: Comparison with intensity-modulated radiotherapy and three-dimensional conformal radio-therapy. *International Journal of Radiation Oncology Biology Physics*, 72(4), 996–1001.

G. Mu, E. Ludlum & P. Xia (2008) Impact of MLC leaf position errors on simple and complex IMRT plans for head and neck cancer. *Physics in Medicine and Biology*, 53(1), 77–88.

I. J. Chetty, B Curran, J.E. Cygler, J.J. DeMacro & G. Ezzell (2007) Report of the AAPM Task Group No. 105: Issues associated with clinical implementation of Monte Carlo-based photon and electron external beam treatment planning. *Medical Physics*, 34(12), 4818–4853.

I. Kawrakow, D. W. O. Rogers & B. R. B. Walters (2004) Large efficiency improvements in BEAMnrc using directional bremsstrahlung splitting. *Medical Physics*, 31(4), 2004, 2883–2898.

L Papiez, D Rangaraj & P Keall (2005) Real-time DMLC IMRT delivery for mobile and deforming targets. *Medical Physics*, 32(9), 3037–3048.

M. H. Rebecca, I. P. N. Smith & C. S. Jarrio (2008) Establishing action levels for EPID-based QA for IMRT. *Journal of Applied Clinical Medical Physics*, 9(3), 16–25.

M. M. Hunter, H. Li & D. A. Low (2008) MLC quality assurance using EPID: A fitting technique with sub-pixel precision. *Medical Physics*, 35(6), 2347–2355.

P. J. Keall, V. R. Kini & S. S. Vedam (2001) Determining parameters for respiration-gated radiotherapy. *Medical Physics*, 28(10), 2139–2146.

P. R. Poulsen, B.l Cho & D. Ruan (2011) Electromagnetic-guided dynamic multileaf collimator tracking enables motion management for intensity-modulated arc therapy. *International Journal of Radiation Oncology Biology Physics*, 79(1), 312–320.

S. H. Levitt, J. A. Purdy & C. A. Perez (2008) *Technical Basis of Radiation Therapy*, Western Europe: Springer Verlag.

U. Mock, D. Georg & J. Bogner (2004) Treatment planning comparison of conventional, 3D conformal, and intensity-modulated photon (IMRT) and proton therapy for paranasal sinus carcinoma. *International Journal of Radiation Oncology Biology Physics*, 58(1), 147–154.

Medicine Sciences and Bioengineering – Wang (Ed.)
© 2015 Taylor & Francis Group, London, ISBN: 978-1-138-02684-1

The estimations for the multifactorial interaction between factors and confidence intervals

Xiao-Dong Wang
Quanzhou Normal University, Quanzhou, China

Jun Tian*
School of Public Health, Fujian Medical University, Fuzhou, China

ABSTRACT: In some researches, the time is a target variable. The factors that may influence the time of an outcome occurring are need to be analyzed. The effect of one factor on the outcome is often modified by another factor because there is an interaction between them, the analysis of which is very important for us to study the mechanism of the effect of the factors on the outcome. This paper proposes the methods used to evaluate the factors influencing the survival time of the patients with cancer, their interactions, and their 95% confidence intervals in the survival analysis.

1 INTRODUCTION

Survival time is the main observation target in the researches on life issues (Elisa, 2013). The connotation of survival time is general. It may be a survival time of patients or animals, and it may be life of the product, or the time of something changed from state to state. Regardless of the field of research, the corresponding data analysis methods are referred to as the survival analyses when the time variable is a main observation target. The survival analysis is widely used in many research areas such as biomedical, industrial, agriculture, forestry, and other industries. In many cases, the survival time is affected by many factors. For example, the survival time of cancer patients can be affected not only by the treatment, but also by the clinical stage, pathological type, nutrition, mental state, and many other factors. It is very important to identify the influence factors of survival time to improving the survival time and patient outcomes.

Let $x_1, x_2, \ldots, x_m$ be m factors affecting the survival time. The observation target is the time of event A in a follow-up study on the objects. If the risk of the event A at time t is denoted as $h(t,x)$, then a model of the relationship between factors and the risk of occurrence of event A can be described using the formula proposed by Cox (1984) as follows:

$$h(t,x) = h_0(t)e^{\beta_1 x_1 + \beta_2 x_2 + \cdots + \beta_m x_m} \tag{1}$$

where $h_0(t)$ is called a base risk, which is the basic incidence rate if $x_1, x_2, \ldots, x_m$ have no effects on survival time. There are m parameters $\beta_1, \beta_2, \ldots, \beta_m$ in the model. Formula (1) is also called proportional hazards model.

If the m factors $x_1, x_2, \ldots, x_m$ take the values $a_1, a_2, \ldots, a_m$, then the risk of the event A of the observed objects must be $h(t,a) = h_0(t)e^{\beta_1 a_1 + \beta_2 a_2 + \cdots + \beta_m a_m}$. On the other hand, if the m factors $x_1, x_2, \ldots, x_m$ take the values $b_1, b_2, \ldots, b_m$, then the risk of the event A of the observed objects must be $h(t,b) = h_0(t)e^{\beta_1 b_1 + \beta_2 b_2 + \cdots + \beta_m b_m}$.

---

*Corresponding author.

In this case, we have

$$RR = \frac{h(t,a)}{h(t,b)} = h_0(t)e^{\beta_1(a_1\,b_1)+\beta_2(a_2\,b_2)+\cdots+\beta_m(a_m\,b_m)} \quad . \tag{2}$$

This value is a relative ratio indicator. It is a multiple of the risk of the event A of the m factors $x_1, x_2, \ldots, x_m$ take the values $a_1, a_2, \ldots, a_m$ and of the risk of the event A of the m factors $x_1, x_2, \ldots, x_m$ take the values $b_1, b_2, \ldots, b_m$. Therefore, the variable RR reflects the impact of various factors on the survival time.

In many cases, the effects on the lifetime of a factor x_i are related to the state of another factor x_j. In these cases, there exists an interaction between x_i and x_j (Mitchell, 2011). Analysis of interactions among factors is considered significant in the study of the influence of factors on the survival time. However, many researches lack this analysis in follow-up studies. In textbooks on the multivariate analysis, the methods used to correctly analyze the interaction among factors are mostly not described. In this paper, we propose a method to analyze the interaction among factors by using the Cox proportional hazards model. This method is applicable to any fields of multivariate data analysis when time is an observed variable.

The organization of the paper is as follows. In Sections 2–4, we describe our new method to analyze the interaction between the factors with Cox proportional hazards model. In Section 2, we give two applicable methods, product term method and dummy variable method to analyze the interaction among the factors. In Section 3, we give an example of the applications of the methods presented in Section 2. Finally, concluding remarks are given in Section 4.

2 METHODS TO ANALYZE THE INTERACTIONS BY USING THE COX MODEL

Let x_1 and x_2 are the two factors affecting the survival time. Without loss of generality, we can assume the two variables are both binary variables taking values 0 or 1. By the definitions of variance and covariance (James, 2012), we know that
If $z = ax_1 + bx_2$, then

$$Var(z) = a^2 Var(x_1) + b^2 Var(x_2) + 2ab Cov(x_1, x_2) \tag{3}$$

If $z = x_1 - x_2$, then

$$Var(z) = Var(x_1) + Var(x_2) + 2Cov(x_1, x_2) \tag{4}$$

where a and b are constants, $Var(x)$ is the variance of x, and $Cov(x, y)$ is the covariance of x and y.

To analyze the interactions between the variables x_1 and x_2, we discuss the following two methods by using the Cox model.

2.1 Product term method

Let $x_3 = x_1 x_2$ is another variable. We will build a Cox model of x_1, x_2, x_3 as follows:

$$h(t,x) = h_0(t) + e^{\beta_1 x_1 + \beta_2 x_2 + \beta_3 x_3}. \tag{5}$$

Let $\beta_1, \beta_2, \beta_3$ be the estimation of the parameters $\beta_1, \beta_2, \beta_3$ in formula (5) according to actual research data: $h(t,x) = h_0(t)e^{\beta_1 x_1 + \beta_2 x_2 + \beta_3 x_3}$.

The amount of modification of x_2 to x_1 can be estimated as follows:

Step 1: Compute the ratio of the risk of $x_1 = 1$ event A occurs to the risk of $x_1 = 0$, when $x_2 = 0$. From formulas (2) and (5), we have:

$$RR_0 = e^{\beta_1} . \tag{6}$$

Step 2: Compute the ratio of the risk of $x_1 = 1$ event A occurs to the risk of $x_1 = 0$, when $x_2 = 1$. From formulas (2) and (5), we have

$$RR_1 = e^{\beta_1 + \beta_3} . \tag{7}$$

Then, the amount of changes caused by x_1 on the survival time due to the different state of x_2 can be expressed as $|RR_1 - RR_0| = |e^{\beta_1 + \beta_3} - e^{\beta_1}|$. It is also called the effect of x_1 on the survival time modified by x_2.

The parameters $\beta_1, \beta_2, \beta_3$ in formula (5) are generally estimated with reference to the research data. Therefore, we have to calculate its 95% confidence interval. If 0 is not contained in this interval, then we can conclude that there is an interaction between x_1 and x_2 (Frank, 2010). The 95% confidence interval of $|RR_1 - RR_0|$ can be expressed as

$$(e^{\beta_1 + \beta_3} - e^{\beta_1}) \pm 1.96\sqrt{Var(e^{\beta_1 + \beta_3} - e^{\beta_1})}. \tag{8}$$

In the preceding formula, $\sqrt{Var(e^{\beta_1 + \beta_3} - e^{\beta_1})}$ can be estimated as follows:

The Taylor expansion of $\sqrt{Var(e^{\beta_1 + \beta_3} - e^{\beta_1})}$ can be written as (Richard, 2010):

$$e^{\beta_1 + \beta_3} - e^{\beta_1} = (e^{\beta_1 + \beta_3} - e^{\beta_1})\beta_1 + (e^{\beta_1 + \beta_3})\beta_3 + +(e^{\beta_1 + \beta_3} - e^{\beta_1})(1 - \beta_1) - (e^{\beta + \beta_3})\beta .$$

If we set $c = (e^{\beta_1 + \beta_3} - e^{\beta_1})(1 - \beta_1) - (e^{\beta_1 + \beta_3})\beta_3$, then c is a constant.

From formula (3), we then have

$$
\begin{aligned}
&Var((e^{\beta_1 + \beta_3} - e^{\beta_1})\beta_1 + (e^{\beta_1 + \beta_3})\beta_3) \\
&= (e^{\beta_1 + \beta_3} - e^{\beta_1})^2 Var(\beta_1) + (e^{\beta_1 + \beta_3})^2 Var(\beta_3) \\
&+ 2(e^{\beta_1 + \beta_3} - e^{\beta_1})e^{\beta_1 + \beta_3} Cov(\beta_1, \beta_3)
\end{aligned} \tag{9}
$$

where $Var(\beta_1)$, $Var(\beta_3)$, and $Cov(\beta_1, \beta_3)$ are the variance and covariance matrices of the parameter estimations.

2.2 Dummy variable method

There are four different combinations of the variables x_1 and x_2 when they take values of 0 and 1: $(0,0);(0,1);(1,0);(1,1)$.

We set three dummy variables z_1, z_2, and z_3 to represent these four combinations:

$$z_1 = \begin{cases} 1 & (x_1, x_2) = (1,1) \\ 0 & \text{otherwise} \end{cases}$$

$$z_2 = \begin{cases} 1 & (x_1, x_2) = (0,1) \\ 0 & \text{otherwise} \end{cases}$$

$$z_3 = \begin{cases} 1 & (x_1, x_2) = (1,0) \\ 0 & \text{otherwise} \end{cases}.$$

Now, the Cox model becomes

$$h(t,z) = h_0(t)e^{\beta_1 z_1 + \beta_2 z_2 + \beta_3 z_3}. \tag{10}$$

We can estimate the parameters $\beta_1, \beta_2, \beta_3$ in formula (8) on the basis of our research data as $\beta_1, \beta_2, \beta_3$. Then we have, $h(t,z) = h_0(t)e^{\beta_1 z_1 + \beta_2 z_2 + \beta_3 z_3}$.

The amount of modification of x_2 to x_1 can be estimated as follows:
Step 1: Because the two cases of $(x_1, x_2) = (1,0)$ and $(x_1, x_2) = (1,1)$ are corresponding to the two cases of $(z_1, z_2, z_3) = (0,0,1)$ and $(z_1, z_2, z_3) = (1,0,0)$, respectively, the ratio of the risk of event A when $(z_1, z_2, z_3) = (1,0,0)$ to the risk of event A when $(z_1, z_2, z_3) = (0,0,1)$ can be computed using formulas (2) and (8) as $RR_1 = e^{\beta_1 - \beta_3}$.
Using formula (4), the 95% confidence interval of RR_1 can be expressed as

$$e^{(\beta_1 - \beta_3) \pm 1.96\sqrt{Var(\beta_1) + Var(\beta_3) - 2Cov(\beta_1, \beta_3)}}. \tag{11}$$

Step 2: Because the two cases of $(x_1, x_2) = (0,0)$ and $(x_1, x_2) = (0,1)$ are corresponding to the two cases of $(z_1, z_2, z_3) = (0,0,0)$ and $(z_1, z_2, z_3) = (0,1,0)$, respectively, the ratio of the risk of event A when $(z_1, z_2, z_3) = (0,1,0)$ to the risk of event A when $(z_1, z_2, z_3) = (0,0,0)$ can be computed using formulas (2) and (8) as $RR_0 = e^{\beta_2}$.
Using formula (4), the 95% confidence interval of RR_0 can be expressed as

$$e^{\beta_2 \pm 1.96\sqrt{Var(\beta_2)}}. \tag{12}$$

We can conclude that there must be an interaction between x_1 and x_2 if the 95% confidence interval of RR_0 and the 95% confidence interval of RR_1 has no intersection. Therefore, the amount of modification of x_2 to x_1 can be evaluated by the difference of RR_1 and RR_2.

3 APPLICATIONS OF THE METHODS

To investigate whether new treatments can improve survival in patients with malignant tumor, we have recorded the treatment methods x_1 ($x_1 = 0$ corresponding to the new treatment method of treatment; $x_1 = 0$ corresponding to a traditional method of treatment) and the lymph node metastases x_2 ($x_2 = 1$ corresponding to lymph node metastasis; $x_2 = 0$ corresponding to no lymph node metastasis), for pathological diagnosis of 63 patients with malignant tumor. We have also made a follow-up observation of their survival time (*time*). If we represent the random event "death" as a random variable *outcome*, then *outcome* = 0 for the patients have not died at the end of the follow-up period, otherwise *outcome* = 1.

The follow-up results for the 63 patients are shown in Table 1.

Table 1. Survival time and its influencing factors of 63 cases of malignant tumor patients.

No.	x_1	x_2	time	out	No.	x_1	x_2	time	out
1	1	0	52	1	33	0	0	120	1
2	0	1	51	1	34	1	1	40	1
3	1	1	35	1	35	0	0	26	0
4	1	0	103	1	36	0	1	120	1
5	0	1	7	0	37	1	1	120	1
6	0	1	60	1	38	0	0	120	0
7	0	1	58	1	39	0	0	3	0
8	1	1	29	1	40	0	0	120	0
9	1	1	70	1	41	0	1	7	0
10	0	1	67	1	42	0	1	18	1
11	0	1	66	1	43	1	1	120	1
12	1	0	87	1	44	0	1	120	1
13	1	0	85	1	45	0	1	15	1
14	0	1	82	1	46	0	0	4	0
15	1	1	76	1	47	1	1	120	1
16	1	1	74	1	48	0	0	16	0
17	1	1	63	1	49	0	1	24	0
18	0	0	101	1	50	0	0	19	0
19	0	0	100	1	51	0	1	120	1
20	1	1	66	1	52	0	0	24	0
21	0	0	93	1	53	0	0	2	0
22	1	1	24	1	54	0	1	120	1
23	1	0	93	1	55	1	1	12	1
24	1	0	90	1	56	0	0	5	0
25	1	1	15	1	57	0	0	120	1
26	0	0	3	0	58	1	1	120	1
27	1	0	87	1	59	0	0	7	0
28	0	0	120	0	60	0	0	40	0
29	0	0	120	0	61	1	1	108	1
30	0	0	120	0	62	0	1	24	1
31	0	1	120	1	63	0	0	16	0
32	1	1	120	1					

We input the data in Table 1 into the computer, and then performed a Cox model fitting by using the process PHREG of statistical package SAS 9.0 (Ron, 2011). We obtained a fitting result of Table 2, and the variance and covariance matrices of parameters of Table 3.

From formula (6) we can see: in the cases of no lymph node metastasis ($x_2 = 0$), the risk of death in patients with traditional method of treatment ($x_1 = 1$) is about $RR_0 = e^{\beta_1} = e^{1.591} = 4.909$ times for those with new treatment method ($x_1 = 0$).

From formula (7) we can see: in the cases of lymph node metastasis ($x_2 = 1$), the risk of death in patients with traditional method of treatment ($x_1 = 1$) is about $RR_1 = e^{\beta_1 + \beta_3} = e^{1.591 + 1.508} = 1.086$ times for those with new treatment method ($x_1 = 0$):

$$| RR_1 - RR_0 | = 4.909 - 1.086 = 3.823.$$

From formula (9) we know

$$
\begin{aligned}
& Var(RR_1 - RR_0) \\
& = (e^{\beta_1 + \beta_3} - e^{\beta_1})^2 Var(\beta_1) + (e^{\beta_1 + \beta_3})^2 Var(\beta_3) \\
& + 2(e^{\beta_1 + \beta_3} - e^{\beta_1}) e^{\beta_1 + \beta_3} Cov(\beta_1, \beta_3) \\
& = 3.823^2 \times 0.366 + 1.086^2 \times 0.493 \\
& + 2 \times 3.823 \times 1.086 \times (-0.365) = 2.899
\end{aligned}
$$

We know that the 95% confidence interval of $| RR_1 - RR_0 |$ must be

$$3.823 - 1.96\sqrt{2.899} : 3.823 + 1.96\sqrt{2.899}.$$

In other words, the 95% confidence interval of $| RR_1 - RR_0 |$ is $0.486 : 7.160$.

Table 2.　Maximum likelihood estimation of the Cox model parameters for 63 cases of patients with malignant tumor.

	Estimations	SE of β	P values
Treatment method x_1	1.591	0.605	0.009
Lymph node metastasis x_2	1.353	0.522	0.009
$x_3 = x_1 x_2$	−1.508	1.702	0.032

Table 3.　Variance and covariance matrix of parameters.

	x_1	x_2	x_3
x_1	0.366	0.201	−0.365
x_2	0.201	0.272	−0.272
x_3	−0.365	−0.272	0.493

4 CONCLUDING REMARKS

This paper has introduced two applicable methods, product term method and dummy variable method, to analyze the interaction between the factors by using the Cox proportional hazards model. An example presented in Section 3 shows that the two methods are very practical.

The result of this application shows that in the case of no lymph node metastasis the new treatment method is better. However, in case of lymph node metastasis, the risk of death with new treatment method is not much lower than that of with the traditional treatment method. Regarding confidence interval, this difference reaches a statistical significance. This shows that there is an interaction between lymph node metastasis and treatment methods. The efficacy of the new treatment method is modified by the severity of the disease.

ACKNOWLEDGEMENTS

This work was supported in part by the Natural Science Foundation of Fujian under Grant 2013J01247, the Fujian Provincial Key Laboratory of Data-Intensive Computing, and the Fujian University Laboratory of Intelligent Computing and Information Processing.

REFERENCES

Cox D.R., Analysis of Survival Data. New York: Chapman and Hall 1984.

Elisa T. Lee, Statistical Methods for Survival Data Analysis, 4th Edition. New York: John Wiley & Sons, Inc. 2013.

Frank E., Jr. Harrell, Regression Modeling Strategies: With Applications to Linear Models, Logistic Regression, and Survival Analysis, New York, Springer-Verlag, 2010.

James T. McClave, Statistics, 12 edition, New York, Pearson, 2012.

Mitchell H. Katz, Multivariable Analysis: A Practical Guide for Clinicians and Public Health Researchers,3 edition, Cambridge, Cambridge University Press, 2011.

Richard Johnsonbaugh, Foundations of Mathematical Analysis, New York, Dover Publications, 2010.

Ron Cody, SAS Statistics by Example, New York, SAS Publishing, 2011.

Medicine Sciences and Bioengineering – Wang (Ed.)

The protection of amyloid precursor protein 17 peptide on diabetic encephalopathy

Duo Zhang & Heng Meng[*]

Affiliated Hospital of Beihua University, Jilin, China

ABSTRACT: Here we use multiple experimental approaches to investigate the effect of APP17 peptide on changes in learning behavior and glycol metabolism in rats. It was found that rats with DE treated by APP17 peptide showed reversed behavioral alternation. The ^{18}F-FDG -PET images and other results all showed that the APP17 peptide could promote glucose metabolism in the brain of the DE rat model. Meanwhile, the insulin signaling was markedly increased as shown by increased phosphorylation of Akt and enhanced GLUT4 activation. No amyloid plaques in the cortex and the hippocampus were detected in either group, indicating that the experimental animals in the current study were not suffering from Alzheimer's disease. These results indicate that APP17 peptide could be used to treat DE effectively.

1   INTRODUCTION

Diabetes mellitus is a group of metabolic diseases in which a person has high blood sugar, either because the pancreas does not produce enough insulin or because cells do not respond to the insulin that is produced (Castilho et al., 2012; Wang et al., 2008). Diabetic encephalopathy (DE) is caused by diabetes (Csibi et al., 2010). The complications of DE include memory loss, dementia, coma, seizures, and finally death. Amyloid precursor protein (APP) is a transmembrane protein with six isoforms in the central nervous system (CNS), of which APP-695 is the most important (Mamelak, 2012; Poisnel *et al.*, 2012). The active domain responsible for this activity has been identified in the 319–335 peptide segment of APP-695 and is known as APP17 peptide. Previous studies reported that APP17 peptide could promote axonal growth, increase synaptic density, and protect neurons from ischemic damage (Zhuang & Sheng, 2002; Shuli et al., 2001). However, little is known about the effects of APP17 peptide on encephalopathy caused by diabetes mellitus. In the present study, we use multiple experimental approaches to investigate the effect of APP17 peptide on changes in learning behavior and glycometabolism in rats.

2   MATERIALS AND METHODS

2.1   *Experimental animals and creation of animal model*

Male Wistar rats (weighing 180–200g) were supplied by the Laboratory Animal Center of Beijing. The animals were divided into three groups: normal controls (CON, n=25), diabetic (DE, n=25), and APP17 peptide-protected group (DE + APP17 peptide, n=25). Rats in the DE +APP17 peptide group were given APP17 peptide for 4 weeks after STZ (Sigma) treatment (0.7 µg per rat, s.c. daily). STZ was prepared before each use at 20 mg/mL in 0.1 M pH4.4 citrate buffer and was injected at 150 mg/kg, i.p., into rats which had been fasted for 12 h prior to receiving the injection. Four days later, nonfasting blood glucose in a tail-vein sample was determined by a glucose analyzer; a value >15 mM/L was accepted as a successfully created diabetic model.

---

*corresponding author

2.2 Learning and memory

Morris water maze tests were performed after training for 12 weeks. After the rats were familiar with the testing environment, normal training was performed from the second day. Orientation test: rats were trained twice per day, one time in the morning and one time in the afternoon. Each training session lasted for 120 sec, and the gap time was 30 s. The training lasted for 4 days. The starting area was randomly selected, and the number of times rats touched the platform in 120 sec was recorded. The platform was removed, and the rats were placed into water at the opposite side of the platform. The percent of residence time in the center area and numbers of times of passing the former platform in 120 sec were recorded.

2.3 In vivo Positron Emission Tomography (PET) scans

PET studies were performed on the rats suffering from diabetes or DE (n=20 per group). PET images were recorded on a high-resolution small-animal PET imaging device with a spatial resolution of 1.35 mm and a field of view (FOV) of 7.6 cm. Brain emission scans were acquired in 3D mode during 60 min after a tail-vein bolus injection MBq of ^{18}F-FDG Standardized uptake values (SUVs) were obtained for each VOI by dividing the mean ^{18}F-FDG activities by the injected dose and the animal weight.

2.4 Harris Hematoxylin and Eosin (H&E) staining

Thirty micron (μm) brain coronal sections were collected from every 200 μm section. The sections were deparaffinized, with two changes of xylene, 10 min each. The sections were rehydrated in 2 changes of absolute alcohol for 5 min each, 95% alcohol for 2 min, and 70% alcohol for 2 min, washed briefly in dH2O, and stained in Harris hematoxylin solution for 8 min. The sections were washed in running tap water for 5 min and differentiated in 1% acid alcohol for 30 sec. The slides were then washed in running tap water for 1min and stained in 0.2% ammonia water or saturated lithium carbonate solution for 30 to 60 sec. The slides were then washed in running tap water for 5 min, rinsed (10 dips) in 95% alcohol, and counterstained in eosin-phloxine solution for 30 sec. The slides were dehydrated in 95% alcohol, 2 changes of absolute alcohol, 5 min each. The slides were cleaned in 2 changes of xylene, 5 min each, and mounted with xylene-based mounting medium. The neurons in CA1 in the hippocampus were observed using an optical microscope.

2.5 IHC staining test

After dissecting tissues at 5 μm and fixed in 4% paraformaldehyde for 10 min, slides were incubated 2 to 3 times in xylene for 10 min each and then incubated twice in 100% ethanol for 2 min each. The slides were hydrated in 95%, 70%, 50%, and 30% ethanol for 2 min each. Slides were placed into buffer containing 5% normal goat serum for 10 min. Slides were incubated in a humidified chamber overnight with primary antibody (rabbit anti-rat Akt/PKB 1 : 500, rabbit anti-rat GLUT4 1 : 1000). They were washed in 5 m in buffer for 3 times and incubated with secondary antibody in a humidified chamber for 30 min. DAB and hematoxylin staining, 5 discontinue brain sections were selected, and 5 fields were selected randomly. The numbers of Akt/PKB and GLUT4 positive cells in CA1 were counted.

2.6 Statistical analysis

Data were expressed as mean ± standard deviation (M ± SD). Group differences in the swimming time in the Morris water maze test and the number of errors in the passageway water maze test were analyzed by SPSS 11.0 using Windows software to conduct two-way analysis of variance (ANOVA, equal variances assumed by S-N-K) on repeated measurements. Other data were analyzed by SPSS 11.0 using Windows software to conduct one-way ANOVA (equal variances assumed by S-N-K). A post hoc test was used to obtain the P values. A $p < 0.05$ was considered significant.

3 RESULTS AND DISCUSSION

3.1 *Memory ability*

The rats of the DE group were polydipsia, polyphagia, polyuria and weight loss, yellowish color, poor spirit of the late, slow-moving symptoms. As shown in Table 1, at the beginning of generating animal model, the values of blood glucose in DE and DE + APP17 peptide groups were much higher than control group on 13th weeks ($p < 0.01$), while the body weight of mice in 3 groups remained the same ($p > 0.05$). After the treatment, the values of blood glucose in DE + APP17 peptide group were decreased, while body weight increased compared with DE group; the difference was significant ($p < 0.05$) (Figures 1(a) and 1(b)). Using the Morris water maze test, the rats treated with APP17 peptide had a prolonged swimming time ($p < 0.05$) and made significantly more errors when compared with the control group ($p < 0.05$). The rats showed reversed behavioral alternation with levels returning close to that of rats in the control group (Figure 1(c)).

3.2 *The APP17 peptide and glucose metabolism in the brain of the DE rat model*

As shown in Table 1, at the beginning of the generation of the animal model, the blood glucose in the DE and DE + APP17 peptide groups was significantly higher than that in the control group ($p < 0.01$), while the body weight of mice in 3 groups remained the same with no significant difference ($p > 0.05$). After the treatment, the blood glucose in the DE + APP17 peptide group decreased, and the body weight significantly increased compared with DE group ($p < 0.05$).

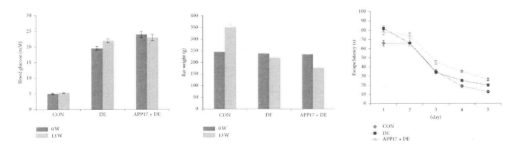

Figure 1. (a) Blood glucose in 3 groups. (b) body weight of mice in 3 groups. (c) The ability analysis of learning and memory of mice in 3 groups.

Table 1. Blood glucose and body weight of mice in 3 groups (x±s, n=1).

Group	Blood (mmol/L)		Body weight (g)	
	0 w	13 w	0 w	13 w
CON	5.40 ± 0.41	5.56 ± 0.35	240.87 ± 5.44	350.32 ± 19.19
DE + APP17	$21.73 \pm 1.53^{**}$	$16.43 \pm 1.12^{**}$	238.97 ± 5.91	$250.58 \pm 15.22^{**}$
DE	$24.28 \pm 1.98^{**}$	$22.96 \pm 1.35^{**\#\#}$	235.00 ± 12.1	$180.02 \pm 14.50^{**\#\#}$

$^*p < 0.05$, $^{**}p < 0.01$ versus CON, $\# p < 0.05$, $\#\# p < 0.01$ versus DE. Different letters represent the significant difference at $p < 0.05$.

41

The mean ^{18}F-FDG activities, corrected for radioactive decay, were evaluated for each VOI on integrated PET images recorded during a 30–60 minute acquisition period. Standardized uptake values (SUVs) were obtained for each VOI by dividing the mean ^{18}F-FDG activities by the injected dose and the animal weight. Regional FDG data were normalized by the FDG uptake within the cerebellum (V. Blanchard, S. Moussaoui, C, 2003). To study glycol metabolism, changes of ^{18}F-FDG–PET images were recorded in the DE rat model. After anatomofunctional combination, cerebral regions such as the cortex, the hippocampus, the striatum, and the cerebellum were outlined on PET images (Figure 2). A significant positive correlation was found between the DE group and DE+APP17 peptide group and the ^{18}F-FDG uptake in the cortex and the hippocampus. Evaluation of glycolmetabolism in animals revealed a decrease of cortical and hippocampal glucose uptake in the DE group compared with the CON group. In the DE+APP17 peptide group, the glucose uptake was increased, as compared with DE group.

3.3 *Expression of Akt/PKB and GLUT4 after treatment of APP17 peptide*

The results of the IHC indicated that, compared with the control group, the number of Akt/PKB positive cells in the hippocampus of the DE group was reduced. In contrast the Akt/PKB positive cells in DE + APP17 peptide group was similar to those in the control group. In the results of western blotting, APP17 acutely stimulated Akt phosphorylation in the group of treatment, compared with control cells (Figure 3). The expression of GLUT4 in membrane was obviously decreased in the rat hippocampal gyrus in DE group ($p < 0.01$). Compared with DE group, the expression of GLUT4 was obviously increased in the rat hippocampal gyrus in DE + APP17 group ($p < 0.05$) (Figure 4).

These results show that glycometabolism plays an important role in the onset and development of neurodegenerative diseases and that the administration of APP17 peptide has neuroprotective effects against the changes induced by abnormal glycometabolism. APP17 peptide may cause these effects through the activation of common intracellular signaling pathways and initiation of

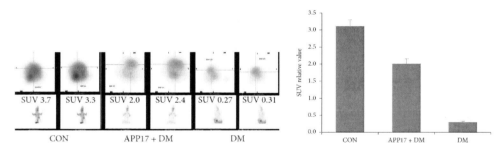

Figure 2. Evaluation of brain glycometabolism in DE activation in animals by PET/CT.

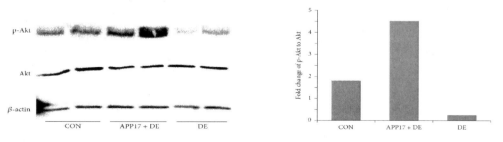

Figure 3. Enhanced insulin-induced Akt the hippocampal gyrus of DE rats with APP17 treatment.

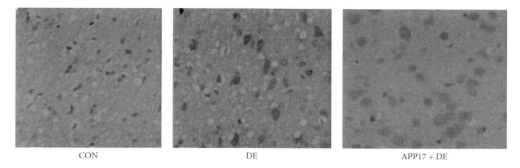

CON   DE   APP17 + DE

Figure 4.   Enhanced GLUT4 expression in the hippocampal gyrus of DE rats with APP17 treatment.

"cross-talk" with neurotrophins. Further investigation is required to determine the mechanism by which APP17 peptide induces neuroprotection in this rat model. This may assist in identifying APP17 peptide as a potential therapeutic for neurodegenerative diseases.

4   CONCLUSION

The results of the current study indicate that APP17 peptide has a comprehensive therapeutic effect on diabetic encephalopathy, particularly through improving glycometabolism.

REFERENCES

A. F. Castilho, J. T. Liberal, F. Ambrosio, "Elevated glucose concentration changes the content and cellular localization of AMP Areceptors in the retina" Neuroscience, vol. 219, 23–32, 2012.

A. Csibi, D.Communi, N. Muller, and S. P. Bottari, "Angiotensin ii inhibits insulin-stimulated GLUT4 translocation and akt activation through tyrosine nitration-dependent mechanisms," PLoS ONE, vol. 5, no.4, Article ID e10070, 2010.

C.-L. Wang, X. Wang, Y. Yu et al, "Type 1 Diabetes attenuates the modulatory effects of endomorphins on mouse colonic motility," Neuropeptides, vol. 42, no. 1, 69–77, 2008.

G. Poisnel, A.S. Herard, N. El Tannir et al, "Increased regional cerebral glucose uptake in an APP/PS1 model of Alzheimer's disease," Neurobiology of Aging, vol. 33, 1995–2005, 2012.

M. Mamelak, "Sporadic Alzheimer's disease: the starving brain," Journal of Alzheimer's Disease, vol. 31, no. 3, Article ID 120370, 459–474.

S. Shuli, Z. Yongmei, Z. Zhijuan, and J. Zhiwei, "β-Amyloid and its binding protein in the hippocampus of diabetic mice: effect of APP17 peptide," NeuroReport, vol. 12, no.15, 3317–3319, 2001.

V. Blanchard, S. Moussaoui, C., "Time sequence of maturation of dystrophic neurites associated with A β deposits in APP/PS1 transgenic mice," Experimental Neurology, vol. 184, no.1, 247–263.

X. M. Zhuang and S. L. Sheng, "Effect of APP17 peptide on the hippocampal neurons ultrastructure and expression of InsR, Ins21 in Type 2 diabetic KKAy mice," Journal of Capital Medical University, vol. 23, no.2, 115–118, 2002 (Chinese).

Medicine Sciences and Bioengineering – Wang (Ed.)
© 2015 Taylor & Francis Group, London, ISBN: 978-1-138-02684-1

The effect of different concentrations of rocuronium bromide used for anesthesia induction on introperative recurrent laryngeal nerve monitoring of the patients with thyroid operation

Peng Chen, Yu-Huan Pan & Feng Liang*
Department of Anesthesiology, China-Japan Union Hospital, Ji Lin University, Changchun, Jilin, China

ABSTRACT: Objective: Evaluate the effect of different concentrations of rocuronium bromide used for anesthesia induction on the thyroid operation introperative recurrent laryngeal nerve monitoring (IONM). Methods: Select 100 cases of thyroid operation patients, male or female, aged from 23 to 67 years old, with the weight from 52 to 84 kg. ASA classification is I or II level. Divide them into five groups randomly: 20 cases in each group. Group I inhale 8% sevoflurane with the oxygen flow being 6 L/min, and adopt video laryngoscope to insert the recurrent laryngeal nerve monitoring special tracheal tube to make the mechanical ventilation 10 seconds later after the end-tidal concentration achieves 2.5%. Group II-V are monitored the level of neuromuscular blockade by TOF-Watch SX accelerometer. After the height of the first muscle twitch response maintains about 100% for three minutes, intravenously inject 0.5, 1, 1.5, 2×ED95 rocuronium bromide. Insert nerve monitoring special tracheal tube after the muscular relaxation achieves maximum suppression. Firstly, we recorded the time from injecting rocuronium bromide to inserting the tube. Secondly, we evaluated endotracheal intubation conditions and then recorded the circumstances of the blood pressure, pulse changes. Adopting NIM-Response 3.0 Nerve Electromyography Monitor to monitor vagus nerve/recurrent laryngeal nerve evoked muscle potential, recording the amplitude of electromyogram signal (μV) every 5 minutes 30 minutes later after the endotracheal intubation is successful. Monitor five groups of signals continuously, and get the stable index of IONM by statistical method. Results: The endotracheal intubation's one-time success rates of the five groups are all 100%. Compared with Group I, the endotracheal intubation condition scores of Group II-V are higher ($P < 0.05$); the stability of IONM signal amplitude of Group I-III meets the monitoring demands. Conclusion: The use of 0.5, 1×ED95 rocuronium bromide during the anesthesia induction period both can improve endotracheal intubation conditions, and don't affect the introperative recurrent laryngeal nerve monitoring. The effect of 1×ED95 rocuronium bromide for induction is the best.

1   INTRODUCTION

Intraoperative recurrent laryngeal nerve monitoring (IONM) technology avoid the damage of intraoperative recurrent laryngeal nerve (Peng Chen, Feng Liang, Zhen-po Su et al, 2012). In the intraoperative recurrent laryngeal nerve monitoring, muscle relaxant is the main interference factor of the determination process (Hui Sun, Xiaoli Liu, Yantao Fu et al, 2010). A study by us in 2012 shows that 1×ED95 rocuronium bromide induction used for thyroid operation under recurrent laryngeal nerve monitoring can provide better endotracheal intubation conditions on the premise of satisfying intraoperative recurrent laryngeal nerve monitoring (Xiuli Meng, Jun Wang, Liping Zhang, 2006). At home and abroad, there are no reports about the effect of different concentrations of rocuronium bromide used for anesthesia induction on

---

*Corresponding Author: Liang Feng, Email: 295253720@qq.com.

intraoperative recurrent laryngeal nerve monitoring of the patients with thyroid operation. This study intends to evaluate the effect of different concentrations of rocuronium bromide used for anesthesia induction on thyroid operation patients intraoperative recurrent laryngeal nerve monitoring.

2 MATERIAL AND METHOD

We will select a time to go on the general anesthesia on the thyroid operation patients of 100 cases, aged from 23 to 67 years old, with the weight from 52 to 84 kg, male or female. ASA classification is I or II level. Divide them into five groups randomly: 20 cases in each group. Intramuscularly inject penehyclidine hydrochloride 1 mg 30 minutes earlier before the anesthesia. Routine monitor ECG, BP, SpO2 after admission, open the venous access, and inject lactated Rnger's solution (infusion rate is 6–8 ml/kg · h). Monitor the expired concentrations of sevoflurane after the induction. Anesthesia induction: Five groups intravenously inject midazolam 2 mg, propofol 2 mg/kg, sufentanil 0.5 ug/kg in turn. After the eyelash reflex disappears, Group I inhale 8% sevoflurane with the oxygen flow being 6 L/min, and adopt video laryngoscope to insert recurrent laryngeal nerve monitoring special tracheal tube to make the mechanical ventilation 10 seconds later after the end-tidal concentration achieves 2.5%.

The patients of Group II-V are monitored the level of neuromuscular blockade by TOF-Watch SX accelerometer. After the height of the first muscle twitch response maintains about 100% for three minutes, intravenously inject 0.5, 1, 1.5, 2×ED95 rocuronium bromide (batch number: H20040423, Organon Company, The Netherlands). Insert nerve monitoring special tracheal tube after the muscular relaxation achieves the maximum suppression. Record the time from injecting rocuronium bromide to inserting the tube, evaluate the conditions of endotracheal intubation. Five groups of patients make the mechanical ventilation after the endotracheal intubation. Ventilatory factors settings: inspiratory to expiratory ratio 1:2, tidal volume 10–12 ml/kg, respiratory frequency 12/min. Anesthesia maintenance: the patients of five groups all inhale sevoflurane-nitrous oxide-oxygen to maintain the depth of anesthesia, maintaining the depth of anesthesia in 1.2 ~ 1.4 MAC. The time from the success of endotracheal intubation to completing the vagus nerve exposure is limited in 30 minutes, endotracheal intubation are completed by the same senior anesthetist. Adopt the score standard of Cooper method (see Table 1) to evaluate the endotracheal intubation conditions, and record the circumstances of the blood pressure, pulse changes. Adopt NIM-Response 3.0 Nerve Electromyography Monitor (Medtronic Xomed Company, USA) to monitor vagus nerve/recurrent laryngeal nerve evoked myogenic potential with 3 mA electric current to stimulate vagus nerve and 1 mA electric current to stimulate recurrent laryngeal nerve. Record the amplitude of electromyogram signal (μV) every 5 minutes 30 minutes later after the endotracheal intubation is successful. Monitor five groups of signals continuously, and get the stable index of IONM by statistical method.

Adopt SPSS19.0 statistics software to analyze, measurement data is showed by mean ± standard deviation ($ x \pm$ s). Repeated measurement data adopts one-way ANOVA of repeated measurement design, enumeration data adopts Chi-square test, ranked data adopts LSD test. $P < 0.05$ means the differences have statistical significance.

Table 1. The score standard of Cooper method endotracheal intubation condition.

Laryngoscope examination	Glottis	Intubation reaction	Score
Impossible	Closed	Cough	0
Difficult	Closed up	Cough slightly	1
General	Active	Slight diaphragm activity	2
Easy	Open	No reaction	3

Note: the total score of 8 ~ 9 is excellent, 6 ~ 7 is great, 3 ~ 5 is general, 0 ~ 2 is poor.

3 RESULTS

The one-time success rates of the endotracheal intubation of five groups are all 100%, but compared with Group I, the scores of the endotracheal intubation condition evaluation of Group II-V are higher ($P < 0.05$); Compared with Group II, the scores of the endotracheal intubation condition evaluation of Group III-V are higher ($P < 0.05$). The scores of the endotracheal intubation condition evaluation of Group III-V don't have obvious differences (see Table 2). Group II-V don't have obvious differences from the induction to endotracheal intubation; Group I-V don't have obvious differences from the induction to the first neurostimulation. DBP, SBP and HR between the groups don't have obvious differences before and after the endotracheal intubation. Statistical analysis shows that the stability of IONM signal amplitude of Group I~III meets the monitoring demands (see Table 3,4).

4 DISCUSSION

In the thyroid operation, adopting intraoperative recurrent laryngeal nerve monitoring (IONM) technology can identify and position recurrent laryngeal nerve, greatly reducing the probability

Table 2. The comparison of five groups endotracheal intubation condition evaluation.

Group	Cooper score	F	P
I	5.20 ± 0.41		
II	5.80 ± 0.62[a]		
III	6.15 ± 0.59[ab]	181.020	< 0.001
IV	8.65 ± 0.59[abc]		

Note: a: Compared with Group I, $P < 0.05$; b: Compared with Group II, $P < 0.05$; c: Compared with Group III, $P < 0.05$;

Table 3. The average of maximum IONM signal amplitude subtracting mimimum IONM signal amplitude of each group (μV, $\bar{x} \pm s$).

Group	The stability of NIM	F	P
I	759.80 ± 566.04		
II	756.55 ± 634.90		
III	483.35 ± 362.17	2.998	0.022
IV	440.05 ± 391.64		
V	385.80 ± 260.36[ab]		

Note: a: Compared with Group I, the difference has statistical significance; b: Compared with Group II, the difference has statistical significance.

Table 4. The average of IONM signal amplitude at five time points (μV, $\bar{x} \pm s$).

Group	The stability of NIM	F	P
I	1788.89 ± 1098.82		
II	2107.80 ± 1161.67		
III	1558.72 ± 726.47	5.797	<0.001
IV	1039.60 ± 579.47[ab]		
V	1033.48 ± 632.25[ab]		

Note: a: Compared with Group I, the difference has statistical significance; b: Compared with Group II, the difference has statistical significance.

of recurrent laryngeal nerve injury. In USA, the usage rate of IONM is 40% -45%. Medtronic Xomed NIM-Response 3.0 Nerve Electromyography Monitor and Special recurrent laryngeal nerve monitoring tracheal tube are the most advanced monitoring facilities. Intraoperatively adopts sevoflurane to maintain the anesthesia, because its blood & air partition coefficent is 0.63, and its anesthesia controllability is good. It has small effects on hemodynamics and neuromuscular junction function, and can eliminate the influence of anaesthetic and hemodynamics factors on recurrent laryngeal nerve monitoring.

The results show that the endotracheal intubation's one-time success rates of the five groups are all 100%. Compared with Group I, the endotracheal intubation condition scores of the patients of Group II-V are higher ($P < 0.05$); Compared with Group II, the endotracheal intubation condition scores of the patients of Group III-V are higher ($P < 0.05$). The scores of the endotracheal intubation condition evaluation of Group III-V don't have obvious differences. It explains that the use of 0.5×ED95 rocuronium bromide can obviously improve the endotracheal intubation condition, while the influence of the use of 1, 1.5, 2×ED95 rocuronium bromide on endotracheal intubation condition don't have obvious differences.

Five groups are all measured vagus nerve/recurrent laryngeal nerve signal (V/R Siganl) 30 minutes later after the endotracheal intubation, but compared with Group I, II, the signal stability of Group IV~V has obvious differences. It explains that evoked electromyogram amplitude of these two groups can't meet the continuous monitoring demands. It points out that the use of 0.5×, 1×ED95 rocuronium bromide both can improve the endotracheal intubation condition, and don't have effect on introperative recurrent laryngeal nerve monitoring. The reasons might be: (1) The acquisition of non-depolarising muscle relaxant ED95 dose is using muscular relaxation monitor to monitor adductor pollicis, different muscle groups have different pharmacodynamics for non-depolarising muscle relaxant. Compared with adductor pollicis, the onset and recovery time of non-depolarising muscle relaxant blocking laryngeal adductor muscle are faster. This may be because, in terms of unit mass, the blood flow of adductor pollicis is less than that of laryngeal muscles, the spreading and eliminating of muscle relaxant in the muscle groups of high blood flow are faster than that in the muscle groups of low blood flow; (2) The clinical effect time of rocuronium bromide used for anesthesia induction has dose correlation. The study shows that the clinical effect time of 2×ED95 rocuronium bromide is 36 minutes, the clinical effect time of 1×ED95 is less than 30 minutes. While our experiment starts from 30 minutes later after the endotracheal intubation, it explains that in the 30 minutes from the conventional operation to nerve exposure, 1.5×ED95 or more dose of rocuronium bromide induction will interfere intoperative recurrent laryngeal nerve monitoring.

To sum up, 0.5×, 1×ED95 rocuronium bromide used in the anesthesia induction period both can improve the endotracheal intubation conditions, and also doesn't influence intraoperative recurrent laryngeal nerve monitoring. The effect of 1×ED95 rocuronium bromide induction is the best.

REFERENCES

Hemmerling TM, Donati F. Neuomuscular blockade at the larynx, the diaphragm and the corrugator su perciliimuscle: a review. *Can J Anaesth*, 2003, 50(8): 779–794.

Hemmerling TM, Schmidt J, Hanusa C et al. Simultaneous determination of neuromuscular block at the larynx, diaphragm, adduvtor polic, orbicularis oculi and corrugator supercilii muscles. *Br J Anaesth,* 2000, 85(6): 856–860.

Hui Sun, Xiaoli Liu, Yantao Fu et al. Application of intraoperative neromonitoring during complex thyroid operation. *Chinese Journal of Practical Surgery,* 2010, 30(1): 66–68.

Peng Chen, Feng Liang, Zhenpo Su et al. The effect of 1×ED95 Rocuronium Bromide used for anesthesia induction on introperative recurrent laryngeal nerve monitoring of the patients with thyroid operation, *Chinese Journal of Anesthesiology*, 2012, 32(5):525–527.

Plaud B, Debenb B, Lequeau F et al. Mivacurium neuromuscular block at the adductor muscles of the larynx and adductor pllicis in humans. *Anesthtsiology,* 1999, 85(1): 77–81.

Sharpe MD, Moote CA, Lam AM, et al. Comparison of integrated evoked EMG between the hypothenar and facial muscle groups following atracurium and Rocuronium administration. *Can J Anaesth,*1991, 38(3): 318–323.

Xiuli Meng, Jun Wang, Liping Zhang. The effect of Atracurium on otologic surgery facial nerve monitoring, *Chinese Journal of Minimally Invasive Surgery,* 2006, 29(2): 137–141.

Medicine Sciences and Bioengineering – Wang (Ed.)
© *2015 Taylor & Francis Group, London, ISBN: 978-1-138-02684-1*

Application and prospect of process control in the modern production of Chinese materia medical

Ming-san Miao, Lin Guo, Shuo Tian, Peng-fei Li & Ling-li Jiang
Henan University of Traditional Chinese Medicine, Zhengzhou, Henan, China

ABSTRACT: Through the analysis of the application and process control method of Chinese materia medical, the characteristics of process control are summarized and corresponding solutions are put forward. This paper aims to improve application methods in process control, to promote popularization and implementation of process control in Chinese materia medical production line and to improve the efficiency and quality of Chinese materia medical production.

1 INTRODUCTION

Process control is to ensure that the production process in a controlled state, to directly or indirectly affect product quality, production, installation, and service process of technology and production process analysis, diagnosis, and monitoring. It is used for chemical industry and has a wide application prospect in the pharmaceutical industry. Process control is proposed on the basis of "medicines quality are produced" cGMP concept and is a new pharmaceutical production model. Compared with the existing "parametric release mode," the model is built on the continuous improvement of the quality control system and is on the understanding of the whole process (Liu, 2011). Chinese Materia Medical (CMM) is an important part of Chinese intangible cultural heritage, and to ensure the quality of CMM products and promote the development of CMM industry are the primary problems. Therefore, perfecting the production process control of CMM is very important.

2 APPLICATION STATUS OF PROCESS CONTROL OF CMM

2.1 *Application of process control in the production of CMM*

2.1.1 *Sliced herbal medicine*
A common process control of sliced herbal medicine includes pretreatment method of washing, cutting, and other control of the processing system method. Combined with the application in Gardenia pretreatment production process of statistical process control in the single variable and multivariable can make the process simplify and monitoring, fault detection, diagnosis, and the corresponding research simplified (Zhou, 2012). Flower and some light or irregular pieces are made into quantitative pills by physical pressing method. It does not change the appearance and inner quality pieces, and does not add any accessories. It avoids pieces that float on the water and is advantageous to pieces of infiltration and compositions. It is innovative, necessity, and feasible (Song, 2012).

2.1.2 *Chinese patent medicine*
Common process control methods include decoction, concentration, and other processes, as well as the content of active component, drying process of moisture, and so on. In view of the online spectrum collection device that is designed by near-infrared (NIR) spectrum technology, online

analysis can fast determine the percolation process of alkaloid and total solids of compound matrine injection and applied to the actual production; it solves the percolation process that lacks technical problems in real-time monitoring, to improve the level of quality control and ensure the stable quality of products (Chen, 2012). Quantitative analysis of model technology combined with the online micro-NIR instrument, not only obtain real-time online information about Chinese medicine powder content, timely evaluation of mixed end, but also detect physical state of powder mixing process in compliance with the quantitative model of the standard, and it has very important practical significance.

2.1.3 *Others*

In addition to sliced herbal medicine and Chinese patent medicine, other products include herbal extracts and health products of traditional Chinese medicine (TCM). The common process control method is a purified, extraction, moisture absorption process with comprehensive supervision on the quality. The automation of the CMM extraction technology can realize the extraction of CMM production operation process and is a key to quality parameters and process conditions throughout the online monitoring, to guarantee quality products and achieve the object of energy cost reduction. Direct analysis in real-time tandem mass spectrometry in the rapid identification of medicine and pieces, real-time of the intermediate or finished products for rapid quantitative analysis with advantage in situ, and direct and rapid detection has strong qualitative ability and advantages. With similar NIR spectroscopy, CMM extract qualitative quality control method can accurately reflect the differences in extracts of Radix scutellariae, honeysuckle, Weeping forsythia, goat horn, and Bear gall powder from batch-to-batch production, and it has been used as a method of the extraction material control.

2.2 *Process control method of CMM*

2.2.1 *Process control method of parameters*

The main process control of sliced herbal medicine is the control of processing parameters. After processing, herbal medicine can remove impurities, do correction of odor, reduce the toxic and side effects, and improve the medicinal effect, so that it has been widely used in clinical treatment. With the help of modern temperature noncontact automatic detection instrument, surface visualization technology can accurately measure and control the processing heating process, and the processing process is strictly quantitative and standardization, which improves the quality and stability of the processed products.

The main CMM industrialization production process is concentrating and drying process. These are multivariable, nonlinear disturbance of large, complex dynamic system (Chen, 2010). Usually, CMM concentration use gas–liquid phase equilibrium evaporation technique. Evaporation not only maintains the characteristic of CMM, but also has strong adaptability to the varieties of CMM, and it is the earliest and most widely used in CMM (Bi, 2013). Production control system and concentrated CMM can improve the production efficiency, product quality, and rate of heat energy, which is of great significance to the integration of automatic control systems of CMM production. Dried herbs can keep the medicinal ingredients intact and not prone to spoilage; it is easy for transportation and storage, and is convenient for pharmaceutical companies cutting, processing, and grinding. With the progress of science and technology, computational fluid mechanics in spray drying process is also used widely.

2.2.2 *Process control method of quality standard*

Quality and resistance of CMM are the dialectical unification relations, where quality is the important guarantee of resistance and resistance is an important expression of quality. The two common securities provide a safe and effective method of CMM.

At present, the analysis method for quality control of CMM and other related methods in our country are mass spectrometry, nuclear magnetic resonance, gas chromatography, high-pressure liquid chromatography (HPLC), and IR, UV Vis, Raman spectroscopies. *Chinese Pharmacopoeia*

2010 edition lists 1063 kinds of CMM, and the composition was determined in 709 kinds by using HPLC and in 24 by using gas chromatography, in 12 by Thin Layer Chromatography Scan (TLCS). Raman spectroscopy can be used for the detection and analysis of CMM biochemical components. NIR technology can realize the online quality control of salvianolic acid B in the purification process.

3   THE CHARACTERISTICS OF PROCESS CONTROL OF CMM

As an emerging production control means, process control of CMM production solves the discrete nature of the production of CMM on one hand. Continuous process control can monitor the crafts quality at the same time, and also merge various optimized crafts parameters, which may help to make the whole production be in its best condition and increase the production efficiency of related products of CMM as well. On the other hand, it may make the process control of CMM production targeted, and so that each process method can be established into appropriate procedures and more optimized process conditions according to the key active ingredients in CMM; as a result, the content of the active ingredients of CMM can be ensured to some degree to ensure efficacy. Additionally, process control has changed the methods of analysis and examination of CMM, from the traditional offline and release mode to online mode. Traditional methods of examinations of quality indicators always have complicated steps and hysteretic feedback, so there is no way to acquire the information of intermediates and the quality of crafts process timely. No matter it is sliced herbal medicine or other related productions of CMM, the problems of production line can be reflected much faster by controlling their production process, which may reduce the losses of raw materials and manpower.

However, current process control of CMM still has some shortcomings as follows: On one hand, the technology of intelligentize and automate in the productive process of CMM develops logging, where few advanced electronic technologies have been applied to the production process of CMM, or the existed technological means cannot meet the needs of multitudinous production, thus the model that truly meets batch control and management in the whole process of pharmaceutical production processes and QMP has not come true. On the other hand, under the influence of the traditional manual production, the crafts of CMM have poor accuracy and relative uncertainty, except for some critical crafts steps have been studied seriously; other crafts, such as infiltration, were not seriously studied and standardized parameters are rare, and these less studied crafts are under manual control and lack of scientific Meanwhile, the components of CMM are more complex, and CMMs have no identified chemical components as chemical medicines, so the control of a single chemical component does not fully indicate that the quality control of the herb has been effectively controlled. Especially in compound preparations such as Chinese patent drugs, the functions of "Sovereign and subject Musa acts" of each herb are different, and disparate extraction methods will affect the efficacy of compatibility of medicines to some extent, so that detecting any one kind of active ingredient cannot reflect the overall effect, which is the fundamental difference in quality standards between CMM and chemical drugs. The developing of process control of CMM is also facing the problem of how to reduce the loss of active ingredients in CMM.

4   SUMMARY

The basic thought of TCM is the overall concept on the basis of which, CMM should pay more attention to the comprehensive and harmonious. Starting from the whole view, the future development direction of CMM production should be on improving the production of CMM on the basis of CMM theory, so that the technology and quality detection control could be continuous, integrated, and intelligent. So the online quality control research and the development of its associated computer system must be the future trend of the development of CMM production.

Online quality control can be approximated as a process analytical technology (PAT). The PAT quality management philosophy is as follows: the quality of the final product is guaranteed by the process analysis, equipment validation, and automatically controlled process parameters. Implementation of standard operating procedures enhances process specification, analysis of each batch of production process in a timely feedback sampling, analysis of data, adjustment of the control parameters, and ensuring the quality of drugs (Yu, 2010).

On the basis of PAT management concept, the process control of the production of CMM can be improved on the basis of three aspects: on one hand, combine with the actual CMM production, enhance the establishment of the process model, strengthen the research and development of related computer program, improve the central control platform (such as distributed control systems), improve the information management system of mass production, make the advanced intelligent, such as computer program, network, intelligent information management system of modern technology, with traditional technology of analyzing and checking to meet timeliness, continuity, scientific in the production and inspection of CMM. The application of object linking and embedding process control technology achieves an NIR analysis online communication method for the two-way data read–write system and automation equipment, and it can be directly used for online analysis and intelligent control of production process (Qin, 2011). On the other hand, we can combine the development of control methods of CMM production with the advantage technology in multisubjects: combine the CMM research of process parameters with physical or other disciplines to standardize the process parameter specification of CMM production. At the same time, for production equipment, increasing the reasonable and the maintainability by reducing the arbitrariness and empirical parameters can ensure the process rigor. Specific detection of effective components of CMM extract can be tested by using enzyme activity, antiviral, antibacterial, anti-inflammatory activity test titer detection method determining uniqueness of the multi-index of CMM can solve the evaluation problem in quality control and effective complexity of CMM, and theoretically, it is superior to qualitative and quantitative analysis of TCM with the current indexes.

China has a rich natural medicaments resource, but CMM products in the international natural medicine market accounted for only 3% to 5% (Zhang, 2013). Process control is automatic intelligent control through the techniques of automation and computer application in pharmaceutical production line. The perfect process control technology used in CMM production line can realize self-examination, self-control, self-correction of the production, and the monitoring of multicomponents of CMM; can ensure the effective ingredients, and improve production efficiency and utilization rate of CMM. In addition, process control—on the basis of the characteristics of wide coverage and multiplication, by applying in the production of CMM—can promote the fusion of CMM and other disciplines of science and technology; opens the way of internationalization, intelligent, and standardization in the production of Chinese traditional medicine, so that the CMM product can enhance share in the international natural medicine market.

REFERENCES

Bi, X.L. & Ni, B. (2013) Technical advances in research of traditional Chinese medicine traditional Chinese medicine intermediate in the preparation of separation. Chin Med JR es Prac, 27(4), 77–81.
Chen, C. & Li, W.L. (2012) An on-line Near-Infrared spectroscopy approach for content determination in the percolation process of compound Kushen Injection. Chin Pharm J, 47(21), 1698–1702.
Chen, Y & Li, Y.E. (2010) Research advances in the complete equipment and automation control technologies of extraction. World Science and Technology Modernization of Traditional Chinese Medicine and Moteria Medica, 12(3), 430–436.
Liu, X.Q. & Tong, Y. (2011) Compound matrine injection alcohol precipitation process optimization and alcohol sedimentation process research.China Journal of Chinese Materia Medica, 36(22), 3108–3133.
Qin.B.D. & Li, L.Q.(2011) Application of OPC technology in near-infrared online intelligent monitoring system in production process of traditional Chinese medicine, Mod Comput, (7), 68–71.

Song, Y.R. & Sheng, R. (2012) Research and manufacture of a new type of quantitative suppressed traditional Chinese medicine. Chin Hosp Pharm J, 32(18), 1456–1459.

Yu, Y. & Zhao, Y.Z. (2010) Traditional Chinese medicine preparation engineering automation and online monitoring technology. Chinese pharmaceutical equipment, (5), 37–42.

Zhou, H.Y. & Bin, X. (2012) Application of statistical process control in pretreatment production process of Gardenia jasminoides. Chinese Journal of Experimental Traditional Medical Formulae, 18(11), 16–18.

Zhang, J.C. & Lin, S.X. (2013) The present situation and development trend of drying technology for Chinese Medicinal Herbs.Guizhou Science, 31(2), 89–93.

Medicine Sciences and Bioengineering – Wang (Ed.)
© 2015 Taylor & Francis Group, London, ISBN: 978-1-138-02684-1

The wireless control system for high-frequency portable X-ray machine based on MCU

Xin Tan, Qian-cheng Liu & Bin-feng Xu
College of Medical Instrument, Guangdong Food and Drug Vocational College, Guangzhou, Guangdong, China

ABSTRACT: In this paper, the objective of the study benefits the medical field—realize the design and development of the control platform of high-frequency portable X-ray machine and wireless control system using C8051F340 MCU and wireless control technology, which can provide the man–machine interaction good for clinicians. It have simple interface, which can perform remote exposure operation in multi environment, multiple operation conditions. It has the characteristics of high efficiency, high definition, high flexible.

1 INTRODUCTION

X machine is an important diagnostic instrument of modern medicine plays a decisive role in many disease diagnoses. In developed countries, clinical X-ray machine has been widely applied to human limbs and organs, which are the common sites of disease diagnosis (Ma Hui, 2011). However, due to limited conditions the domestic use of portable diagnostic X-ray machine is little, largely influenced by the particular environment on the accuracy of diagnosis. The operator is away from the radiation hazards and will lengthen the cable, which will not only affect the portability of the system but also bring about new problems such as power consumption, interface management, and system costs. Wireless control system is the use of wireless communication to complete the inspection work in remote control X-ray machines. This not only improves the portability of the system but also reduces the harm of rays on field staff (SUO Dan, HAN Yan & YANG Guang, 2010).

In this paper, by analyzing the development status of domestic and foreign literature and technical documents and the current wireless control system, proposed in the portable X-ray machine on the main control platform design using C8051F340 microcontroller and wireless control technology, the portable X-ray machine remote control design is discussed. The paper then studies the theories of SCM control technology, LCD touch screen display technology, and wireless remote control technology; the design and implementation of control system can be used for ensuring high frequency of portable X-ray machine control platform and remote exposure.

2 SYSTEM DESIGN

According to the need of function of the system, the high frequency of portable X-ray machine wireless control system design enables low cost, high versatility, and high reliability; the overall system structure is shown in Figure 1.

The wireless control system is mainly composed of a transmitting module, a receiving module, and an LCD touch screen module. The transmitting module is mainly based on the control signal to encode encoder, and the control signal to the built-in radio transmitting apparatus to send out. The receiving module receives the control signal using the radio signal–receiving apparatus, and the signal is decoded and then transmitted to the microcontroller for processing; after single-chip

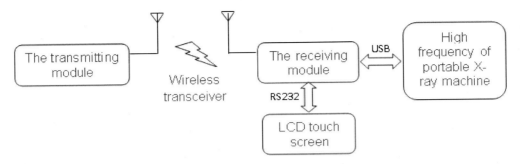

Figure 1. The overall system structure diagram.

processing, controlling frequency portable X-ray machine settings, and preparation and exposure operation, at the same time, the state information is displayed on the LCD screen through the interactive interface so as to achieve the purpose of remote control.

3 THE HARDWARE SYSTEM DESIGN

3.1 Select the wireless communication mode

Wireless communication technology is a mode of information transmission in free space by using the electromagnetic wave signal; according to the technical form, it can be divided into two categories: one is based on cellular access technologies, such as cellular digital packet data, general packet radio transmission technology, and EDGE; the second is based on LAN-based techniques, such as WLAN, Bluetooth IrDA, Home-RF, and micropower short-range wireless communications technology. The wireless control system designed in this paper is based on short-distance wireless communication, so it mainly uses second ways for remote control (PAN Gao-Feng, XUE Jun, XIE Yong & LIANG Sheng, 2012).

In the system of wireless control system used by wireless transceiver chip codec to achieve remote control, the main consideration is whether the infrared communication technology is relatively mature and the development cycle is short, as well as strong directivity and low cost. Thus, the system uses the Princeton Technology Corporation's PT2262 as the wireless communications sending and encoder chip. PT2262 is an RF remote control transmitter chip with address and data encoding function, which uses a low-power CMOS process manufacturing low-cost generic codec circuit. The transmitting chip PT2262-IR carrier oscillator, encoder, and transmitter are integrated in one unit, and the emitter circuit is very simple (Gou Yangen, 2006).

3.2 The transmitting module

The transmission module using Silicon Labs' C8051F340 microcontroller, microcontroller with on-chip power on reset, VDD monitor, voltage regulator, and watchdog and clock oscillator on-chip system devices are able to work independently. It is worth mentioning that for use in MCU development the United States Keil Software Inc. has produced the microcontroller development system Keil C51. The tool is obviously advantageous in function, structure, readability, and maintainability, so to be able to develop the control program in a convenient and fast manner (WANG Xiao-ning, 2009).

According to the system design requirements, the need to put the remote control instruction of X-ray machine were encapsulated by C8051F340 single chip microcomputer, encoded and transmitted through the PT2262-IR code chip. Therefore need to I/O port and PT2262-IR code chip MCU A0-A11 pins connected. For each address, the data type determines the status pin and the output from the output terminal D-out is encoded and transmitted through an infrared emission.

The encoded D-out output is modulated on a 38-kHz carrier; OSC1, OSC2, and the external resistor determine the carrier frequency, and the general resistance can be selected in the range of 430k–470k.

3.3 The receiving module

The receiving module uses Silicon Labs' C8051F340 microcontroller as the control unit. The decoding chip is PT2272; it is a chip to decode the encoded signal. The encoder chip PT2262 is used by the address code, data code, and synchronization code to form a complete code. The decoding chip receives the signal, the address code after two relatively checked, VT pin output high level. At the same time, the corresponding data foot also outputs the high level; if the sending end has been holding down the button, the code chip will continuum emission. When the transmitter does not press the button, PT2262 does not switch on the power and the 17 foot is low, so the 315-MHz high-frequency emission circuit does not work. When a button is pressed, PT2262 works with electricity its 17-foot output-modulated serial data signal. When the 17 pin is high, the 315 MHZ oscillation circuit work and transmit the high frequency signal. When the 17 pin is low, 315 MHz oscillation circuit to stop oscillation, so high frequency transmitting circuit is controlled by the output digital signal of the 17 pin of PT2262. The C8051F340 microcontroller controls commands through the parallel port cable receiver chip decoder and then sends instructions via the USB port to a high-frequency portable X-ray machine in order to achieve remote control. The receiving module circuit is shown in Figure 2.

3.4 Touch LCD monitor

The touch LCD monitor communicates via an RS232 serial port with the C8051F340 MCU, which forms the receiving module. When the system commands work in the remote control mode, single-chip wireless receiver and decoded through the RS232 serial port to send to the LCD monitor. The display will coordinate the response button or parts display, indicating the current operating status of the portable X-ray machine. When the portable X-ray machines operating in local mode touch the corresponding position of the LCD screen, it will coordinate instruction in accordance with the instruction format sent to the microcontroller through the RS232 serial port. The MCU program will process the data and respond to the corresponding coordinate values of operating instructions to the X-ray machine, in order to achieve complete local operating procedures (ZHANG Tao, 2012).

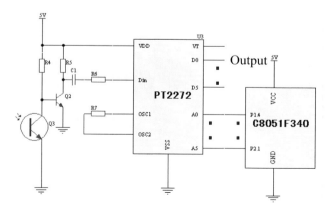

Figure 2.   The receiving module circuit diagram.

4 THE SOFTWARE SYSTEM DESIGN

4.1 The wireless transmitting program and the receiving program

The wireless transmission program and the receiving program design use a modular design. The software is mainly composed of the main program, a send control command subroutine, a receive control command subroutine, coding and decoding subroutines, delay subroutines, interrupt service routines, and other components. Based on the aforementioned design of each program module, the software realizes the sending and receiving control commands and the system has some practical value. Main workflow software development using the Keil C51 software development environment, using C language modular programming, allows great convenience for system debugging. The main program flowchart of sending and receiving modules is shown in Figure 3.

4.2 LCD interactive interface program

LCD interactive interface program also be written using C language, because the LCD screen instruction has been solidified in the integrated control module of the screen, so the program focused on the design coordinate values through the serial port to get through serial port to send control commands, a rectangular area on the screen corresponding anti-color and receiving X-ray machine feedback instruction The functional structure of the interactive interface includes wireless control, parameter storage, preparation/exposure control, LCD display control functions, and communication management functions (TANG Jingnan & SHEN Guoqin, 2008).

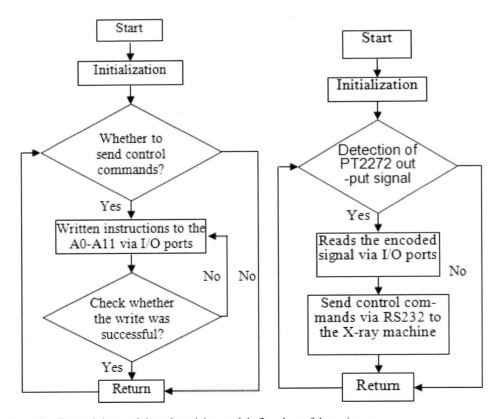

Figure 3.   Transmitting module and receiving module flowchart of the main program.

5 CONCLUSION

Development and manufacture of high frequency portable X-ray machine wireless control system based on C8051F340, with good economic and social benefits to improve the convenience of operation and the diversity of applications of X-ray machine. System testing to is done to verify feasibility and design reasonable products that meet the design requirements. Although the use of infrared wireless transmission technology can effectively reduce cost, the distance and direction of infrared transmission may make the received signal unstable in certain complex environments. This can be solved by increasing the transmission power or by RF transmission mode in the follow-up work. System design effectively protects the operator from radiation hazards while reducing the design cost. The application of this system will have broad prospects.

REFERENCES

Gou Yangen. (2006) *Design and implementation of a short-range wireless USB control system*. [Lecture] University of Electronic Science and Technology of China, June.

Ma Hui. (2011) Development of portable X-ray machine. *Telecommunication Engineering*, 241, 275.

PAN Gao-Feng, XUE Jun, XIE Yong, LIANG Sheng. (2012) Design and Implementation of a Remote Control System Based on Wireless Bridge, *Telecommunication Engineering*, 52(7):1174–1177.

SUO Dan, HAN Yan, YANG Guang. (2010) The Remote Control System for Portable X-Ray Machine based on Wireless Local Area Network, *Non-Destructive Testing*, 32(3):209–213.

TANG Jingnan, SHEN Guoqin. (2008) *MCS-51 single chip C language development and examples*. Beijing, Posts & Telecom press.

WANG Xiao-ning. (2009) USB Data Collection System Based on MCU C8051F340, *Chinese Medical Equipment Journal*, 30(7):111–113.

ZHANG Tao. (2012) Design and Implementation of Man-Machine Interface of Wireless Control System, *Chinese Journal of Liquid Crystals and Displays*, 25(6):841–845.

Medicine Sciences and Bioengineering – Wang (Ed.)
© *2015 Taylor & Francis Group, London, ISBN: 978-1-138-02684-1*

Bisimulation-based consistency checking on syndrome Tan-Yu-Bi-Zu in rheumatoid arthritis between textbook and clinical practice

Guang Zheng*, Ling-Ru Wang, Huan-huan Shi & Rong Li
School of Information Science-Engineering, Lanzhou University, Lanzhou, China

Miao Jiang
Institute of Basic Research in Clinical Medicine, China Academy of Chinese Medical Sciences, Dongzhimen, Beijing, China

Ai-Ping Lu
Institute of Basic Research in Clinical Medicine, China Academy of Chinese Medical Sciences, Dongzhimen, Beijing, China
Hong Kong Baptist University Schools of Chinese Medicine, Kowloon Tong, Kowloon, Hong Kong

ABSTRACT: Checking the consistency of knowledge items between textbook and clinical practice is very important for Traditional Chinese Medicine (TCM). In this study, focused on syndrome Tan-Yu-Bi-Zu in Rheumatoid Arthritis (RA), consistency checking is done through bisimulation, which is an equivalence relationship/method in formal methods. As a result, on syndrome Tan-Yu-Bi-Zu most knowledge items in the textbook can be simulated by the clinical practice, e.g., syndrome, symptom, herbal formula, and herbal medicine. What is more, in clinical practice there are also variations based on TCM's basic rules. In brief, bisimulation is a proper method for consistency checking between TCM textbook and clinical practices.

1 INTRODUCTION

Checking the consistency of knowledge items between textbook and clinical practice is very important for Traditional Chinese Medicine (TCM). In the clinical practice of TCM, when facing different patients of rheumatoid arthritis different doctors may prescribe different Chinese herbal formulas according to their different therapeutic methods and understanding of the patients' constitutions (Zhongying Zhou *et al.*, 2007; Zheng Guang *et al*, 2010). Although effective in many clinical cases, TCM is very flexible and hard to master (Zhongying Zhou *et al.*, 2007; Zhongjia Deng *et al.*, 2008) according to its nature of personal medical treatment. Thus, checking the consistency of knowledge items between textbook and clinical practice is very important for clinical reference and medical research (Zheng Guang *et al.*, 2010).

Rheumatoid Arthritis (RA) is a chronic, systemic inflammatory disorder that may affect many tissues and organs but principally attacks flexible (synovial) joints (J. Zhao *et al.*, 2012; G. Chen *et al.*, 2012; A. P. Lu *et al.*, 2011; C. Zhang *et al.*, 2011). According to the textbook of internal medicine of TCM (Zhongying Zhou *et al.*, 2007), syndrome Tan-Yu-Bi-Zu is an important one in RA, which is believed to be caused by phlegm static and impediment (WHO Health organization, 2007).

When checking the consistency of knowledge items of syndrome Tan-Yu-Bi-Zu in RA between textbook and clinical practice, the formal method of bisimulation is employed (Zheng Guang *et al.*, 2010; Zheng Guang *et al.*, 2011; Zheng Guang *et al.*, 2007; Zheng Guang *et al.*, 2009). Bisimulation is an equivalence relationship/method in formal methods that can be used to compare the consistency of a system's description and its behaviors (Zheng Guang *et al.*, 2011; Robin Milner, 1989).

---

*Corresponding author: forzhengguang@163.com

Knowledge items from textbook can be taken as the system's description, and knowledge items from clinical practice, which are extracted from clinical literatures with the text mining technique (Sam Schmidt *et al.*, 2008) of data slicing algorithm (Zheng Guang & Guo Hongtao *et al.*, 2011; Zheng Guang & Jiang Miao *et al.*, 2011), can be taken as behaviors of the system.

As a result, most of the items in textbook on syndrome Tan-Yu-Bi-Zu can be bisimulated by clinical practice. However, in clinical practice there are variations based on the basic rules of traditional Chinese medicine, e.g., syndrome, symptom, herbal formula, and herbal medicine. What is more, these variations are all based on the basic rules of traditional Chinese medicine according to specified clinical situations.

In brief, bisimulation is a proper method to check the consistency between TCM textbook and clinical practices. By checking the consistency of knowledge items on syndrome Tan-Yu-Bi-Zu between textbook and clinical practice, some new knowledge items can be extracted and demonstrated, which might be a good reference for both clinical practice and medical research.

2 MATERIAL AND METHODS

2.1 *Data collection*

The knowledge items of textbook are taken from the Internal Medicine of traditional Chinese medicine, which is the kernel textbook of traditional Chinese medicine (Zhongying Zhou *et al.*, 2007). The knowledge items of clinical practice are extracted from the literature database of SinoMed (http://sinomed.cintcm.ac.cn/index.jsp). The dataset was downloaded from SinoMed with the query term "rheumatoid arthritis" on November 22, 2012. This dataset contains 15,900 records of literatures. In this dataset, each record/paper is tagged with a unique ID. All the data are stored and pretreated for text mining (Zheng Guang *et al.*, 2011; Sam Schmidt *et al.*, 2008). As RA's data for syndrome "Tan-Yu-Bi-Zu" is not rich, then, as on the primary herbal formula of Shuang-He-Tang associated it tightly, the text mining process turned to data set of Shuang-He-Tang for further rich associated information.

2.2 *Data mining*

Data slicing algorithm is a powerful tool in constructing associated rules in traditional Chinese medicine (Sam Schmidt *et al.*, 2008; Zheng Guang *et al.*, 2011). There are several steps in this algorithm: (1) Extract information from a dataset, e.g., keyword lists of syndrome, symptom, herbal formula, disease, and Chinese herbal medicine. (2) Construct the network on the syndrome, symptom, herbal formulas, and herbal medicines associated with them.

2.3 *Bisimulation*

2.3.1 *Definition*

In theoretical computer science, a bisimulation is a binary relation between state transition systems, associating systems that behave in the same way in the sense that one system simulates the other and vice versa. Two systems are intuitively bisimilar if they match each other's moves (Zheng Guang *et al.*, 2009; Zheng Guang *et al.*, 2011; Robin Milner, 1989).

Definition 1: Given a labeled state transition system $(S, \wedge, \rightarrow)$, a bisimulation relation is a binary relation R over S (i.e., $R \subseteq S \times S$) such that both R^{-1} and R are simulations.
Equivalently, R is a bisimulation if for every pair of elements p, q $\in$ S with $(p, q) \in R$, $\forall \alpha \in \wedge$:

$\forall$ p$'$ $\in$ S, p $\xrightarrow{\alpha}$ p$'$ implies that there is a q$'$ $\in$ S such that q $\xrightarrow{\alpha}$ q$'$ and $(p', q') \in R$;

$\forall$ q$'$ $\in$ S, q $\xrightarrow{\alpha}$ q$'$ implies that there is a p$'$ $\in$ S such that p $\xrightarrow{\alpha}$ p$'$ and $(p', q') \in R$;

Given two states p and q in S, p is bisimilar to q, written as p $\sim$ q, if there is a bisimulation R such that $(p, q) \in R$.

The bisimilarity relation "~" is an equivalence relation. Furthermore, it is the largest bisimulation relation over a given transition system.

2.3.2 *Bisimulation process*

In the bisimulation process, there are four steps in the consistency checking on knowledge items of textbook and text mining, which is demonstrated in Figure 1:

Step 1: This is the initialization step of bisimulation. In this step, both textbook and text mining started from the root point of "rheumatoid arthritis";

Step 2: This is the second step of bisimulation. In this step, syndrome Tan-Yu-Bi-Zu is mined out from clinical literatures and then bisimulated with the knowledge items from textbook;

Step 3: In this step, the bisimulation is focused on symptoms, disease, herbal formulas, and herbal medicines associated with syndrome Tan-Yu-Bi-Zu. This is the main part in bisimulation;

Step 4: This step is focused on the consistency checking between the bisimulated items from textbook and text mining.

3 FIGURE

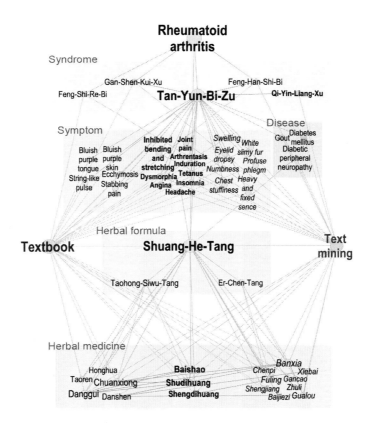

Figure 1. Network bisimulation of RA syndrome Tan-Yu-Bi-Zu on knowledge items of textbook and text mining.

4 RESULTS

By merging the results of textbook and text mining, RA's bisimulation on Tan-Yu-Bi-Zu is demonstrated in Figure 1. In Figure 1, the bisimulation process is divided into 5 steps:

Step 1: Bisimulation of syndromes associated with RA. All the four syndromes associated with RA from textbook are mined out. Besides, another syndrome of Qi-Yin-Liang-Xu (dual deficiency of Qi and Yin) is also mined out, which is associated with syndrome Tan-Yu-Bi-Zu;

Step 2: Bisimulation of disease syndrome Tan-Yu-Bi-Zu and formula Shuang-He-Tang.

Step 3: Bisimulation of symptoms. According to the classification of symptoms, they are divided into three groups. The central group in bold font mainly focuses on symptoms associated with joints, which are also the main symptoms in RA. The left group in normal font mainly focuses on symptoms associated with syndrome Yu (phlegm static), whereas the right group in italic font mainly focuses on symptoms associated with syndrome Bi-Zu (phlegm impediment).

Step 4: Bisimulation of herbal formula associated with syndrome Tan-Yu-Bi-Zu. There are also two knowledge points that cannot be simulated by text mining clinical literatures. They are the relationship between herbal formulas Shuang-He-Tang, Taohong-Siwu-Tang, and Er-Chen-Tang. In the theory of TCM herbal formula, the name Shuang-He-Tang means merging two formulas (i.e., Taohong-Siwu-Tang and Er-Chen-Tang), which can facilitate memorization and clinical usage (Zhongjia Deng *et al.*, 2008).

Step 5: Bisimulation of herbal medicines. Herbal medicines are listed in three columns. The central group in bold font focuses on the therapeutic effects associated with joint symptoms, i.e., inhibited bending and stretching, dysmorphia, angina, joint pain, and so on. The left groups in normal font are the medicines for symptoms associated with syndrome Tan-Yu (phlegm static). The right groups in italic font are the medicines for symptoms associated with syndrome Bi-Zu (phlegm impediment).

5 CONCLUSION AND DISCUSSION

For the normalization and modernization of traditional Chinese medicine, it is very important to check the consistency of knowledge items between textbook and clinical practices with respect to the flexibility of TCM. In this study, the associated results are shown in Figure 1. By analyzing the consistency, we reach the conclusion that clinical practice implies more knowledge items than those existing in the textbook. (1) **Major syndromes can be found for bisimulation:** For RA's syndrome of Tan-Yu-Bi-Zu, Feng-Han-Shi-Bi, Shi-Re-Bi-Zu, and Gan-Shen-Kui-Xu can be bisimulated. (2) **Most of the symptoms on syndrome Tan-Yu-Bi-Zu can be bisimulated.** (3) **New diseases found associated with Shang-He-Tang:** As shown in the gray part tagged "Disease" in Figure 1, besides RA diabetes, gout, and diabetic peripheral neuropathy are found associated with Shuang-He-Tang. This may indicate some new therapeutic effect of this herbal formula. (4) **Bisimulation rate on herbal medicine is high:** As shown in Figure 1, of all 12 herbal medicines 9 can be bisimulated.

ACKNOWLEDGMENTS

This work was partially supported by the National Science Foundation of China (No. 81072982), Gansu Science Foundation (No. 1208RJZA249) and HKBU project (RC-IRMS/12-13/02, SDF13-1209-P01).

REFERENCES

A. P. Lu, et al. (2011), Clinical Chinese medicine study on rheumatoid arthritis in the evidence-based medicine times. *Zhongguo Zhong Xi Yi Jie He Za Zhi*, vol. 31, pp. 1161–3 [Accessed Sep 2011].
C. Zhang, et al. (2011), Evidence-based Chinese medicine for rheumatoid arthritis, *J Tradit Chin Med*, vol. 31, pp. 152–7.

Guang Zheng, Miao Jiang, Xiaojuan He1, Jing Zhao, Hongtao Guo, Gao Chen, Qinglin Zha, and Aiping Lu (2011). Discrete derivative: a data slicing algorithm for exploration of sharing biological networks between rheumatoid arthritis and coronary heart disease. [Online] Available from: BioData Mining 2011, 4:18. http://www.biodatamining.org/content/4/1/18.

G. Chen, et al. (2012), A network-based analysis of traditional Chinese medicine cold and hot patterns in rheumatoid arthritis. *Complement Ther Med*, vol. 20, pp. 23–30 [Accessed Feb-Apr 2012].

J. Zhao, et al. (2012), Expert Consensus on the Treatment of Rheumatoid Arthritis with Chinese Patent Medicines. *Altern Complement Med* [Accessed Aug 6 2012].

Robin Milner (1989), Communication and Concurrency, Prentice Hall.

Sam Schmidt, Peter Vuillermin, Bernard Jenner, Yongli Ren, Gang Li, Yi-Ping Phoebe Chen (2008), Mining Medical Data: Bridging the Knowledge Divide, *Proceedings of eResearch Australasia*.

WHO Health organization (2007). *WHO International Standard Terminologies on Traditional Medicine in the Western Pacific Region*, ISBN 978 92 9061 2484. WHO Library Cataloguing in Publication Data.

Zheng Guang, Guo Hongtao, Guo Yuming, He Xiaojuan, Li Zhongxian, Lu, Aiping (2011). Two dimensions data slicing algorithm, a new approach in mining rules of literature in traditional Chinese medicine. *Communications in Computer and Information Science,* v 237 CCIS, pp. 161–174, Emerging Research in *Artificial Intelligence and Computational Intelligence-International Conference, AICI 2011, Proceedings.*

Zheng Guang, He Xiaojuan, Jiang Miao, Lu Aiping (2010). Goal based bisimulation for testing therapies in traditional Chinese medicine. 2010 IEEE International Conference on Bioinformatics and Biomedicine Workshops, BIBMW 2010, p 603–608, 2010 IEEE International Conference on Bioinformatics and Biomedicine Workshops, BIBMW 2010.

Zheng Guang, Jiang Miao, Lu Cheng, Guo Hongtao, Zhan, Junping; Lu Aiping (2011), Exploring the biological basis of deficiency pattern in rheumatoid arthritis through text mining. BIBMW 2011, pp. 811–816.

Zheng Guang, Li Lian; Chen Wenbo, He Anping, Wu Jinzhao (2009). Process algebra with chaos executing policy for unhealthy systems, *Journal of Computers*, v 4, n 1, pp. 86–93.

Zheng Guang, Li Shaorong, Wu Jinzhao, Li Lian (2007). A non-interleaving denotational semantics of value passing CCS with action refinement. [Lecture] Lecture Notes in Computer Science (including subseries Lecture Notes in Artificial Intelligence and Lecture Notes in Bioinformatics), v 4613 LNCS, p 178–190, 2007, Frontiers in Algorithmics - First Annual Inter-national Workshop, FAW 2007, Proceedings.

Zheng Guang, Wu Jinzhao, Lu Aiping (2011). Stochastic process algebra with value-passing and weak time restrictions. *Journal of Software*, v 6, n 5, pp. 769–782.

Zhongjia Deng, et al. (2008.) *Formulae of Chinese Medicine.* China Press of Traditional Chinese Medicine. ISBN 7-80156-322-0 (in Chinese).

Zhongying Zhou, et al. (2007) *Internal Medicine of Traditional Chinese Medicine.* China Press of Traditional Chinese Medicine. ISBN 978-7-80156-313-2 (in Chinese).

67

Medicine Sciences and Bioengineering – Wang (Ed.)

Farrerol improves the blood pressure, plasma biochemical indices and aortic media thickness in spontaneously hypertensive rats

Xiao-jiang Qin
School of Pharmaceutical Science, Shanxi Medical University, Taiyuan, Shanxi, China

Xiao-min Hou
Department of Pharmacology, Shanxi Medical University, Taiyuan, Shanxi, China

Tai-gang Liang & Qing-shan Li*
School of Pharmaceutical Science, Shanxi Medical University, Taiyuan, Shanxi, China

ABSTRACT: Farrerol, a flavonoid considered to be the major bioactive component in a traditional Chinese herb, "Man-shan-hong", which is the dried leaves of Rhododendron dauricum L. Our previous study found that farrerol possesses vasoactive effects. Therefore, we postulated that Farrerol may have potential antihypertensive activity. In this study, we examined this hypothesis by evaluating the effects of farrerol on the systolic blood pressure, heart rate and body weight in the Spontaneously Hypertensive Rats (SHR) and its normotensive Wistar-Kyoto rats (WKY) control strain of 12 weeks of age for a duration of 20 weeks. Aortic media thickness were examined as they are the cardiovascular parameters that are directly associated with increased blood pressure. Plasma biochemical indices were also performed to assess whether these parameters were affected. These results showed that farrerol significantly improved blood pressure and plasma biochemical index and reduced aortic media thickness, which suggests that farrerol is a potential candidate drugs to prevent the development of hypertension.

1 INTRODUCTION

Hypertension is one of the most common chronic illnesses effecting more than 1 billion people worldwide and is a major risk factor for coronary artery, heart failure, stroke and renal failure (Plehm, R. *et al.*, 2007). By the year 2025, the global prevalence of hypertension is projected to increase to 29.2% in adult population (Kearney, P. M. *et al.*, 2005). It is well established that reduction in blood pressure is associated with decreased cardiovascular morbidity and mortality.

Currently, antihypertensive drugs include thiazide diuretics, beta blockers, Angiotensin-Converting Enzyme inhibitors, angiotensin receptor blockers and calcium channel blockers and so on. Global estimates suggest that less than 35% of hypertensives are able to achieve their target systolic and diastolic blood pressure with these drugs (Thoenes, M. *et al.*, 2009).

Farrerol, a typical natural flavanone, has been isolated from Rhododendron dauricum L., and has been extensively used to alleviate symptoms associated with bronchial asthma in China (Qin, X. *et al.*, 2014). Accumulating evidence suggested that farrerol possesses many biological properties, including antibechic, antibacterial, anti-inflammatory effects, and an inhibitory effect on vascular smooth muscle cells (VSMCs) proliferation (Li, Q.-y. *et al.* 2011). Furthermore, our previous study showed that farrerol presents a strong anti-atherosclerosis activity in VSMCs and exhibited a significant cytoprotective activity against hydrogen peroxide (H_2O_2)-induced injury in

---

*Corresponding author: Qingshan Li PhD; E-mail: sxlqs2012@163.com; Tel: 86-351-4690322

human umbilical vein endothelial cells, indicating its potential to treat and prevent cardiovascular diseases (Li, Q.-y. *et al.* 2011). The purpose of this study is to clarify the role of farrerol as a potential anti-hypertension agent and the mechanisms.

2 METHODS

2.1 *Animal grouping and medicine*

WKY and SHR aged 12 weeks were obtained from breeding pairs purchased from Vital River Laboratory Animal Technology Co. Ltd. Rats were housed at a temperature of 21–25°C in individual cages and freely fed a regular pellet diet.

They were divided into four groups of eight animals each: (1) WKY (control group), (2) SHR (untreated), (3) SHR treated with farrerol, and (4) SHR treated with verapamil. Farrerol and verapamil were administered during 8 weeks as a dose of 50 mg/kg/day dissolved in the drinking water, respectively. The dosage and duration of administration were calculated considering the maximum therapeutic dose in humans and based on previous studies, the concentrations being adjusted according to daily water consumption and body weight in order to ensure correct dosage. Verapamil was purchased from Sigma Company.

2.2 *Blood pressure measurement*

Systolic blood pressure and the heart were measured once every week at 8 Am in a quiet room. After staying in a box at 29 ± 1°C for 10 min, the tail systolic blood pressure was measured using a blood pressure monitor. Body weight was measured on the same day that blood pressure was measured.

2.3 *Aorta tissue sampling and measurements in plasma*

At the end of the experimental period, all animals were fasted overnight before killing. They were anesthetized with pentobarbital (50 mg/kg i.p.) and plasma samples were taken from the abdominal aorta, centrifuged at 3000 rpm and 4°C for 20 min, and plasma was quickly frozen in liquid nitrogen. Rats were killed by decapitation, then the aorta was quickly removed and washed out with cold Krebs-Ringer buffer. The adhering fat and connective tissue were removed. Samples of the aorta were frozen and stored at −80°C until use.

Superoxide dismutase (SOD), Malonaldehyde (MDA), Nitric oxide (NO), Nitricoxide synthase (NOS), Endothelin (ET), Angiotensin II (Ang II), Lnterleukin-6 (IL-6) and Tumor necrosis factor-α (TNF-α) were measured in plasma using a quantitative sandwich enzyme immunoassay (commercial ELISA kits).

2.4 *Statistical analyses*

Data were analyzed with GraphPad Prism 6 software. All data are presented as means $\pm$ SD. One way or two-way ANOVA followed by Bonferroni's multiple comparison test (where indicated) was used for statistical comparisons. Results were considered statistically significant when $P < 0.05$.

3 RESULTS

3.1 *Effect of farrerol treatments on systolic blood pressure, heart rate and body weight*

Systolic blood pressure levels of SHR were higher than those of WKY (119 ± 5 mmHg in WKY vs. 190 ± 6 mmHg in SHR, $P < 0.01$), while administration with verapamil or farrerol for 8 weeks significantly decreased systolic blood pressure levels of SHR (190 ± 6 mmHg in

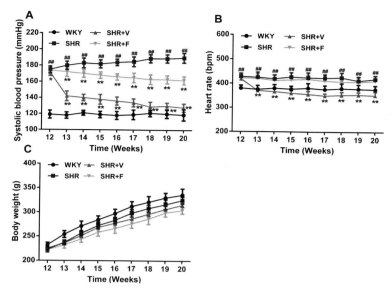

Figure 1. Time course of effect of farrerol on systolic blood pressure and heart rate.

Note: The graphs show the effect of farrerol on the systolic blood pressure (SBP) and heart rate (HR) in SHR and WKY rats from 12–20 weeks of age. Each point represents means ± SD ($n = 6$). Two-way ANOVA was used for statistical comparisons between the different treated groups on the SBP and HR changes over the whole duration of treatment. *$P < 0.05$; **$P < 0.01$, compared with SHR.

SHR vs. 128 ± 5 mmHg in verapamil-treated SHR, $P < 0.01$ or 162 ± 5 mmHg in farrerol treated SHR, $P < 0.01$) (Figure 1A).

After 8 weeks of treatment (from 12–20 weeks of age), the heart rate of verapamil treated SHR was significantly lower ($P < 0.01$) than that of farrerol treated SHR group and untreated SHR group (Figure 1B).

The body weights gained in treated animals over the 8 weeks treatment period were not significantly different from that of untreated animals (Figure 1A).

3.2 *Plasma biochemical indices*

Our experiments were observed the relationship of oxidant stress, inflammatory factor and endothelial function occurs with hypertension through testing the changes of SOD, MDA, NO, NOS, ET, Ang II, IL-6 and TNF-α from plasma of SHR after application of farrerol.

Plasma levels of MDA, ET, Ang II, IL-6 and TNF-α, were significantly higher in SHR than in WKY, SHR+Farrerol, and SHR+Verapamil group; While plasma levels of SOD, NO and NOS, were significantly lower in SHR than in WKY, SHR+Farrerol, and SHR+Verapamil group (Figure 2).

3.3 *Effect of farrerol treatment on the aorta*

The finding was observed Nuclei size were significantly lower in the farrerol and verapamil treated SHR group than SHR untreated groups, farrerol clearly modified the phenotype of vascular smooth muscle cells and increased nuclei number.

Morphological differences in the aortic parameters of treated and control SHR, and control WKY rats, respectively. One-way ANOVA showed that treatments with farrerol and verapamil had a significant effect on the aortic indices ($P < 0.05$) in the SHR (Figure 3 and Figure 4).

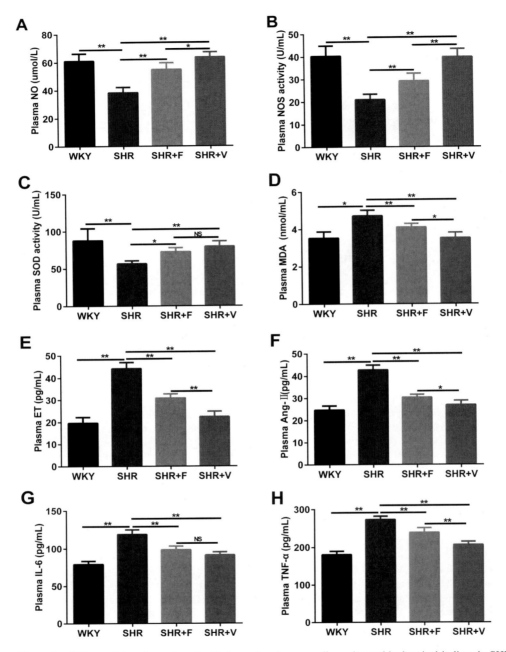

Figure 2. Effects of chronic treatment with farrerol and verapamil on plasma biochemical indices in SHR and WKY.

Note: Each value represents as means ± SD, $n = 8$. The statistical analysis used the Anova with Dunnet's post hoc test. $*P < 0.05$, $** P < 0.01$.

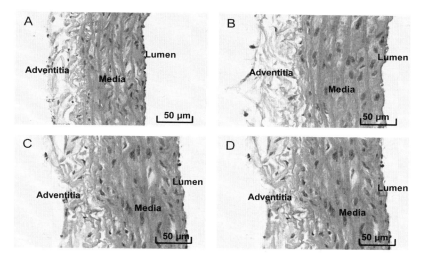

Figure 3.   Effects of farrerol on morphological changes in aorta in SHRs and WKY rats.

Note: A: WKY+C group; B: SHR+C group; C: SHR+F group D: SHR+V group. WKY: Wistar Kyoto; SHR: Spontaneously hypertensive rat; F: Farrrerol; V: Verapamil.

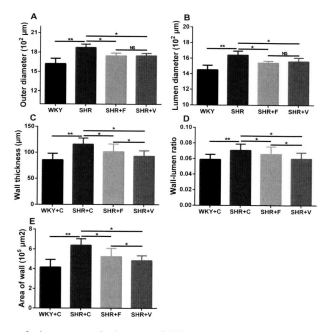

Figure 4.   Changes of microstructure in the aorta of different group in SHR and WKY.

Note: A: Outer diameter; B: Lumen diameter; C: Wall thickness; D: Wall-lumen ratio; E: Area of wall. The statistical analysis used the Anova with Dunnet's post hoc test. Data are expressed as means $\pm$ SD. ($n = 7$–10). *$P < 0.05$, **$P < 0.01$.

4 SUMMARY

Taken together, our results demonstrated that farrerol can effectively improve blood pressure in the treatment of hypertension. Farrerol also reduce the risk of cardiovascular disease associated with hypertension by improving the plasma biochemical indices, and vascular smooth muscle hypertrophy induced by hypertension. Furthermore, the antihypertension effect of farrerol may be related with antioxidation, endothelium function and inhibition of inflammatory cytokines. Thus our results suggest that farrerol may be a possible therapeutic agent for the treatment of hypertension diseases.

REFEFENCES

Kearney, P. M.; Whelton, M.; Reynolds, K.; Muntner, P.; Whelton, P. K.; He, J., Global burden of hypertension: analysis of worldwide data. The Lancet 2005, 365(9455):217–223.

Li, Q.-y.; Chen, L.; Zhu, Y.-h.; Zhang, M.; Wang, Y.-p.; Wang, M.-w., Involvement of estrogen re-ceptor-β in farrerol inhibition of rat thoracic aorta vascular smooth muscle cell proliferation. Acta Pharmacologica Sinica 2011, 32(4):433–440.

Plehm, R.; Barbosa, M. E.; Bader, M., Animal models for hypertension/blood pressure recording. In Cardiovascular Disease, Springer: 2007, pp 115–126.

Qin, X.; Hou, X.; Zhang, M.; Liang, T.; Zhi, J.; Han, L.; Li, Q., Relaxation of Rat Aorta by Farrerol Correlates with Potency to Reduce Intracellular Calcium of VSMCs. International journal of mole-cular sciences 2014, 15(4):6641–6656.

Thoenes, M.; Neuberger, H.; Volpe, M.; Khan, B.; Kirch, W.; Böhm, M., Antihypertensive drug therapy and blood pressure control in men and women: an international perspective. Journal of hu-man hypertension 2009, 24(5):336–344.

Medicine Sciences and Bioengineering – Wang (Ed.)
© 2015 Taylor & Francis Group, London, ISBN: 978-1-138-02684-1

Application of neck elastic tourniquet in thyroid surgery

Yan-Ming Li, Wen-Jing Sun & Song Yan*
Nursing college, Beihua University, Jilin province, China

ABSTRACT: This article evaluates the effect of postoperative thyroid neck elastic tourniquet involved in increasing the comfort level, reducing the amount of bleeding, and improving the satisfaction of clients. A total of 120 thyroid surgery patients in our hospital were randomly divided into an experimental group and a control group. Patients used the neck elastic tourniquet in the experimental group, and patients were given oppression using 0.5-kg-heavy sandbags in the control group. The results show that comfort and satisfaction in the experimental group was significantly more than that in the control group ($P < 0.05$); blood loss in the former was significantly less than that in the control group ($P < 0.05$). The neck elastic tourniquet used in thyroidectomy can effectively reduce postoperative bleeding of neck and improve comfort and satisfaction of patients.

1 INTRODUCTION

Postoperative bleeding is one of the complications of thyroid surgery, occurring postoperatively within 48 h; the incidence is 0.3%–1.0%. It is related to postoperative bleeding with not complete intraoperative bleeding (Weiping yang & Tanglei shao, 2012), postoperative severe coughing, nausea, vomiting, and frequent neck movement. The cervical area space is small, and 50 mL of bleeding can cause tracheal compression symptoms; greater than 100 mL of bleeding can significantly compress the trachea, cause breathing difficulty, cause choking, and endanger the patient's life (Shaoyi lu et al., 2008). In order to reduce bleeding, the incision after surgery is oppressed by sandbags. The incision after surgery is often used sandbags oppression; this method has a certain hemostasis effect, but patients feel uncomfortable with pressure and limited neck mobility. Recently, a neck elastic tourniquet developed by our hospital was applied postoperatively in thyroid patients and it not only reduced postoperative bleeding but also increased the comfort level.

2 MATERIALS AND METHODS

2.1 Subject choice

The study considered 120 cases of thyroid surgery patients in our university-affiliated hospital from January 2012 to May 2013, which included 68 cases of males and 52 cases of females. Their ages ranged from 25 to 76 years old. The average age was 42.8. There were 25 cases of hyperthyroidism, 39 cases of bilateral nodular goiter, and 16 cases of thyroid carcinoma, and none of them had diabetes or cardiovascular disease. The 104 cases with subtotal thyroidectomy and 16 cases with thyriodectomy are placed the rubber drainage tube after operation. Then, we randomly divided them into an experimental group and a control group, each group consisting of 60 cases. Data were analyzed between the two groups, and the difference was not statistically significant ($P > 0.05$).

---

*Corresponding author

2.2 Production and use of neck elastic tourniquet

2.2.1 Materials
A piece of cotton cloth, specification is 50 cm × 20 cm; four elastic bands, specification is 5 cm × 3 cm; two pairs of Velcro, specification is 5 cm × 3 cm; and two plastic sheets, specification is 9 cm × 3 cm.

2.2.2 Production methods
The neck elastic tourniquet consists of three parts, including the inner layer and outer layer of cervical anterior as well as cervical posterior. First, the cotton cloth is cut. It is sewn into a 9 cm × 5 cm rectangular cloth in double piece as the posterior, and the two upper and lower edges are cut concavely. Two sets of the double layers rectangular cloth with 13 cm × 9 cm as the inner layer and outer layer of cervical anterior respectively. The edge near the jaw and the bottom edge are cut concavely. The plastic sheets are placed on the both sides on with inner layer of cervical anterior which is playing supporting roles to prevent curve. A bag is sewed in the outer layer of cervical anterior which can placed airbags, water bags, ice bags to make the stress balance.

The areas of overlap between anterior, inner, and outer layers should be sewn with the Velcro, and the three parts of the neck elastic tourniquet should be connected with elastic (Figure 1).

2.2.3 Using methods
Put the tourniquet around the neck; fix the Velcro in the overlapping parts of the anterior portion. According to the patient's neck circumference, adjust the tightness to appropriate pressure, but it should not restrict breathing.

2.3 Research methods

The control group is given 0.5-kg-weighing sandbags for oppression on the incision with conventional nursing after operation. The experimental group is using the neck elastic tourniquet on the incision with conventional nursing after operation. The effects of the two methods were observed and compared.

2.4 Observed indicators

After 48 h, observe the two groups of patients in terms of postoperative bleeding, comfort level, and satisfaction.

2.5 Statistical analysis

SPSS17.0 software was used for statistical analysis, measurement data were used for t test, and data were counted using $\chi 2$ test.

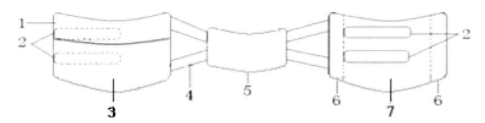

Figure 1.   Neck stretch tourniquet.

1. Anterior outer; 2. Velcro fastener; 3. Outer cloth bag; 4. Elastic bands; 5. Back of the neck; 6. Plastic sheet; 7. Anterior inner.

2.6 Interpretation of the results

2.6.1 Assessment standards for amount of bleeding

The method of calculating the amount of bleeding was the sum of drainage of wound dressings and exudation. Specifications for the dressing of 30 cm × 30 cm, about fully soaked in bleeding, were 20 mL (Jinying liu & Caixia wang, 2005).

2.6.2 Assessment standards for comfort level

According to the patient's feelings, they can be divided into comfortable, more comfortable, general comfortable, and uncomfortable (Liumin *et al.*, 2003).

2.6.3 Evaluation standards for satisfaction

Used the self-designed "patient satisfaction questionnaire" before discharge, which is divided into three grades of satisfied, more satisfied, and dissatisfied (Hongjuan liu, 2005).

3 RESULTS

3.1 Comparison of postoperative bleeding

After 48 hours postoperatively, the amount of bleeding of the experimental group was 48.3 ± 3.5 ml and that of the control group was 77.5 ± 5.6 mL. In t test, there was significant difference between the two groups ($t = 4.25$, $P < 0.05$).

3.2 Comparison of comfort

Judging from Table 1, the patient's comfort level of the experimental group was better than that of the control group and the difference was statistically significant ($\chi2 = 14.69$, $P < 0.05$).

3.3 Comparison of satisfaction

A total of 120 copies of questionnaires were distributed to the patients. The response rate was 100%. The satisfaction difference between the two groups was statistically significant ($\chi2 = 11.43$, $P < 0.05$) (Table 2).

4 DISCUSSION

Thyroid surgery is the most basic treatment of hyperthyroidism, thyroid adenoma, thyroid cancer, and other thyroid diseases, but the blood circulation of thyroid is rich and the function and anatomical structure are very complex. Intraoperative and postoperative bleeding can happen and can be life threatening. Patients who have little bleeding that have not obvious symptoms, patients have massive bleeding can appear cervical massive fluid drainage, dyspnea, cyanosis with mouth and

Table 1. Comparison of the comfort level of the two groups.

Groups	n	Comfortable		More comfortable		General comfortable		Uncomfortable	
		n	%	n	%	n	%	n	%
Experimental group	60	32	53.3	18	30	8	13.3	2	3.3
Control group	60	15	25	14	23.3	17	28.3	14	23.3

Table 2. Comparison of satisfaction of the two groups.

Groups	n	Satisfied		More satisfied		Dissatisfied	
		n	%	n	%	n	%
Experimental group	60	42	70	13	21.7	5	8.3
Control group	60	28	46.7	11	18.3	21	35

so on (Hongmei jiang, 2013). The ways to prevent bleeding are not only gentle operation but also proper observation and nursing.

The sandbag compression method has some effect on reducing the bleeding after operation, but the compression strength cannot be controlled. Patients often feel tightness and discomfort when using it. The sandbags easily fall off when patients turn over, sit up, or leave the bed for some activity, so it cannot play any role in continued oppression.

A neck elastic tourniquet uses a cotton cloth as the main material; it is very soft, comfortable, and simple to use and can play a role in continued oppression hemostasis to reduce postoperative bleeding. The amount of bleeding is statistically different between the control group and the experimental group.

The neck elastic tourniquet has elastic bands at both of its ends, which have a certain scale. It can effectively adjust the intensity of oppression to avoid restrictions on breathing. The neck elastic tourniquet does not affect the patient's eating and activity. Compared with the control group, it can significantly improve patient's comfort and satisfaction and embodies the concept of human care.

REFERENCES

Hongjuan Liu. (2005) Application of clinical pathways for elderly patients with acute myocardial in farction rehabilitation care. *Nurse Education Magazine*, 20(7):607.
Hongmei Jiang. (2013) Thyroid surgery nursing and observation. *Jilin Medical*, 34(19):3895.
Jinying Liu, Caixia Wang. (2005) Complicated by bleeding and postoperative nursing of choking prevention of hyperthyroidism thyroid function. *Modern Medicine and Health*, 21(18):2522.
Liu Min, Zhaomei Li, Peishan Wang, etc. (2003) Application of multi-functional heart-shaped pillow after cardiothoracic surgery. *QiLu Nursing Magazine*, 9(3):161–162.
Shaoyi Lu, Fanglin, Li Zhe, etc. (2008) Clinical analysis of postoperative wound bleeding of thyroid. *Journal of Clinical Surgery*, 16(10):666.
Weiping Yang, Tanglei Shao. (2012) Prevention of bleeding and treatment of thyroid surgery. Chinese *Journal of Practical Surgery*, 32(5):377.

Medicine Sciences and Bioengineering – Wang (Ed.)
© 2015 Taylor & Francis Group, London, ISBN: 978-1-138-02684-1

To explore the famous TCM doctor Wang Xing-Kuan's rule of prescriptions for coronary heart disease on the basis of association rule

Hou-wu Gong, Yi Wen, Jin-yang Li, Hao-yu Qu, Xiong Du, Lei Jiang, Jun-feng Yan* & Jin-ru Fan
Hunan University of CM, Changsha, Hunan, China

ABSTRACT: Objective: To explore Wang Xing-Kuan's rule of prescriptions for Coronary Heart Disease (CHD). Methods: In this study, 267 medical records were collected from the outpatient departments of the first affiliated hospital of the Hunan University of Traditional Chinese Medicine (TCM) by using a digital camera. Then, we standardized the terminology of herbs and established Excel database. Finally, the descriptive statistics of prescription and the association rules of herbs were analyzed using Weka 3.6 software. Results: (1) Clinical herbal formulae mainly include cathartic and tonic herbs. (2) The credibility of combination of herbs is always higher than 0.90, which were the combination between danshen root or Chinese thorowax root with the tonifying qi yin herbs or the eliminating phlegm and blood-stasis-removing herbs. (3) The credibility of combination of similar herbs which is always higher than 0.65, which were used in treatment of heart and liver, such as debark peony root with golden thread are used to treat heart, turmeric root tuber with Chinese thorowax root are used to regulate liver. (4) The herbs that Prof. Wang used to treat CHD are quite mild and the dosage of herbs is normal, not less or more. Conclusion: Results indicate that liver–heart conjunction treatment, catharsis and tonic in combination, and using mild herbs are Wang Xing-Kuan's rule of prescriptions for CHD.

1 INTRODUCTION

Wang Xing-Kuan is the second, third, fourth, and fifth batches' senior instructor of inheriting the academic experience of old Chinese medicine experts, and the national old Chinese tradition studio expert. As a famous TCM doctor of Hunan province, he is also the first tenured professor, medical academic leader, chief physician, and PhD supervisor of the first affiliated hospital of the Hunan University of TCM.

With the guidance of advanced theory of "Collection of Experiences of Famous Physicians in the Ming Dynasty," "Chambers and the Secret Record," and his 50 years of clinical experience, Prof. Wang advocated liver-heart conjunction treatment to treat coronary heart disease (CHD).

Some academic papers and writings introduced the case analyses and the academic experiences (ZENG Y et al., 2012). However, these were lacking systematic analysis and research. Therefore, this study found the individual herbs and their combinations showing positive outcomes in patients with CHD, by using the data mining technology and statistical analysis in the cases of CHD treated by Prof. Wang in the last one year.

---

*Correspondence to: Dr. YAN Jun-feng, E-mail: teacheryan@qq.com.

2 METHOD

2.1 *Cases source*

We took the photos from medical records of the CHD patients who were treated by Prof. Wang in the first affiliated hospital of the Hunan University of Chinese medicine during August 1, 2012 to July 31, 2013.

2.2 *Diagnostic criteria*

The diagnostic criteria of CHD are on the basis of clinical diagnosis and treatment guidelines, Cardiovascular (ZENG Y, GE Z & TONG J, 2012).

2.3 *Inclusion criteria*

(1) In accordance with the preceding CHD diagnostic criteria. (2) Patients who were using TCM decoction.

2.4 *Exclusion criteria*

(1) According to the ICD-10 diagnostic criteria, CHD is the secondary diagnosis. (2) High blood pressure is out of control (resting blood pressure within 1 week ≥ 160/100 mmHg). (3) Accompanied by severe arrhythmia, combined with heart failure (NYHA Classes III and IV).

2.5 *Data preprocessing*

Firstly, we input the original case data that captured by digital camera to excel database. The database mainly includes the basic information (name, gender, age, etc.), traditional Chinese and Western medicine diagnosis, prescriptions, and so on. Then, we standardized 123 kinds of herbs by reference to the Pharmacopoeia of China.

2.6 *Database establishment*

After finishing the disposal of original case data, we established database by ordering the family name of patients. Follow-up records were included in the case data, so that each patient had its unique case data. The database included 143 effective cases and 267 diagnoses. The mean age of the patients was 58.47 (range 31–85 years) and 74 patients were female, 62 patients were male (another 7 people's basic information is unknown), 5 patients were affected by simple CHD. The condition of CHD complicated with other diseases is as follows: hypertension (100 cases), cervical spondylosis (44 cases), chronic gastritis (25 cases), arrhythmia (23 cases), chronic cardiac insufficiency (17 cases), chronic bronchitis (16 cases), lacunar infarction (15 cases), diabetes mellitus (10 cases), and so on.

2.7 *Association rules analysis*

Data mining is a process of extracting effective information from numerous data. The major methods were: descriptive statistics, frequent item-set, relational analysis, fuzzy clustering analysis, and so on. Descriptive statistics is a kind of frequency analysis that can find some statistical regularity. In this study, we adopted frequency analysis and association rules to explore Wang Xing-Kuan's rule of prescriptions for CHD. Using the data-mining software Weka 3.6, we can get frequency statistics on herbs, the rules between herbs (set minimum support to 10%, set minimum confidence interval to 90%) and commonly used similar herb (set minimum support to 3%, set minimum confidence to 50%) by a priori algorithm.

Note: The database establishment and statistical analysis were done by two persons in separate computers, and the results were checked by the third person.

3 RESULT

3.1 *Commonly used herbs*

The top 26 most frequently used herbs (frequency is equal or greater than 50) in the CHD treatments are listed in Table 1 which shows that Prof. Wang used cathartic and tonic herbs to treat CHD.

3.2 *Two-itemset association analysis*

On the basis of the two-itemset association analysis, we got 8 two-itemset association results (see Table 2). The couplet medicines that Prof. Wang usually used are Chinese magnoliavine fruit with golden thread, white ginseng with golden thread, processed pinellia tuber with snakegourd peel, golden thread with snakegourd peel, and golden thread with processed pinellia tuber. The herbs that are from Shengmai San and Xianxiong Decoction reflect the synergy of qi-tonifying herb (white ginseng, Chinese magnoliavine fruit), yin-tonifying herb (golden thread), eliminating phlegm and dispersing blood stasis herbs (snakegourd peel, processed pinellia tuber), and channel ushering herb (golden thread).

3.3 *Commonly used herbs analysis*

To do in-depth analysis of Prof. Wang's rule of prescriptions for CHD, we analyzed the association of commonly used herbs as shown in Table 3 which shows Prof. Wang's treatment of CHD by liver–heart conjunction treatment. White ginseng, Chinese magnoliavine fruit, and debark peony root with golden thread are used to tonify qi yin (confidence = 100%), processed pinellia tuber, golden thread with snakegourd peel, longstamen onion bulb with danshen root, milkvetch root with radix glycyrrhizae preparata, and honey-fried radix polygalae with Chinese arborvitae kernel are used to treat heart. Turmeric root tuber with Chinese thorowax root, tall gastrodia tuber, *Tribulus terrestris* with gambir plant nod, and abalone shell are used to regulate liver. Poria cocos with bitter apricot seed are used to diffuse the lung (confidence ≥ 0.65).

Table 1. Top 26 most frequently used herbs.

Herb	F	Rate (%)	Herb	F	Rate (%)
Danshen root	238	89.14	Gambir plant nod	109	40.82
Snakegourd peel	234	87.64	Chinese arborvitae kernel	99	37.08
Processed pinellia tuber	230	86.14	Abalone shell	97	36.33
Radix ophiopogonis	228	85.39	Bitter apricot seed	86	32.21
Golden thread	228	85.39	Honey-fried radix polygalae	78	29.21
Chinese magnoliavine fruit	208	77.90	Milkvetch root	72	26.97
Chinese thorowax root	203	76.03	Poria cocos	69	25.84
White ginseng	200	74.91	Turmeric root tuber	65	24.34
Tall gastrodia tuber	179	67.04	Largehead atractylodes rhizome	63	23.60
Radix glycyrrhizae preparata	175	65.54	Sanqi	55	20.60
Poria with hostwood	144	53.93	Spine date seed	52	19.48
Kudzuvine root	129	48.31	Longstamen onion bulb	51	19.10
Tribulus terrestris	114	42.32	Debark peony root	50	18.73

Table 2. Two-itemset association analysis of herbs.

Left herbs	F		Right herbs	F	Confidence
Chinese magnoliavine fruit	208	==>	Golden thread	207	0.99
White ginseng	200	==>	Golden thread	196	0.98
Processed pinellia tuber	230	==>	Snakegourd peel	222	0.97
Golden thread	228	==>	Snakegourd peel	218	0.96
Golden thread	228	==>	Processed pinellia tuber	218	0.96
Snakegourd peel	234	==>	Processed pinellia tuber	222	0.95
Processed pinellia tuber	230	==>	Golden thread	218	0.95
Snakegourd peel	234	==>	Golden thread	218	0.9

Table 3. The association of commonly used similar herbs.

Efficacy	Left herbs	F		Right herbs	F	Confidence
Tonify qi yin	White ginseng, Chinese magnoliavine fruit, debark peony root	41	==>	Golden thread	41	1.00
Eliminate phlegm and disperse blood stasis	Processed pinellia tuber, golden thread	218	==>	Snakegourd peel	213	0.98
Activate blood and dredge collaterals	Longstamen onion bulb	51	==>	Danshen root	49	0.97
Sooth liver and promote circulation of qi	Turmeric root tuber	65	==>	Chinese thorowax root	60	0.92
Benefit qi and tonify asthenia	Milkvetch root	72	==>	Radix glycyrrhizae preparata	53	0.74
Stabilize liver yang	Tall gastrodia tube, *Tribulus terrestris*	114	==>	Gambir plant nod, abalone shell	81	0.71
Nourish heart and tranquilize mind	Fushen, honey-fried radix polygalae	49	==>	Chinese arborvitae kernel	35	0.71
Diffuse the lung	Poria cocos	69	==>	Bitter apricot seed	45	0.65

4 DISCUSSION

After using association rule in analyzing 123 herbs that were collected from outpatient departments of the first affiliated hospital of the Hunan University of TCM, we can know that Prof. Wang uses cathartic and tonic herbs to treat CHD. The efficacy of cathartic herbs are to activate blood and dredge collaterals (e.g., danshen root, longstamen onion bulb), sooth liver and promote circulation of qi (e.g., Chinese thorowax root, turmeric root tuber), eliminate phlegm and disperse blood stasis (e.g., snakegourd peel, processed pinellia tuber), disperse lung qi (e.g., bitter apricot seed), dredge governor vessel (e.g., kudzuvine root), ushere channel (e.g., golden thread), and stabilize liver yang (e.g., tall gastrodia tuber, gambir plant nod, *Tribulus terrestris*, abalone shell). The efficacy of tonic herbs are tonify heart and Qi Yin (e.g., white ginseng, Radix Ophiopogonis, Chinese magnoliavine fruit, debark peony root), nourish heart and tranquilize mind (e.g., poria with hostwood, Chinese arborvitae kernel, honey-fried radix polygalae, spine date seed), benefit qi, and tonify asthenia (e.g., milkvetch root, Poria cocos, largehead atractylodes rhizome, Poria cocos, liquorice root, radix glycyrrhizae preparata).

When the confidence is equal or greater than 0.90, the combination of herbs always is ShengmaiXianxiong Decoction with danshen root or Chinese thorowax root. It reflects the synergy of activating blood and dredging collaterals herbs, soothing liver-qi stagnation herbs, tonifying qi yin herbs, eliminating phlegm, and dispersing blood stasis herbs.

When the confidence is equal or greater than 0.65, white ginseng, Chinese magnoliavine fruit, debark peony root with golden thread are used to tonify qi yin (confidence = 100%), processed pinellia tuber, golden thread with snakegourd peel, longstamen onion bulb with danshen root, milkvetch root with radix glycyrrhizae preparata, honey-fried radix polygalae with Chinese arbor-vitae kernel are used to treat heart. Turmeric root tuber with Chinese thorowax root, tall gastrodia tuber, *Tribulus terrestris* with gambir plant nod, abalone shell are used to regulate liver. Poria cocos with bitter apricot seed are used to diffuse the lung (confidence ≥ 0.65).

In addition, there are few herbs that are highly potent in the 123 kind of herbs, even those with blood stasis merely use danshen root, sanqi, turmeric. Herbs that has blood-breaking efficacy, like zedoray rhizomeis, leech, pangolin scales, are seldom used. The dosage analysis shows that the herbs dosage in the treatment of CHD conforms with the prescribed dosage in Chinese pharmacopoeia. So, we can conclude that the characteristic of herbs used by Prof. Wang to treat CHD is mild.

5 CONCLUSION

In conclusion, liver-heart conjunction treatment, catharsis and tonic in combination, and using mild herbs is Wang Xing-Kuan's rule of prescriptions for CHD. The clinic curative effect of this rule is obvious. It also shows the rationality of the viscera holistic concept of TCM.

ACKNOWLEDGEMENTS

This study was supported by Programmes of Innovation platform open fund in Hunan province universities under Grant 13 k076 and the diagnosis of TCM open fund in the Hunan University of CM under Grants 2013ZYZD08 and 2013ZYZD25.

REFERENCE

ZENG Y, GE Z, TONG J, et al. Treatment of Cough Variant Asthma from Liver[J]. Chinese Archives of Traditional Chinese Medicine, 2012, 11: 060.

Medicine Sciences and Bioengineering – Wang (Ed.)
© 2015 Taylor & Francis Group, London, ISBN: 978-1-138-02684-1

Apprehending big data of TCM from the perspective of the complexity of the symptoms

Hou-wu Gong, Jin-hua Lu, Heng Chen, Yi Wen, Wen-chen Liu,
Xiong You & Jun-feng Yan*
Hunan University of CM, Changsha, Hunan, China

ABSTRACT: On the basis of 'The Big Data Describe the Chart of Modern TCM,' clinical symptoms in Traditional Chinese Medicine (TCM) are taken as an example, the complexity of TCM data is discussed, and the big data of TCM from the perspective of the complexity of the symptoms are apprehended.

1 INTRODUCTION

The view in paper *The Big Data Describe the Chart of Modern TCM* is very impressive to us. In this paper, a technological paradigm of clinical symptoms in Traditional Chinese Medicine (TCM) was mentioned as follows: "...To clinical problems as the drive, the data as the guide, with the aid of data model, the new conception of the modern TCM chart has been depicted..." (III. Liu Baoyan, 2013). It is quite clear that the core value of the modern TCM chart is the big data. Nowadays, the TCM big data include not only the vast ancient medical books, but also a large number of research literatures, the dynamic updates, and the clinical records of multimedia.

Compared with the traditional data warehousing applications, the big data analysis has the features of massive amounts of data and complex query analysis, and so on. The characteristics of big data could be summarized as four V's (volume, variety, value, and velocity)—the four characteristics: massive volume, various data types, low density value but high commercial value and high-speed velocity. Clearly, the complexity of the data is the bottleneck of the information construction in TCM. Considering the complexity of the data, the big data of TCM is required to be normalized and standardized. That may become simple data accumulation which is low value without the standardization and normalization.

For a number of reasons, many terms in the TCM have standardization problems, such as abstracted statements, multiple nomenclatures, vagueness between intension and extension, staggered contents, and so on. The TCM Data has the features as follows. The terms are difficult to handle among the modern data and a large number of the ancient Chinese. For the nonstandard nomenclature, polysemy and synonym are very common in TCM, and that make the difficulty of data cleaning. The data are mostly qualitative, lack of quantitative expression, and it hampers computer program in processing. There are a large number of unstructured data and it is hard to structure analysis. The TCM data content is the combination of humanities and natural science that is against the application of logical deduction and general data analysis tools (I. Cui Meng, Li Haiyan & Lei Meng, 2013).

The differentiation of diagnosis is primarily according to the clinical symptoms in TCM. We suggest that the complexity of the TCM data is largely embodied in clinical symptoms. The following is the analysis and discussion in the complexity of symptoms.

---

*Correspondence to: Dr. YAN Jun-feng, E-mail: teacheryan@qq.com

It is summarized by Wang Zheyu into the following four aspects. The accuracy of the symptoms depending on the doctor's knowledge and experience, and there is a strong subjectivity. The variables of the symptoms just can be measured using discrete numerical method, such as no, light, medium, and heavy. There is a complex correlation among various variables of the symptoms. There is nonunified standard in the differentiation from symptoms to syndrome (V.Wang Zheyu, Jia Zhenhua & Wu Yiling, 2008).

With the development of the research on the complexity of symptoms, ten attributes of the symptoms unit and nine relationships among symptoms were found in TCM, and the quantification of symptoms had launched the research by scholars.

2 TEN ATTRIBUTES OF THE SYMPTOMS UNIT

How many symptoms are in TCM? It is hard to answer, because currently the definition standards of the symptoms are not established in TCM.

Zhang Qiming, a professor at the Institute of TCM Clinical Basic Medical in China Academy of Traditional Medical Sciences, proposed the new concept of symptoms units on the basis of the previous medial case database research. Symptoms unit is defined as the smallest independent symptoms in section and nature, 462 feature symptoms units are selected, and these units have a single form and limited number (IX. Zhang Qiming, Wang Yiguo & Zhang Lei, 2010).

With the definition of attribute and concept in philosophy and logic, Yu Donglin (VIII. Yu Donglin, Zhang Qiming & Zhang Lei, 2011) proposed six inherent attributes and four occasional attributes in the symptoms unit. The inherent attributes include observers, instruments, objects, perspectives, observed results, and the normal biological phenomenon which the symptoms unit corresponds to. The occasional attributes include derived section, derived nature, limiting factor, and associated symptoms. It should be noted that the symptoms unit is an entity concept, and the content should have multiple attributes.

3 NINE RELATIONSHIPS AMONGST THE SYMPTOMS

Using the statistical method to study syndromes in TCM, researchers usually designed symptoms as observed indexes. From the statistical point of view, symptoms must be independent variable, and extension cannot contain or overlap each other.

Zou Aiyun (XII. Zou Aiyun & Zhang Qiming, 2013) identified 2751 symptoms from the medical cases in the history of Song, Yuan, Ming and Qing dynasties, modern times, and college textbooks. The relationships among the symptoms were analyzed using a logic method. According to the viscera-state doctrine, the symptoms were categorized into four aspects: 1) symptoms represented the disease of viscera function; 2) symptoms represented the disease of ten pathways in human body; 3) symptoms represented the disease of inner viscera; and 4) symptoms represented the disease of external form. Among these symptoms, there are: six concept relationships, namely the same relationship, inclusive relationship, cross relationship, contrary relationship, contradictive relationship, and disparate relationship; two judgment relationships, namely the essential judgment and relation judgment; and one causal relationship.

4 THE RESEARCH OF QUANTIFICATION OF SYMPTOMS IN TCM

The measurement of TCM quantitative diagnosis (XI. Zhu Wenfeng, 2008) has made significant progress in the research in this decade. With the development of the quantitative diagnosis, the quantification of the symptoms gradually becomes the research hotspot, and applied to clinical diagnosis, curative effect evaluation, certificate, and so on.

By collecting and reading the related literature (IV. Liu Guoping, 2008, VII. You Song, 2002, X. Zhou Xiaoqing & Liu Jianxin, 1992), the quantification of the symptoms were summarized into four kind of methods: the grading scored method, weighting method, 100-mm-scale method, and weighted-integral method. The symptoms were quantified with light degree, medium degree, and heavy degree or scored according to certain criteria as The Delphi method and the fuzzy mathematics method. It can be seen that, scholars adopted different quantitative methods arbitrarily with different criterions.

The author proposes that, the quantitative classification standard should be established, according to the group investigation like multiple-center and large samples. It is useful for the objective of the Chinese medicine diagnosis with the objectivity and universality. It will be an achievement for studying TCM with the integrated methods from qualitative to quantitative, and the method was advocated by academician Qian Xuesen.

Syndrome system reflected high dimensions with various factors while collecting the patient symptoms. To build a platform for the later research, we attempted to find the symptoms of the national standard for the symptoms encoding and the database design. Unfortunately, there were not related national standards.

In the textbooks of "The Diagnostics of TCM Symptoms and Differentiation" (VI. Yao Naili, 2005), there are 623 items compiled ordering by the common symptoms such as internal medicine, gynecology, pediatrics, surgery, dermatology, and ENT in TCM. Obviously, the dimensions of data are too high for statistics with this standard, coupled with demographic characteristics and examination index.

These high dimensions of the syndrome made problems in data mining that we made on patients with coronary heart disease (CHD). The samples came from 143 CHD patients who were treated from January 1, 2012 to August 30, 2013 by Prof. Wang Xingkuan, a famous TCM doctor in the first affiliated hospital of the Hunan University of TCM. These samples included 145 symptoms, 36 syndrome factors, 54 pathogenesis, 73 therapies, and 123 herbs. Each variable were binary variables as absent or not. Using the data-mining method, we attempted to explore diagnosis rules of Prof. Wang. In this case, the dimensions number far exceeded the number of cases in data processing. At last, while using Weka 3.6 software to analysis the association rules of symptoms, the computer prompted memory corruption error for high dimensions.

The complexity of the syndrome is due to the high dimension and higher order. The high dimension of syndrome represents various factors of the syndrome system. There are nine kinds of factors involved in this system: pathogenesis, etiology, illness, disease, pathology, attempt, symptoms, pathogenic relationship, and physical state. Each type of factors contained secondary factors. The high order of syndrome represents the complexity of the relationship among various factors. On the basis of Bayesian network technology, Guo Lei, Wang Xuewei & Wang Yongyan (2006) carried out the research on the correlation of syndrome factors at lung diseases. The results indicated that the correlations were very complex, the correlations contained both linear and nonlinear, and they were intertwined. The syndrome factors had a complex network structure, and the correlations presented typical nonlinear features.

Nowadays, the development of medical science has been out of the experience medicine, and the evidence-based medicine will be the right direction. Thus, the numerous clinical research data is bound to form a "big data of traditional Chinese medicine." As the rule in data mining, high-quality decision inevitably depends on the quality data. The TCM big data will no longer be the simple data accumulation, and each research will no longer be the "information islands," after standardization and normalization of the symptoms. With the improvement of the utilization, the TCM big data will provide great convenience to TCM personnel, and promote the development of the TCM informatization.

ACKNOWLEDGMENTS

The authors acknowledge the contribution of YAN Jun-fen, Female, MD, Professor of Computer Science, Master Instructor, Main Research: Medicine Informatics and Data Mining.

E-mail: teacheryan@qq.com; Innovation platform open fund in Hunan province universities (NO:13 k076) and the diagnosis of traditional Chinese Medicine open fund in Hunan University of CM (NO:2013ZYZD08,2013ZYZD25).

REFERENCES

Cui Meng, Li Haiyan, Lei Meng. "Age of Big Data" and "Knowledge-intensive" data of TCM [J]. Intelligence Magazine of TCM, 2013,37(3):1–3.

Guo Lei, Wang Xuewei, Wang Yongyan. The Complexity of the Syndrome with High-dimension and Higher-order [J]. Journal of Chinese medicine, 2006,21(2):76–78.

Liu Baoyan. The Technological Paradigm of Clinical Symptoms in TCM [J]. Journal of Traditional Chinese Medicine, 2013,54(6):451–455.

Liu Guoping, Wang Yiqin. Retrospect and Prospect on Quantitative Method Research of Symptoms [J]. Journal of Jiangsu Chinese Medicine, 2008,40(10):124–126.

Wang Zheyu, Jia Zhenhua, Wu Yiling. Hidden Variables Analysis of Syndromes Data with Non-guide in TCM [J]. Journals of Mathematical Statistics and Management, 2008,27(5):938–944.

Yao Naili. The Diagnostics of TCM Symptoms and Differentiation [M]. Beijing: People's Medical Publishing House, 2005.

You Song. The Quantitative Method of TCM Symptoms [J]. Journal of Beijing University of Chinese Medicine, 2002,25(2):13.

Yu Donglin, Zhang Qiming, Zhang Lei. Ten Attributes of the Symptoms Unit [J]. Journal of the modernization of Chinese Medicine, 2011,13(5):816–820.

Zhang Qiming, Wang Yiguo, Zhang Lei. Connotation of Smallest Independent Symptoms [J]. Journal of Beijing University of Chinese Medicine, 2010,33(1):5–10.

Zhou Xiaoqing, Liu Jianxin. The Quantitative Diagnosis of TCM Symptoms [J]. Journal of Liaoning Chinese Medicine, 1992,19(6):11.

Zhu Wenfeng. Differentiation of Syndrome Element [M]. Beijing: People's Medical Publishing House, 2008.

Zou Aiyun, Zhang Qiming. Nine Relationships amongst the Symptoms [J]. Journal of Beijing University of Chinese Medicine, 2013,36(4):224–226.

Medicine Sciences and Bioengineering – Wang (Ed.)
© *2015 Taylor & Francis Group, London, ISBN: 978-1-138-02684-1*

A method to measure the trans-lamina cribrosa pressure difference in rabbits

Feng Zhao, Chuan Wang, Zheng Wei, Zhi-hang Liu & Bao-qing Xu
Key Laboratory for Biomechanics and Mechanobiology of the Ministry of Education, School of Biological Science and Medical Engineering, Beihang University, Beijing, China

Di-ya Yang, Ke-gao Liu & Ning-li Wang
Beijing Tongren Eye Center, Beijing Tongren Hospital, Capital Medical University Beijing, China

Yu-bo Fan*
Key Laboratory for Biomechanics and Mechanobiology of the Ministry of Education, School of Biological Science and Medical Engineering, Beihang University, Beijing, China

ABSTRACT: Primary Open-Angle Glaucoma (POAG) is the most common form of glaucoma and its etiology remains unknown. Recent research suggests that abnormal rising of Trans-lamina Cribrosa Pressure Difference (TCPD) caused by decrease of cerebrospinal fluid (CSF) pressure may be the pathogenesis of POAG. However, the TCPD (intraocular pressure minus CSF pressure of optic nerve subarachnoid space) had not been directly measured, but was calculated clinically as difference of intraocular pressure (IOP) minus lumbar CSF pressure instead. In this paper, an IOP and CSF pressure-measuring device was developed and validated. Accuracy was obtained through a water-column pressure-measuring experiment with the maximum absolute error of 0.4 mmH$_2$O. Then the TCPD of three adult New Zealand White rabbits was measured (4.19 ± 0.52 mmHg). This method might help to research the relationship between the increase of TCPD and primary open-angle glaucoma.

1 INTRODUCTION

Glaucoma is the second leading cause of blindness worldwide. It is estimated that there will be 79.6 million people with glaucoma in 2020 (Quigley & Broman, 2006). Glaucoma is a kind of progressive optic neuropathy with characteristic optic nerve damage and visual loss, whose main risk factor is the level of intraocular pressure (IOP) elevation (Weinreb & Khaw, 2004). However, the pathogenesis of primary open-angle glaucoma (POAG) remains unclear, which accounts for 74% of the total number of glaucoma patients (Quigley & Broman, 2006). Currently, the mainstream theory concerning POAG is mechanical or pressure-related suggesting that IOP can induce optic nerve damage through biomechanical or structural factors (Fechtner & Weinreb, 1994). Nevertheless, it was observed clinically that about 90% people with ocular hypertension did not have nerve optic damage and visual loss in five years (Kass *et al.*, 2002), whereas around one-third to one-half of glaucoma with normal IOP still got progressive visual loss (He *et al.*, 2006).

Recent researches suggest that abnormal rising of trans-lamina cribrosa pressure difference (TCPD) caused by decrease of cerebrospinal fluid (CSF) pressure may be pathogenesis of POAG. In 1979, Yablonsky *et al.* reduced the intracranial pressure of experimental animals by ventricular drainage, which brought about glaucomatous optic nerve damage after three weeks. A retrospective study found that the patients of control group without glaucoma had significantly higher intracranial pressure (13.0 ± 4.2 mmHg) than patients with POAG (9.2 ± 2.9 mmHg) ($P < 0.00005$) (Berdahl *et al.*, 2008). A prospective study found that the TCPD of patients with

---

*Corresponding author. Email: yubofan@buaa.edu.cn

normal tension glaucoma (6.6 ± 3.6 mmHg) was significantly higher than that of nonglaucoma group (1.4 ± 1.7 mmHg) ($P < 0.001$) (Ren et al., 2010).

However, the TCDP (IOP minus CSF pressure of optic nerve subarachnoid space) has not been directly measured so far, but calculated clinically as difference of IOP minus lumbar CSF pressure instead. Consequently, the relationship between TCPD and primary open-angle glaucoma cannot be studied directly. The goal of this study was the development and validation of a method to measure the TCDP in rabbits.

2 METHODS

2.1 An IOP and CSF pressure measuring device

An IOP and CSF pressure measuring device was developed to acquire the TCPD of rabbits, which consisted of four primary parts: a microfeeding device, two pressure sensors, a data acquisition card, and a computer (Figure 1). A microfeeding device was designed in CAD software (SolidWorks 2010, Dassault Systemes). It ensured that probe could be punctured gradually in 20 μm through dura mater encephali into optic nerve subarachnoid space to measure the CSF pressure behind lamina cribrosa. Pressure sensors (HY133, Beijing Huayuzhanyekeji Limited Liability Company) were connected to the probe by catheter: one for measuring IOP and another for CSF pressure. The measuring range of pressure sensor is 0 to 10 kPa (0–75 mmHg) and the accuracy is 0.1% (0.075 mmHg or 1.02 mmH$_2$O). Power supply (12–24 V direct current) and signal output (4–20 mA current) of the pressure sensor shared a circuit. The signal from sensor was acquired and amplified by a data acquisition card (USB7660, ZTIC, Beijing). The data acquisition card was connected to a computer with USB interface and controlled by customized software written in LabVIEW8.5 with functions including data acquisition, displaying, processing, analysis, and storage.

2.2 Accuracy evaluation

Accuracy of the pressure measuring device was evaluated by measuring the pressure of five water columns with different heights ranging from 100 to 600 mm. The actual pressure of water columns were measured using a ruler with accuracy of 0.1 mmH$_2$O, which is better than pressure sensor (1.02 mmH$_2$O). For the reliability, the amount of zero drift in 1200s was assessed and the maximum of drift was gained.

2.3 Application on rabbits

Three adult New Zealand white rabbits with weight of 2 to 2.3 kg were used in the experiments. Animal treatment and care were in accordance with the Regulations for the Administration of

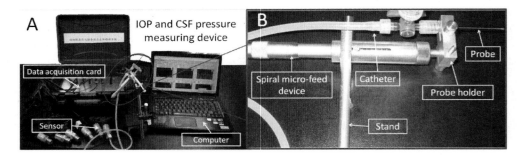

Figure 1.   (A) IOP and CSF pressure measuring device. (B) Microfeeding device.

Affairs Concerning Experimental Animals promulgated by Decree No. 2 of the State Science and Technology Commission of China and the Guiding Principles for the Care and Use of Animals approved by Beijing Government. All protocols were approved by the Animal Care Committee of Beihang University, China. Rabbits were anesthetized by injecting 1% of pentobarbital sodium (3 ml/kg) into the ear-edge veins.

Pressure sensors were calibrated before experiments. A probe was punctured into the anterior chamber of rabbit through cornea to measure the IOP. For CSF pressure of optic nerve subarachnoid space, first, the eye of rabbit was fixed by eye thimble and stitches. Second, the lateral wall of eye was opened and lateral rectus and superior rectus were cut off for fully exposure of optic nerve. Then, a probe was punctured gradually into optic nerve subarachnoid space. IOP, CSF, and TCPD were measured and displayed simultaneously. Average value of 50 to 100s was calculated as results when the value achieved stability.

3 RESULTS

Accuracy evaluation showed that maximum absolute error was 0.4 mmH$_2$O and maximum relative error was 0.124%. For number one sensor, mean error was -0.3 ± 0.07 mmH$_2$O (-0.4 to 0.2 mmH$_2$O) and relative error was 0.09% $\pm$ 0.01% (0.073%–0.107%). For number two sensor, mean error was -0.2 ± 0.23 mmH$_2$O (-0.4 to 0.2 mmH$_2$O) and relative error was 0.09% $\pm$ 0.03% (0.044%–0.124%). The maximum of zero drift in 1200s were 9.5×10^{-4} mmH$_2$O and 7.5×10^{-4} mmH$_2$O, respectively. Consequently, the device has good accuracy and excellent reliability for continuous measurement of rabbits' IOP and CSF pressure.

Results of the rabbit experiment are presented in Table 1. The IOP of the rabbits was 15.50 $\pm$ 0.43 mmHg, the CSF pressure of optic nerve subarachnoid space was 11.31 $\pm$ 0.09 mmHg, and TCPD was 4.19 $\pm$ 0.52 mmHg.

4 DISCUSSION

The purpose of this study was to introduce a method to measure the TCPD of rabbit. The IOP of rabbits was found as 15.50 $\pm$ 0.43 mmHg, which was extremely similar with Zhang et al. (2014) and within the range of previously published data (15–19 mmHg). The CSF pressure of optic nerve subarachnoid space and TCPD were found as 11.31 $\pm$ 0.09 mmHg and 4.19 $\pm$ 0.52 mmHg, respectively. True TCPD had not been measured directly before, which was calculated as difference of IOP minus lumbar CSF pressure. Nevertheless, CSF pressure distribution is not entirely consistent in different chambers, which means that the CSF pressure of optic nerve subarachnoid space might be represented by lumbar CSF pressure (Killer et al., 2009).

In conclusion, this study would likely provide an accurate and reliable method to measure the TCPD of rabbits in vivo. This might be helpful to further research focusing on the relationship between the increase of TCPD and POAG. On the other hand, this study may contribute to research the relationship among the CSF pressure of optic nerve subarachnoid space, lumbar CSF pressure, and intracranial pressure.

Table 1. The TCPD of rabbits (mmHg).

	1	2	3	Mean $\pm$ SD
IOP	15.00	15.75	15.75	15.50 $\pm$ 0.43
CSF-P	11.41	11.27	11.25	11.31 $\pm$ 0.09
TCPD	3.59	4.48	4.50	4.19 $\pm$ 0.52

IOP: intraocular pressure; CSF-P: cerebrospinal fluid pressure; TCPD: trans-lamina cribrosa pressure difference.

ACKNOWLEDGEMENTS

This work was supported by the National Nature Science Foundation of China under Grants 11072021 and 31200725, the National Science & Technology Pillar Program of China under Grant 2012BAI22B02, and SRTP of Beihang University.

REFERENCES

Berdahl, J. P., Allingham, R., & Johnson, D. H. (2008). Cerebrospinal fluid pressure is decreased in primary open-angle glaucoma. *Ophthalmology*, 115(5), 763–768.

Fechtner, R. D., & Weinreb, R. N. (1994). Mechanisms of optic nerve damage in primary open angle glaucoma. *Survey of ophthalmology*, 39(1), 23–42.

He, M., Foster, P. J., Ge, J., Huang, W., Zheng, Y., Friedman, D. S., & Khaw, P. T. (2006). Prevalence and clinical characteristics of glaucoma in adult Chinese: a population-based study in Liwan District, Guangzhou. *Investigative ophthalmology & visual science*, 47(7), 2782–2788.

Kass, M. A., Heuer, D. K., Higginbotham, E. J., Johnson, C. A., Keltner, J. L., Miller, J. P., & Gordon, M. O. (2002). The Ocular Hypertension Treatment Study: a randomized trial determines that topical ocular hypotensive medication delays or prevents the onset of primary open-angle glaucoma. *Archives of ophthalmology*, 120(6), 701–713.

Killer, H. E., Jaggi, G. P., & Miller, N. R. (2009). Papilledema revisited: is its pathophysiology really understood?. *Clinical & experimental ophthalmology*, 37(5), 444–447.

Quigley, H. A., & Broman, A. T. (2006). The number of people with glaucoma worldwide in 2010 and 2020. *British Journal of Ophthalmology*, 90(3), 262–267.

Ren, R., Jonas, J. B., Tian, G., Zhen, Y., Ma, K., Li, S., ... & Wang, N. (2010). Cerebrospinal fluid pressure in glaucoma: a prospective study. *Ophthalmology*, 117(2), 259–266.

Weinreb, R. N., & Khaw, P. T. (2004). Primary open-angle glaucoma. *The Lancet*, 363(9422), 1711–1720.

Yablonski, M. E., Ritch, R., & Pokorny, K. S. (1979, January). Effect of decreased intracranial pressure on optic disk. In *INVESTIGATIVE OPHTHALMOLOGY & VISUAL SCIENCE* (pp. 165–165). 227 EAST WASHINGTON SQ, PHILADELPHIA, PA 19106: LIPPINCOTT-RAVEN PUBL.

Zhang, H., Yang, D., Ross, C. M., Wigg, J. P., Pandav, S., & Crowston, J. G. (2014). Validation of rebound tonometry for intraocular pressure measurement in the rabbit. *Experimental eye research*, 121, 86–93.

Medicine Sciences and Bioengineering – Wang (Ed.)
© *2015 Taylor & Francis Group, London, ISBN: 978-1-138-02684-1*

miRNAs and targets that underlie glomerular development

Xian Wu*, Yan-fang Ding* & Jin-yao Zhao
Dalian Medical University, Dalian, Liaoning, China

Gordon Guo
Department of Radiation Oncology, University of Manitoba, Winnipeg, Canada

Yong-qi Li, Tian-bai Li Jin-liang Wang & Shi-ying Cui
Dalian Medical University, Dalian, Liaoning, China

ABSTRACT: MicroRNAs (miRNAs) are small, naturally occurring, and noncoding RNAs that regulate gene expression at post-transcript stage. Although miRNAs have been implicated in the regulation of diverse biologic processes, little is known about miRNAs and targets that underlie in the kidney and glomerular development. Here we define the miRNA and target expression pattern in glomerular development from embryonic stage to mature stage by using miRNA, mRNA array, bioinformatics, and molecular techniques. The results indicate that in comparison to developed glomeruli, miRNAs are differently expressed in developing glomeruli, and therefore, this could clearly separate subtype of immature and mature glomeruli. The targets predicted from miRNAs were further compared with genes that were analyzed from mRNA array data. A total of 1264 genes, whose function being relevant to cellular development, was shared in both miRNA and mRNA data. Finally, miR-222 and target gene *NPM1* were validated by quantitative real-time polymerase chain reaction (qRT-PCR), immunohistochemistry (IHC), and Western Blotting (WB). Our data indicate that miRNA and target gene profiles may not only aid in discriminating between different stages of glomerular development, but may also represent novel therapeutic targets for innate and acquired kidney glomerular disease.[1]

1 INTRODUCTION

In the past few years, a major breakthrough in biology is the discovery of miRNAs. As a consequence, with the identification of hundreds vertebrate miRNAs, it has been predicted that a significant proportion of all transcripts may be regulated by miRNAs (Zhao, 2012). Emerging data suggest a critical role of miRNAs in the regulation of development and diseases (He, 2004). Recent studies showed that miRNAs are essential in kidney development and glomerular diseases (Ambros, 2004; Pasquinelli, 2006), and miR-191, -192, -194, -204, -215, and -216 are reported to be highly and quite exclusively expressed in the adult kidney (Khella, 2013 & Nagpal, 2014). Loss of function of miR-23a, -24, and -26b might lead to rapid glomerular and tubular injury (Jacqueline, 2008). However, the miRNAs that underlie in glomerular development are largely unknown.

Glomerulus develops from metanephrogenic tissue via S-shaped, capillary loop, and mature stages. Previously, we developed a method that allowed us to isolate glomerulus from each of the major developmental stages (Cui, 2005). The first mature glomerulus appears at E13–14 in mouse, and 18%–20% of mature glomeruli are developed at birth, but all mature glomerulus are completely developed until their postnatal days 20–22. The proper development and preservation of this structure throughout life is essential and important to prevent serious kidney disease.

---

*Contributed equally

Abnormal glomerular development leads to a broad spectrum of kidney diseases and related syndromes, afflicting millions of people per year worldwide (Yi, 2010). A better understanding of the mechanisms of glomerular development may lead to the identification of new targets for therapeutic intervention and to the development of safer treatment modalities.

In this article, we define the profile of miRNA expression and target genes in glomerular development from embryonic stage to mature stage.

2 MATERIAL AND METHODS

2.1 *Kidney dissection and glomerular isolation*

Kidneys were dissected and glomeruli were isolated from 108 embryos at E18.5 and 12 mice at postnatal 4 weeks (4W). The procedure of glomerular isolation from embryos was described previously (Cui, 2005). Briefly, the embryo/mouse was microperfused with Hanks Balanced Salt Solutions (HBSS) buffer through the heart under a dissecting microscope. The kidneys were minced into pieces and collagenase A and deoxyribonuclease I in HBSS (Hanks Balanced Salt Solutions) buffer were added. After the digestion, glomeruli were isolated with a magnetic particle concentrator.

2.2 *Total RNA isolation, miRNAs labeling, and data analysis*

RNAs were extracted from glomeruli and 10 µg of total RNA was labeled using the mercury labeling kit, which was performed at the microarray facility (Duke University, USA). All samples were co-hybridized to printed arrays that contained a 592 Ambion mirVana miRNA Set2 probe and 1140 Invitrogen's NCode multispecies miRNA probes. The hybridized arrays were scanned on a GenePix 4000B scanner, and expression data were generated using the GenePix Pro software (Molecular Devices, Sunnyvale, California).

2.3 *mRNA array and data analysis*

Affymetrix GeneChip Mouse Genome 430 2.0 Array (Santa Clara, CA) were used for RNA array analysis, which was performed at the microarray facility (The Hospital for Sick Children, Toronto, Canada). For array hybridization, RNA was amplified using the affymetrix two-cycle kit, and the data analysis was performed using Microsoft Excel program. The genes whose expression was either up- or down-regulated at least twofold between E18.5 and 4W glomeruli were chosen for further analysis by Affymetrix GCOS, SpotFire, and Array assist programs.

2.4 *miRNA targets prediction in comparison with mRNA data*

To identify individual genes that are likely to be important for glomerular development, we used three programs: (1) miRBase (http://microrna.sanger.ac.uk/), (2) MicroCosm (http://www.ebi.ac.uk/enright-srv/microcosm/htdocs/targets/v5/), and (3) miRanda (http://www.microrna.org/microrna/getGeneForm.do) to predict miRNA targets. The list of targets predicted from miRNAs was further compared with the genes that were generated from mRNA array data.

2.5 *Quantitative real-time PCR*

Reverse transcription was performed using High-Capacity cDNA Reverse Transcription Kits according to the manufacturer's instruction. Real-time PCR for the *NPM1* gene was performed using the SYBR GREEN PCR kit. For the real-time PCR reaction, 2 µg of total RNA was subjected to cDNA synthesis and amplified over 40 PCR cycles. The threshold cycle (C_t) was calculated by the instrument's (Agilent Technologies Stratagene Mx3000P) software.

2.6 Immunohistochemistry and western blotting

To demonstrate the targets in protein level, *NPM1* was checked by both immunohistochemistry (IHC) and western blotting (WB). The primary antibody (Ab) used was anti-NPM1 (1:200 dilution), and secondary Ab was biotin-related anti-rabbit (Vectastain Kit; Burlingame, CA). After 3,3′-diaminobenzidine(DAB, 3,3N-Diaminobenzidine Tertrahydrochloride) development, samples were counterstained with hematoxylin, and photographed.

3 RESULTS

3.1 Qualification test of miRNA and mRNA array samples

On the basis of entire expression level of miRNAs, GeneSpring GX 73.1 software was used to verify the distribution of the samples by microarray. The results of the PCA plot of samples from glomerulus at E18.5 are clearly separated from 4 W. All samples of the expression level of glomerulus at 4 W located on the second PCA, which separated from the samples of E18.5 glomeruli that distributed on the first PCA, suggesting batch variance is criterion. After amplification with the Affymetrix two-cycle kit, the quality of mRNA array samples was evaluated by an ethidium bromide–stained gel and electropherogram of RNA to confirm the integrity of RNA purified from isolated glomeruli. Scatter plot of the microarray database showed signal/separated detection of gene expression from 4W isolated glomeruli compared with E18.5.

3.2 miRNA expression profiles and unique miRNAs of glomerular development

In the developing glomeruli, 374 miRNAs were considered detectable, whereas 129 were detectable in the mature glomeruli. The most abundant miRNAs in both developing and mature glomeruli were let-7 family and miR-16, -24, -22, and -497. Sixty-nine unique miRNAs were detected with significant fold changes (less than twofold), of which 48 were found to be downregulated, 21 upregulated in 4W compared with E18.5 glomeruli. Among the unique miRNAs, miR-29a, -222, -497, -22, -145, -24, -143 and let-7b, -7c, -7e were preferentially expressed in the mature glomeruli, and miR-542–3p, -199b, -338, and -19a were most highly expressed in developing glomerulus. Interestingly, miR-542–3p and miR-1 are highly expressed in glomeruli at E18.5 and disappeared at 4W, suggesting an important role in developing glomeruli. miR-29a, -222, -24, and -143 have no expression at developing glomerulus, but highly expressed at mature glomerulus, implying an important role in maintaining glomerular function after 4W.

3.3 miRNA targets prediction and comparison with mRNA array data

The targets prediction of miRNAs showed that 1463 were targeted on the biological function of cell development. Of which, 633 were targeted on the cell differentiation/proliferation cycle and 766 on the signal transduction. When the targets predicted from miRNA data were compared with mRNA array results, a total of 76 miRNAs and 1264 genes was shared in both data. The targeted genes from let-7 family (let-7b, 7c, 7e) were further analyzed, of which 567 were identified to regulate the function related to cell proliferation and differentiation, suggesting let-7 family might play an important role in glomerular development.

3.4 Validation of key miRNA and target genes

To demonstrate the utility of this profile, we examined the expression of miR-222 and target gene *NPM1* that were differently expressed in glomeruli of E18.5 from 4W. We, first, validated their reciprocal expression by qRT-PCR. The results showed that the expression of miR-222 was 2.7 times higher in glomeruli at 4W than E18.5, which confirmed the data obtained by miRNA array analysis. Whereas, *NPM1* levels were 4.5 times higher in glomeruli at E18.5 than 4W, which

Table 1. Key miRNAs generated from miRNA array.

No.	Systematic	miRNA name	Fold Change 4W vs. E18.5	No.	Systematic	miRNA name	Fold Change 4W vs. E18.5
1	2154	mmu-miR-29a	65.27	29	2264	mmu-miR-422b	4.55
2	1198	mmu-miR-222	56.55	30	SM10337	rno-miR-221	4.55
3	1431	mmu-let-7b	17.44	31	1017	mmu-miR-191	4.46
4	1870	mmu-miR-497	17.27	32	SM10056	mmu-miR-107	4.29
5	1022	mmu-miR-22	15.23	33	SM10438	mmu-let-7e	4.27
6	2198	dre-miR-145	14.67	34	1196	rno-miR-151*	3.9
7	SM10606	mmu-miR-145	14.4	35	1063	mmu-miR-99b	3.56
8	1044	mmu-miR-24	14.03	36	1310	dre-miR-29a	3.2
9	1268	mmu-let-7c	13.38	37	1064	mmu-miR-100	2.86
10	SM11050	rno-let-7b	12.1	38	2143	mmu-miR-140*	2.81
11	1955	dre-miR-192	11.67	39	1076	rno-miR-151	2.71
12	SM10436	mmu-let-7c	11.3	40	1005	mmu-miR-320	2.64
13	1995	hsa-miR-497	10.98	41	SM10633	mmu-miR-187	2.26
14	1415	mmu-miR-143	10.6	42	2186	mmu-miR-685	2.07
15	1113	dre-miR-23b	10.58	43	1098	mmu-miR-296	−2.62
16	1114	mmu-miR-23a	10.1	44	SM10660	mmu-miR-1	−4.37
17	1931	dre-miR-23a	9.87	45	2065	dre-miR-202	−4.74
18	2238	dre-miR-143	9.57	46	SM10850	mmu-miR-298	−5.81
19	2305	dre-miR-27d	8.89	47	2859	mmu-miR-301b	−6.58
20	SM10576	mmu-miR-143	8.75	48	2842	mmu-miR-763	−6.76
21	1168	mmu-miR-145	7.14	49	SM10094	mmu-miR-338	−6.8
22	1428	mmu-let-7a	6.95	50	SM10649	mmu-miR-19a	−6.9
23	1421	mmu-let-7e	6.66	51	SM10316	mmu-miR-379	−6.99
24	SM10401	mmu-miR-126–5p	6.26	52	1176	mmu-miR-199b	−7.52
25	SM10203	mmu-miR-22	5.87	53	SM10526	mmu-miR-199b	−7.87
26	1851	rno-miR-422b	4.76	54	SM11298	mmu-miR-291b-3p	−11.55
27	1018	mmu-miR-193	4.7	55	SM11302	rno-miR-542–3p	−36.9
28	2302	dre-miR-27e	4.68	56	SM11299	rno-miR-1	−54.95

Table 2. The key miRNAs and targets predicted by three softwares.

miRNA	Fold change	Target symbol	MicroCosm			miRanda			TargetScan	
			MicroCosm	score	P value	miRanda	mirSVR score	PhastCons score	TargetScan	P_{CT}
miR-143	9.45	Npm1	YES	16.67	0.0317	NO	—	—	NO	—
miR-23a	8.55	Npm1	NO	—	—	YES	−0.6727	0.7171	NO	—
miR-126p	6.26	Npm1	YES	16.56	0.0405	YES	−0.7551	0.7171	NO	—
miR-222	56.55	Npm1	YES	17.01	0.0181	YES	—	—	NO	—

was consistent with the targets predicted from miRNA data and mRNA array results. Consequently, *NPM1* expression, upregulated in glomeruli at E18.5, was validated at protein levels by IHC (Figure 1A) and WB (Figure 1B). *NPM1* was highly expressed in the podocyte precursors of the S-shaped body of glomerular in early developing stage, and podocytes of the capillary loop stage

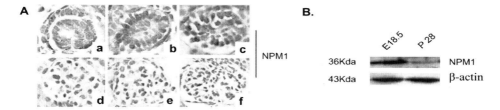

Figure 1. NPM1 high expression in the immature glomeruli was validated by IHC (A) and WB (B).

of glomerular in developing stage, except for proximal tubule cells, at E18.5. Whereas, there was a poor staining of *NPM1* in the mature developed glomeruli at 4W. The quantitative analysis by WB further demonstrated that *NPM1* was 3–4 times lower in glomeruli at 4W than E18.5.

4 CONCLUSION

In this study, we defined the expression pattern of miRNAs and target genes in glomerular development from embryonic stage to mature stage. miRNAs and target genes are differently expressed in developing and developed glomeruli, as observed in both miRNA and mRNA microarrays. The profiles of key miRNAs and target genes were predicted by three bioinformatics software and confirmed by qRT-PCR. The reciprocal expression of miRNA and its target was validated by quantitative and qualitative analysis at both gene and protein levels. This study may advance to better understand the novel therapeutic targets for innate and acquired kidney glomerular disease.

ACKNOWLEDGMENTS

This work was supported by National Basic Research Program of China 973 Program No. 2012CB517600 (No. 2012CB517603).

REFERENCES

Ambros, V. (2004) The functions of animal microRNAs. *Nature*, 431:350–355.

Cui S, C Li, (2005) Rapid Isolation of Glomeruli Coupled with Gene Expression Profiling Identifies Downstream Targets in Pod1 Knockout Mice. *J Am Soc Nephrol*, 16(11):3247–3255.

He, L.Hannon, GJ. (2004) MicroRNAs: small RNAs with a big role in gene regulation. *Nat Rev Genet*, 5:522–531.

Ho Jacqueline, Kar Hui Ng, (2008) Podocyte-specific loss of functional microRNAs leads to rapid glomerular and tubular injury. *J Am Soc Nephrol*, 19: 2069–2075.

Khella HW, Bakhet M, (2013) miR-192, miR-194 and miR-215: a convergent microRNA network suppressing tumor progression in renal cell carcinoma. *Carcinogenesis*, 34(10):2231–2239.

Nagpal N, Kulshreshtha R. (2014) miR-191: an emerging player in disease biology. *Front Genet*, 5:99.

Pasquinelli AE, (2006) Demystifying small RNA pathways. *Dev Cell*, 10:419–424.

Yi Tingfang, Kunrong Tan, (2010) Regulation of embryonic kidney branching morphogenesis and glomerular development by KISS1 receptor (Gpr54) through NFAT2- and Sp1-mediated Bmp7 expression. *J Biol chem*, 285(23):17811–17820.

Zhao JY, Cui S. (2012) Synchronous detection of miRNAs, their targets and down-stream proteins in transferred FFPE sections: Applications in clinical and basic research. *Methods,* 2012 Oct; 58(2):156–163.

Medicine Sciences and Bioengineering – Wang (Ed.)
© 2015 Taylor & Francis Group, London, ISBN: 978-1-138-02684-1

Performance research of a single cell as a microreactor by microchip electrophoresis with laser-induced fluorescence

Chu-ting Liang, Yue Sun*, Yue-qing Rong, Shu-mei Wang & Sheng-wang Liang
School of Traditional Chinese Medicine, Guangdong Pharmaceutical University, Guangzhou, China

ABSTRACT: In this article, performance of a single cell as a microreactor was studied by microchip capillary electrophoresis with Laser-Induced Fluorescence (LIF) detector. The reaction of FITC and amino acids was chosen as the analysis model system. Three amino acids with positive, neutral, and negative charge, respectively, and FITC were mediated into cells through liposome. Reaction of amino acids and FITC in single cell and in flask at various times were detected, respectively. It was observed that both the reaction speed and efficiency of the cells are much higher than in conventional reactor.

1 INTRODUCTION

Cell is the basic building block of living organisms. Such a "nano" environment raises questions about the applicability of bulk chemical assays toward understanding cellular processes. Chiu *et al.* (1999) first used liposome as biomimetic containers to study fast chemical reaction kinetics that are inaccessible in traditional bulk turbulence mixing technique. Kulin *et al.* (2003) used optical method to manipulate and fuse giant liposomes as reaction containers to evaluate chemical and biomolecular kinetics. Karlsson *et al.* (2000) developed a single-cell-sized unilamellar liposome as microreactor to observe the chemical intercalation reaction between T2-phage DNA and YOYO-1. However, the intracellular reaction is much more complex than in lipid.

Visualization of biologically relevant molecules and activities inside living cells is the main method to study cellular progress (Johnsson, 2007), but optical technique requires a high cost, including instrument and fluorescent dyes, and cannot obtain an accurate quantitative result. The traditional assay of group of cells contents always led to a big error accompanied with a long and tedious process, including crushing, centrifugation, and extraction. The micrometer channel dimensions of microfluidic chips are ideally suited for sample introduction, manipulation, reaction, separation, and detection of single cells. In recent years, there have been many reports on the separation of the intracellular contents (Gu *et al.*, 2011) of single cell in microfluidic chip.

The aim of this study was to have a rough understanding about the character of a single cell as a microreactor by comparing the reaction speed inside and outside a cell. Obviously, a rapid reaction is difficult to test, so the derivatization reaction of amino acids by FITC was chosen, which often needs a long time to finish (Zinellu *et al.*, 2009). Moreover, reaction of FITC and amino acids is not an intrinsic cellular bioreaction, so the difference in reaction in vivo and in vitro would be just owing to the closed and tiny physical surrounding of a single cell, because of which the complexity of the study was greatly reduced. High concentration of FITC and amino acids were delivered into cells through liposome, and the reaction extent was obtained by a series of single-cell analysis in microchip capillary electrophoresis (CE) with a LIF detector. A real-time detection of the reaction in flask was also tested by microchip CE. The results showed an astonished difference in reaction in flask and in a single living cell. The study can offer valuable insights into an in vivo reaction in cell.

---

*Email: sunyuesdzb@163.com

2 MATERIALS AND METHODS

2.1 *Chemicals*

Phosphatidylcholines was obtained from the Chemical Factory of East China Normal University (Shanghai, China). PBS, which consisted of 0.9% NaCl, 0.2% Na_2HPO_4, and 0.01% NaH_2PO_4 (pH 7.6), was used for washing and preserving cells. Hydroxypropyl methylcellulose (HPMC) was purchased from Sigma (St. Louis, MO, USA), and a PBS-HPMC solution (0.4% HPMC in PBS) was used as medium for the cell suspension. A 10 mM sodium dodecyl sulfate (SDS) solution, which was used as the medium for cell lysis as well as the working electrolyte for CE separation, was prepared by dissolving the surfactant in 10 mM borate buffer (pH 9.2). Fluorescein isothiocyanate (FITC) was purchased from Aldrich (St. Louis, MO, USA). RPMI-1640 medium was obtained from GibcoBRL (Gaithersburg, MD, USA). A 1.0×10^{-3} M stock solution of amino acids (Shanghai Biochemical Reagents, China) was prepared by dissolving appropriate amounts of amino acids in water. All chemicals of analytical grade and Millipore purified water were used throughout.

2.2 *Apparatus*

JY98-3D Ultrasonic Homogenizers (Ningbo Xinzhi Scientific Instruments, Ningbo, China) was used for producing nanometer-sized liposome. The microchip CE experiments were carried out on a ZDMCI6-1 microfluidic chip detector (Hangzhou Meijing Electronic Company, Hangzhou, China) equipped with a multiterminal high-voltage power supply (0–3000 V), and a confocal microscope LIF system with a 488-nm argon-ion laser was used for detection, and the emitted light up 500 nm can be connected to amplifier. The microchip used in this study is same as described in the work by Sun *et al.* (2006).

2.3 *Liposome preparation and characterization*

Liposomes containing 10^{-4} M of each kind of amino acids and 10^{-4} M FITC, respectively, were prepared by a sonication method (Sun *et al.*, 2006). The concentration of nonencapsulated substrates (C_1) in the dialysate can be determined by microchip CE-LIF. Assuming the original amino acids concentration as C_0, the volumes of the original liquid and the dialysate were V_0 and V_1 (mL), respectively. The encapsulation yield was calculated from the formula $(C_0V_0 - C_1V_1)/C_0V_0$. The numbers of the vesicle (n) were estimated from: $C_0 \times 4/3\pi r^3 \times n = (C_0V_0 - C_1V_1)$, where r (cm) is the vesicle average radius.

2.4 *Intracellular delivery of amino acids and FITC mediated by liposomes*

200 μL of HepG2 cells (5×10^5 cells per mL) was seeded in a 96-well plate in RPMI-1640 medium, and cultured for 24 hours in RPMI-1640 medium supplemented with 100 U mL^{-1} penicillin, 100 μg mL^{-1} streptomycin, and 10% fetal bovine serum in a humidified atmosphere of 95% air and 5% CO_2 at 37°C. The cells were then washed with PBS two times, and incubated with 1.0 mL FITC-encapsulated liposomes and 1.0 mL amino acids–encapsulated liposomes freshly added for 2 hours. After incubation, the cells were washed with PBS two times to remove excessive liposome, and were resuspended and diluted in PBS-HPMC solution to obtain a cell population of 1.2×10^5 cells per mL.

2.5 *Procedure for single-cell analysis on microchip*

80, 80, and 50 μL working electrolyte solutions were added to the reservoirs B, BW, and SW, respectively. Then, 100 μL cell suspension (1.2×10^5 cells per mL) was added to the reservoir S as described previously. When a single cell was introduced, docked, and lysised under visualization as described in the work by Sun *et al.* (2006), the chip was then shifted from the channel-crossing viewing position to the detection point and the laser beam was refocused; and the data acquisition and processing system were activated to record the electropherograms.

2.6 *Determination of reaction kinetic in flask by microchip electrophoresis*

The reaction of FITC and amino acids in a flask containing PBS medium and alkaline surrounding (pH 9.2) was compared with the reaction in cell. The final concentration of all the reagents was 10^{-4} M, and the separation electrical potentials were same as used in single-cell analysis. The 1200 V separation potential is used after 60 seconds of injection.

3 RESULTS AND DISCUSSION

3.1 *Characterization of liposomes*

Using the particle size analyzer, the average diameter of liposomes encapsulated with amino acids was measured to be 125 nm, and liposomes encapsulated with FITC was 122 nm. All liposomes were stable within a week and began to aggregate after a week. The amino acids in dialysate were derivatized by FITC for 15 hour in pH 9.2. Then, the encapsulation yields of amino acid liposomes were calculated to be 38%, 48%, and 42% for Arg, Tyr, and Glu, respectively. The encapsulation yields of FITC liposomes were calculated to be 46%.

3.2 *Reaction of FITC and amino acids in cell*

To avoid the interference generated from intracellular amino acids and proteins, a quant of amino acids far beyond the normal levels of intracellular amino acids and the same concentration of FITC were mediated into cells by liposomes. After incubation of liposomes with cells for 2, 4, 6, and 8 hours, respectively, a consecutive injection of 5 cells was detected by microchip CE-LIF. Electrophoresis of two consecutive single-cell analysis results is shown in Figure 1. As shown in Figure 1, just after 2 hours of incubation of liposomes with cells, only one peak was obtained in single-cell analysis electropherogram, and the average migration time of the emerged peaks (34.2 seconds) with a reproducibility of 1.4% RSD for five consecutively injected cells, agreed well with that obtained using the FITC standard (34.0 seconds). According to the report (Sun *et al.*, 2006), the mediation time need 2 hours, so it was inferred that FITC and amino acids were mediated into cells, but the reaction between them did not occur or the reaction products were too little to be detected. After a next standing time of 2 hours, new peaks were obtained and became higher

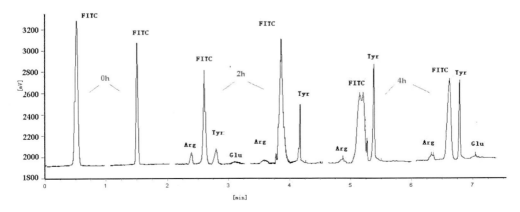

Figure 1.   Reaction of FITC and amino acids in cell at different times.

101

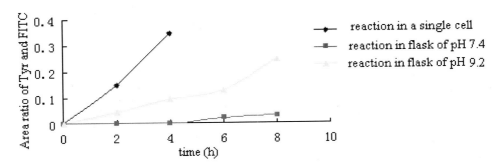

Figure 2.   Comparative results of reaction in cell and in flask.

in single-cell electropherogram. The new peaks were identified as Arg, Tyr, and Glu also by means of comparing the relative migration times of amino acid standard solution. The average retention time of Arg, Tyr, and Glu was 16.0, 45.0, and 56.8 seconds, respectively, with the reproducibility of 6.6%, 1.9%, and 6.0% RSD, respectively, for five consecutively injected cells.

It is impossible to get a time and concentration relationship of FITC and amino acids mediated by liposomes in a same single cell with the current method. In addition, the introduced amount of FITC and amino acids were different between cells because of the cellular heterogeneity (Shoemaker et al., 2005). However, we observed that the area ratio of Tyr and FITC is basically same at a series of consecutive single-cell analysis results after the same reaction time. So, the peak area ratio of Tyr and FITC was used to label the reaction extent. Another thing to be noticed was that not all Glu peaks could be found in each single-cell electropherogram, as shown in Figure 1, which maybe owing to the big difference of molecular polarity and encapsulation yields of Glu and FITC. After a stay time of 8 hours for amino acids and FITC in cell, many disordered peaks appeared in the electropherogram of single cell, maybe because native intracellular amino acids and proteins were derivatized by FITC.

3.3   Reaction of FITC and amino acids in flask

PBS of pH 7.4 and borate buffer of pH 9.2 were used separately in flask to make a comparison with the reaction in cell, for pH plays a critical role in the function of the cell. In addition, reagent concentration is an important factor for reaction speed, so a final concentration of 10^{-4} M of FITC and amino acids in flask were used, which was higher than mediated into cells. The reaction was detected once every 2 hours by microchip CE-LIF. The results are shown in Figure 2. It was demonstrated that in conventional reactor, little amino acids were derivatized by FITC in neutral solution, consistence with previous reports (Zinellu et al., 2009). In flask, the reaction speed is obviously faster in pH 9.2 than in pH 7.4, but still lower than in cell.

4   CONCLUSION

Microchip CE-LIF can be used to detect the cell performance as a microreactor. Although the reaction rate constant was not directly derived, but the ratio of Tyr and FITC could already prove an amazing speed and efficiency in cell compared with the extracellular responses. This result will help to understand more cellular process.

ACKNOWLEDGMENT

This study was supported by the National Natural Science Foundation of China under project no. 81001600.

REFERENCES

Chiu, D. Tl, C. F. Wilson, F. Rytsen, A. Strömberg, C.Farre, A. Karlsson, S. Nordholm, A. Gaggar, B. P. Modi, A. Moscho, R. A. Garza-López, O. Orwar, and R. N. Zare. (1999) Chemical transformations in individual ultrasmall biomimetic containers. *Science* 283: 1892–1895.

Gu S. Q., Y. X. Zhang, Zhu Y, et al. (2011) Multifunctional picoliter droplet manipulation platform and its application in single cell analysis. *Anal Chem*, 83: 7570–7576.

Johnsson N, Johnsson K (2007) Chemical tools for biomolecular imaging. *ACS Chem Bio* 2: 31–38.

Karlsson M, Nolkrantz K, Davidson M J, et al. (2000) Electroinjection of colloid particles and biopolymers into single unilamellar liposomes and cells for bioanalytical applications. *Anal Chem* 72: 5857–5862.

Kulin S, Kishore R, Helmerson K, et al. (2003) Optical manipulation and fusion of liposomes as microreactors. *Langmuir* 19: 8206–8210.

Li X J, Chen Y, Li P C H. (2011) A simple and fast microfluidic approach of same-single-cell analysis (SASCA) for the study of multidrug resistance modulation in cancer cells. *Lab on a Chip* 11: 1378–1383.

Shoemaker G L, Lorieau J, Lau L H, et al. (2005) Multiple sampling in single-cell enzyme assays using CE-Laser-Induced fluorescence to monitor reaction progress. *Anal Chem* 77: 3132–3137.

Sun Y, Lu M, Yin X F (2006) Intracellular labeling method for chip-based capillary electrophoresis fluorimetric single cell analysis using liposomes. *J Chromatogr A* 1135: 109–114.

Zinellu A, Sotgia S, Bastianina S, et al. (2009) Taurine determination by capillary electrophoresis with laser-induced fluorescence detection: from clinical field to quality food applications *Chessa. Amino Acids* 36: 35–41.

Medicine Sciences and Bioengineering – Wang (Ed.)
© *2015 Taylor & Francis Group, London, ISBN: 978-1-138-02684-1*

Linear correlation analysis method of normality test for medical statistical data

Ming Lei* & Jia Zuo

Jilin Economic Radio Station, Mathematics College, Beihua University, Jilin City, China

ABSTRACT: A new method of normality test for original data is studied in this paper. Variable X represents the midpoint of class, and variable Y represents the probability unit; by using linear correlation analysis method, the normality for data of X and Y is tested. The result obtained by this method is correct. This method is simple, rapid, and easy to master, and the conclusion is reliable.

1 INTRODUCTION

In clinical experiments and basic medical research, we often need to introduce a new index; we must do the normality test according to the collected data based on the new index, because if the data does not meet normal distribution it cannot be described by mean and standard deviation and in the process of analyzing data we cannot use t-test, u-test, or variance analysis method to do statistical processing. Therefore, we must conduct normality test on original data to judge whether it is a normal distribution (Fang, J. Q, 2008).

There are many methods for conducting normality test for data, but they are all so tedious that they are not easy for nonstatistical professionals to master. I consider that using linear correlation analysis method to test normality for data is simple and rapid and is easy for statistical professionals to master.

2 MATERIAL AND METHOD

2.1 *Material*

All the original data determined by all kinds of indexes can stand as original material for the normality test. For example, in order to study the change of platelet average volume and its significance, to compare the platelet average volume in different populations, we should first think if the index of platelet average volume belongs to normal distribution data in different populations. This needs normality test. The material is the value of platelet average volume (MPV) with 382 normal people. Its original data has been sorted to be frequency material; see columns ① and ② of Table 1.

2.2 *Method*

To calculate the midpoint of class (the average of lower limit values for the class and the adjacent class) for the material, which has been sorted to be a frequency table (Ma, B. R., 2006), the values are listed in column ③; the cumulative absolute frequencies (order accumulation of frequencies of classes) are listed in column ④. To calculate cumulative relative frequency (the percentage of cumulative absolute frequencies of classes divided by total number) by cumulative absolute

---

*bhdxlm@163.com

frequency, they are listed in column ⑤. To check the corresponding probability unit of cumulative relative frequency from percentage p and probability unit comparison table, please see Table 2 in column ⑥. The probability unit of the last class is taken as 7.8130 according to the percentage 99.75%. The midpoint of class at column ③ is taken as variable X, and the probability unit at

Table 1. Normal distribution test of platelet average volume (MPV).

MPV ①	Frequency ②	Midpoint of class ③	Cumulative absolute frequency ④	Cumulative relative frequency (%) ⑤	Probability unit ⑥
4.9–	4	5.3	4	1.1	2.7010
5.7–	15	6.1	19	5.0	3.3551
6.5–	17	6.9	36	9.4	3.6829
7.3–	40	7.7	76	20.2	4.1654
8.1–	67	8.5	143	37.5	4.6813
8.9–	75	9.3	218	57.1	5.1790
9.7–	59	10.1	277	72.5	5.5978
10.5–	48	10.9	325	85.1	6.0404
11.3–	21	11.7	346	90.6	6.3171
12.1–	18	12.5	364	95.3	6.6766
12.9–	14	13.3	378	98.9	7.2990
13.7–14.5	4	14.1	382	100.0	7.8130

Table 2. Comparison between percentage p and probability unit.

%	Probability unit	%	Probability unit	%	Probability unit	%	Probability unit
1	2.6737	26	4.3567	51	5.0251	76	5.7063
2	2.9463	27	4.3872	52	5.0502	77	5.7388
3	3.1192	28	4.4172	53	5.0753	78	5.7722
4	3.2493	29	4.4466	54	5.1004	79	5.8064
5	3.3551	30	4.4756	55	5.1257	80	5.8416
6	3.4452	31	4.5041	56	5.1510	81	5.8779
7	3.5242	32	4.5323	57	5.1764	82	5.9154
8	3.5949	33	4.5601	58	5.2019	83	5.9542
9	3.6592	34	4.5875	59	5.2275	84	5.9945
10	3.7184	35	4.6147	60	5.2533	85	6.0364
11	3.7735	36	4.6415	61	5.2793	86	6.0803
12	3.8250	37	4.6681	62	5.3055	87	6.1264
13	3.8736	38	4.6945	63	5.3319	88	6.1750
14	3.9197	39	4.7207	64	5.3565	89	6.2265
15	3.9636	40	4.7467	65	5.3853	90	6.2816
16	4.0055	41	4.7725	66	5.4125	91	6.3408
17	4.0458	42	4.7981	67	5.4399	92	6.4051
18	4.0846	43	4.8236	68	5.4677	93	6.4758
19	4.1221	44	4.8490	69	5.4959	94	6.5548
20	4.1584	45	4.8743	70	5.5244	95	6.6449
21	4.1936	46	4.8996	71	5.5534	96	6.7507
22	4.2278	47	4.9247	72	5.5828	97	6.8808
23	4.2612	48	4.9498	73	5.6128	98	7.0537
24	4.2937	49	4.9749	74	5.6433	99	7.3263
25	4.3255	50	5.0000	75	5.6745	99.75	7.8130

column ⑥ is taken as variable Y; to do linear correlation analysis for variables X and Y, calculate the correlation coefficient r, by taking degree of freedom as 1. Test level is taken as $\alpha = 0.10$ to infer the statistical conclusion, namely, if $r < 0.988$ and $p > 0.10$ the data does belong to normal distribution and if $r \geq 0.988$ and $p \leq 0.10$ the data belongs to normal distribution (Dong, S. F, 2008).

In the process of linear correlation analysis, if we have a dual variable calculator we can directly calculate r value when variable X and variable Y can be directly input to the calculator; if we use a single variable calculator, then it needs to separately calculate the mean ($\bar{X}$) and standard deviation (S_x) of X and the mean ($\bar{Y}$) and standard deviation (S_y) of Y, as well as the sum of the two variables' products ($\sum XY$ is the sum of the two variables' products in each class), and then calculate r value by the following formula:

$$r = \frac{\sum XY - n\bar{X}\bar{Y}}{(n-1)S_x S_y} \tag{1}$$

where n is the class number of data (Luo, J. H. & Xu, T. H, 2008).

3 RESULTS

When calculated by dual variable calculator for this data (Table 1), we get $r = 0.998$. Clearly, the data belongs to normal distribution.

4 DISCUSSION

This method is simple, rapid, and easy to master, and the conclusion is reliable.

Table 2 is a tool table in this paper; it only lists the probability units when the percentage is an integer. When the cumulative relative frequency is in decimal, we can check the probability unit of its integer part and then add the product of the corresponding decimal multiplied by the difference of adjacent probability unit and this probability unit. For example, when the third class in the data, namely, the class's cumulative relative frequency, is 9.4% and the platelet average volume is 6.5, its corresponding probability unit is the sum of the probability unit (3.6592) for 9% and the product of the difference of probability unit (3.7184) for 10% and probability unit for 9% multiplied by 0.4, namely, $3.6592 + (3.7184 - 3.6592) \times 0.4 = 3.6829$. The cumulative relative frequency of the final class must be 100%, but 100% has no probability unit and the probability unit of this class is uniformly taken as 7.8130 for 99.75%.

REFERENCES

Dong, S. F. (2008) Biostatistics. Beijing, Science Press.
Fang, J. Q. (2008) Health Statistics. 6th Edition. Beijing, People's Medical Publishing House.
Luo, J. H. & Xu, T. H. (2008) Medical Statistics. Beijing, Science Press.
Ma, B. R. (2006) Medical Statistics. 4th Edition. Beijing, People's Medical Publishing House.

Medicine Sciences and Bioengineering – Wang (Ed.)
© 2015 Taylor & Francis Group, London, ISBN: 978-1-138-02684-1

A comparative study on the application of three-dimensional ultrasound to breast intraductal lesion

Sheng-nan Liu, Guang Sun[1] & Yan-xi Liu
Mammary Surgery of China-Japan Union Hospital of JiLin University, JiLin Province Breast Diseases Institute, Changchun, JiLin, China

ABSTRACT: To investigate the diagnostic values of three-dimensional (3D) ultrasound for breast intraductal lesion methods, patients with ecstatic mammary duct, who were diagnosed by high-frequency ultrasound, were examined with 3D ultrasound. Comparison and analyses of these results are presented, combined with the results of pathology and FDS. From that, we concluded that 3D ultrasound should be the first choice or an effective diagnostic method for the diagnosis of breast intraductal lesion.

1 INTRODUCTION

With further research on breast cancer, a close relevance exists between mammary intraductal lesion and breast cancer diagnosis method on breast intraductal lesion obtained during the development (Surry, K. J. M., Mills, G. R., & Bevan, K., 2007). At present, the high-frequency ultrasound and fiberoptic ductoscopy (FDS) are treated as conventional diagnostic methods, especially FDS has become an important diagnostic method, but it has deficiencies in the diagnosis of intraductal lesion. This article analyzes the relevant information of 762 patients with mammary duct expansion from 2012 to 2013 in our hospital through contrast and analysis of the endoscopy and pathological results including high-frequency ultrasound, three-dimensional (3D) ultrasound, and FDS. It explored the value of 3D ultrasound in the diagnosis of mammary intraductal lesion.

2 METHODS AND MATERIAL

2.1 *Material*

This study was performed on 762 female patients with ecstatic mammary duct. They were 24–76 years old (mean 43.6 years). Of which, 627 patients (group 1) did not have nipple discharge, while 135 patients (group 2) had. All of them were admitted in China-Japan Union Hospital of Jilin University. The 2D (two-dimensional) and 3D images were obtained using Mylab60 ultrasound system (Esaote Medical Systems, Italy). FDS (FVS-6000MI, Blade, China) was used in this study, including optical fibers, cold light source, and a medical image graphic workstation.

2.2 *Methods*

When high-frequency ultrasound examination is made, the patient should supine, fully exposing breast and axillaries. With her nipple as center, radically full scanning is made. We need to check its inner diameter size and the place of expansion in order to decide whether duct expansion exists or not, and describe ultrasonographic features of intraluminal abnormal changes, whether the echo

---

[1]Corresponding author is Guang Sun. E-mail: guangsun2013@163.com

of the intraductal expansion is clear or not. Meanwhile, to understand the situation of blood flow, at last to observe lymph node in drainage area, then real-time 3D ultrasound is applied, adjusting the sampling frame size accordingly, automatically acquiring data, selecting the best direction of observation for 3D reconstruction imaging and power Doppler image, and recording the ultrasonic characteristics of abnormal changes. Before performing FDS, the prone patient is disinfected and draped. Eye probe dilators with outer diameters of 0.72 mm and length of 6.5 mm were used to dilate the lactiferous duct after adding 0.5–1 mL of 2% lidocaine to discharging nipple orifice. The fiberscope was then inserted into the duct orifice. The discharging nipple orifice and its branches were observed in succession and the positions as well as the feature of the lesions were recorded.

3 RESULTS

3.1 Pathology /FDS in evaluation of inconclusive high-frequency ultrasound and 3D ultrasound findings in group

The detection rate of high-frequency ultrasound in mammary duct ectasia, intraductal proliferative lesion, duct carcinoma in situ, intraductal papilloma, and intraductal papillary carcinoma is 0.80%, 0.32%, 0%, 1.12%, and 0%, respectively, and of 3D ultrasound is 1.43%, 0.80%, 0.16%, 1.75%, and 0.16%, respectively, in group 1 (Table 1). Pathology in evaluation of inconclusive high-frequency ultrasound, 3D ultrasound, and FDS findings in group 2 is shown in Table 2. In mammary duct ectasia, the diagnosis rate of FDS is 100%, high-frequency ultrasound is 78.12%, 3D ultrasound is 90.62%.

In intraductal proliferative lesions, the diagnosis rate of FDS is 95.23%, high-frequency ultrasound is 33.33%, and 3D ultrasound is 71.42%. In duct carcinoma in situ, the diagnosis rate of FDS is 85.71%, high-frequency ultrasound is 28.57%, and 3D ultrasound is 57.14%. In intraductal papilloma, the diagnosis rate of FDS is 92.85%, high-frequency ultrasound is 57.14%, and 3D ultrasound is 78.57%. In intraductal papillary carcinoma, the diagnosis rate of FDS is 83.33%, high-frequency ultrasound is 16.67%, and 3D ultrasound is 50.00%.

Table 1. Pathology/FDS in evaluation of inconclusive high-frequency ultrasound and 3D ultrasound findings in group 1.

Pathology/FDS	High-frequency ultrasound	3D ultrasound
Ecstatic mammary duct only	613	600
Mammary duct ectasia	5	9
Intraductal proliferative lesions	2	5
Duct carcinoma in situ	0	1
Intraductal papilloma	7	11
Intraductal papillary carcinoma	0	1
Total	627	627

Table 2. Pathology in evaluation of inconclusive high-frequency ultrasound, 3D ultrasound, and FDS findings in group 2.

	Case	High-frequency ultrasound	3D ultrasound	FDS
Galactophoritis	55	0	0	55
Mammary duct ectasia	32	23	29	32
Intraductal proliferative lesions	21	7	15	20
Duct carcinoma in situ	7	2	4	6
Intraductal papilloma	14	8	11	13
Intraductal papillary carcinoma	6	1	3	5

3.2 Image of high-frequency ultrasound, 3D ultrasound, and FDS

Appearances of mammary duct ectasia on high-frequency ultrasound, 3D ultrasound, and FDS (Figure. 1). a. Mammary ectatic duct, caliber 1.9–3.5 mm, glabrous tube wall, echoless lumens, with anechoic areas of multifarious size. b. Echo uneven lumens, not smooth tube wall. c. Mammary ectatic duct, some of which express cystic dilatation, not smooth tube wall, a spot of white floccules float in lumens, and white floccules also attached to tube wall.

Appearance of intraductal papilloma on high-frequency ultrasound, 3D ultrasound, and FDS (Figure. 2). a. Unclear hypoechogenic mass in ectatic mammary duct. b. Ectatic mammary duct, clear hypoechogenic mass in lumens, regular appearance. c. Lesion is located on the connection between main-duct and first branch-duct, pink mass of regular appearance, of no hemorrhagic tendency.

Appearance of intraductal papillary carcinoma on high-frequency ultrasound, 3D ultrasound, and FDS (Figure. 3). a. Echo mass not homogeneous and unclear in ectatic mammary duct, with echo attenuation on backside. b. Ectatic mammary duct, unclear hypoechogenic mass in lumens, irregular appearance. c. Irregular mass, with shaggy nodes on it, ectatic mammary duct, thickening and spastic tube wall with fresh hemorrhage and remote hemorrhage.

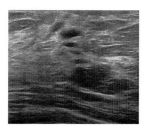 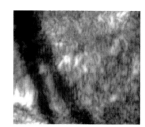 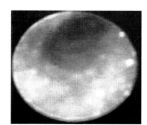

a. High-frequency ultrasound   b. 3D ultrasound   c. FDS

Figure 1. Appearances of mammary duct ectasia.

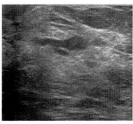 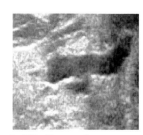 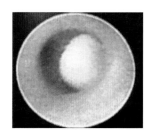

a. High-frequency ultrasound   b. 3D ultrasound   c. FDS

Figure 2. Appearances of intraductal papilloma.

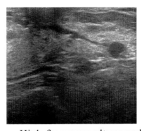 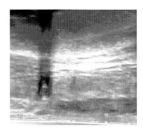 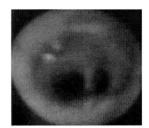

a. High-frequency ultrasound   b. 3D ultrasound   c. FDS

Figure 3. Appearances of intraductal papillary carcinoma.

4 DISCUSSION

With the rapid development of computer science and technology, the huge progress has been made on 3D ultrasound (Badve S, Wiley E, & Rodriguez N, 2003), which at present has entered the stage of clinical application. 3D ultrasound not only keeps all information about 2D ultrasound (YH Hsiao, YL Huang, SJ Kuo, WM Liang, ST Chen, & DR Chen, 2009) but also provides a more intuitive 3D shape space. On one hand, it display space structure and the infringement level of lesions and surrounding tissues and organs (Chang Jung Min, Moon Woo Kyung, & Cho, Nariya, 2011), on the other hand, it can be arbitrarily cut, and the internal structure information of lesions can be known. 3D ultrasound at the same time also has special 3D color power angiography imaging technology, therefore it makes the lost information of blood flow inside lesions caused by blood flow direction more clear, more fully and intuitively shows the blood vessels within lesions and its internal situation and more truly reflects the angiogenesis in lesion, which makes diagnosis and differential diagnosis more convincing (Chen, Dar-Ren, & Lai, Hung-Wen, 2011). 3D ultrasound can provide detailed basis for the breast lesions diagnosis and the differential diagnosis of benign and malignant tumor. In this study, for intraductal proliferative lesions, duct carcinoma in situ, intraductal papilloma, and intraductal papillary carcinoma, high-frequency ultrasound images can display that there is ecstatic mammary duct or not. Whether the catheter has abnormal echo or not, the 3D ultrasound can clearly show the lesions form in catheter cavity, and can also present vividly infiltrating duct condition, which is of great help for differentiating benign and malignant lesions.

4.1 *Pathology /FDS in evaluation of inconclusive high-frequency ultrasound and 3D ultrasound findings in group 1 (Table 1)*

The detection rate of high-frequency ultrasound in mammary duct ectasia, intraductal proliferative lesions, duct carcinoma in situ, intraductal papilloma, and intraductal papillary carcinoma is 0.80%, 0.32%, 0%, 1.12%, and 0%, respectively, and that of 3D ultrasound is 1.43%, 0.80%, 0.16%, 1.75%, and 0.16%, respectively.

4.2 *Pathology in evaluation of inconclusive high-frequency ultrasound, 3D ultrasound, and FDS findings in group 2 (Table 2)*

In intraductal proliferative lesions, the diagnosis rates of FDS, high-frequency ultrasound, 3D ultrasound are 95.23%, 33.33%, and 71.42%, respectively. In duct carcinoma in situ, the diagnosis rate is 85.71%, 28.57%, and 57.14%, respectively. In intraductal papilloma, the diagnosis rate is 92.85%, 57.14%, and 78.57%, respectively. In intraductal papillary carcinoma, it is 83.33%, 16.67%, and 50.00%, respectively. Contrasted with FDS, in high-frequency ultrasound and 3D ultrasound, the possibility of misdiagnosis and missed diagnosis exists, but significant difference can be recognized among them. Therefore, 3D ultrasound applied in the diagnosis of breast intraductal lesion is better than high-frequency ultrasound.

4.3 *FDS has become an important method for the diagnosis of breast intraductal lesions*

At present, FDS has become an important method for the diagnosis of breast intraductal lesions, which not only can observe lesion directly and locate them, but also can directly get biopsy under the microscope, at the same time has a certain therapeutic effect, but FDS is not perfect. The FDS is an invasive examination, if the pressure is made too much during the operation or fiber optic stabbing of the conduit wall, swelling, bleeding, and infection may appear. For complicated breast lesions or special anatomical structure of lesions, FDS is of limited value. For example, Badve et al. reported it is unlikely that FDS, which can visualize only the first few divisions of the ducts, would be able to identify lesions located in these distal ducts and lobules.

Indication of FDS needs to be perfect. In this study, the first set of contrast shows that for the patients with no nipple discharge, there is a breast intraductal lesion. Without ultrasound help, FDS shows missed diagnosis and misdiagnosis but ultrasonic especially 3D ultrasound, to some extent, makes up for the lack of FDS. 3D ultrasound has the advantages of being noninvasive, repeatable, and providing real-time dynamic imaging; especially, for the areas that are inaccessible for the FDS, 3D ultrasound can provide valuable information.

To sum up, in this article, through the valued research on 3D ultrasound applied in the diagnosis of mammary intraductal lesions, the 3D ultrasound can be used as a kind of effective diagnosis method preferring for or screening of breast intraductal lesions.

REFERENCES

Badve S, Wiley E, & Rodriguez N, (2003) Assessment of utility of ductal lavage and ductoscopy in breast cancer retrospective analysis of mastectomy specimens. *Mod Pathol*, 16(3): 206.

Chang Jung Min, Moon Woo Kyung, & Cho Nariya, (2011) Radiologists' performance in the detection of benign and malignant masses with 3D automated breast ultrasound (ABUS). *European Journal of Radiology*, 78(1): 99–103.

Chen Dar-Ren & Lai Hung-Wen, (2011) Three-dimensional ultrasonography for breast malignancy detection. Expert opinion on medical diagnostics, 5(3): 253–61.

Surry KJM, Mills GR, & Bevan K, (2007) Stereotactic mammography imaging combined with 3D US imaging for image guided breast biopsy, *Medical Physics*, 34(11): 4348–4358.

Hsiao YH, Huang YL, Kuo SL, Liang WM, Chen ST, & Chen DR, (2009) Characterization of benign and malignant solid breast masses in harmonic 3D power Doppler imaging. *Eur J Radiol*, 71: 89–95.

Medicine Sciences and Bioengineering – Wang (Ed.)
© 2015 Taylor & Francis Group, London, ISBN: 978-1-138-02684-1

Roles of different ionic currents in the automaticity of central and peripheral sinoatrial node

Hong Zhang, Xiao Zheng, Wei Zhao & Dan Zhao
School of Electrical Engineering, Xi'an Jiaotong University, Shannxi, Xi'an, China

Xin Huang
Cardiology Department, First Hospital, Xi'an Jiaotong University, Shannxi, Xi'an, China

ABSTRACT: As the electrical source of hearts, the sinoatrial node (SAN) plays a significant role in rhythmic firing. Ca^{2+} and K^+ currents as well as the hyperpolarization-activated funny current, I_f, contribute to the production of action potential. The aim of this study is to determine the effect of these currents on automaticity of the central and peripheral SAN at the tissue level. Based on a mathematical model addressing central and peripheral SAN cells in coupling with an atrial model, a one-dimensional fiber with a gradual heterogeneity of SAN was developed. Graphic Processing Unit technology was used to accelerate the computation of the tissue model. The results demonstrated that the decrease in L-type Ca^{2+} current, I_{CaL}, and rapidly activated K^+ current, I_{Kr}, could bring about the cessation of rhythmic firing. T-type Ca^{2+} current, I_{CaT}, and hyperpolarization-activated funny current, I_f, had effects on sinus rates, but their downregulations had little impact on automatic diastolic depolarization. Therefore, I_{CaL} and I_{Kr} played key roles in determining the spontaneous activities of central and peripheral SAN cells.

1   INTRODUCTION

Sinoatrial node cells (SANCs) are the leading pacemakers of the heart. They spontaneously exhibit slow diastolic depolarization to a threshold for firing, thereby periodically initiating action potentials to set the rhythm of the heart. The Ca^{2+} current I_{Ca}, K^+ current I_K, and hyperpolarization-activated funny current I_f have been reported to contribute to spontaneous rhythmic firing (Chen *et al.*, 2010). I_{Ca} can be separated into two kinetically different components, L-type (I_{CaL}) and T-type (I_{CaT}) currents. I_K also includes slowly and rapidly activated components, I_{Ks} and I_{Kr}, respectively. Recordings from intact SAN revealed the heterogeneity in action potential from the central to the peripheral SANCs (Zhang *et al.*, 2001; Dobrzynski *et al.*, 2005). However, the roles of these currents for rhythmic depolarization in the center and periphery are not very clear at the tissue level. Therefore, in the present paper a one-dimensional tissue model coupling SAN with an atrium was developed to evaluate the effects of these currents on the electrical behavior and automaticity of SAN by a computer simulation method.

2   METHOD

Zhang's model (Zhang *et al.*, 2000) was chosen to develop a tissue in which a region of SAN was coupled to an adjoining atrium (Hilgemann *et al.*, 1987). Equation 1 with the no-flux boundary conditions was used to describe the electrical behavior of the developed fiber:

$$\nabla \bullet (\sigma V) = A_m (C_m \frac{\partial V}{\partial t} + I_{ion})$$

$$(\nabla V)|_{x=0} = (\nabla V)|_{x=ls+la} = 0 \tag{1}$$

where V is the transmembrane potential, C_m is the membrane capacitance, t is the time, I_{ion} is the total ionic current, and x is the spatial coordinate. σ Denotes tissue conductivity. A_m denotes the cell surface to volume ratio. Further, l_s and l_a represent the lengths of SAN and atrium, respectively. To simulate heterogeneity within the SAN region, an exponential form reported by Garny *et al.* (2003) was used.

To investigate the roles of I_{CaL}, I_{CaT}, I_{Ks}, I_{Kr}, and I_f in automaticity of central and peripheral SANCs, a factor C x was introduced to alter the conductance of each current. Here, the subscript x denotes CaL, CaT, Ks, Kr, and f.

The operator splitting technique (Zhang *et al.*, 2010) was used to split Equation 1 into two parts, in which calculation of the behavior of each single cell was allowed to be seperated from calculation of the electrical diffusion between adjacent cells. The accelerating technique with Graphic Processing Unit was used to compute the tissue model. The CUDA code was programmmed and performed on a personal computer with nVIDIA GeForce GTX550Ti.

3 RESULTS

3.1 *Action potential propagation*

Figure 1 displays electrical propagation along the fiber. As inspected, with presence of the atrium, the leading pacemaker site located at the upper central SANC and the excitation gradually propagated to the lower periphery and activated the atrial cells. Compared with the periphery, the central SANC was characterized by decreased maximum diastolic potential and upstroke velocity, as well as long action potential duration (APD) and cycle length (CL).

3.2 *Effects of ionic currents*

Figure 2 shows action potentials of central and peripheral SANCs corresponding to different ratios of C_CaL and C_CaT. As shown in Figure 2(a) and 2(b), when C_CaL was decreased to 0.85 times its control condition (C_CaL = 1.0) both amplitude and CL of the action potential were reduced. When C_CaL continued to drop to 0.5, SANCs could not be fired again and lost their automaticity completely. Figure 2(c) and 2(d) exhibits the effects of I_{CaT} on rhythmic firing. As shown, CL changed with the decrease of C_CaT. But opposite to I_{CaL}, the reduction of I_{CaT} prolonged CL rather than shortening it. Thus, the firing rate became slow after I_{CaT} was decreased. Besides, the complete block of I_{CaT} did not induce the cessation of spontaneous firing.

Figure 3 shows the effect of I_{Kr} and I_{Ks} on sponstaneous activity in the center and periphery. In Figure 3(a) and 3(b), when I_{Kr} was completely blocked (C_Kr = 0) central and peripheral SANCs lost their automaticity completely. The resting potentials stayed at about −25 mV and −65 mV for central and peripheral SANCs, respectively. When C_Kr was elevated to 0.5, the central SANC started to oscillate with a very small amplitude. In contrast, the peripheral SANC exhibited rhythmic firing with normal amplitude. Additionally, in this case CLs of central and peripheral SANCs were prolonged compared with the control condition (C_Kr = 1), indicating a slow firing rate at small I_{Kr}. Therefore, I_{Kr} showed significant effect on automaticity for both central and peripheral SANCs, which was especially remarkable for the center. Figure 3(c) and (d) displays the effect of I_{Ks}. The results demonstrated that for either the center or the periphery the change in I_{Ks} only brought a slight difference in CL even in the situation of completely blocking I_{Ks}. Thus, I_{Ks} showed little impact on rhythmic firing and sinus rate for both the center and the periphery.

Figure 4 displays action potentials of the central and peripheral SANCs at different values of C_f. As shown, for both cell types the decrease in C_f caused prolongation of CL, thus slowing spontaneous activity. Compared with the control condition (C_f = 1), after C_f was halved the firing rate of the center and the periphery decreased about 2.8% and 3.7%, respectively. After complete blocking (C_f = 0), their firing rate decreased about 5.2% and 4.9%, respectively. Additionally, complete blocking of I_f did not cause the complete cessation of rhythmic firing.

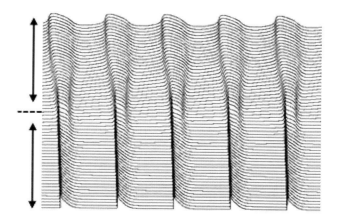

Figure 1.   Electrical propagation along the fiber.

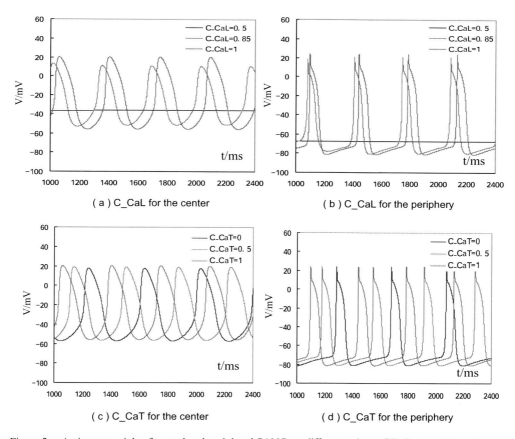

Figure 2.   Action potentials of central and peripheral SANCs at different values of C_CaL and C_CaT.

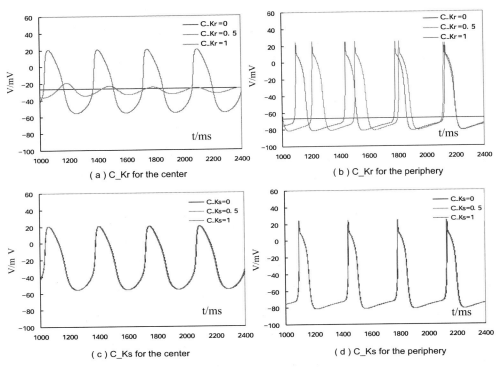

(a) C_Kr for the center

(b) C_Kr for the periphery

(c) C_Ks for the center

(d) C_Ks for the periphery

Figure 3.   Action potentials of central and peripheral SANCs at different values of C_Kr and C_Ks.

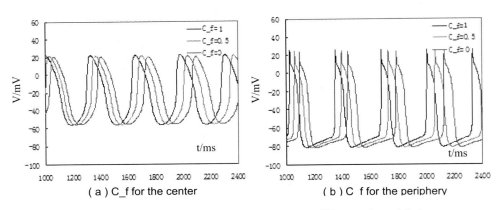

(a) C_f for the center

(b) C_f for the periphery

Figure 4.   Action potentials of the central and peripheral SANCs at different values of C_f.

4   DISCUSSION AND CONCLUSIONS

So far, efforts have been devoted to revealing mechanisms of sponstaneous firing in SANCs. There is still some controversy about the initiation of automatic diastolic depolarization (Chen et al., 2010). In fact, a variety of ionic currents participates in and contributes to the production of an action potential. Because an intact SA node can reflect the reality more accurately than a single SANC, in the present paper effects of five major ionic currents on automaticity were investigated at the tissue level. The results showed that I_{CaL} played a much more important role in depolarization in the SA node than that in the ventricule. When it was downregulated, spontaneous activity of the SANC ceased. Besides, downregulation of I_{CaL} shortened CL, thus increasing the pacemaking rate. This phenomenon was consistent with other reports (Kodama *et al.*, 1997) in which the shortening of APD was considered as the cause of rate increment. In contrast, the effect of I_{CaT} on automaticity was not so significant as I_{CaL} although its reduction slowed the pacemaking rate. I_{CaT} has a low activation threshold ($\sim$$-60$ mV); its activation was suggested as an additional mechanism contributing to the late diastolic depolarization. So, complete blocking of I_{CaT} did not cause a pause in rhythmic firing.

K$^+$ current is mainly responsible for the repolarization of an action potential. Because down-regulation of I_{Kr} made the absolute value of membrane voltage smaller than the maximum voltage required for diastolic depolarization, the currents responsible for spontaneous depolarization could not be activated, leading to the cessation of rhythmic firing after I_{Kr} was reduced. Because the contribution of I_{Ks} to repolarization is not so great as that of I_{Kr}, I_{Ks} played a less significant role in the determination of SA node properties.

I_f has long been considered as the most important ionic channel involved in sponstaneous activity and rate regulation of SA node (Baruscotti *et al.*, 2005). Consistent with the report, in the present paper results showed that downregulation of I_f caused a slowdown of pacemaking rate. However, rhythmic firing was not found to be paused by the complete blocking of I_f. Therefore, in contrast, I_{CaL} and I_{Kr} played the key role in determining the spontaneous activity. I_{CaT} and I_f had effects on the pacemaking rate, but their downregulation did not cause the cessation of rhythmic firing.

ACKNOWLEDGEMENTS

This work was supported by the National Natural Science Foundation of China (Nos. 81271661 and 30870659), Health Foundation of Shaanxi province in China (08D23), Scientific Research Foundation for Returned Overseas Chinese Scholars, State Education Ministry (SRF for ROCS), and Fundamental Research Funds for the Central Universities.

REFERENCES

Baruscotti, M., Bucchi, A. & DiFrancesco, D. (2005) Physiology and pharmacology of the cardiac pacemaker ("funny") current. *Pharmacology & Therapeutics*, 107(1), 59–79.

Chen, P.S., Joung, B., Shinohara, T., Das, M., Chen, Z.H. & Lin, S.F. (2010) The Initiation of the heartbeat. *Circ J*, 74(2), 221–225.

Dobrzynski, H., Li, J., Tellez, J. & Greener, I.D. (2005) Computer three-dimensional reconstruction of the sinoatrial node. *Circ*, 111(7), 846–854.

Garny, A., Kohl, P., Hunter, P.J., Boyett, M.R. & Noble, D. (2003) One-dimensional rabbit sinoatrial node models: benefits and limitations. *J Cardiovasc Electrophysiol*, 14(10 Suppl), S121–S132.

Hilgemann, D.W. & Noble, D. (1987) Excitation-contraction coupling and extracellular calcium transients in rabbit atrium: reconstruction of basic cellular mechanisms. *Proc R Soc Lond B Biol Sci*, 230(1259), 163–205.

Kodama, I., Nikmaram, M.R., Boyett, M.R., Suzuki, R., Honjo, H. & Owen, J.M. (1997) Regional differences in the role of the Ca^{2+} and Na$^+$ currents in pacemaker activity in the sinoatrial node. *Am J Physiol Heart Circ Physiol*, 272, H2793–H2806.

Zhang, H. , Holden, A.V. & Boyett, M.R. (2001) Gradient model versus mosaic model of the sinoatrial node. *Circ*, 103(4), 584–588.

Zhang, H., Holden, A.V., Kodama, I. & Honjo, H. (2000) Mathematical models of action potentials in the periphery and center of the rabbit sinoatrial node. *Am J Physiol Heart Circ Physiol*, 279(1), 397–421.

Zhang, H., Joung, B., Shinohara, T., Mei, X., Chen, P.S. & Lin, S.F. (2010) Synergistic dual automaticity in sinoatrial node cell and tissue models. *Circ J*, 74(10), 2079–2088.

Medicine Sciences and Bioengineering – Wang (Ed.)
© 2015 Taylor & Francis Group, London, ISBN: 978-1-138-02684-1

Effect of using six sigma in improving service efficiency in endoscopy departments

Hsueh-Ling Ku

Cathay General Hospital, Taipei, Taiwan
National Central University, Taoyuan, Taiwan
Taipei Medical University College of Nursing, Taipei, Taiwan

Chia-Long Lee[*]

Cathay General Hospital, Taipei, Taiwan

ABSTRACT: Purpose: This study evaluates the difference in service time before and after the implementation of the six sigma initiative in Endoscopy Departments (EDs). Nursing staff in ED used structured data collection forms to record data from six processes checkpoints for endoscopy patients in a medical center during the enrollment period. Methods: This study enrolled 115 patients in the baseline group (from May 1, 2012 to May 15, 2012) and 123 patients in the posttest group (from August 1, 2013 to August 17, 2013). The differences in service efficiency were compared using the t-test and the chi-square test. Results: The analyses demonstrated that staying time reductions of 50.2 ± 10.4 and 47.5 ± 11.0 minutes in ED ($p < .05$) were achieved in the baseline and posttest groups, respectively. Moreover, turnaround time was reduced by 11.4 ± 3.2 and 5.3 ± 1.3 minutes ($p < .05$) and employee overtime was reduced by 128 ± 46.6 and 30.0 ± 36.7 minutes in the baseline and posttest groups, respectively ($p < .05$). Conclusions: The study concludes that the six sigma technique can effectively reduce a patient's staying time in ED, improve turnaround time of ED, and significantly reduce staff overtime. This study provides empirical results for use by managers in peer hospitals and endoscopy departments and for administrative purposes.

1 INTRODUCTION

Taiwan started the National Health Insurance (NHI) system in 1995; the National Health Insurance Bureau extended the implementation on case payment in 1997 to control the growing medical expenses. However, hospital administrations have been admitting more patients and strengthening medical service quality for their survival. On being admitted to hospitals, most surgical patients are subject to the mode of clinical pathway, which means that they are put into standard procedure since their arrival and go through examinations, treatment, surgery, and recovery until discharge. The studied hospital is located at downtown Taipei; it is a general hospital that has been operating for 30 years. It has 747 beds. Therefore, most of the endoscopy processes need to be put on waiting. To ensure the smoothness of service flow for patients and for avoiding the traffic, endoscopy departments serve as important gatekeepers for patients. Therefore, to provide a safe medical environment, improve the flow of patients and reduce idle time, and ensure that the patients enter the endoscopy departments at the earliest schedule, as well as maximizing the efficiency of endoscopy departments, is our focus on improvement.

---

[*]cghleecl@cgh.org.tw

2 METHODS

This study collected daily groups of patients as subjects who simultaneously underwent endoscopy from endoscopy departments. Given the fact that service to the examination patients is offered in a single usage basis rather than repeated usage, the study was designed to collect individual cases for pre- and postimprovements to make comparisons. The total number of patients interviewed from March 25, 2012 to May 15, 2012, two weeks in the preimprovement stage, was 115; a total of 123 patients were interviewed from June 27, 2013 to August 7, 2013, at two weeks in the postimprovement stage. The study included the time of endoscopy departments processed in the examination, total process time for the patients in the endoscopy departments, turnover time, and level of quality of Six Sigma and the measurement. The improvement measures of Six Sigma management (M.D. Carrigan, D. Kujawa, 2006; C. Caldwell, J. Brexler & T. Gillem, 2005; E. Maniago, B. Ardolic & J.E.D. Peana, 2005; V.K. Sahney, 2003, R.E. Stafford, B. Lanham, 2005; D. Young, 2004) were followed. The study applied the tool's five steps by implementing and measuring Six Sigma and its DMAIC in the improvement process: (i) D, (Define). Collect information to produce the endoscopy departments process diagram, which is based on the total activity processes of the patient examined, and use the examining chart to record the patient's each operation processing time of medical activity and the causes of any delays. (ii) M, (Measure). Review daily cases of time recordings on the checklist by the responsible nursing staff in endoscopy departments and the causes for delays and incompleteness. (iii) A, (Analysis). Then make a thorough investigation on the critical reasons applying the 80/20 rule to find the potential variables that affect the quality of the result, and consequently decide on the priority of improvement areas. (iv) I, (Improvement). Identify the best improvement programs through brainstorming by members, group discussions, benchmark learning, and literature reviews to compare time of present value and time of expected value using Failure Mode and Effect Analysis, FMEA. This is to calculate the risk index in accordance with the occurring frequency, level of risk, and difficulty of detection. The total score of the risk index is set at 300 and weighted; the total weighted score exceeding 180 is categorized into the improvement target group and is subject to pre- and postimprovements at a random base. Other measures include educating members to reach consensus on patient-focused care processes, disclosing and announcing regular and periodic examination results through the ways of education, and discussion for gathering and collating the common views of each subdivision manager to enhance the awareness of compliance to the standard endoscopy procedures. (v) C, (Control). Apply the statistical tool in process management (Six Sigma) to validate the improvement outcome and to conduct meetings to discuss, improve, and learn from the cases that had extended waiting times. Also, remove members and factors contributing to failure to achieve the goal through the utilization of endoscopy departments' information system with a real-time-based feedback system among endoscopy departments and a centralized control station; apply PACE and Intercom system promptly and publish the improvement results regularly as long-term tracking references, thereby making improvements in long-term, continuous practice.

3 RESULTS

3.1 *Frequency analysis*

The surgical department accounted for most of the pre- and postimprovements of collected cases in the intervention of Six Sigma management; due to the various levels of complexity of diseases, it makes substantial difference for time consumption between simple and complicated examinations. The analyses demonstrate that staying time achieved reductions of 50.2 ± 10.4 and 47.5 ± 11.0 minutes in ED ($p < .05$). Moreover, turnaround time was reduced by 11.4 ± 3.2 and 5.3 ± 1.3 minutes ($p < .05$) and employee overtime was reduced by 128 ± 46.6 and 30.0 ± 36.7 minutes in the baseline and posttest groups, respectively ($p < .05$).

3.2 *Analysis for defect*

With respect to the sources of a defect and its improvement measures, Failure Mode and Effect Analysis (FMEA) was utilized to analyze the current value and expected value and conducted the comparison of pre- and postimprovements in the aspects of defect level, frequencies, and level of complexity to detect. In order to assess the systemic risk factor of FMEA, the total score of preimprovement risk index was 300 and 180 was set as the threshold for improvement target; the postimprovement reduced the index to 100. Out of the entire FMEA process improvement measures, it was measured with the elimination of critical attributes as the performance reference; the critical attribute analysis showed that the late arrival of endoscopists was the most serious and frequent factor (the improvement measures are to advance the meeting time, closing meeting on time, as well as interdepartmental cooperation efforts), which was followed by the late arrival of anesthesiologists (the improvement measures were fine-tuning shift arrangements and increasing anesthesiologist manpower during peak hours) and late arrival of patients (improvement measures were utilizing the real-time-based feedback system with the computer-based endoscopic information interface and integration of floor to strengthen communications).

4 CONCLUSIONS

The effective utilization of endoscopy departments' scheduling, constant monitoring, reduction of anesthesia time, shortening of the occupation time for patients, and improving the productivity of staff would enhance the efficiency of endoscopy departments. This study aimed at a frequency analysis of all the variables to calculate the numbers of allocation of each variable, times of means and standard deviation, quality level of Six Sigma, etc., so as to comprehend the application of Six Sigma in the intervention of examination patients of pre- and postprocess managements in the endoscopy departments in the hospital and to minimize the variation of turnover time and time required before examination for next-in-line patients. Six kinds of medical care characteristics including security, validity, needing, proper, timeliness, fairness that IOM defines were achieved in this study, which met the patients' expectation on quality of medical care. In the entire endoscopic procedures, the structure, processing, and results are the critical focus (L. Caramanica, J.A. Cousino & S. Petersen, 2003; M.A. Makary, J.B. Sexton, J.A. Freischlag & E.A. Millman, etc., 2006). To avoid complications and contingencies during the examination or surgery in delaying the medical intervention, the primary goal for medical staff was to be engaged in building a safe medical environment and offering timely service. Therefore, the improvement in this study depended on good surveillance and prompt intervention.

REFERENCES

Carrigan MD, Kujawa D. Six Sigma in health care management and strategy. Health Care Manag (Frederick). 2006; 25:133–41.
Caldwell C, Brexler J, Gillem T. Lean-Six Sigma for Healthcare: A Senior Leader Guide to Improving Cost and Throughput. Milwaukee: ASQ Quality Press, 2005: 195.
Caramanica L, Cousino JA, Petersen S. Four elements of a successful quality program. Alignment, collaboration, evidence-based practice, and excellence. Nurs Adm Q 2003; 27:336–43.
Maniago E, Ardolic B, Peana JED. Patient Flow: Utilizing the Six Sigma Approach to Reduce Emergency Department Overcrowding. Proceedings of the 2005 Research Forum Educational Program. Washington Convention Center, 2005: 22–6.
Makary MA, Sexton JB, Freischlag JA, Millman EA, Pryor D, Holzmueller C, Pronovost PJ. Patient safety in surgery. Ann Surg 2006; 243: 628–35.
Sahney VK. Generating management research on improving quality. Health Care Manage Rev. 2003; 28: 335–47.
Stafford RE, Lanham B. Six Sigma Methodology Enhances Patient Safety by Improving Glycemic Control in the ICU. Proceedings of the 34th Critical Care Congress. Phoenix: Society of Critical Care Medicine, 2005: 298.
Young D. Six Sigma black-belt pharmacist improves patient safety. Am J Health Syst Pharm. 2004; 61:1988.

Medicine Sciences and Bioengineering – Wang (Ed.)
© *2015 Taylor & Francis Group, London, ISBN: 978-1-138-02684-1*

Research progress in induced liver cancer model of rats

Di-fei Cao*, Yao Sun, Lei Wang, Dong-kai Wang, Qiong Wu, Yao Li, Guo-qing Huang, Jin-hai Zhao, Wan-Ying Hou & Yang Jiang
Institute of Advanced Technology, Heilongjiang Academy of Sciences, Harbin, China

ABSTRACT: HCC is a common clinical malignancy, with the characteristics of short duration and high mortality. HCC is always a hot spot for clinical research and basic research, but the mechanism of liver cancer has not been fully elucidated. As a good model for simulating liver cancer in the human body, the rat model can be built to conduct research on the physiological aspects and cellular and molecular pathogenesis of the disease. Therefore, it can be a new method for liver cancer treatment. A review on the research progress of induced liver cancer is discussed in this paper.

1 INTRODUCTION

Hepatocellular carcinoma (HCC) is one of the malignant tumors with the highest incidence rate in China. In recent years, the incidence rate of HCC has been rising, and it already ranks second among the malignant tumors in China (WU Meng-chao, 1998). The occurrence and development of HCC is caused by many factors, and the pathogenesis of HCC is still not clear; meanwhile, no safe and effective treatment measures have been summarized. Understanding the pathogenesis is the important basis of liver cancer treatment. An experimental animal model of cancer is built to simulate human cancer expression, which can be divided into spontaneous tumor, inducible, transplantation, and transgenic animal (WeiHong, 2001). The etiology and pathogenesis of HCC model in rats is important for liver cancer research. In this paper, research progress on HCC model in rats is reviewed.

2 THE ROUTE OF ADMINISTRATION

There are mainly two routes: oral administration and injection. Oral administration includes automatic oral drug delivery and forced intragastric administration. Automatic oral drug delivery intake is through drinking water or food, and intragastric administration is via carcinogen gavage. For injection, a carcinogen is injected and administered intraperitoneal injection is the most common way. According to the cancer-inducing agent, different injection sites as well as different methods will be selected (Shao Chengwei *et al*, 2002).

---

*Brief introduction of the author: CAO Di-fei (1981–), female, Harbin person, doctor degree, assistant research fellow, engaged in the research of anticancer drugs.

3 TYPES OF CANCER-INDUCING AGENTS

Plenty of cancer-inducing agents can be used, and they are discussed in the following subsections.

3.1 Diethylnitrosamine (DEN)

(1) Induced rats HCC model: The rats were given DEN water intragastrically (10 mg/kg of rats' weight, 0.25% concentration) once a week, and 0.025% DEN water was supplied for the rest of the time. It took about 4 months before liver cancer was induced and 5 to 6 months before the inducing rate reached over 80%; 0.05% DEN in drinking water could also be used, which would take 8 months to induce HCC (Jiang Youchun et al, 2001). (2) Solt-Farber-induced cancer model (Solt DB et al, 1977): According to the weight, single intraperitoneal injection of 200 mg/kg of DEN was given to the rats on the first day, and a diet with 2-acetylaminofluorene (2-AAF), 0.02% DEN started 2 weeks later. Two-thirds hepatectomy was done at the end of the third week, and at the end of the fourth week the standard diet was recovered. Foci of altered hepatocytes in the liver appeared in the fourth week with microscope observation. (3) Male Wistar rats of 200 g were selected and given 200 mg/kg DEN intraperitoneal injection plus 0.05% DEN drinking water, and it took 12 weeks to induce cancer (Zhang Xinli et al, 2001). (4) The same rats as in (3) were used, which were supplied with DEN water for free drinking, and it took 16 weeks to induce cancer (Jin Xinglin et al, 2009).

3.2 AflatoxinB1 (AFB1)

Inducing methods: (1) Cancer-inducing rate reached 100% in 3 months when fed AFB1 4–5 g continuously for 6 weeks. The minimum dose for AFB1 was 0.001–0.005 g/day in this method (Ressolinovitch SD et al, 1972). (2) AFB1 dissolved in dimethyl sulfoxide (DMSO) was injected intraperitoneally 400 g/kg once daily. The AFB1 injection was stopped after 14 consecutive days and a diet with 0.015% 2-AAF took its place, which lasted for 30 days (subtotal removal on the twenty-first day of the experiment); A short-term experimental model of HCC induced by AFB1 could also be constructed by a single injection of 0.75–1.5 mg/kg AFB1, which was followed by administration of 2-AAF combined with subtotal removal 14 days later. (Wolf M, 2008); (3) 2% DEM water solution and 0.004% AFB1 DMSO solution were alternately given to rats by gavage for 7 weeks to induce rat liver cancer (Zheng Jianming et al, 2000).

3.3 O-aminoazotoluene (OAAT)

Inducing methods: (1) About 2 -3 drops of 1% OAAT benzene solution were smeared on the skin between scapulae once every other day, about 100 times in all. Tumor nodules could appear 2 months after administration and it took more than 7 months before mouse liver tumor was induced, with an inducing rate of 55% or so (Yang Fuchun et al, 2004). (2) About 2.5 mg OAAT dissolved in vegetable oil, subcutaneous injection for 4 times, with an interval of 2 weeks, was used to induce liver cancer. The method is used for etiology, occurrence, pathogenesis, and genetics research (Giavazzi R et al, 1986).

3.4 P-dimethylaminoazobenzene (DAB)

Inducing methods: (1) Generally, 0.06% of DAB was added to the diet of rats, with a limitation in the intake of vitamin B2 at the same time (no more than 1.5–2 mg/kg of body weight), and liver cancer induction will occur in 4–6 months (Xu Yuyin & Chen Li, 2011).

3.5 2-Acetylaminofluorene (2-AAF)

Inducing methods: (1) About 0.05% of 2-AAF was added to the diet of rats, and after 21 days canceration appeared. Cell degeneration, hyperplasia nodules of varying sizes, and cancer nests nodule formation were observed with microscope. This method is also applicable to rabbit, dog, chicken, and other animals (DangShuangshuo & YuanLichao, 2004).

4 SUMMARY

Rat hepatoma model will improve continuously with the development of liver cancer treatment means and increasing thorough of clinical basic research. With the use of molecular biology techniques, the possible development direction of the rat hepatoma model includes: establishing the rat model with a variety of biological characteristics which is more suitable for liver cancer, as well as the establishment of new stable model, the reduction or elimination of individual differences in order to improve the feasibility and accuracy of the experiment, and finding a more suitable way to build the model.

ACKNOWLEDGMENT

Fund Project: Key project of the Heilongjiang Academy of Sciences youth fund (2013–03).

REFERENCES

DangShuangshuo, YuanLichao. (2004) Research status of liver cancer model. Abstract of the latest medical information, 3(1): 968–970.
Giavazzi R, Jessup JM, Campbell DE, et al. (1986) Experimental nude mouse model of human colorectal cancer liver metastases. Nat Cancer Inst, 77(6): 1303–1308.
JiangYouchun, DongQinan, XiaoBangliang, et al. (2001) Studies on Liver Cancer Induced by Non-necrotizing Dose of Diethylnitrosamine in Rats. Journal of West China University of Medical Sciences, 32(4): 555–558.
JinXinglin, QianChangshi, DuXichen, et al. (2009) Pathologic and morphologic study on modified DEN-induced hepatocarcinoma model in rats. China Journal of Modern Medicine, 19(17): 2593–2596.
Ressolinovitch SD, Mihailovich N, Wogan GN, et al. (1972) AflatoxinB1, a hepatocarcinogen in infant mouse. Cancer Res, 32(11): 2289–2291.
ShaoChengwei, TianJianming, WangPeijun, et al. (2002) Two Methods of Making Liver Cancer Model in Rats: A Comparative Study. *Journal of Clinical Radiology*, 21(12): 985–987.
Solt DB, Medline A, Farber E. (1977) Rapid emergency of carcinogen-induced hyperplastic lesion in a new model for the sequential analysis of liver carcinogenesis. Am J Patho, 88(3): 595–618.
WeiHong. (2001) Medical Laboratory Animal Science. In: BianXiuwu (eds.) Tumor animal model. 2nd edition Cheng du: Sichuan Science and Technology Publishing House: 421–4.
Wolf M. (2008) Influence of matrigel on biodistribution studies in cancer research. Pharmazie, 63(1): 43–48.
WU Meng-chao. (1998) Advances in diagnosis and treatment of primary liver cancer. Journal of Chinese Journal of Surgery, 36(9): 515–518.
XuYuyin, ChenLi. (2011) Methods to establish the animal model of liver cancer. Journal of Clinical and Experimental Pathology, 27(4): 405–408.
YangFuchun, ZhengShushen, JiangTianan. (2004) Study on modified DEN-induced hepatocarcinoma model in rats. Chinese Medical Journal, 84(23): 2018–2019.
ZhangXinli, ShiJingquan, BianXiuwu. (2001) Quantitative study on morphologies features and proliferative activity during DEN-induced hepatocarcinogenesis in rats. Journal of Third Military Medical University, 23(3): 304–307.
Zheng Jianming, Tao Wenzhao, Zheng Weiqiang, et al. (2000) Establishment of the orthotopic transplantation tumor model from the subcutaneous model of human hepatocellular carcinoma in nude mice. Journal of Second Military Medical University, 21(5): 456–459.

Medicine Sciences and Bioengineering – Wang (Ed.)
© 2015 Taylor & Francis Group, London, ISBN: 978-1-138-02684-1

The study of gray matter lesions in multiple sclerosis via proton magnetic resonance spectroscopy

Jun Ma
Department of CT and MRI, Affiliated Hospital of Beihua University, Jilin city, Jilin province, China

Zhao-hui Wang*
Department of Neurology, Affiliated Hospital of Beihua University, Jilin city, Jilin province, China

ABSTRACT: By combining metabolic and anatomical images, ^{1}H-MRS can be used in the early diagnosis and prognosis of MS more sensitively, and especially in preventing the emergence of cognitive decline and disability in MS patients. This noninvasive treatment may play an important role in the detection of MS disease.

1 INTRODUCTION

Multiple Sclerosis (MS) is an autoimmune demyelinating disease in the central nervous system. Gray matter lesions, which emerge in the early course of the disease, are important causes of neurological dysfunction in patients with MS progression. Recently, some studies have shown the occurrence of lesions of axonal and gray matter in MS, suggesting the existence of nondemyelinating damage (Li YX, 2008; Li MZ, 2008). In order to improve the early diagnosis of multiple sclerosis and prevent cognitive decline and emergence of disability in MS patients, the gray matter lesions in MS were examined by magnetic resonance spectroscopy (^{1}H-MRS).

2 MATERIALS AND METHODS

2.1 Clinical data

A total of 32 cases of MS patients with gray matter damage in the affiliated hospital of Beihua University were selected (ranging from 8 to 52 years old, a male to female ratio of 0.86, and mean age of 32.5 years), which meet the McDonald diagnostic criteria for MS. In these MS patients, clinical symptoms of hemiparesis, numbness, dizziness and ataxia, unilateral or bilateral optic nerve damage, decreased vision, and periorbital pain were detected. Further, 20 healthy adult volunteers without any central nervous system diseases and clinical manifestations were selected as the normal control group (NC). Before the ^{1}H-MRS examination, all patients and volunteers signed an informed consent form.

2.2 Methods

Conventional MRI examination was used to detect differences in gray matter between MS group and normal group. In this study, MRI examination was conducted by Siemens Novous 1. 5T superconducting MRI machine. For MRI examination, routine horizontal, sagittal, and coronal

---

*Corresponding author. E-mail: gxg8222@gmail.com.

scans were used, and standard head coil was utilized as the transmitter and receiver coil. For ¹H-MRS analysis, point-resolved spectroscopy and chemical shift selective saturation water suppression method were used to collect the signal. The metabolite spectrum was obtained from SUN Aw3.0 workstation and Functool software, including concentrations of aspartate (NAA), creatinine (Cr), choline (cho), and so on.

2.3 Data acquisition

The Expanded Disability Status Scale (EDSS) score of MS patients was obtained according to the degree of impairment (Gao, 2007). The curves of NAA, Cho, Cr, MI, Lip, and Lac were obtained, and the areas under the peak were calculated. The results were expressed as mean ± SD (standard deviation). The relevant test between the ratio of NAA to Cr, Cho to Cr, and EDSS scores were analyzed using spearman. A probability of $P < 0.05$ was considered statistically significant.

3 RESULTS

Compared with health volunteers, all MS patients showed brain atrophy and reduced surface area of gray matter. There are different degrees of atrophy in deep gray matter in MS such as the thalamus, caudate nucleus, putamen, etc. Moreover, more remarkable gray matter atrophy was found in MS patients with cognitive disabilities than in MS patients without cognitive disabilities. The damage of gray matter in MS usually occurs in the basal ganglia and thalamus, and the damage of each lobe in brain and hippocampus was also detected with concurrent lesions of sac and semioval center. The detection rate of gray matter lesion was higher by unenhanced FLAIR sequence.

¹H-MRS examination indicated reduced NAA and increased Cho and MI in the damage zone of gray matter, while decreased NAA and significant increase in inositol in normal-appearing white matter (NAWM) were detected in MS patients. The NAA to Cr ratio decreased significantly in acute plaque lesions than in chronic plaque. With the development of MS disease, NAA levels and NAA to Cr ratio decreased in chronic lesions, whereas these indexes reach normal level in acute plaque. The Cho/Cr levels were lower in chronic lesions than in acute lesions, which showed a trend of returning to normal level. The differences of NAA/Cr, Cho/Cr, and mI/Cr between the control group and the focus groups in NAWM area of MS patients were statistically significant ($P < 0.05$) (shown in Table 1).

In this study, we also found that compared with the control group MS patients had a relatively smaller thalamus and lower level of NAA. According to the concentration of NAA in MS patients and healthy people, we speculate that if the NAA concentration decreases by more than 25% there may be gray matter lesions in MS patients. Moreover, the ratio of NAA to Cr in the plaque of MS patients was far lesser than that in the NAWM group, suggesting that NAA to Cr value is an indicator of disease activity (shown in Figure 1).

Table 1. ¹H-MRS measurements of gray matter lesions in multiple sclerosis.

	NAA/Cr	Cho/Cr	NAA/ Cho	mI/Cr	Lac/Cr
MS	1.46 ± 0.12	1.29 ± 0.15	1.31 ± 0.18	0.56 ± 0.07	0.33 ± 0.12
NAWM	1.64 ± 0.15	1.20 ± 0.08	1.50 ± 0.12	0.48 ± 0.05	0.28 ± 0.11
NC	1.93 ± 0.04	1.08 ± 0.10	1.67 ± 0.04	0.40 ± 0.03	0.17 ± 0.02

Note: MS: multiple sclerosis; NAWM: normal-appearing white matter; NC: normal control.

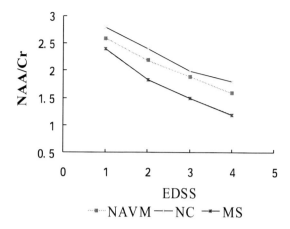

Figure 1. Correlation analysis between NAA/Cr value and EDSS score.

4 DISCUSSION

The pathogenesis of gray matter lesions is mainly attributed to the apoptosis of neuronal and transected dendrites and axons. Demyelinating damages in cortex, basal ganglia, thalamus, and hypothalamus were detected. Significantly decreased number of neurons was observed in cortex lesions, suggesting that demyelination of gray matter and neuronal loss may lead to disability and cognitive impairment in MS patients (Wang, 2009). MRI studies indicated that the characteristics of gray matter lesions were focal injury, diffuse tissue abnormalities, and irreversible tissue atrophy. The gray matter lesions that appeared earlier had an effect on the cerebral cortex and the basal ganglia. And the progress of gray matter lesions was faster than white matter in the short term, which reflects the progress of MS disease and determines the ultimate brain gray matter atrophy disability (Hu, 2010).

However, conventional brain MRI was not sensitive enough to detect the small cortical lesions. Moreover, the poor contrast with the normal area caused by extended relaxation time and low specificity caused by volume effect of cerebrospinal fluid and dual echo MRI scan made things worse (Chen, 2010). Proton magnetic resonance spectroscopy (^{1}H-MRS) can analyze the metabolites in living tissue quantitatively. N-acetyl aspartate (NAA) is the best indicator of neuronal loss, creatine (Cr) can be used as a myelin disintegration marker, choline (Cho) and Mi (inositol) cause increase in gliosis, and Lac (lactic acid) is associated with elevated inflammatory response, suggesting that ^{1}H-MRS can be more sensitive to detect MS disease in the early course and provide clues for the detection of MS dysfunction (Caramanos Z, 2009).

In this study, the reduced NAA in MS and NAWM suggested that MS lesions caused a wide range of changes in the brain. The results also showed that lactate (Lac) level in MS patients was higher than that in the control group, indicating a potential marker for MS diagnosis. We also found that relatively small thalamic volume in MS patients may be associated with neuronal atrophy. Moreover, our results showed that the demyelination of hypothalamic neurons was positive relative to the axonal damage in NAWM. As it is known that neuronal injury and demyelination can reflect the inflammation of gray matter, the progress of disease and treatment efficacy could be examined by measuring changes in whole-brain NAA concentration. Many changes in neuronal degeneration can explain cognitive impairment in MS patients (Filippi, 2011). The results showed that NAA/Cr value was negative relative to the degree of clinical disability, suggesting an indicator of disease.

5 SUMMARY

In short, by combining metabolic and anatomical images ^{1}H-MRS can be used in the early diagnosis and prognosis of MS more sensitively, and especially in preventing the emergence of cognitive decline and disability in MS patients. This noninvasive treatment may play an important role in the detection of MS disease.

ACKNOWLEDGMENT

This work was supported by the Project of Technology Department of Jilin city (No. 201233120).

REFERENCES

Caramanos Z, DiMaio S, Narayanan S, et al. (2009). H-MRSI evidence for cortical gray matter pathology that is independent of cerebral white matter lesion load in patients with secondary progressive multiple sclerosis. *Journal of the Neurological Sciences.* 282(1):72–79.

Chen SL, Luo MY, Chen SQ, et al. (2010) Analysis of 1H magnetic resonance spectroscopy in multiple sclerosis. *Clinical Radiology.* 29(1):18–21.

Filippi M, Rocca MA. (2011) The role of magnetic resonance imaging in the study of multiple sclerosis: diagnosis, prognosis and understanding disease pathophysiology. *Acta Neurologica Belgica.* 111(2):89–98.

Gao BT, Hu XQ, Sun CL, et al. (2007) The clinical and imaging features of multiple sclerosis with damage of cerebral gray matter. *Stroke and Nervous Diseases.* 14(5):299–301.

Hu B, Yang Y, Zou Y, et al. (2010) Clinical application of magnetic resonance spectroscopy and diffusion tensor imaging in multiple sclerosis. *New medicine.* 41(10):640–643.

Li MZ, Gui SG, Liu DR, et al. (2008) Study of 1H magnetic resonance spectroscopy in multiple sclerosis. *Practical Clinical Medicine.* 9(9):99–101.

Li YX, Chu SG, Li ZX, et al. (2008) Magnetic resonance imaging and diffusion tensor imaging of gray matter damage in multiple sclerosis. *Chinese Journal of Radiology.* 42(7):709–713.

Wang F, Yu CS, Li CC. (2009) Progress on MRI investigation on multiple sclerosis. *Chinese Journal of Medical Imaging Technology.* 25(11):2132–2134.

Medicine Sciences and Bioengineering – Wang (Ed.)
© 2015 Taylor & Francis Group, London, ISBN: 978-1-138-02684-1

The optimization of scan parameters on head and neck in children by somatom definition flash

Jun Ma, Jing Ma, Yan Wang & Xiao-mei Mu
Department of CT and MRI, Affiliated Hospital of Beihua University, Jilin city, Jilin province, China

Fan-li Kong[*]
School of Basic Medical Sciences, Beihua University, Jilin city, Jilin province, China

ABSTRACT: Our study showed that Hyun-speed Flash dual-source CT for CTA examination of head and neck in children not only provides a lot of information on anatomy and function but also reduces the radiation dose. This quick and easy examination method increases the accuracy of diagnosis and improves repeatability and will play an important role in clinical diagnosis.

1   INTRODUCTION

The radiation dose of CT scan for children is a hot topic in clinical research. The emergence of dual-source CT with two balls and a detector tube system give some hope in reducing the radiation dose in CTA (Feng Y, 2011). In this study, the second generation of Siemens Somaton Definition Flash (DSCT) was used in CTA scan for children with head and neck. During the process of CTA scanning, we follow the three principles of International Commission on Radiological Protection (ICRP) (Huang HY, 2011) to optimize the CTA scan parameters for children's head and neck.

2   MATERIALS AND METHODS

2.1   Clinical data

A total of 120 cases of children in the affiliated hospital of Beihua University were selected (ranging from 2 to 14 years old, male to female ratio of 1.07, and mean age of 5 years). The clinical symptoms of these children include dizziness, headache, physical activity not working, aphasia, convulsions, decreased vision, and so on. Children who were sensitive to iodinated contrast agents or had serious dysfunction of heart and kidney were excluded. The body weights of children were restricted (boys: 5–40 kg; girls: 4–35 kg). The scan parameters were fixed as follows: tube voltage 80/Sn 140 kV and fusion coefficient 0.6; tube current adjusted (Care Dose 4D) open.

2.2   Scan methods

Before scanning, family members signed informed consent forms. The children were treated with chloral hydrate (0.5 mL/kg), and a trocar was embedded in the right front elbow of each child to establish intravenous access. The contrast agent iopromide (1.5–2.0 mL/kg) was injected intravenously with a flow rate of 4 mL/s. Using DSCT and keeping the patient supine, the scanning ranged from the aortic arch to the base of the skull. The supine patient was detected via DSCT with the scanning range from the aortic arch to the base of the skull. Enhanced scanning was performed with scanning software (Bolus Tracking). The trigger point was located at the fourth

---

[*]Corresponding author. E-mail: gxg8222@gmail.com.

vertebra in the neck near the internal carotid artery, and the trigger threshold was set at 100 Hu, followed by the injection of 40 mL saline with a flow rate of 4.5 mL/s. Scan parameters were as follows: 0.33 s/turn, collimation 64 × 0.6 mm, voltages 140 kV and 80 kV, tube current adjusted (Care Dose 4D) open, currents of double tube fixed at 27–40 mAs and 114–140 mAs, pitch 0.9, and FOV adjusted according to the size of individual children. The thickness of the reconstruction layer was 1.0 mm, and the reconstruction interval was 0.75 mm.

2.3 *Image reconstruction and imaging evaluation*

The collected image data was processed by Syngo CT Workplace workstation. Fusion images were obtained with 80 kVp and 140 kVp at a ratio of 0.6 by Somaton definition flash dual-source CT (40% of 80 kVp, 60% of 140 kVp, equivalent to 120 kVp). Four groups of images were obtained: group I consisted of 140-kVp images, group II was equivalent to 120-kVp images, group III contained 80-kVp (I26) images, and group IV had 80-kVp (D26) images. All processed images were treated with VR, MIP, MPR, and CPR. Images of carotid bifurcation of the carotid artery and thoracic inlet, the noise of the basilar artery, and the signal to noise ratio of CNR were analyzed quantitatively. The radiation doses of CTDIvol, DLP, and ED were calculated. CTDIvol, DLP, and ED were calculated. The blood vessels displayed clearly and vascular wall was smooth was excellent, slightly rough vessel wall and continuous wall was well, and serious arrhythmia or missing vascular edge segments was regarded as poor result.

2.4 *Statistical analysis*

The image was read via a double-blind method. SPSS19.0 software was used in statistical analysis. The radiation dose of indicators was ±s, and $P < 0.05$ was considered statistically significant.

3 RESULTS

As shown in Table 1, there was difference in arterial CT values between groups I, II, III, and IV when reducing the voltage, indicating increased CT value as the lower voltage. There was difference in background noise between group III, group IV, and the control group, indicating significantly elevated background noise in group IV. There was no significant difference in SNR and CNR values between groups II, III, and I ($P > 0.05$). No significant impact was detected in image reconstruction by 80 kVp (I26).

As shown in Table 2, there was no significant difference in image quality between groups I, II, and III ($P > 0.05$), and the reconstructed image quality and the diagnostic yield in group IV 80 kVp (D26) were lower than those in the other groups ($P < 0.05$).

As shown in Table 3, compared with group I volume CT dose index in groups II, III, and IV decreased by 34%, 58%, and 36%, respectively, and the effective length and effective doses decreased by 24%, 54%, and 29%, respectively. Compared with group IV, the volume CT dose index in group III decreased by 35% and the effective length and effective doses decreased by 34%.

4 DISCUSSION

Children are more sensitive to radiation than adults. In order to avoid inducing thyroid cancer in children, CTA examination of head and neck needs more consideration to prevent the damage caused by x-ray radiation. Hyun-speed Flash dual-source CT system with two tubes can work independently, while using different sexual energy imaging (Qiu J, 2010). Due to the high-sensitivity detector, only a small radiation dose can be used to obtain high-quality images. Moreover, with the help of Care Dose 4D software Hyun-speed Flash dual-source CT can automatically adjust

Table 1. Quantitative analysis of the reconstructed image quality.

Group	Thoracic inlet	Carotid artery bifurcation	Basilar artery
I			
CTvalue (HU)	395.10 ± 422	382.10 ± 2.62	357.10 ± 2.02
Noise	14.25 ± 0.23	14.62 ± 0.22	15.25 ± 0.63
SNR	23.06 ± 2.05	26.35 ± 3.14	28.17 ± 2.08
CNR	24.05 ± 3.06	26.78 ± 2.86	28.15 ± 2.32
II			
CT value (HU)	428.02 ± 4.01	425.05 ± 6.32	368.08 ± 3.62
Noise	14.28 ± 0.28	14.85 ± 0.72	15.36 ± 0.66
SNR	25.05 ± 1.15	27.09 ± 3.26	29.25 ± 2.18
CNR	22.32 ± 2.03	25.75 ± 2.05	26.72 ± 1 26
III			
CT value (HU)	435.10 ± 5.69	430.05 ± 4.07	429.10 ± 6.22
Noise	14.26 ± 0.36	14.82 ± 0.25	15.32 ± 0.72
SNR	28.16 ± 2.26	32.17 ± 2.21	35.08 ± 1.03
CNR	27.75 ± 0.25	31.72 ± 1.06	33.63 ± 1.37
IV			
CT value (HU)	438.04 ± 4.62	432.07 ± 2.54	428.06 ± 4.33
Noise	15.55 ± 0.25	15.62 ± 0.28	15.78 ± 0.68
SNR	20.15 ± 1.32	21.17 ± 2.23	22.02 ± 2.32
CNR	20.32 ± 1.06	20.78 ± 1.03	21.75 ± 2.28

Table 2. The assessment of image quality.

Image quality	I	II	III	IV
Excellent	118	102	88	50
Good	2	18	32	22
Poor	0	0	0	48
Diagnostic yield(%)	100	100	100	60

Table 3. Comparison of the radiation dose.

Data	I	II	III	IV	P
CTDI (mGy)	9.92 ± 0.22	6.45 ± 0.32	4.12 ± 0.12	6.32 ± 0.21	<0.05
DLP (mGy/cm)	220.51 ± 2.61	168.63 ± 1.21	102.11 ± 0.36	155.21 ± 2.62	<0.05
ED (msv)	5.06 ± 0.03	3.86 ± 0.06	2.34 ± 0.02	3.56 ± 0.02	<0.05

the output tube current and tube size according to each child to achieve the goal of ensuring high quality of images at low radiation doses. The advanced dual-source CT image reconstruction technique can detect the vessels of head and neck and display abnormal structures of the nervous system more accurately, providing a basis for surgical positioning (Ma GL, 2011).

The results showed that Hyun-speed Flash dual-source dual-energy CT has many advantages such as overcoming the problem of image registration caused by moving, reducing the radiation dose, improving the stability of the inspection and the efficiency of reconstruction, displaying more peripheral vascular, and detection and removal of calcium plaque in detail.

Our results indicated that good images were obtained by SAFIRE reconstruction using a low radiation dose. It is good iterative algorithm combined the raw data and image First, the algorithm iterates the original data field to remove various artifacts and then iterates the image to remove noise and artifacts portion. This algorithm can improve the image quality and reduce the radiation dose of 54%–60%, which has been approved by the FDA (Shi MG, 2012).

5 SUMMARY

In conclusion, our study showed that Hyun-speed Flash dual-source CT for CTA examination of head and neck in children not only provides a lot of information on anatomy and function but also reduces the radiation dose. This quick and easy examination method increases the accuracy of diagnosis and improves the repeatability and will play an important role in clinical diagnosis.

ACKNOWLEDGMENT

This work was supported by the Project of Technology Department of Jilin city (No. 201233120).

REFERENCES

Feng Y, Xue JP, Li YH. (2009) Evaluation of vascular disorders in head and neck with dual-source CT angiography. *Chinese Computed Medical Imaging*. 15(5):431–437.
Huang HY, Pu H, Tao KY, et al. (2011) Optimal scanning parameters of dual resource CT angiography in intracranial and cervical arteries. *Practical Journal of Clinical Medicine*. 8(1):49–52.
Ma GL, Wang W, Zhang YC. (2011) The clinical application of low-dose helical CT scans of children. *Chinese Journal of Radiological Medicine and Protection*. 31(1):111–114.
Qiu J. (2010) Clinical Progress of Low-dose CT Scan in Children. *Medical Recapitulate*. 16(16):2500–2502.
Shi MG. (2012) CT entering low dose imaging times. *China Medical Devices*. 27(1):39–43.

Medicine Sciences and Bioengineering – Wang (Ed.)
© *2015 Taylor & Francis Group, London, ISBN: 978-1-138-02684-1*

Development of thoracic impedance detection system based on embedded

Xiao-yuan Yan, Tao Chen, Shu-mei Gao & Yi-lin Song[*]
School of Mechanical & Electrical Engineering, Heilongjiang University, Harbin, China

ABSTRACT: In order to realize the noninvasive detection of Cardiac Output (CO), the impedance detection system for human body is designed and developed in this paper. The ECG detection circuit is also designed and the ECG is detected as the reference signal. The experimental results show that the stability of the developed system is good and it is suitable for the detection of the human thoracic impedance.

1 INTRODUCTION

As one of the important indicators of diagnosis and treatment of cardiovascular disease, cardiac output is detected in many instances. At present, the monitoring of cardiac output is mainly used in serious patients, but the importance of monitoring of cardiac output in the family will also be increased gradually with the improvement of people's living standard. The methods for measuring cardiac output or stroke volume, such as Fick method, heat dilution method, echocardiography and electrical impedance cardiography, have been developed (Zhao Zhe et al., 2010). Among all the methods, the thoracic impedance method, because of its non-invasive and good stability, gets more medical researchers or medical institutions recognition, and related detecting equipment has been used in clinical. In this paper, the design of detection system based on the theory of the thoracic impedance method is introduced, and the detecting experiment of the impedance cardiography (ICG) is carried out.

This design applies the PWM function of MCU of PIC series to produce a square wave signal with the frequency of 50 kHz. Then, the signal is converted to a sine wave with the same frequency by using a signal process circuit, and is imposed on electrodes placed on the surface of the human skin as an excitation signal of the thoracic impedance detection. The detection electrodes located in the anterior median line are used to detect the potential difference for calculating the electrical impedance between electrodes.

2 METHOD

2.1 *The thoracic impedance method*

The thoracic impedance method is based on the thorax cylinder model of Nyboer and the formula for estimating stroke volume (SV) of Kubieck (Lin Zhenheng et al., 2008). A pair of excitation electrodes placed on the neck and the abdomen is used to impose constant sinusoidal current (50 kHz, $2mA_{rms}$), and a pair inner electrodes that should be placed more than 3 cm apart from each current electrode as the detection electrodes is used to detect the change of output voltage, so the potential difference before and after blood inflow into the aorta is measured.

---

[*] Corresponding author

With the above thorax cylinder model, the impedance changes before and after blood inflow into the arteries can be analyzed, and the formula of stroke volume is deduced, see the formula (1). Then the cardiac output can be calculated by using the product of heart rate and stroke volume.

$$SV = \rho_b \left(\frac{L}{Z_0} \right)^2 (\frac{dZ}{dt})_{min} T_s \qquad (1)$$

Where ρ_b is the blood resistivity associated with hematocrit (HCT) and given as 150Ω cm in normal healthy subjects, L is the distance between detection electrodes, and T_s is the ventricular ejection time.

In the actual detection, the electrical impedance is usually converted to electrical admittance for the calculation of CO, such as formula (2). Compared formula (1) with formula (2), it can be found that the calculation formula represented by the electrical admittance does not contain the total electrical admittance Y_0, which makes CO easy get and the calculation accuracy improve.

$$SV = \rho_b L^2 Y_b = \rho_b L^2 \times dY / dt|\max \times T_s \qquad (2)$$

Studies have found that the CO obtained by this method varies as the subject's age and weight. And the measured values in most cases are slightly lower than the normal range (Yolanda et al., 2011). The stability of this method is better, and the results are basically identical under different positions such as lying down and standing. Besides, it also has an acceptable repeatability under the mild to moderate aerobic activity (Martin et al., 2012). The experimental results show that the band electrodes can make the thoracic current distribution more uniform. However, it can also make a certain influence on human body for a long time use, and be easy to cause the complication, such as dermatitis. So the spot electrodes are used in this research.

3 DEVELOPMENT OF THE SYSTEM

The system structure diagram of thoracic impedance detection system is shown in Figure 1. The system mainly consist of 6 parts, such as electrodes, the sine wave generator circuit, the impedance detection circuit, ECG detection circuit, MCU control and display. The electrodes are divided into excitation electrodes and detection electrodes. The sine wave generator circuit is designed to produce a sine wave (50 kHz, 2 mA$_{rms}$) as input of the excitation electrodes. The impedance detection circuit and the ECG detection circuit are used to get signals from detection electrodes. The detection signal obtained will be displayed on display unit.

3.1 *The sine wave generator circuit*

The principle of the sine wave generator circuit is shown in Figure 2. In order to achieve the detection of human body thoracic electrical impedance, the 50 kHz sine signal with constant current is needed. In this research, the method that the square wave is generated by the PWM function of MCU, and then it is transformed into sine wave is adopted. The generated square wave is shown in Figure 3 and the sine wave is shown in Figure 4.

3.2 *The thoracic impedance detection circuit*

The thoracic impedance detection circuit is mainly used to detect the following two signals: the basal thoracic electrical impedance Z_0 and the pulsatile electrical impedance ΔZ between

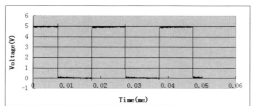

Figure 1.　The system block diagram.

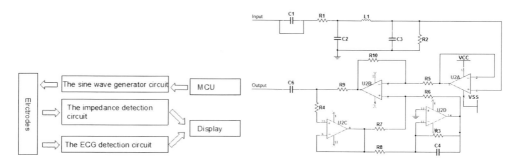

Figure 2.　The sine wave generator circuit.

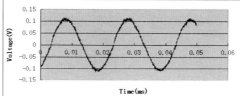

Figure 3.　The square wave.

Figure 4.　The sine wave.

the detection electrode and the reference electrode when the two excitation electrodes impose sinusoidal current I (50 kHz, 2 mA$_{rms}$). So the low frequency signal and the high frequency signal are extracted by the filter circuit, respectively. Because the excitation signal is alternating, it is needed to have the rectifying part in the detection circuit. Based on the principle of thoracic impedance method, the formula (1) or (2) can be used to calculate the cardiac output of the body if the measurement data is obtained. In addition, through the detection of electrical impedance Z_0 and ΔZ in different positions, the thoracic impedance Z_0 (Z_0-map) and ΔZ distribution (ΔZ-map) can be mapped. It can provide the basis for further study of the best spot electrode array.

3.3　ECG detection circuit

The Electrocardiogram (ECG) reflects the electrical activity process of cardiac excitement, and it has important reference value for the research of heart functions and other pathological mechanism. In this research, as a reference signal ECG is also detected. The ECG detection circuit is mainly composed of the preamplifier circuit, the filter circuit, the trap circuit, and the post amplifier circuit.

General human ECG amplitude is about 20 μV ~ 5 mV and the width of frequency band is 0.05 Hz~100 Hz. Because of the ECG signal being derived from living, there is a strong background noise and interference in the signal (S.De Ridder & X.Neyt, 2011). In this development the magnification of the preamplifier circuit and the post amplifier circuit are set to 20 times and 50 times, respectively. In addition, in order to remove the power line interference, the trap circuit with the center frequency of 50 Hz is added. Also, ECG is a weak low frequency non-stationary signal, so the characteristics such as high input impedance, low noise, low drift, the ability of voltage amplification are required and the integrated instrumentation amplifier INA128 is chosen.

3.4 *The other parts of the system*

Electrode is the key element in the electrical impedance detection, so its performance can also cause certain influence on the detection. In the actual experiments, the medical disposable ECG spot electrode is used. For the placement of spot electrodes, the research showed that the thoracic impedance changes in gradient when the two excitation electrodes are placed on the back of the ear and the lower abdomen (near the waist bone), and the detection electrodes are placed on the middle of the clavicle and the sword convex near the anterior median line. The control part of system is a PIC18F4520 MCU. Using the pulse width modulation function of MCU in the design, the 50 kHz square wave signal at the CCP1 pin by setting up appropriate parameters with software is easy gotten. The signal is shown in Figure 3. The signal acquisition and display section is performed by NEC recorder in this research.

4 EXPERIMENTAL RESULTS AND ANALYSIS

4.1 *The Z_0 and ΔZ*

Before the experiment of thoracic impedance detection, the positions of every spot electrode must be determined. According to the research of our group, the detection effect is the best when the spot electrodes are placed on the anterior median line in the thoracic electrical impedance measurement (Akira Ikarashi et al., 2007). Therefore, in the actual experiment, the detection electrodes are attached on the anterior median line, and the results of the multiple potions are recorded simultaneously. In order to reduce the influence of respiration on the experimental results, the subjects are required lying on the bed and hold their breathing in the process of actual measurement. The subjects of this experiment are six healthy young men, aged from 21 to 26. The waveform of ΔZ shown in Figure 5 is obtained. At the same time, the electrical impedance Z_0 of each position is detected and their scatter plot is shown in Figure 6.

From the Figure 5 it is seen that as the spot electrode gets closer and closer to the location of sword convex, the pulsatile component (ΔZ) becomes smaller and smaller. And it can be also found that the pulsatile component changes periodically with the beat of the heart, compared with the ECG signal. Through measuring the value of the electrical impedance in each position many times, the averages of Z_0 are calculated and their trend diagram of the changing is drawn, just shown in Figure 6. It can be seen from the diagram that the electrical impedance Z_0 on the anterior median line from position 1 to 6 presents a gradual step-down trend, and it almost changes linearly. The results further confirm our previous results.

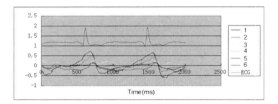
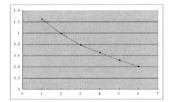

Figure 5. ΔZ waveform obtained by six electrodes.   Figure 6. The trend diagram of the changing of electrical impedance Z_0.

5 CONCLUSION

A human thoracic impedance detection system is developed in this paper. By using the PWM function of MCU, the square wave signal is gotten, and it is further turned to the constant current sine wave signal by a circuit. The excitation electrodes are imposed sinusoidal current, the detection electrode and the reference electrode are used to detect the voltage changes between the two electrodes by the thoracic impedance detection circuit, and the parameters Z_0 and ΔZ are obtained. The results are properly displayed on the display device. Experimental results show that the system has good linearity and stability.

ACKNOWLEDGEMENT

This work was partly supported by the Ministry of Human resources and Social Security, China (2007 Return Project for High-level Overseas Talent).

REFERENCES

Akira Ikarashi, Masamichi Nogawa, Shinobu Tanaka, et al. (2007) Experiment and numerical study on optimal spot-electrodes arrays in transthoracic electrical impedance cardiography. *Proceedings of the 39th Annual International Conference of IEEE EMBS, 23–26 August 2007,* Lyon, pp. 4580–4583.216.

Lin Zhenheng, Huang Yuanqing & Yang wei. (2008) The research of new Kubieck model of stroke volume. *Journal of Xiamen University*, 47(5), 677–680.

Martin G. Schultz, Rachel E.D. Climie, Sonja B. Nikolic, et al. (2012) Reproducibility of cardiac output derived by impedance cardiography during postural changes and exercise. *Artery Research*, 6(2), 78–84.

S.De Ridder & X.Neyt. (2011) Comparison between EEMD,Wavelet and FIR Denoising: influence on event detection in impedance cardiography. *The 33rd Annual International Conference of IEEE EMBS, Oct 30th-Sept 2rd 2011*, Boston, pp. 806–809.

Yolanda Ballestero, Jesu's Lopez-Herce, Javier Urbano, et al. (2011) Measurement of cardiac output in children by bioreactance. *Pediatric Cardiology*, 32(4), 469–472.

Zhao Zhe, Wang ling, Pan Songxin, et al. (2010) Measurement principles and development of cardiac output monitoring . *Chinese Journal of Biomedical Engineering*, 29(4), 619–626.

Medicine Sciences and Bioengineering – Wang (Ed.)
© *2015 Taylor & Francis Group, London, ISBN: 978-1-138-02684-1*

Altered functional connectivity of the entorhinal cortex in mild cognitive impairment

Ya-qin Zhang
Key Laboratory for NeuroInformation of Ministry of Education, School of Life Science and Technology, University of Electronic Science and Technology of China, Chengdu, China

Yong Liu
LIAMA Center for Computational Medicine, National Laboratory of Pattern Recognition, Institute of Automation, Chinese Academy of Sciences, Beijing, China

Chun-shui Yu
Department of Radiology, Tianjin Medical University General Hospital, Tianjin, China

Tian-zi Jiang
Key Laboratory for NeuroInformation of Ministry of Education, School of Life Science and Technology, University of Electronic Science and Technology of China, Chengdu, China
LIAMA Center for Computational Medicine, National Laboratory of Pattern Recognition, Institute of Automation, Chinese Academy of Sciences, Beijing, China
The Queensland Brain Institute, The University of Queensland, Brisbane, Australia

ABSTRACT: Entorhinal cortex (ERC) is a primary area of dysfunction in Alzheimer's Disease (AD). Its involvement in Mild Cognitive Impairment (MCI), which is considered to be a transitional state between normal aging and early AD, is not well understood. The present study investigated altered functional connectivity of the ERC in MCI. The ERC mainly exhibited decreased connectivity with the default mode network and increased connectivity with the lateral temporal cortex. Our research provided new knowledge of the MCI mechanisms and biomarkers for clinical diagnosis.

1   INTRODUCTION

Alzheimer's Disease (AD) is the most common cause of dementia in the elderly (Liu *et al.*, 2014). Between normal aging and early AD, mild cognitive impairment (MCI) is considered to be a transitional state with a high risk for developing AD (Berchtold *et al.*, 2014). Histological and imaging studies have convergently implicated that the entorhinal cortex (ERC) is a primary area of dysfunction in AD (Moreno *et al.*, 2007; Whitwell *et al.*, 2007; Braak & Del Tredici, 2012; Khan *et al.*, 2014). However, affection of the ERC in MCI is not well understood. Using resting-state functional magnetic resonance imaging (rs-fMRI), the present study investigated disrupted functional connectivity of the ERC in MCI patients.

2   MATERIALS AND METHODS

2.1   *Subjects*

Eighteen patients with MCI and twenty-one healthy controls (HC) were recruited after signed a written, informed consent form. The study was approved by the ethics committee of Xuanwu Hospital. The diagnosis of MCI was according to standard criteria (Petersen *et al.*, 1999; Petersen *et al.*, 2001; Choo *et al.*, 2007) and a Clinical Dementia Rating (CDR) score of 0.5. HC have a CDR score of 0. Demographics and clinical characteristics of the participants are summarized in Table 1.

Table 1. Demographics and clinical characteristics.

	HC (n = 21)	MCI (n = 18)	*P*-value
Gender (M/F)	7/14	10/8	0.163
Age(year)	65.0 ± 8.1	70.2 ± 7.9	0.055
MMSE	28.5 ± 1.4	21.9 ± 5.0	<0.001
CDR	0	0.5	—

Note: Pearson chi-squared test was used for gender comparison; Two-sample two-tailed *t* test were used for age and MMSE comparisons. MMSE: mini-mental state examination; CDR: clinical dementia rating.

2.2 Data acquisition

All images were acquired on a 3-T MR scanner (Magnetom Trio, Siemens, Germany). Sagittal T1-weighted MR images were collected using a magnetization-prepared rapid gradient-echo sequence (Repetition time (TR) = 2000 ms, echo time (TE) = 2.6 ms, flip angle (FA) = 9°, matrix = 256 × 224, field of view (FOV) = 256 mm × 224 mm, 176 continuous sagittal slices with 1 mm thickness). The rs-fMRI data were acquired by an echo planar imaging sequence (TR/TE = 2000/30 ms, FA = 90°, matrix = 64 × 64, FOV = 220 mm × 220 mm, slice thickness = 3 mm with interslice gap = 1 mm). During scanning, participants were instructed to keep their eyes closed and move as little as possible.

2.3 Data analysis

Preprocessing of rs-fMRI data was carried out by AFNI (http://afni.nimh.nih.gov/afni) and FSL (http://www.fmrib.ox.ac.uk/fsl). The first 10 images were discarded to allow the signal stabilization. The remaining 170 images were first corrected for within-scan acquisition time differences between slices and then realigned to the first volume to correct for interscan head motions. After that, the realigned images were spatially smoothed with a Gaussian kernel of 6 × 6 × 6 mm³ to decrease spatial noise. The rs-fMRI waveform of each voxel was temporally band-pass filtered (0.01 Hz < f < 0.08 Hz) and the linear drift of signal was removed. Subsequently, we spatially registered the filtered images to the Montreal Neurological Institute (MNI) space and resampled them to 2 × 2 × 2 mm³. Besides, several sources of spurious or regionally nonspecific variance were removed by regression of nuisance variables: six parameter rigid body head motion (obtained from motion correction), the signal averaged over the whole-brain, the signal averaged over the lateral ventricles, and the signal averaged over a region centered in the deep cerebral white matter.

Masks of the ERC were defined by the Brodmann atlas (Brodmann, 1909) for each hemisphere separately (Figure 1). For each subject, mean time series was extracted from the ERC and then Pearson correlations with other brain voxels were computed. The Fisher's z transform was applied to normalize the original correlation maps. After that, a two sample *t*-test ($p < 0.01$, AlphaSim corrected; with age and gender treated as covariates) between MCI and HC was performed on these maps to determine regions with significantly different connectivity to the ERC.

3 RESULTS

As illustrated in Figure 2, the left ERC exhibited decreased functional connectivity with the left angular gyrus, right superior frontal gyrus, left middle cingulate gyrus, right precuneus and

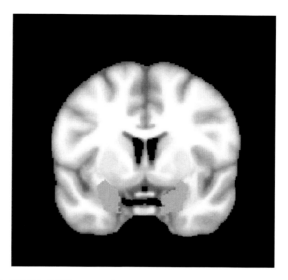

Figure 1. Masks of the ERC in MNI space. The ERC regions were defined by combining the ventral ERC (BA 28) and dorsal ERC (BA 34) together. BA: Brodmann area.

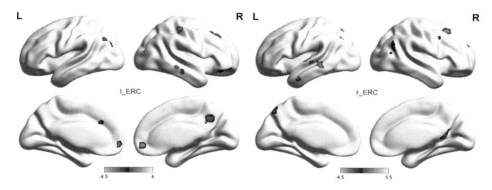

Figure 2. Significant differences of functional connectivity between MCI and HC groups, with a corrected statistical threshold of $p < 0.01$. Hot and cold colors represent increased and decreased functional connectivity in the MCI group compared with HC group, respectively.

bilateral medial prefrontal cortex in MCI group. Increased functional connectivity was found in the right postcentral gyrus and right posterior middle temporal gyrus. Compared with HC, MCI patients showed decreased connectivity between right ERC and left superior parietal lobe, left intraparietal sulcus, right superior frontal gyrus, right angular gyrus and right retrosplenial cortex. Left anterior middle temporal gyrus and left posterior temporal cortex had advanced connectivity with the right REC in MCI stage.

4   DISCUSSION

The present study assessed altered functional connectivity of the ERC in MCI patients. Compared with HC, regions of the default mode network (DMN) demonstrated decreased connectivity. Increase functional connectivity was mainly observed in lateral temporal cortex.

145

Disrupted connectivity of the DMN has been widely reported in AD patients (Mevel *et al.*, 2011; Wu *et al.*, 2011; Vergara & Behrens, 2013). Recent studies revealed that the DMN is also involved in MCI stage (Binnewijzend *et al.*, 2012; Cha *et al.*, 2013), which is consistent with our research. Furthermore, impairment in connectivity within the DMN is suggested to be associated with decline in memory (Wang *et al.*, 2013; Dunn *et al.*, 2014). The anterior temporal area and lateral posterior temporal cortex are the hubs of semantic processing (Hickok & Poeppel, 2007; Turken & Dronkers, 2011). Increased connections might reflect a compensatory recruitment to maintain semantic performance. This may be supported by the previous evidence that MCI impairs episodic memory while sparing semantic system (Balthazar *et al.*, 2007).

5   SUMMARY

In this study, disrupted functional connectivity of the ERC in MCI was investigated. The ERC mainly exhibited decreased connectivity with DMN and increased connectivity with lateral temporal cortex. Our research provided new knowledge of the MCI mechanisms and biomarkers for clinical diagnosis.

REFERENCES

Balthazar M.L., Martinelli J.E., Cendes F. & Damasceno B.P. (2007) Lexical semantic memory in amnestic mild cognitive impairment and mild Alzheimer's disease. Arq Neuropsiquiatr, 65(3A), 619–622.

Berchtold N.C., Sabbagh M.N., Beach T.G., Kim R.C., Cribbs D.H. & Cotman C.W. (2014) Brain gene expression patterns differentiate mild cognitive impairment from normal aged and Alzheimer's disease. Neurobiol Aging, 35(9), 1961–1972.

Binnewijzend M.A., Schoonheim M.M., Sanz-Arigita E., Wink A.M., van der Flier W.M., Tolboom N., Adriaanse S.M., Damoiseaux J.S., Scheltens P., van Berckel B.N. & Barkhof F. (2012) Resting-state fMRI changes in Alzheimer's disease and mild cognitive impairment. Neurobiol Aging, 33(9), 2018–2028.

Braak H. & Del Tredici K. (2012) Alzheimer's disease: pathogenesis and prevention. Alzheimers Dement, 8(3), 227–233.

Brodmann K. (1909) Vergleichende Lokalisationslehre der Gro hirnrinde: Springer.

Cha J., Jo H.J., Kim H.J., Seo S.W., Kim H.S., Yoon U., Park H., Na D.L. & Lee J.M. (2013) Functional alteration patterns of default mode networks: comparisons of normal aging, amnestic mild cognitive impairment and Alzheimer's disease. Eur J Neurosci, 37(12), 1916–1924.

Choo I.H., Lee D.Y., Youn J.C., Jhoo J.H., Kim K.W., Lee D.S., Lee J.S. & Woo J.I. (2007) Topographic patterns of brain functional impairment progression according to clinical severity staging in 116 Alzheimer disease patients: FDG-PET study. Alzheimer Dis Assoc Disord, 21(2), 77–84.

Dunn C.J., Duffy S.L., Hickie I.B., Lagopoulos J., Lewis S.J., Naismith S.L. & Shine J.M. (2014) Deficits in episodic memory retrieval reveal impaired default mode network connectivity in amnestic mild cognitive impairment. Neuroimage Clin, 4 473–480.

Hickok G. & Poeppel D. (2007) The cortical organization of speech processing. Nat Rev Neurosci, 8(5), 393–402.

Khan U.A., Liu L., Provenzano F.A., Berman D.E., Profaci C.P., Sloan R., Mayeux R., Duff K.E. & Small S.A. (2014) Molecular drivers and cortical spread of lateral entorhinal cortex dysfunction in preclinical Alzheimer's disease. Nat Neurosci, 17(2), 304–311.

Liu Y., Yu C., Zhang X., Liu J., Duan Y., Alexander-Bloch A.F., Liu B., Jiang T. & Bullmore E. (2014) Impaired long distance functional connectivity and weighted network architecture in Alzheimer's disease. Cereb Cortex, 24(6), 1422–1435.

Mevel K., Chetelat G., Eustache F. & Desgranges B. (2011) The default mode network in healthy aging and Alzheimer's disease. Int J Alzheimers Dis, 2011 535816.

Moreno H., Wu W.E., Lee T., Brickman A., Mayeux R., Brown T.R. & Small S.A. (2007) Imaging the Abeta-related neurotoxicity of Alzheimer disease. Arch Neurol, 64(10), 1467–1477.

Petersen R.C., Doody R., Kurz A., Mohs R.C., Morris J.C., Rabins P.V., Ritchie K., Rossor M., Thal L. & Winblad B. (2001) Current concepts in mild cognitive impairment. Arch Neurol, 58(12), 1985–1992.

Petersen R.C., Smith G.E., Waring S.C., Ivnik R.J., Tangalos E.G. & Kokmen E. (1999) Mild cognitive impairment: clinical characterization and outcome. Arch Neurol, 56(3), 303–308.

Turken A.U. & Dronkers N.F. (2011) The neural architecture of the language comprehension network: converging evidence from lesion and connectivity analyses. Front Syst Neurosci, 5 1.

Vergara E.F. & Behrens M.I. (2013) [Default mode network and Alzheimer's disease]. Rev Med Chil, 141(3), 375–380.

Wang Y., Risacher S.L., West J.D., McDonald B.C., Magee T.R., Farlow M.R., Gao S., O'Neill D.P. & Saykin A.J. (2013) Altered default mode network connectivity in older adults with cognitive complaints and amnestic mild cognitive impairment. J Alzheimers Dis, 35(4), 751–760.

Whitwell J.L., Przybelski S.A., Weigand S.D., Knopman D.S., Boeve B.F., Petersen R.C. & Jack C.R., Jr. (2007) 3D maps from multiple MRI illustrate changing atrophy patterns as subjects progress from mild cognitive impairment to Alzheimer's disease. Brain, 130(Pt 7), 1777–1786.

Wu X., Li R., Fleisher A.S., Reiman E.M., Guan X., Zhang Y., Chen K. & Yao L. (2011) Altered default mode network connectivity in Alzheimer's disease—a resting functional MRI and Bayesian network study. Hum Brain Mapp, 32(11), 1868–1881.

Medicine Sciences and Bioengineering – Wang (Ed.)
© *2015 Taylor & Francis Group, London, ISBN: 978-1-138-02684-1*

Sedative and hypnotic effects of *Schisandra* polysaccharides

Chun-mei Wang, Wei-jing Sun, He Li, Jing-hui Sun, Hao Jia,
Jian-guang Chen & Xin-tian Fan*
College of Pharmacy, Beihua University, Jilin, China

ABSTRACT: The aim of this study was to investigate the sedative and hypnotic effects of *Schisandra* polysaccharide. 40 ICR mice, weighing 20 ± 2 g, half male and half female, were randomly divided into 4 groups, namely, control (distilled water), high-dose *Schisandra* polysaccharide, moderate-dose *Schisandra* polysaccharide, and low-dose *Schisandra* polysaccharide groups. The mice were orally given *Schisandra* polysaccharide continuously for 7 days. After the last administration, effects of *Schisandra* polysaccharide on autonomic activities of the mice were observed using an independent activity recorder; effects of *Schisandra* polysaccharide on the sleep number, sleep latency, and sleep time of mice treated with a subthreshold dose of sodium pentobarbital were observed. The results showed that *Schisandra* polysaccharide could significantly reduce the number of autonomic activities, increase the sleep number, shorten the sleep latency, and prolong the sleep time of mice treated with the threshold dose of sodium pentobarbital, indicating that *Schisandra* polysaccharide has a sedative and hypnotic effect in mice.

1 INTRODUCTION

Sleep disorders and the number of sleep-deprived people are increasing steadily, which seriously harms human health. Currently available drugs used for the treatment of insomnia in the clinic mostly induce hangover, tolerance, dependence, and other adverse reactions in varying degrees. Therefore, finding safe and effective sedative-hypnotic drugs is of great significance. *Schisandra* (*Schisandra Chinensis Baill*) has been recorded in the first division of Pharmacopoeia of the People's Republic of China. It is described as a Chinese herbal medicine that has a tranquilizing effect and is worthy of development. It has been proved that both *Schisandra* itself and its extracts have sedative and hypnotic effects (Huo Shuangyan, *et al*, 2005, Wang Wenwen, 2008), but there has been no in-depth study on the sedative and hypnotic effects of its specific ingredients. It is the first to investigate in sedative and hypnotic effects of *Schisandra* polysaccharide.

2 MATERIALS

2.1 *Experimental animals*

ICR mice weighing 20 ± 2 g provided by the Changchun Yisi Experimental Animal Research Center were raised in separate cages; they ate and drank freely at 20°C–25°C for 5 days to adapt to the environment.

---

*Professor Fan Xintian is the corresponding author of this article, and his e-mail address is fanxintian@126.com.

2.2 *Drugs and reagents*

Schisandra polysaccharide with a purity of 50% was provided by the Food Science and Engineering Laboratory, College of Forestry, Beihua University. Sodium pentobarbital (batch number: 090919) was purchased from the Beijing Chemical Reagent Company.

3 METHODS

3.1 *Animal grouping and administration*

40 ICR mice were randomly divided into four groups, including control group (distilled water), high-dose *Schisandra* polysaccharide group (300 mg/kg), moderate-dose *Schisandra* polysaccharide group (150 mg/kg), and low-dose *Schisandra* polysaccharide group (75 mg/kg). Mice in each *Schisandra* polysaccharide group were orally administered the corresponding doses of *Schisandra* polysaccharide 2 times every morning and evening, and those in the control group were given the same volume of distilled water in the same way. The administration volume was 0.1 mL/10 g, and the agents were administered consecutively for 7 days. 8 Hours prior to the last administration, all the mice underwent fasting.

3.2 *Effects of* Schisandra *polysaccharide on autonomic activities of mice*

40 Minutes after the administration, mice in each group were placed in an autonomic activity recorder. After they adapted to the environment for 5 minutes, autonomic activities of mice in each group were recorded, including the number of autonomic activities and standing up within 5 minutes.

3.3 *Effects of* Schisandra *polysaccharide on the sleep of mice treated with the subthreshold dose of sodium pentobarbital*

The subthreshold dose of sodium pentobarbital determined by the preexperiment was 37.5 mg/kg. At 40 min after the last administration (the peak effect appeared at the first 10-15 minutes after the last administration), mice in each group were given sodium pentobarbital (37.5 mg/kg) as an intraperitoneal injection, and then the number of mice who could not show righting reflex for more than 1 minute within 30 minutes and the sleep latency of the mice were recorded.

3.4 *Effects of* Schisandra *polysaccharide on the sleep of mice treated with the threshold dose of sodium pentobarbital*

At 40 min after the last administration, mice in each group were given sodium pentobarbital (49.5 mg/kg) as an intraperitoneal injection, and then the time to fall asleep and the time to wake up of mice were recorded.

3.5 *Statistical analysis*

SPSS 13.0 software was applied for statistical analysis. All the data were described as mean ± standard deviation. Multiple group comparisons were conducted with one-way ANOVA, and $P < 0.05$ meant a significant difference.

4 RESULTS

4.1 *Effects of* Schisandra *polysaccharide on autonomic activities of mice*

Compared with the control group, the moderate-dose and high-dose *Schisandra* polysaccharide groups could significantly reduce the number of independent activities of mice ($P < 0.05$, $P < 0.01$). The results are shown in Figure 1.

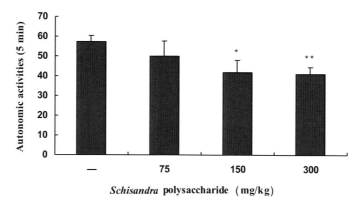

Figure 1. Effects of *Schisandra* polysaccharide on autonomic activities of mice (mean ± standard deviation, $n = 10$).

Note: Compared with those in the control group: $*P < 0.05$, $**P < 0.01$.

4.2 *Effects of* Schisandra *polysaccharide on the sleep of mice treated with the subthreshold dose of sodium pentobarbital*

Compared with the control group, *Schisandra* polysaccharide could increase the number of sleeping mice treated with the subthreshold dose of sodium pentobarbital and shorten the sleep latency ($P < 0.05$, $P < 0.01$). The results are shown in Figure 2.

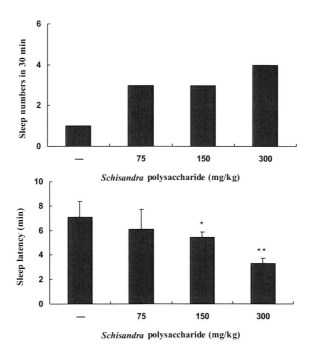

Figure 2. Effects of *Schisandra* polysaccharide on sleep number and latency of mice treated with the subthreshold dose of sodium pentobarbital (mean ± standard deviation, $n = 10$).

Note: Compared with those in the control group: $*P < 0.05$, $**P < 0.01$.

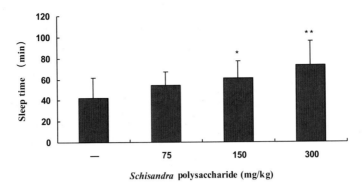

Figure 3. Effects of *Schisandra* polysaccharide on the sleep time of mice treated with the threshold dose of sodium pentobarbital (mean ± standard deviation, $n = 10$).

Note: Compared with those in the control group: $*P < 0.05$, $**P < 0.01$.

4.3 *Effects of* Schisandra *polysaccharide on the sleep time of mice treated with the threshold dose of sodium pentobarbital*

Compared with the control group, moderate-dose and high-dose *Schisandra* polysaccharide could significantly prolong the sleep time of mice treated with the threshold dose of sodium pentobarbital ($P < 0.05$, $P < 0.01$). The results are shown in Figure 3.

5 DISCUSSION

The measurement of autonomic activity is a simple experimental method commonly used to study neuropsychiatric drugs (Chang Cui, *et al*, 2008), and the autonomic activity experiment is an important indicator to evaluate the stimulant state of central nervous system (CNS) in mice. It is reported that the number of autonomic activities is positively correlated with the cerebral cortex excitability in mice (Nan Du & Li-En wang, 2008). In this study, effects of different doses of *Schisandra* polysaccharide on autonomic activities in mice were examined indirectly to explore the polysaccharide's effects on cortical excitability. The results showed that *Schisandra* polysaccharide could reduce the number of autonomic activities in mice, indicating that it has a sedative effect through inhibiting cerebral cortex excitability.

Sodium pentobarbital with a wide range of inhibition on CNS, one of barbiturates, with the increase in dosage, can show different effects. It can shorten REMS and extend NREMS, potentiate the process of CNS depression, and prolong sleep time (Wang Yanwu & Heli, 2010). Therefore, barbiturates have been used for the establishment of experimental models of animals (Zhu Kunjie & Fen Shuyi, 2006). In this experiment, the synergistic effects of threshold/subthreshold doses of sodium pentobarbital with *Schisandra* polysaccharide on the induction of sleep were studied by observing the sleep number, sleep latency, and sleep time of mice. The results showed that *Schisandra* polysaccharide could increase the sleep number, sleep latency, and sleep time in mice treated with threshold/subthreshold doses of sodium pentobarbital, indicating that *Schisandra* polysaccharide has a significant hypnotic effect.

ACKNOWLEDGMENT

This research work was supported by a project of Jilin province's education department (No. 2013-185).

REFERENCES

Huo Shuangyan, Chen Xiaohui, Li Kang, et al. (2005) Sedative and hypnotic effects of *Schisandra*. *Journal of Shenyang Pharmaceutical University*, 22(2), 126–127.

Wang Wenwen, Yang Liuqing. (2008) Sedative and hypnotic effects of each extract of Fructus Schisandrae in mice. *Journal of Jiangsu University (Medical Science)*, 18(2), 122–123.

Chang Cui, Song Lingling, Yang Hongtu, et al. (2008) Study on the sedative and hypnotic effects of Wuweizi Ningshen Oral Liquid in different ratios of drugs. *China Pharmacist*, 8(11), 884–886.

Nan Du, Li-En wang. (2008) Augmentative effect of tetrandrine on pentobarbital hypnosis mediated by 5-HT1A and 5-HT2A/2V receptors in mice. *Journal of Chinese Pharmaceutical Sciences*, 17(3), 192–196.

Wang Yanwu, Heli. (2010) Study on the improvement of Bailing Shuimian Capsule on sleeping function. *Journal of Applied Preventive Medicine*, 16(1), 49–50.

Zhu Kunjie, Fen Shuyi. (2006) Observation on sedation and hypnosis of diazepam and pentobarbital on two kinds of mice. *Progress in Modern Biomedicine*, 6(8), 44–45.

Medicine Sciences and Bioengineering – Wang (Ed.)
© *2015 Taylor & Francis Group, London, ISBN: 978-1-138-02684-1*

Three polymorphisms in Programmed cell Death 1 Ligand (PD-L1) gene are not associated with Aplastic Anemia (AA) in Chinese Han populations

Zhi-jun Ming[1]
Department of Pharmacology, College of Pharmaceutical Science, Suzhou, China

Yi-guo Jiang[1]
Department of Pharmacology, College of Pharmaceutical Science, Suzhou, China
Affiliated Children's Hospital, Soochow University, Suzhou, China

Miao Miao
Department of Hematology, First Affiliated Hospital, Suzhou, China

Wei-peng Wang & Yi Zhang
Department of Pharmacology, College of Pharmaceutical Science, Suzhou, China

Xue-guang Zhang* & Yu-hua Qiu*
Medical Biotechnology Institute, Suzhou, China

ABSTRACT: Three PD-L1 Single-Nucleus Polymorphisms (SNPs) were selected to study the association with AA. It was found that the three PD-L1 SNPs had no obvious differences between AA group and normal control. The polymorphism distribution in rs7042084 and rs12002985 did not exist in the Chinese population. Our results indicated that polymorphisms of three PD-L1 genes might not be involved in the genetic background of AA patients in the Chinese population.

1   INTRODUCTION

Aplastic Anemia (AA) is a heterogeneous disease characterized by the failure of bone marrow hematopoiesis, which results in varying degrees of pancytopenia with a markedly hypocellular bone marrow (Young, 2000). More researchers realized that AA might be an immune-mediated disease (Dufour *et al*, 2009). The dysfunction of T cells might be the reason for the pathogenesis of AA (Solomou *et al*, 2007).

Programmed cell Death 1 (PD-1) and its Ligands (PD-L1) are negative costimulatory molecules that can inhibit T-cell proliferation and downregulate immune responses (Fife *et al*, 2009). Studies showed that the PD-L1/PD-1 pathway could contribute to the development of many autoimmune diseases. PD-1 SNPs have been associated with several autoimmune disorders such as systemic lupus erythematosus (SLE) (Prokunina *et al*, 2002), type 1 diabetes (T1D) (Ni *et al*, 2007), rheumatoid arthritis (RA) (Prokunina *et al*, 2004 & Kong *et al*, 2005), multiple sclerosis (MS) (Kroner *et al*, 2005), and ankylosing spondylitis (AS) (Lee *et al*, 2006). PD-L1 SNPs have also been reported with several autoimmune disorders such as grave's disease (GD) in Japanese populations (Hayashi *et al*, 2008) and AS in a Chinese population (Yang *et al*, 2011). Three PD-L1 SNPs were associated with autoimmune Addison's disease (AAD) in the United Kingdom and a Norwegian population and also associated with GD in a United Kingdom population (Mitchell *et al*, 2009).

---

[1] These authors equally contributed to the paper.
* Corresponding author. E-mails: smbxuegz@public1.sz.js.cn; qyh820@126.com. Fax: 0086-512-65880020.

Our previous study had showed that SNPs of PD-1 (rs11568821, rs2227981, rs10204525, and rs2227982) were not associated with AA (Ming *et al*, 2012), whereas the polymorphism of PD-1 (rs36084323) was associated with AA (Wu *et al*, 2013). As one ligand of PD-1, PD-L1 might usually play an important role in PD-1/PD-L1 negative regulation pathways, but whether the polymorphisms of PD-L1 gene would also be associated with AA was not known. In the present study, three PD-L1 SNPs in 196 normal controls and 200 AA patients were detected and compared in a Chinese Han population.

2   MATERIAL AND METHODS

2.1   *Study subjects and sample collection*

A total of 200 patients with AA (116 females and 84 males) with a mean age of 31.9 ± 17.0 years were recruited into the study from the Department of Hematology, First Affiliated Hospital of Soochow University, China. The diagnosis of AA was established on the basis of the WHO diagnostic criteria for AA. The control group was made up of 196 normal individuals who underwent a health examination in the Health Center of the First Affiliated Hospital of Soochow University. They had no previous medical history and no abnormal laboratory results. All the subjects and controls were of Chinese origin and were matched for age and sex. Samples were obtained from subjects after they provided written informed consent. This study was carried out with the approval of the East ethics committee of the First Affiliated Hospital of Soochow University.

2.2   *Polymorphism genotype of PD-L1 gene*

Genomic DNA was extracted from the peripheral blood of each subject according to standard protocols (Genomic DNA kit; Qiagen). The eight genetic polymorphisms of PD-L1 were directly genotyped by PCR (Biometre, Germany). PCR was performed in a reaction volume of 15 μL containing 8 μL of Premix Taq (Takara, Japan), 1 μL of allele-specific primer and common primer, 1 μL of genomic DNA, and 5 μL of double-distilled water (ddH2O) to make up a final volume of 15 μL. The PCR system was as follows: initial denaturation at 95°C for 10 min, which was followed by 35 cycles of denaturation at 95°C for 30 sec, annealing for 30 sec, and extension at 72°C for 1 min, followed by a final extension at 72°C for 10 min. Primer sequences were designed by us. The primers, product length, and annealing temperature are shown in Table 1. The PCR products (5 μL) were analyzed on 1.5% agarose gels (Biowest, Spain). Ten to fifteen percent of all samples were regenotyped blind for each assay to ensure fidelity of genotyping (99% for each SNP).

Table 1.   The primers, product length, and annealing temperature of three PD-L1 SNPs.

Locus/rs	Primer name	Sequence (5–3)	Fragment size	Annealing temperature
rs2297137	Allele-specific primer	aggcattccactgttcaagag		
		aggcattccactgttcaagaa		
	Common primer	ccagctggttgcaactaatgcaaga	231bp	54°C
rs7042084	Allele-specific primer	gaacctattcttccagtactgg		
		gaacctattcttccagtactgt		
	Common primer	aatagtggcattacctgagccagta	717bp	62°C
rs12002985	Allele-specific primer	gtgatgccagtactgtgtaac		
		gtgatgccagtactgtgtaag		
	Common primer	cagttagaaccaccaagtcccatat	595bp	55°C

2.3 Statistical analysis

The genotype frequency and allelic frequency distributions in the polymorphisms in both AA patients and controls were analyzed by the χ2 method. SPSS Version 10.0 software was used to analyze the data. A P-value that was less than 0.05 was considered statistically significant. Allelic frequencies were expressed as a percentage of the total number of alleles. Odds ratios (ORs) were calculated from genotype frequencies and allelic frequencies with 95% confidence interval (95% CI). Adherence to the Hardy-Weinberg equilibrium constant was tested using the test with one degree of freedom.

3 RESULTS

The allele frequencies of three PD-L1 SNPs are shown in Table 2. The results showed that polymorphisms of the three PD-L1 genes in AA patients and controls were not significantly associated (see Table 2). The polymorphism distribution in rs7042084 and rs12002985 did not exist in the Chinese population.

Table 2.   Genotype and allele frequencies of PD-L1.

SNP rs number	AA patients (%)	Controls (%)	P-value	OR (95% CI)
rs2297137				
Genotype				
AA	52 (26%)	60 (32.61%)		
AG	96 (48%)	72 (39.13%)		
GG	52 (26%)	52 (28.26%)	0.188	
Allele				
A	200 (50%)	192 (52.17%)		
G	200 (50%)	176 (47.83%)	0.547	1.091 (0.822−1.448)
rs7042084				
Genotype				
TT	120 (100%)	120 (100%)		
TG	0 (0%)	0 (0%)		
GG	0 (0%)	0 (0%)	—	
Allele				
T	240 (100%)	240 (100%)		
G	0 (0%)	0 (0%)	—	—
rs12002985				
Genotype				
GG	0 (0%)	1 (%)		
CG	0 (0%)	0 (%)		
CC	120 (100%)	120 (100%)	0.318	
Allele				
G	0 (0%)	2 (0.83%)		
C	240 (100%)	240 (99.17%)	0.158	0.992 (0.98−1.003)

4 DISCUSSION

PD-L1 gene SNPs indicated excellent candidate alleles for autoimmune diseases because of their negative function in T-cell regulation and in the maintenance of peripheral tolerance. The human PD-L1 gene, which is located on chromosome 4p24, is composed of 7 exons and 6 introns. It encodes a 290-amino acid type I transmembrane protein designated PD-L1, a member of the B7/CD28 family. According to the NCBI SNP database, there are 417 known polymorphism loci in human PD-L1 gene. For most of them, the association with diseases and biological function are not confirmed. Many studies have showed that polymorphisms of PD-L1 are associated with autoimmune diseases in different populations.

Our result showed that three PD-L1 polymorphisms were not associated with AA. The polymorphism distribution of PD-L1 rs12002985 and rs7042084 could not be found in the Chinese Han population in our study. To our knowledge, this is the first time that the association of PD-L1 gene polymorphisms with AA in a Chinese population is reported. PD-L1 genetic polymorphisms might not be involved in the pathogenesis of AA. More polymorphism distributions of PD-L1 genes will be further investigated.

ACKNOWLEDGMENTS

This work was supported by a grant from the National Natural Science Foundation of China (NSFC 81373236) and the Priority Academic Program Development of Jiangsu Province (PAPD).

REFERENCES

Young, N.S. (2000) Hematopoietic cell destruction by immune mechanisms in acquired aplastic anemia. *Semin Hematol*, 37:3–14.

Dufour, C., Ferretti, E., Bagnasco, F., Burlando,O., Lanciotti, M., Ramenghi, U., Saracco, P., Van Lint, M.T., Longoni, D. & Torelli, G.F. (2009) Changes in cytokine profile pre- and post-immunosuppression in acquired aplastic anemia. *Haematologica*, 94:1743–1747.

Solomou, E.E., Rezvani, K., Mielke, S., Malide, D., Keyvanfar, K., Visconte, V., Kajigaya, S., Barrett, A.J. & Young, N.S. (2007) Deficient CD4+ CD25+ FOXP3+ T regulatory cells in acquired aplastic anemia. *Blood*, 110:1603–1606.

Fife, B.T., Pauken, K.E., Eagar, T.N., Obu, T. & Wu, J. (2009) Interactions between PD-1 and PD-L1 promote tolerance by blocking the TCR-induced stop signal. *Nat Immunol*, 10:1185–1192.

Prokunina, L., Castillejo-López, C., Oberg, F., Gunnarsson, I., Berg, L., Magnusson, V., Brookes, A.J., Tentler, D., Kristjansdóttir, H. & Gröndal, G. (2002) A regulatory polymorphism in PDCD1 is associated with susceptibility to systemic lupus erythematosus in humans. *Nat Genet*, 32:666–669.

Ni, R., Ihara, K., Miyako, K., Kuromaru, R., Inuo, M., Kohno, H. & Hara, T. (2007) PD-1 gene haplotype is associated with the development of type 1 diabetes mellitus in Japanese children. *Hum Gene*, 121:223–232.

Prokunina, L., Padyukov, L., Bennet, A., de Faire, U., Wiman, B., Prince, J., Alfredsson, L., Klareskog, L. & Alarcón-Riquelme, M. (2004) Association of the PD-1.3A allele of the PDCD1 gene in patients with rheumatoid arthritis negative for rheumatoid factor and the shared epitope. *Arthritis Rheum*, 50:1770–1773.

Kong, E.K., Prokunina-Olsson, L., Wong, W.H., Lau, C.S., Chan, T.M., Alarcón-Riquelme, M. & Lau, Y.L. (2005) A new haplotype of PDCD1 is associated with rheumatoid arthritis in Hong Kong Chinese. *Arthritis Rheum*, 52:1058–1062.

Kroner, A., Mehling, M., Hemmer, B., Rieckmann, P., Toyka, K.V., Mäurer, M. & Wiendl, H. (2005) A PD-1 polymorphism is associated with disease progression in multiple sclerosis. *Ann Neurol*, 58:50–57.

Lee, S.H., Lee, Y.A., Woo, D.H., Song, R., Park, E.K., Ryu, M.H., Kim, Y.H., Kim, K.S., Hong, S.J. & Yoo, M.C. (2006) Association of the programmed cell death 1 (PDCD1) gene polymorphism with ankylosing spondylitis in the Korean population. *Arthritis Res Ther*, 8:163.

Hayashi, M., Kouki, T., Takasu, N., Sunagawa, S. & Komiya, I. (2008) Association of an A/C single nucleotide polymorphism in programmed cell death-ligand 1 gene with Graves' disease in Japanese patients. *Eur J Endocrinol*, 158:817–822.

Yang, Q., Liu, Y., Liu, D., Zhang, Y. & Mu, K. (2011) Association of polymorphisms in the programmed cell death 1 (PD-1) and PD-1 ligand genes with ankylosing spondylitis in a Chinese population. *Clin Exp Rheumatol*, 29:13–18.

Mitchell, A.L., Cordell, H.J., Soemedi, R., Owen, K., Skinningsrud, B., Wolff, A.B., Ericksen, M., Undlien, D., Husebye, E. & Pearce, S.H. Programmed death ligand 1 (PD-L1) gene variants contribute to autoimmune Addison's disease and Graves' disease susceptibility. *J Clin Endocrinol Metab*, 94(2009):5139–5145.

Ming, Z.J., Hui, H., Miao, M., Qiu, Y.H. & Zhang, X.G. (2012) Polymorphisms in PDCD1 gene are not associated with aplastic anemia in Chinese Han population. *Rheumatol Int*, 32:3107–3112.

Wu, Z., Miao, M., Qiu, Y., Qin, Z., Wang, J., Jiang, Y., Ming, Z. & Zhang, X. (2013) Association between polymorphisms in PDCD1 gene and aplastic anemia in Chinese Han population. *Leuk Lymphoma*, 54:2251–2254.

Medicine Sciences and Bioengineering – Wang (Ed.)
© *2015 Taylor & Francis Group, London, ISBN: 978-1-138-02684-1*

Quantitative relationship between mental fatigue and sustained attention: A CPT study

Yi-xuan Lv

School of Biological Science and Medical Engineering, Beijing University of Aeronautics and Astronautics, Beijing, China

Yi Xiao

National Key Laboratory of Human Factors Engineering, China Astronaut Research and Training Center, Beijing, China

Qian-xiang Zhou*

School of Biological Science and Medical Engineering, Beijing University of Aeronautics and Astronautics, Beijing, China

ABSTRACT: To study the influence of mental fatigue on sustained attention, we studied performance and subjective rating in two tasks: mental-fatigue-inducing task (2-back) and sustained attention [Continuous Performance Task (CPT)]. Fourteen healthy male volunteers participated in this experiment who were required to perform 2-back task for 120 min. Before and after the 2-back task, they finished CPT task as well (10 min). The results showed that the performance was significantly decreased and the levels of mental fatigue were significantly increased. Furthermore, linear regression analysis was used to achieve the quantitative relationship among the 2-back, the subjective rating, and the CPT task.

1 INTRODUCTION

Mental fatigue was a gradual and cumulative process and may lead to reduced efficiency, change in behavioral performance, and impaired cognitive ability (Lal and Craig, 2001). For mental fatigue studies, it is important to induce mental fatigue statement. 0-/2-back was used to represent a lower/higher mental load task, which could be performed without/with working memory (Shigihara Y *et al*, 2013) and may reveal the mechanism of mental fatigue. 2-back task has been successfully applied to induce mental fatigue to examine their neural mechanisms (Tanaka, M *et al*, 2014). Sustained attention is also called vigilance, refers to focus on a special event, while excluding the distracting things (Wang S *et al*, 2013). Continuous Performance Task (CPT) is the most widely used to evaluate sustained attention (Shalev L *et al*, 2011). CPT is a simple task which requires participants to concentrate on a continuous stream of stimuli and to press a prespecified key when the target was presented on the computer screen. Many researchers illustrated that mental fatigue would impair sustained attention, but the quantitative relationship, to the best of our knowledge, is still unclear. The object of this research was to evaluate the effects of mental fatigue on sustained attention, and establish a quantitative relationship between them.

---

*Qian-xiang Zhou. Address: School of Biological Science and Medical Engineering, Beijing University of Aeronautics and Astronautics, Beijing 100191, China. E-mail address: zqxg@buaa.edu.cn.

2 MATERIAL AND METHODS

2.1 Participants and experimental design

Fourteen healthy male volunteers from the Beijing University of Aeronautics and Astronautics participated in the experiment. Their age ranged from 21 to 35 years (28.3 ± 4.3, mean $\pm$ SD). All of them were right-handed, nonsmoker, no personal or familiar history of psychiatric or color blindness. Subjects were required to have a regular sleep prior to their test day. Before starting the experiment, all the participants gave informed written consent. Each participant was asked to attend a practice before the formal experiment to ensure that everyone was familiar to the tasks. Experiment included two tasks, mental-fatigue-inducing task (2-back) and sustained attention-evaluating task (CPT). Before and after the 120 min mental-fatigue-inducing task, participants performed CPT for 10 min and finished the questionnaire. The experiment conducted in a quiet lab.

2.2 Mental-fatigue-inducing task

Stimuli were the white numbers "0–9" which presented in a central location on a black background computer screen. Participants were required to judge whether the letter presented on the screen was the same as the one presented two trials back. If it was same, pressed the "F" key, but if it was not, pressed the "J" key, and performed the task as correctly and as quickly as possible. Each stimulus was presented on the screen for 500 ms, and stimulus onset asynchrony (SOA) was 1500–3000 ms. Both stimuli and SOAs were selected randomly. The couple target numbers (e.g., 3-X-3) represented 33% of the total stimuli. To evaluate the change of mental fatigue, the task duration was divided into pre-10 min and post-10 min. Percentage correct was measured.

2.3 Sustained attention-evaluating task

A modified CPT was designed by E-prime 2.0 to evaluate sustained attention. Stimuli were the three colors (red, green, and blue) number "0–9" which presented in random location on a black background computer screen. Each stimulus was presented on the screen for 500 ms, and stimulus onset asynchrony (SOA) was 1500–3000 ms. Both stimuli and SOAs were selected randomly. The targets were red "3" and green "9," which represented 15% of the total stimuli, respectively. Participants were instructed to press the space bar as soon as possible, and to withhold responses to all other stimuli. Reaction times (RTs) and percentage error were obtained. A response was regarded invalid, if RT was <100 ms and excluded from the analysis.

2.4 Subjective rating

A subjective fatigue questionnaire proposed by the Japanese Association for Industrial Health (JAIH) in 1971 was used in this experiment (Park, J et al, 2001). Participants were required to rate the levels of their attention, sleepiness, and fatigue on a scale from 1 (minimum) to 10 (maximum).

3 RESULT

3.1 Mental-fatigue-inducing task

The changes of pre-10 min and post-10 min in this task performance are shown in Figure 1. Comparing pre- and post-10 min, 2-back correct (%) was significantly decreased ($p = .009$).

3.2 Subjective rating

Participant's subjective rating before and after the mental fatigue task is shown in Figure 2. After the 2-back task, subjective levels of attention ($p = .000$), sleepiness ($p = .000$), and fatigue ($p = .000$) were notably increased.

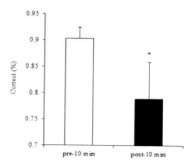

Figure 1.   2-back performance

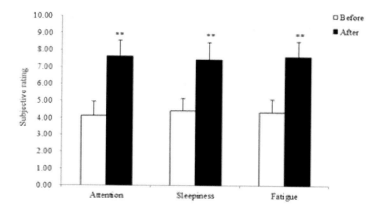

Figure 2.   Subjective rating

3.3   *Sustained attention-evaluating task*

Task performances before and after the mental-fatigue-inducing task are shown in Figures 3 and 4. After the 2-back task, the RT and the error (%) were markedly increased ($p = .018$, $p = .023$, respectively).

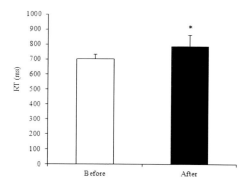

Figure 3.   CPT performance-RT

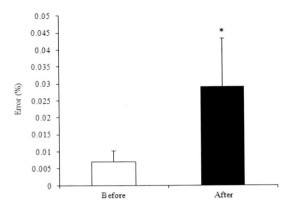

Figure 4.   CPT performance-error (%)

3.4   *Linear regression analyses*

When the correlation coefficient between subjective questionnaire scores (fatigue item, as independent variable x) and the CPT performance outcome (error %, as dependent variable y) was $R_1 = 0.553$ ($p = .002$), the results of a linear regression analysis showed that the slope was 0.006, the y-intercept was –0.016, namely the regression equation is $y = 0.006x - 0.016$ ($R_1^2 = 0.306$) (Figure 5). When the correlation coefficient between 2-back performance outcome (correct %, as independent variable x) and the CPT performance outcome (RT-ms, as dependent variable y) was $R_2 = -0.754$ ($p = .000$), the results of a linear regression analysis showed that the slope was –784.696, the y-intercept was 1410.643, namely the regression equation is $y = -784.696x + 1410.643$ ($R_2^2 = 0.569$) (Figure 6).

4   DISCUSSION

Different inducing factors may lead to different types of mental fatigue, such as work memory, sleep restriction/deprivation, and a long-term, monotonous performance of some simple/mental tasks. To clarify the mechanism of mental fatigue, the inducing method should include one inducing factor and simultaneously abandon the others. The 2-back task required work memory and

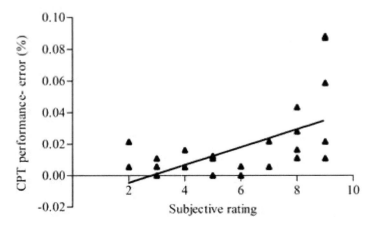

Figure 5.   Relationship between subjective rating and CPT performance, [error (%)]

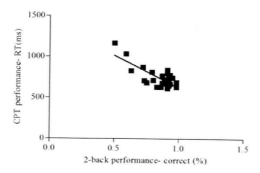

Figure 6. Relationship between 2-back performance [error (%)] and CPT performance [RT (ms)].

higher mental load to induce mental fatigue. Compared with the 2-back task, 0-back is a lower mental load, more monotonous task, and no work memory task, which may induce another type of mental fatigue. Although these two types of mental fatigue have been illustrated (Shigihara Y *et al*, 2013), the effects on sustained attention require further study.

5 SUMMARY

Mental fatigue would impair the sustained attention. Results showed that performing 120-min 2-back task influenced the sustained attention, for the RT and the error (%) of CPT performance was significantly increased. The quantitative relationship among subjective rating, 2-back performance, and the CPT performance could suggest the real condition.

ACKNOWLEDGEMENTS

This work was supported by the Technology Foundation of National Science under Grant A0920132003; the Natural Science Foundation of China under Grants 31170895 and 71201148; the opening foundation of the Science and Technology on Human Factors Engineering Laboratory, Chinese Astronaut Research and Training Center under Grant HF2013-K-06; the National Basic Research Program of China (973 program) under Grant 2011CB711003; the foundation of the National Key Laboratory of Human Factors Engineering under Grants HF2011-Z-Z-A-01, HF2011-Z-B-02, HF2011-Z-Z-B-02, and HF2012-Z-B-02; and China Manned Space Medical Engineering Advanced Research Project under Grant 2012SY54B1701.

REFERENCES

Lal, S. K., & Craig, A (2001) A Critical Review of the Psychophysiology of Driver's Fatigue. *Biological Physiology* 55, 173–194.
Park, J., Kim, Y., Chung, H. K., & Hisanaga , N (2001) Long Working Hours and Subjective Fatigue Symptoms. *Industrial health*, 39(3), 250–25.
Shalev, L., Ben-Simon, A., Mevorach, C., Cohen, Y., & Tsal, Y (2011) Conjunctive Continuous Performance Task (CCPT)—A Pure Measure of Sustained Attention. *Neuropsychologia*, 49(9), 2584–2591.
Shigihara Y, Tanaka M, Ishii A, et al (2013) Two Types of Mental Fatigue Affect Spontaneous Oscillatory Brain Activities in Different Ways. *Behavior Brain Function*, 9(2):1–12.
Tanaka, M., Ishii, A., & Watanabe, Y (2014) Neural Effects of Mental Fatigue Caused by Continuous Attention Load: A Magnetoencephalography Study. *Brain research*, 1561, 60–66.
Wang S, Yang Y, Xing W, et al (2013) Altered Neural Circuits Related to Sustained Attention and Executive Control in Children with ADHD: An Event-related fMRI Study. *Clinical Neurophysiology*, 124(11): 2181–2190.

Medicine Sciences and Bioengineering – Wang (Ed.)
© *2015 Taylor & Francis Group, London, ISBN: 978-1-138-02684-1*

Standardized development of the thyroid operation anesthesia under neuromuscular electric monitoring

Peng Chen, Yu-huan Pan, Jia Zhao & Yang-dong Han*
Department of Anesthesiology, China-Japan Union Hospital, Ji Lin University, Changchun, Jilin, China

ABSTRACT: Intraoperative recurrent laryngeal nerve monitoring (IONM) is a revolutionary technology that is developed and successfully used for the thyroid operation intraoperative identifying and positioning recurrent laryngeal nerve in recent years. In the recurrent laryngeal nerve-monitoring determination, anesthesia is the main interference factor. This paper retrospectively summarizes 3029 cases of thyroid operation anesthesia under recurrent laryngeal nerve monitoring in our hospital from September, 2011 to November, 2013, aiming at exploring the standardized development of the thyroid operation anesthesia under neuromuscular electric monitoring.

1 MATERIAL AND METHOD

General data: Of 3029 cases, there are 2568 female and 461 males, aged from 19 to 71 years old, with the weight from 37 to 109 kg. Among these, there are 2313 thyroid cancer operation cases, 738 second operation cases, 189 third operation cases, 213 preoperative concurrent recurrent laryngeal nerve injury cases, and 11 nonrecurrent recurrent laryngeal nerve cases. ASA classification is Level I or Level II.

Anesthesia Method: Patients are intramuscularly injected 1 mg of penehyclidine hydrochloride 30 minutes earlier to the operation. The venous access is opened and the ECG, NIBP, $SpO2$, and $PetCO2$ are continuously monitored after admission. Midazolam 2 mg, propofol 2 mg/kg, sufentanil 0.5 mg/kg, and rocuronium bromide 0.3 mg/kg (batch number: H20040423, Organon Company, the Netherlands) are intravenously injected after implanting the shoulder pad (Figure 1). After 5 minutes, the recurrent laryngeal nerve-monitoring special tracheal tube (Medtronic Xomed Company, USA) is inserted. In this group, there are 576 cases adopting the conventional laryngoscope cooperating with beroptic laryngoscope to intubate and position in the early stage. All the other cases use the video laryngoscope to intubate and position. The score standard of Cooper method is adopted to evaluate the endotracheal intubation conditions and record the circumstances of the blood pressure and pulse changes. Anesthesia maintenance adopts sevoflurane—oxygen inhalation to maintain, maintaining the depth of anesthesia in 1.4–1.6 MAC (Monitored Anesthesia Care) during the operation. NIM-Response 2.0 or NIM-Response 3.0 Nerve Electromyography Monitor is used to monitor nerve electromyogram signals during the operation. After the operation, the anesthesia is reduced. Once the depth of anesthesia achieves 0.1 MAC, the respiration is manually controlled. When the patient opens his/her eyes and recovers autonomous respiration, the tracheal tube is removed. Observing for 15 minutes, when the general state of the patient achieved stable, the patient is sent back to the thyroid surgery recovering room. The patient is under postoperation follow-up for 24 hours.

---

*Corresponding Author: Han Yangdong, Email: 295253720@qq.com.

2 RESULTS

All the patients are inserted special monitoring tracheal tube successfully. The endotracheal intubation conditions of the patients are satisfactory, and the endotracheal intubation reactions are minimal. All the patients are measured vagus nerve/recurrent laryngeal nerve signal (V/R signal) amplitude, and the continuity of the signals meet the monitoring demands. The operations of all the patients are successfully completed. Intraoperative adverse events include: 227 cases of bucking and air way resistance increasing during the endotracheal intubation; 167 cases need adjustment of the tracheal tube position, among these, 129 cases being too deep, 38 cases rotating; in 19 cases the signals are not stable as intraoperative oral secretion is high; in 147 cases intraoperative body movement or hemodynamics are not stable; 1 case of oral mucosa injury, hemorrhage; 176 cases of sore throat when making the postoperation follow-up; 234 cases of pharyngeal discomfort; 19 cases of postoperative hoarseness and arytenoid dislocation; 3 cases of aspiration pneumonia; 21 cases of xerophthalmia; 21 cases of the patients' neck region behind the ears being numb and discomfortable; 49 cases of conjunctival hyperemia.

3 DISCUSSION

The incidence of the thyroid disease has been rising in recent years. Recurrent laryngeal nerve injury is a common complication of the complicated thyroid operation. Intraoperative recurrent laryngeal nerve monitoring (IONM) is a revolutionary technology that can reduce the probability of recurrent laryngeal nerve injury (Dralle H, Sekulla C, Lorenz K et al, 2008 & Sturgeon C, Sturgeon T, Angelos P, 2009). In the recurrent laryngeal nerve-monitoring determination, anesthesia has been the main interference factor. This paper summarizes the experience that our hospital develops the thyroid operation anesthesia under neuromuscular electric monitoring in recent years, aiming at exploring the standardized development of the thyroid operation anesthesia under neuromuscular electric monitoring.

1. The key point of the thyroid IONM anesthesia is the anesthesia induction period; the difficulty is the correct usage of the nondepolarizing muscle relaxant and the placement of IONM tracheal tube.

The use and the residue of muscle relaxant will interfere the monitoring results of the nerve electromyogram signals (Horne Sk, Gal TJ, Brennan JA, 2007 & Peng Chen, Feng Liang, Zhenbo Su, 2012), bringing about a false positive result that recurrent laryngeal nerve continuity breaks off, so the thyroid specialists do not use less muscle relaxant.

In other countries, because patients are relatively fewer, and the professional anesthesiologists are enough, the common method involves the use of nondepolarizing muscle relaxant or no muscle relaxant induction to solve this problem. In China, as the amount of the patients are large and the professional anesthesiologists are lacking, the inherent disadvantage of using nondepolarizing muscle relaxant induction and the operational difficulties of the no muscle relaxant induction attribute to less use of this method by anesthesiologists. Our experience is to recommend on using rocuronium bromide for anesthesia induction, the specific dosage is $1 \times$ ED95 rocuronium bromide, and it can slightly add the dosage of the general anesthetics and acesodyne on the basis of the conventional dosage or only the conventional dosage. In one study, we compared the nerve electromyogram signal amplitude obtained from using $1 \times$ ED95 rocuronium bromide induction with that obtained from inhaling sevoflurane induction. The results show that although the signal amplitude obtained from $1 \times$ ED95 rocuronium bromide induction is lower, it can completely meet the operation requirements, and it can meet the anesthesiologists' muscular relaxation demand of the endotracheal intubation (Xiuli Meng, Jun Wang, Liping Zhang, 2006).

On the placement of IONM tracheal tube: (1) we recommend placing at the position first, then making the endotracheal intubation, because in the traditional method the endotracheal intubation is first, then the position, which may cause the inward shift of the tracheal tube during the positioning process. It results in the tracheal tube being too deep, making the measurement of the signal inaccurate. (2) In the laryngoscope field, we recommend the use of video laryngoscope. Otherwise, we recommend labeling the monitoring tracheal tube first, then the endotracheal intubation. The vertical line of the labeled line should maintain in the central position, and the horizontal line of the labeled line should join with the vocal cord. Fiberoptic bronchoscopy shall be used to position (Figure 3).

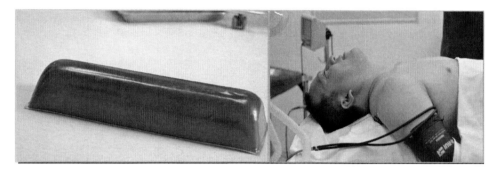

Figure 1.

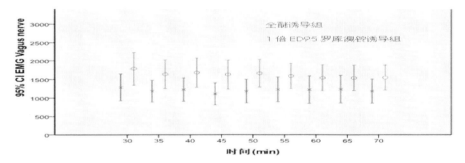

Figure 2.

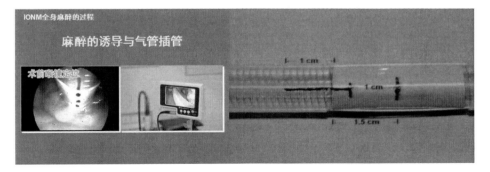

Figure 3.

2. The rule in the anesthesia maintenance period: because the request of thyroid operation on muscular relaxation is extremely low, the thyroid operation under recurrent laryngeal nerve monitoring need not use muscle relaxant as far as possible, so we recommend to not use muscle relaxant in the whole anesthesia maintenance period, except for the anesthesia induction period. It suggests that the departments which have the end-tidal air-monitoring condition use sevoflurane to maintain and the depth of anesthesia is in 1.4–1.6 MAC or so. Because this depth not only meets the anesthesia and analgesia requirements, but also can produce certain centrally acting muscle relaxation effect, and have no influence on monitoring signals (Meng Xiuli, Wang Jun, Zhang Liping, 2006). If no end-tidal air-monitoring facilities, it can use general anesthesia or intravenous inhalational anesthesia. The rule is that the anesthesia depth should not be too shallow in the anesthesia maintenance period and should be steady as far as possible.

3. In the postanesthetic recovery period, it should recover the patients spontaneously; decrease the complications of anesthesia such as dysphoria. Our experience is: not reduce the anesthesia before completing the operation, and pull in shoulder pad, dress the wound after the operation. On gradually reducing the anesthesia depth, after 10 minutes, the anesthesia depth can go down to 0.1 MAC or so in general. In this process, especially when the anesthesia depth is about 0.2–0.3 MAC, it must not have any movements that stimulate the patients, or it will be easy to cause dysphoria. When the anesthesia depth is achieved below 0.1 MAC, the respiration is manually controlled. When the autonomous respiration recovery is satisfactory, after the patients' recovery, remove the tracheal tube and encourage the patients to cough. If the patients appear coughing or recovering the autonomous respiration before the anesthesia depth goes down to 0.1 MAC, it can directly turn to the manual control and assisted respiration, but it should not stimulate the patients or too big tidal volume manual control, to avoid iatrogenic injuries such as sore throat and throat discomfort.

4. The special circumstances and their handle in the perioperative period:

    (1) Signal disappearing: Among the thyroid operation under recurrent laryngeal nerve monitoring, the surgeons care the most about the stability of the signal. The signals decreasing or disappearing, except for the operation reason, the common reasons are: the excessive use of nondepolarizing muscle relaxant, tracheal tube shifting (too deep, too shallow or rotating), loop electrode falling off, mechanical malfunction, and so on, among which the first three are most common.

    (2) The reason of the signal's instability might be related to following: the influence of airway secretions, for example, the patients are always in the light anesthesia state, not using anticholinergic drugs before the operation, the length of the operation are too long, all these factors can make the patients' oral secretions increase, influence the conduct of the nerve electromyogram signals, causing the signal acquisition not stable; the incorrect use of electrosurgical generator, sounding electrode can induce other muscle groups to produce bioelectrical signals, superimpose with the recurrent laryngeal nerve electromyogram signals, resulting in the unsteady signals.

    (3) The common reason that patients cough, airway resistance increase during the endotracheal intubation process is the shallow anesthesia. It suggests that the thyroid operation anesthesia induction period under recurrent laryngeal nerve monitoring should adopt deep anesthesia. The recommended dosage: intravenously inject midazolam 2 mg, propofol 2 mg/kg, sufentanil 0.5 mg/kg to induce. Besides, because the modes of Medtronic Xomed Company's tracheal tube are more single, it might not have appropriate tracheal tube. If the sizes are small, be careful that the cuff pressure should not be too large, to avoid cuff convex influencing the tube inner diameter and causing compression injury on tunica mucosa tracheae.

    (4) The intraoperative body movement or hemodynamics are not stable, because the anesthesia depth is not stable. In the anesthesia induction period, the direct inhibition of intravenous anesthesia drugs on the myocardium and the too long fasting time result in the relatively deficiency of the patients' circulation volume before the anesthesia. It can result in the lower

170

blood pressure after the induction. Some anesthesiologists are accustomed to adopting the method of reducing the anesthesia to gain relatively "satisfactory" hemodynamics index; during the operation, because the maintenance period does not use muscle relaxant, considering the misgivings "not enough anesthesia," it might make the anesthesia too deep. To recover hemodynamics index as quickly as possible after making the anesthesia too deep, the anesthesia should be reduced quickly. These two circumstances in the clinical anesthesia might result in intraoperative body movement or hemodynamics being not stable, so we recommend using end-tidal air monitoring or BIS(bispectral index) monitoring to maintain the stable anesthesia depth. If not aware of the conditions, experienced anesthesiologists should do the anesthesia management, especially be careful that not reduce the anesthesia too early whereby the patients would recover slowly before completing the operation.

(5) The common reason of postoperative hoarseness and arytenoid dislocation is the incorrect use of video laryngoscope. Generally, video laryngoscope is not zero degree mirror, and compared with the usually used laryngoscope, it might have certain visual deviation. One case of this group had pharyngeal side wall mucosa injury, hemorrhage, because of the incorrect use of video laryngoscope. The use of video laryngoscope should be trained before go into the practical operation. Besides, that the modes of recurrent laryngeal nerve-monitoring tracheal tube produced by Medtronic Xomed Company are not enough might be one of the reasons. Our experience is encouraging the patients to cough immediately when removing the tracheal tube might have good therapeutic effect. Besides, the following day after the operation, the fiber bronchoscope check by the department has important significance on discovering and treating the arytenoid dislocation in time.

(6) Conjunctival hyperemia, xerophthalmia: Because of the long time of operation, the head operation, the improper bedding of the sterile sheets, may result in patients' hypophasis, causing conjunctival hyperemia or xerophthalmia, especially being careful about the catacleisis circumstance of the patients after the anesthesia who have done double eyelid surgery before. 21 cases of this group postoperatively happened xerophthalmia, among these, 17 cases are the patients who have done double eyelid surgery before, so we recommend using eye paste or smearing the spongarion.

(7) Facial numbness: Mostly caused by too long hypsokinesis of head, it should reduce the operation time as far as possible. Make the explanation work preoperatively and go on the preoperative train.

To sum up, the thyroid operation anesthesia under neuromuscular electric monitoring can adopt the anesthesia scheme that uses $1 \times$ ED95 rocuronium bromide cooperating with deep anesthesia induction, intraoperatively inhaling sevoflurane to maintain the anesthesia depth. It should strengthen the thorough understanding of this technology, strengthen postoperation follow-up, and be good at discovering the problem, communicating with the specialists in time, accumulating experience together.

REFERENCES

Dralle H, Sekulla C, Lorenz K, et al. Intraoperative monitoring of the recurrent laryngeal nerve in thyroid surgery. *World J Surg*, 2008, 32(7):1358–1366.

Horne Sk, Gal TJ, Brennan JA. Prevalence and Patterns of intraoperative nerve monitoring for thyroidectomy. *Otolaryngol Head Necksurg*, 2007;136:952–956.

Peng Chen, Feng Liang, Zhenpo Su et al. The effect of 1×ED95 Rocuronium Bromide used for anesthesia induction on introperative recurrent laryngeal nerve monitoring of the patients with thyroid operation, *Chinese Journal of Anesthesiology*, 2012, 32(5):525–527.

Sturgeon C, Sturgeon T, Angelos P. Neuromonitorine in thyroid surgery, attitudes, usage patterns and predictors of use among endocrinesurgeons. *WOrld J Surg* 2009;33:417–425.

Xiuli Meng, Jun Wang, Liping Zhang, The effect of Atracurium on otologic surgery facial nerve monitoring, *Chinese Journal of Minimally Invasive Surgery*, 2006, 29(2):137–141.

Medicine Sciences and Bioengineering – Wang (Ed.)
© *2015 Taylor & Francis Group, London, ISBN: 978-1-138-02684-1*

The effect of different concentrations of vecuronium bromide used for anesthesia induction on intraoperative recurrent laryngeal nerve monitoring of patients with thyroid operation

Peng Chen, Yu-Huan Pan & Feng Liang*
Department of Anesthesiology, China-Japan Union Hospital, Ji Lin University, Changchun, Jilin, China

ABSTRACT: Objective: Evaluate the effect of $1 \times$ ED95 or two times of vecuronium bromide used for anesthesia induction on the thyroid operation intraoperative recurrent laryngeal nerve monitoring. Methods: Select 117 cases of thyroid operation patients, male or female, aged 23–67 years old, with a weight of 52–84 kg. The ASA classification is level I or II. Adopt the method of the table of random numbers, and randomly divide them into three groups: Group I ($n = 39$), Group II ($n = 40$), Group III ($n = 38$). Intravenously inject midazolam 2 mg, propofol 2 mg/kg, and sufentanil 0.5 ug/kg in turn. After the eyelash reflex disappears, intravenously inject vecuronium bromide 0.05 mg/kg to Group I and vecuronium bromide 0.1 mg/kg to Group II. After 5 minutes, insert recurrent laryngeal nerve monitoring special tracheal tube; Group III inhales sevoflurane, and recurrent laryngeal nerve monitoring special tracheal tube is inserted when the end-tidal concentration achieves 4%. After the endotracheal intubation, make the mechanical ventilation, inhaling sevoflurane–nitrous oxide–oxygen to maintain the anesthesia. Record the endotracheal intubation condition scores of each group. Adopt nerve electromyography monitor to monitor recurrent laryngeal nerve–evoked myogenic potential. When the operation continues to the 30-minute time point, record the amplitude of the evoked myogenic potential every 5 minutes until the operation continues to the 70-minute time point; monitor SBP, DBP, and HR during the experimental process. Results: During the experimental process, SBP, DBP, and HR are all maintained in the normal ranges. The one-time success rates of endotracheal intubation of the three groups are all 100%, but compared with Group III the endotracheal intubation condition evaluations of Groups I and II are higher ($P < .05$); Groups I and III all get effective nerve electromyogram signals at each time point, and compared with Group III the nerve electromyogram signals of Group I decrease at each time point ($P < .05$), but the electromyogram signals can meet the monitoring demands. The patients of Group II lose signal at the 30-minute time point, and the recurrent laryngeal nerve–evoked electromyogram signals at the 35-, 40-, and 45-minute time points cannot meet the monitoring demands. Conclusion: $1 \times$ ED95 vecuronium bromide used for the anesthesia induction of thyroid operation patients not only does not only provide satisfactory endotracheal intubation condition but also does not influence intraoperative recurrent laryngeal nerve monitoring.

1 INTRODUCTION

Thyroid operation adopts intraoperative neuromonitoring (IONM) for recurrent laryngeal nerve monitoring. It can give early warning about the distance between the operative site and the recurrent laryngeal nerve and avoid the damage of the intraoperative recurrent laryngeal nerve. The use of a nondepolarizing muscle relaxant during anesthesia induction is the main interference factor in the IONM determination process. Studies have shown that only $2 \times$ ED95 dose of nondepolarizing

---

*Corresponding author: Liang Feng, E-mail: 295253720@qq.com.

muscle relaxant during the anesthesia induction can interfere with intraoperative recurrent laryngeal nerve monitoring (Hui Sun, Xiaoli Liu, Yantao Fu et al, 2010 & Xiuli Meng, Jun Wang, Liping Zhang, 2006). Vecuronium bromide is the most widely used nondepolarizing muscle relaxant at home. This study intends to evaluate the effect of different concentrations of vecuronium bromide used for anesthesia induction on intraoperative recurrent laryngeal nerve monitoring of thyroid operation patients.

2 MATERIAL AND METHOD

This study has got approval from our hospital ethics committee, and the patients and family members have signed informed consent forms. We will select a time to apply general anesthesia on the thyroid operation patients of 117 cases, aged 23–67 years old, weighing 52–84 kg, male or female. The ASA classification is level I or II. Adopt the method of the table of random numbers, and randomly divide them into three groups: Group I ($n = 39$), Group II ($n = 40$), and Group III ($n = 38$). Intramuscularly inject penehyclidine hydrochloride 1 mg 30 minutes before anesthesia. Routinely monitor ECG, BP, SpO2, and the inspired and expired concentrations of sevoflurane after admission; open the venous access; and inject lactated Ringer's solution (infusion rate is 6–8 mL/kg×h). Anesthesia induction: the three groups are intravenously injected midazolam 2 mg, propofol 2 mg/kg, and sufentanil 0.5 ug/kg in turn. After the eyelash reflex disappears, Group I is intravenously injected 1 × ED95 vecuronium bromide 0.05 mg/kg (batch number: H20040423, Organon Company, The Netherlands) and Group II is intravenously injected 2 × ED95 vecuronium bromide 0.1 mg/kg (batch number: H20040423, Organon Company, The Netherlands). After 5 minutes, use a video laryngoscope to insert recurrent laryngeal nerve monitoring special tracheal tube (Medtronic Xomed Company, USA) for mechanical ventilation; Group III inhales 8% sevoflurane, with the oxygen flux 6 L/min. Use a video laryngoscope to insert recurrent laryngeal nerve monitoring special tracheal tube for mechanical ventilation 10 seconds after the end-tidal concentration achieves 4%. Ventilatory factors settings: inspiratory to expiratory ratio 1:2, tidal volume 10–12 mL/kg, and respiratory frequency 12/min. Anesthesia maintenance: the patients of the three groups all inhale sevoflurane–nitrous oxide–oxygen to maintain the depth of anesthesia; the depth of anesthesia is maintained in 1.2–1.4 MAC. Complete the vagus nerve exposure 30 minutes after the success of endotracheal intubation. Endotracheal intubations are completed by the same senior anesthetist.

Adopt the score standard of Cooper method to evaluate the endotracheal intubation conditions, see Table 1. Adopt the NIM-Response 3.0 Nerve Electromyography Monitor (Medtronic Xomed Company, USA) to monitor recurrent laryngeal nerve–evoked myogenic potential. With 1-mA electric current to stimulate, record electromyogram signal amplitude (μV) every 5 minutes after the nerve exposure, monitoring nine groups of signals continuously. Record the circumstances of blood pressure and pulse changes at the same time.

Adopt SPSS16.0 statistics software to analyze; measurement data are showed by mean ± standard deviation ($\bar{x} \pm s$). Repeated measurement data adopt variance analysis of repeated measurement design, enumeration data comparison adopts Chi-square test, and ranked data adopt rank-sum test. $P < 0.05$ means the differences have statistical significance.

Table 1. The score standard of Cooper method endotracheal intubation condition.

Laryngoscope examination	Glottis	Intubation reaction	Score
Impossible	Closed	Cough	0
Difficult	Closed up	Cough slightly	1
General	Active	Slight diaphragm activity	2
Easy	Open	No reaction	3

Note: The total score of 8 to 9 is excellent, 6 to 7 is great, 3–5 is general, 0–2 is poor.

3 RESULTS

The one-time success rates of endotracheal intubation of three groups are all 100%, but compared with Group III the endotracheal intubation condition evaluations of Groups I and II are higher ($P < 0.05$) and Groups I and II do not have obvious differences. Groups I and III all get effective nerve electromyogram signals at each time point, and compared with Group III the nerve electromyogram signals of Group I decrease at each time point ($P < 0.05$), but the recurrent laryngeal nerve–evoked electromyogram signals can meet the monitoring demands. The patients of Group II lose signal at the 30-minute time point, and the recurrent laryngeal nerve–evoked electromyogram signals at 35-, 40-, and 45-minute time points cannot meet the monitoring demands. The intraoperative DBP, SBP, and HR are all in the normal range, see Tables 2 and 3.

4 DISCUSSION

In a thyroid operation, IONM has been the supplementary means of identifying recurrent laryngeal nerve standard. In USA, the usage rate of IONM is 40%–45% (Hemmerling TM, Donati F, 2003 & Sharpe MD, Moote CA, Lam AM, et al, 1991). Medtronic Xomed NIM-Response 3.0 Nerve Electromyography Monitor and special recurrent laryngeal nerve monitoring tracheal tube are the most advanced monitoring facilities, so this study on intraoperative recurrent laryngeal nerve monitoring adopts Medtronic Xomed NIM-Response 3.0 Nerve Electromyography Monitor and special recurrent laryngeal nerve monitoring tracheal tube. Intraoperatively adopts sevoflurane to maintain the anesthesia, because its blood and air partition coefficient is 0.63. It has small effects on hemodynamics and neuromuscular junction function and can eliminate the influence of anesthetic and hemodynamics factors on recurrent laryngeal nerve monitoring.

The results of this study show that the following: The one-time success rates of the endotracheal intubation of the three groups are all 100%, but compared with Group III the endotracheal intubation condition evaluations of Groups I and II are higher ($P < 0.05$); Groups I and II do not have obvious differences. Groups I and III all get effective nerve electromyogram signals at each time point, and compared with Group III the nerve electromyogram signals of Group I decrease at each time point ($P < 0.05$), but the electromyogram signals can meet the monitoring demands. The patients of Group II lose signal at the 30-minute time point, and the recurrent laryngeal nerve–evoked electromyogram signals at 35-, 40-, and 45-minute time points cannot meet the monitoring demands. Note: $1 \times ED95$ vecuronium bromide used for the anesthesia induction not only does not provide better endotracheal intubation condition but also does not influence thyroid

Table 2. The comparison of endotracheal intubation condition evaluations of the three groups.

Group	N	Excellent	Great	General	Poor
I	39	34 (87%)	5 (12%)	0	0
II	40	37 (92%)	3 (7%)	0	0
III[ab]	38	24 (63%)	9 (23%)	5	0

Note: Compared with Group I, [a]$P < 0.05$; compared with Group II, [b]$P < 0.05$.

Table 3. The comparison of recurrent laryngeal nerve electromyogram signal amplitudes (μV) of the three groups (μV, $\bar{x} \pm$ s).

Group n	30 min	35 min	40 min	45 min	50 min	55 min	60 min	65 min	70 min
I ($n = 39$)	1103 ± 8400	1196 ± 687	1155 ± 1004	1109 ± 846	1258 ± 847	1326 ± 879	1407 ± 951	1466 ± 1046	1426 ± 981
II ($n = 40$)	—	101 ± 69^a	165 ± 103^a	168 ± 91^a	487 ± 38^a	646 ± 257^a	989 ± 362^a	1291 ± 401^a	1320 ± 387
III ($n = 38$)	1795 ± 1140^{ab}	1687 ± 969^{ab}	1657 ± 116^{ab}	1528 ± 879^{ab}	1606 ± 108^{ab}	1598 ± 1107^b	1507 ± 1109^b	1493 ± 936^b	1432 ± 879

Note: Compared with Group I, [a]$P < 0.05$; compared with Group II, [b]$P < 0.05$.

intraoperative recurrent laryngeal nerve monitoring. The reasons might be as follows: (1) The acquisition of nondepolarizing muscle relaxant ED95 dose is using a muscular relaxation monitor to monitor adductor pollicis, and different muscle groups have different pharmacodynamics for nondepolarizing muscle relaxant. Compared with adductor pollicis, the onset and recovery time of the nondepolarizing muscle relaxant blocking the laryngeal adductor muscle are faster. This may be because, in terms of unit mass, the blood flow of adductor pollicis is less than that of laryngeal muscles, and the spreading and elimination of muscle relaxant in the muscle groups of high blood flow are faster than that in the muscle groups of low blood flow (Plaud B, Debenb B, Lequeau F, et al, 1999 & Hemmerling TM, Schmidt J, Hanusa C, et al, 2000 & Jun Tang, 1997). (2) The dose of vecuronium bromide used in the anesthesia induction period is less and shortens the time of clinical effect. The study shows that the clinical effect time of $2 \times$ ED95 vecuronium bromide is 40–50 minutes and the clinical effect time of $1 \times$ ED95 is less than 30 minutes, but it needs at least 30 minutes from the moment of endotracheal intubation to intraoperative recurrent laryngeal nerve monitoring.

To sum up, $1 \times$ ED95 vecuronium bromide used in the anesthesia induction period not only does not provide better endotracheal intubation condition but also does not influence thyroid intra-operative recurrent laryngeal nerve monitoring.

REFERENCES

Hemmerling TM, Donati F. Neuromuscular blockade at the larynx, the diaphragm and the corrugator super-cilii muscle: a review. *Can J Anaesth*, 2003, 50(8): 779–794.

Hemmerling TM, Schmidt J, Hanusa C, et al. Simultaneous determination of neuromuscular block at the larynx, diaphragm, adductor pollicis, orbicularis oculi and corrugator supercilii muscles. *Br J Anaesth,* 2000, 85(6): 856–860.

Hui Sun, Xiaoli Liu, Yantao Fu et al. Application of intraoperative neuromonitoring during complex thyroid operation. *Chinese Journal of Practical Surgery,* 2010, 30(1): 66–68.

Jun Tang. The effect of muscle relaxant on different muscles. *Foreign Medical Sciences (Anesthesiology and Resuscitation)*, 1997, 19(4):200–203.

Palohe MP, Wilson RC, Edmonds HL Jr, et al. Comparison of neuromuscular blockade in upper facial and hypothenar muscles. *J Clin Monit,* 1988, 4(4): 256–260.

Plaud B, Debenb B, Lequeau F, et al. Mivacurium neuromuscular block at the adductor muscles of the larynx and adductor pollicis in humans. *Anesthesiology,* 1999, 85(1): 77–81.

Sharpe MD, Moote CA, Lam AM, et al. Comparison of integrated evoked EMG between the hypothenar and facial muscle groups following atracurium and vecuronium administration. *Can J Anaesth,* 1991, 38(3): 318–323.

Xiuli Meng, Jun Wang, Liping Zhang. The effect of Atracurium on otologic surgery facial nerve monitoring, *Chinese Journal of Minimally Invasive Surgery,* 2006, 29(2): 137–141.

Medicine Sciences and Bioengineering – Wang (Ed.)
© 2015 Taylor & Francis Group, London, ISBN: 978-1-138-02684-1

Study on the determination of anticancer drug nedaplatin in a spectrophotometer

Juan Peng, Jian He, Qing-kun Wang & Shao-ping Pu
Kunming Gui Yan Pharmaceutical Co. Ltd., Kunming, China

ABSTRACT: Determine the anticancer drug nedaplatin in silver, the acid condition, TMK solution, and the silver ions red complex. Color depth is positively related to the amount of silver; in 0–25 µg/25 mL, good linear relationship is shown. The maximum absorption wavelength is 540 nm, and the molar absorptive is $\varepsilon540 = 9.1 \times 104$ L·mol^{-1}cm^{-1}. Determination of nedaplatin samples can be applied under this condition. The results and the original absorption spectra are consistent.

1 INTRODUCTION

Nedaplatin (254 S, CDGP) is a kind of platinum development Japan Shionogi & Co. the antitumor drugs, listed in Japan in 1995. Nedaplatin in head and neck tumor with more than 40% efficiency, better than cisplatin, efficacy and cisplatin on lung cancer, esophageal cancer has on the efficiency of more than 50%, 20% higher than cisplatin, effective rate of cervical cancer has been more than 40%. Nedaplatin has good curative effect, is less toxic, and has the side effects of a new generation of platinum anticancer drugs. It is highly soluble in water; all kinds of animal tumors, in a wide range of dosage, showed better effect with nedaplatin. Renal toxicity and animal digestive organ toxicity are low. Europe and the United States and other countries have put silver on monitoring index (Cacas, 2014). Nedaplatin of the silver ion is introduced in the production process, in order to reduce Nedaplatin toxicity. Control and determination of silver in silver products in the production process is very important and necessary. Silver-controlled anticancer drugs have been reported (Cacas, 2010, Cacas, 2009), but the silver Nedaplatin in platinum anticancer drugs was determined by spectrophotometry and was not reported in the literature.

2 EXPERIMENTAL SECTION

2.1 *Instruments and reagents*

Instruments: Japan Shimadzu UV-2450UV spectroscopy. ZEEnit700 atomic absorption spectrometer.

Reagent: 1 TMK solution: concentration is 1.3×10^{-5} M/mL ethanol solution; under brown bottle storage, it can be stored for one week. 2 silver standard solutions: formulated with pure silver nitrate analysis, liquid reserve is 1 µg/mL when used with a 0.1 N dilution of 10 µg/mL.

2.2 *Experimental principles*

A TMK solution and the silver ions red complex are used; color depth is related to the silver content. The analysis can be colorimetric. In 0–25 µg/25 mL, good linear relationship is shown.

2.3 Experimental methods

Draw 10 µg/mL standard solution of silver in 1 mL, 25 mL volumetric flask; add 1 mL of 0.1 N nitric acid and add 1 mL of TMK solution with shaking. Use water to dilute to scale, and shake. In spectrophotometer curettes, with 1 cm than to do, reagent blank absorbance Determination of absorbance.

3 RESULTS AND DISCUSSION

3.1 Silver complex absorption spectrum

According to the experimental method, draw 10 µg/mL standard solution of silver in 1 mL, 25 mL volumetric flask; add 1 mL of 0.1 N nitric acid and add 1 mL of TMK solution with shaking. Use water to dilute to scale, and shake. In spectrophotometer cuvettes, with 1 cm than to do, reagent blank absorbance determination reference.

Results are shown in Figure 1 that the maximum absorption wavelength is 540 nm, thus 540 nm is chosen as the actual measuring wavelength.

3.2 Chromomeric agent selections

The TMK solution and the silver ions in the acidic conditions form a red complex. Color depth is related to the silver content, and the analysis can be colorimetric. In 0–25 µg/25 mL, good linear relationship is shown. See Figure 2.

3.3 The influence of pH

Experiments show that the silver complexes have a stable absorbance in the pH range of 3 to 4; the experiment was performed at pH 3.2.

3.4 Effect of the dosage of TMK

When the dosage of TMK was 0.8–1.2 mL, complexes of high absorbance and stability were obtained. Method is chosen to join 1 ml volume.

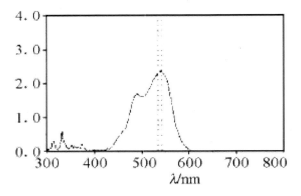

Figure 1.   The Ag TMK absorption spectra of the complexes.

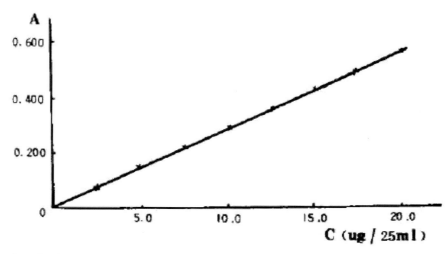

Figure 2. Absorbance and concentration of silver.

3.5 *Standard curves*

Experiments show that the silver content of Bill's law is in accordance with the 0–25 μg/25 mL range (see Figure 2). The molar absorptive is calculated as $_{\varepsilon 540} = 9.1 \times 10^4$ L·mol^{-1}cm^{-1}. The calibration curve linear regression equation is given as A = 0.025 × Cag + 0.002.

The correlation coefficient is given as follows: r = 0.999.

3.6 *Stability of the chromomeric agent*

Ag–TMK complexes colored completely in 5 minutes, and in 1 hour they were stable. Afterward, the absorbance gradually decreased.

3.7 *Sample analysis*

Determination of the steps that take 0.1 nedaplatin in a 50-mL beaker, Join 1:1 10 ml heated and dissolved nitrate. After cooling, a quantitative filter paper is dissolved in a 250-mL volumetric flask. With the same concentration of dilute nitric acid to scale, shake. At the same time, keep reagent blank. Draw a certain volume (silver containing about 1 μg/mL) placed in a 25-mL volumetric flask for the standard test method for observing color and measuring the absorbance.

Detection of drawing: learn and test the same volume of reagent blank solution in a 25-mL volumetric flask, adding 0, 1, 2.5, 5, 7.5, 10, 15, and 20 μg of silver standard solution, test solution. A method is applied to in accordance with the above operation. The analysis results are as follows:

The above results show that nedaplatin silver meets the European and United States Pharmacopoeia standards. This method is validated in 10 batches with a pass rate of 100%.

Table 1. Analytical results of samples of silver.

Samples	The actual amount	Measured	Adding quantity	The measured total	Recovery rate	RSD%
	ZEEnit700	/μg • g^{-1}	/μg • g^{-1}	/μg • g^{-1}		
1	2.15	2.11	5	7.17	100.3	2.7
2	1.01	0.98	5	5.96	99.2	2.6
3	3.19	3.11	5	8.16	99.6	2.5

CONCLUSIONS

Under the acidic condition, after silver with TMK solution reaction of nedaplatin sample handling in the form a red complex, color depth are related with the silver content which can be colorimetric. In the range 0–25 µg/25 mL, good linear relationship is shown. Determination of nedaplatin can be applied to the sample.

REFERENCES

HeJian etc. patent no. 200910094394.0 (already authorized) China's patent.
Li xue jie et al Guangzhou Huagong 2010, 38 (12).
EDQM Publication European Pharmacopoeia 8.2 supplement 07/2014.

Medicine Sciences and Bioengineering – Wang (Ed.)
© *2015 Taylor & Francis Group, London, ISBN: 978-1-138-02684-1*

Species and plant morphology and biological characteristics of Banlangen (*Radix isatidis*) in China

Gang Chen, Su-ping Wang & Xiang Huang
Wuhan Institute of Agricultural Sciences, Wuhan, China

Juan Hong & Mi-hong Ge
Wuhan Institute of Agricultural Sciences, Wuhan, China
College of Resources and Environment, Huazhong Agricultural University, Wuhan, China

Li-hong Zhang & Lei Du
Wuhan Institute of Agricultural Sciences, Wuhan, China

ABSTRACT: Banlangen (*Radix isatidis*) is an herbal medicine, and it grows in various parts of China. It can be classified into North *Radix isatidis* and South *Radix isatidis*. Different regions have different varieties; these species are different in terms of shape and biological characteristics with geographical variation. With the rising demand of users all over the world, more and more popularly used herbal plants are now grown in agricultural fields. This article provides a brief review on the morphological and biological characteristics of wild and cultivated varieties of *Radix* in China, so as to provide some reference for *Radix* planting.

1 INTRODUCTION

Banlangen (*Radix isatidis*) includes North *Radix isatidis* and South *Radix isatidis*. North *Radix isatidis* is derived from the root of a kind of cruciferous plant—*Isatis tinctoria* L.—and Daqing grass (*Isatis indigotica* Fort); South *Radix isatidis* is derived from the rhizomes and root of Acanthaceae cusia (*Strobilanthes blume* S. L.). *Isatis tinctoria* L. belongs to the cruciferous family, including about 30 species worldwide. *Isatis tinctoria* L. is mainly distributed in the Mediterranean Sea east of Central Asia and Iran spit blue region of its distribution center eastward up to Sakhalin and Japan, as well as North and Central and North America; there are six varieties, with three distributed in northern China, including Hebei, Beijing, Heilongjiang, and Henan (Li, 2001).

South *Radix isatidis* originated in the Assam region of northern India. There are 115 varieties, 1 variant, and an introduced species, which is widely cultivated in subtropical southern China, including Fujian, Taiwan, Guangdong, Guangxi, and Zhejiang (Deng, 2007). Both North and South *Radix isatidis* have good medicinal value. For instance, *Folium isatidis* S. (Dyers Woad Leaf) is effective against influenza and herpes simplex virus (Fang, 2005; Wang, 2006). Extensive research has been conducted on *Radix isatidis* in terms of its medical value and action mechanisms (Peng, 2005; Xie et al., 2011), chemical composition (Ye, 2011), and extraction of active ingredients (Chen et al., 2011). At the same time, some progress has also been made in the breeding of *Radix isatidis*, such as using 0.05%–0.3% concentration of colchicine solution for growing seedlings to obtain tetraploid plants (Qiao et al., 1989), and studies indicated that the induction effect varied with concentration of colchicine and processing times; with the same concentration the induction rate increased with processing time, whereas the induction rate increased with increasing concentration of colchicine given the same time (Duan et al., 2006). In the past decade, tissue culture method has also been successfully applied to breed *Radix isatidis* (Zhang et al., 2006; Wang et al., 2008; Tu et al., 2009; Zhang et al., 2009; Li et al., 2011).

In the past, most of the species of medicinal materials were originally obtained from wild sources. However, with the rising demand of users all over the world, more and more commonly used herbal plants are now being grown in agricultural fields (Leung and Cheng, 2008). Meanwhile, overharvest of wild medicinal plants enhances the extinction of wild plant species so that agricultural cultivation of these wild species becomes more important (Wang and Xiao, 2000). In recent years, the cultivated area of *Radix isatidis* has been significantly expanded in China. However, the cultivation of Banlangen (*Radix isatidis*) at a large scale may not guarantee high yield and quality as many factors are involved, such as place of cultivation, soil quality, climate change, harvest procedures, storage conditions, etc. (Tang *et al.*, 2004). The efficacy of herbs is also affected by soil, water, and management practices. Herbal plants are vulnerable to different forms of pollutions like pesticides, fertilizers, heavy metals, and other toxic elements (Cheng, 2012). It is believed that medicinal function is embodied by herbs and the formation of the herbs is impacted by environmental conditions, including temperature, precipitation, topography, and soil quality (Tang *et al.*, 2010). Studies on the cause of distinction in antiendotoxic activation of *Radix isatidis* from different cultivated populations showed that pharmacological activity varied in germplasm sources cultivated in the same environment (Liu & Qiao, 1999), indicating that germplasm difference is the primary factor that affects the quality of *Radix isatidis*. However, the difference in activity intensity between different populations and off-site cultivation is related to environmental factors (Liu & Qiao, 1999). This paper attempts to provide a brief account of recent progress in plant morphology and biological characteristics of different varieties and the effects of main environmental factors on the growth and quality of *Radix isatidis* in China and elsewhere.

2 PLANT MORPHOLOGY AND BIOLOGICAL CHARACTERISTICS OF *RADIX ISATIDIS*

There are significant differences in biological characteristics and plant morphology between different varieties of *Isatis tinctoria* L. (songlan). *Isatis tinctoria* L. is a biennial herbaceous plant mainly produced in Hebei, Beijing, Heilongjiang, Henan, Jiangsu, and Gansu. It usually consists of a deep taproot (up to 5–8 mm in diameter) with sallow skin, an upright stem 40-90 cm high, and alternate leaves (larger basal leaves and leaves oblong with petiole). The leaves of *Isatis tinctoria* L. is 3.5–11 cm long and 0.5–3 cm wide, with an obtuse apex, and the leaf margins has obvious serrulate. There is no significant difference between lower and upper epidermal cells of leaves. There are no apparent differences between palisade tissue and spongy tissue, and the vascular bundles of the main vein are well developed (Ye, 2006). *Isatis tinctoria* L. has wide racemes; its flowers are small without involucres, only 3 to 4 mm in diameter with slender pedicels, and each flower has four green sepals and four yellow petals with obovate. It includes six stamens and one oblong pistil. Silique oblong with midrib in a flat wing shape include only one seed. From late April to early May, seeds begin to rapidly accumulate substances, and the grain weight can grow to maximum at 7.41 g in the end of May (Ye, 2006). The reducing sugar and soluble sugar content accumulate rapidly in the early growing stage, reach the peak in mid-April, and then reduce gradually after first sharply decreasing with increasing starch content. The yield and quality of *Isatis tinctoria* vary in the harvesting season; the quality of seeds is usually better when harvested in spring than in autumn. Bolting and flowering of *Isatis tinctoria* is caused by vernalization, and low-temperature treatment of seedlings and seeds can result in advance bolting (Ye, 2006).

Isatis indigotica Fort is mainly distributed in the Yangtze River Basin, China, and there are some cultivation species in Jiangsu and Gansu provinces that are similar to *Isatis tinctoria* L. in plant morphology and biological characteristics. However, its leaves and fruit morphology display a slight difference, with lower part of the leaf being ear shaped and top of the fruit being obtuse with concave block or full truncate. A series of physiological changes occur during the growth of *Isatis indigotica* Fort.

The seeds can quickly absorb water, which can be divided into three stages, namely, a rapid water absorption and a slow water absorption, followed by a slowly spit water period. Seeds begin to rapidly absorb water after being soaked for 2 h, reaching 73.3% of the total amount of water absorption (Bai et al., 2009). At the germination stage, the content of GA_3 reaches its peak, and the content of ABA starts to decline after the seeds are soaked for 24 h to 48 h. α-Amylase and protease are activated and the stored substances start to be decomposed and utilized after 96 h, and then the seeds begin to germinate (Luo, 2003). *Isatis indigotica* Fort plants have obvious midday depression during growth, and the net photosynthetic rate of tetraploid is higher than that of diploid (Guo et al., 2008). The growth peak period of leaves of *Isatis indigotica* Fort is in early July and then the vegetative growth starts to slow down, and the growth peak period of roots is from mid-July to September (Wu, 2008). The leaf area reaches maximum in 20 days after transplanting, and net photosynthetic rate (*Pn*), photochemical efficiency (Fv/Fm), and potential photochemical activity (Fv/F0) attain the highest level after 25 days of transplanting. Its respiration and membrane permeability are then enhanced and various assimilates are exported from the leaves. At the late growth stage, a large quantity of assimilates are transported to the roots, and the dry matter accumulation dynamic follows an "S" curve (Luo, 2003). Some important medicinal ingredients of *Radix isatidis*, such as indigo, indirubin, and polysaccharides, are mostly distributed in the leaves, with the base leaves having the highest content, and only a small portion is stored in the roots, stems, and flowers at the florescence stage. The total amounts of indigo and indirubin are higher at the flowering stage. During this period, more polysaccharide is accumulated in the roots (Tang *et al.*, 2011). The content of active ingredients changes greatly during different growth periods. The peak of its accumulation appears after the vegetative growth stage (Gong, 2005). A rapid accumulation trend occurs in mid-August (Ruan *et al.*, 2010). The contents of indigo and indirubin in leaves include two accumulation peaks in mid-July and mid-September, and the highest level occurs in mid-September (Wu, 2008). Therefore, the leaves should be harvested in mid-July and mid-September, respectively. The biosynthesis peaks of indigo and indirubin in the root of *Isatis indigotica* Fort appear in mid-July and early October, respectively, and the highest level occurs in early October. According to the yield and the concentrations of main active ingredients, the best season of harvest for roots should be early October (Wu, 2008). It must be pointed out that the optimal harvest time varies with the geographical environment.

There are obvious differences in physiological characteristics even for the same species when they are from different geographical locations. Studies have shown that photosynthetic pigment content and net photosynthetic rate display obvious differences among the different populations of *Isatis indigotica* Fort. Photosynthetic pigment content in populations that have leaves with wax and brassica populations is generally greater than those of Shandong, Shanxi, and Sichuan (Guo *et al.*, 2008); intraspecific variation and ecological environmental differences lead to different cultivated populations of *Isatis tinctoria* L. with significantly different microscopic morphologies, accumulation of secondary metabolites, and isozymes (Wang, 1999; Wang, 2000; Dong, 2006).

Baphicacanthus cusia (Nees) is perennial herbaceous and shrubby, with erect stems up to more than 1 m. It has obvious internode with wane and the leaf is opposite with 1 to 2 cm petiole, and its shape is oblong or ovate-oblong, or oval-lanceolate; leaves is oblong to ovate-oblong or oval-lanceolate, apex acuminate, base attenuate, margin shallowly serrate, 5 to16 cm long and 2.5 to 6 cm wide. Studies on *Baphicacanthus cusia* in Fujian province of China showed that there are nonglandular hairs, glandular hairs, and glands scales cover on the root, stem, and leaf external (Huang, 2009). The inflorescence growth at the top stem, spicate the bracts like leaf is length of 1 to 2 cm, caducous, 5 sepals (4 small and1 large) are full crack, corolla funnel-shaped, 5-lobed, 4 stamens and 2 strong. It is located in the upper part of the corolla tube; ovary superior, style slender. One boll contains four seeds. Spring and autumn are the seasons that *Baphicacanthus cusia* gains strong growth; its vegetative stage is in the spring and summer, and reproductive stage emerges in autumn. Its florescence is from the end of November to the end of next February, and the fruit period is from February to the end of March (Du, 2008).

The medicinal ingredient content of *Baphicacanthus cusia* also varied in different growth stages and parts. The contents of indirubin and indigo reach the maximum value in November, so it is the best period for extracting the two substances (Huang et al., 2009). The contents may be determined during the harvest period or season. Studies showed that the content of indirubin shows a trend of reducing with the growth years (Chen, 2011) and the content of indirubin is the greatest in leaves, followed by stems, and lowest in roots (Du, 2008), which is similar to that of *Isatis indigotica* (Tang et al., 2011).

3 CONCLUSIONS

The aforementioned studies focuses on the distribution of *Radix isatidis* varieties in different regions in China and the different biological characteristics of different species; we know that different geographical environments bring obvious effects on the morphology and biological properties of *Radix isatidis*, and they also influence medicinal ingredient content. Additional research should focus on the influence of geographical environmental factors on the growth of *Radix isatidis* and its mechanisms, for example, soil, microclimate, and exogenous nutrients. Such research can establish a sound plant management system to meet the needs of growth of *Radix isatidis* in different regions so that high yield and quality of *Radix isatidis* can be ensured.

ACKNOWLEDGMENTS

The project has been funded by the Wuhan Institute of Agricultural Sciences, and the conditions for learning and research including laboratory, instrument, and learning resources and so on have been provided by the University of Florida.

REFERENCES

Bai, L. D., X. H. Sha, Di-Li-Ti-Ni-Ya-Zi, and Y. H. Guo. 2009. Studies on water absorption characteristics and the germination conditions of *Isatis indigotica* seeds. *Guihaia* 29(6): 836–838.
Chen, X. Q. 2011. Study on key cultivation technologies of *Baphicacanthus cusia* (Nees) Bremek. Guangzhou University of Chinese Medicine: *Master's degree thesis*.
Cheng, K. F., P.C. Leung. 2012. Safety in Chinese Medicine Research. *Open Journal of Safety Science and Technology* 2: 32–39.
Deng, Y. F. 2007. Taxonomic studies on the genus *Strobilanthes blume* S. L. (Acanthaceae) from China. *Kunming Institute of Botany: Doctoral Dissertation*.
Dong, J. Z., S Liang, and W. Qin. 2006. Active ingredient content difference on roots, leaves of *Isatis indigotica* (Radix, Daqingye) from different regions. *Journal of Applied Ecology* 17(9): 1613.
Du, P. X. A research on biological characteristics of *Baphicacanthus cusia*. 2008. *Guangzhou University of Traditional Chinese Medicine: Master's degree thesis*.
Duan, Y. Z., Y. Q. Chen, and F. R. Chai. 2006. A study on induction polyploidy in Isatica Indicago by colchicine treatment. *Journal of Tangshan Teachers College* 28(2): 21–23.
Guo, Q. H., K. C. Wang, X. Q. Tang, and Y. Zhang. 2008. Photosynthetic characteristics of *Isatis indigotica* Fort in autumn. *Jiangsu Journal of Agricultural Sciences* 24(4): 485–491.
Huang, Y. Z. 2009. Fujian study of medicinal plants-*Radix Isatidis*. *University of Fujian Agriculture and Forestry: Doctoral Dissertation*.
Huang, Y. Z., D. R. Pan, Z. C. Wang, W. J. Ning, and Y. F. Zhou. 2009. Effects of different growing period on *Baphicacanthus cusia (Nees)* bremek medicine constituents. *Chinese Agricultural Science Bulletin* 25(16): 75–78.
Leung, P. C., and K. F. Cheng. 2008. Good Agricultural Practice (GAP)-Does it ensure a perfect supply of medicinal herbs for research and drug development? *International Journal of Applied Research in Natural Products* Vol.1(2), pp. 1–8, June/July.
Li, G. Q., Z. T. Wang, X. B. Li, and G. J. Xu. 2001. Isozyme analysis and its systematic significance of *Isatis indigotica* genus. *Journal of Plant Resources and Environment* 10(4): 22–28.
Li, T., W. Y. Lin, and Z. Z. Wang. 2011. Anther culture and haploid induction from *Isatis indigotica* (Cruciferae). *Plant Diversity and Resources* 33(2): 225–228.

Liu, S., C. Z. Qiao, and Y. Wang. 1999. Research on cause of distinction in antiendotoxic activation of *Radix isatidis* from different cultivated populations. *Journal of Chinese Materia Medica*. Volume 24, Issue 7: 398–340.

Luo, L. J. 2003. Yield and quality formation and regulation of Isatis Indigotica Fort. *China Agricultural University, a master's degree thesis*.

Qiao, C. Z., M. S. Wu, F. B. Dai, X. Cui, and Y. Li. 1989. Studies on polyploid breeding of *Isatidis Indigotica* Fort. *Acta Batanica Sinica* 31(9): 678–683.

Ruan, H. S., and L. Cao. 2010. Study on the indirubin contents of changes in *Isatis tinctoria* L. at different growing seasons. *Journal of Anhui Agri. Sci* 38(5): 2328–2329.

Tang, S. H., H. J. Yang, and L. Q. Huang. 2010. Discuss on effect of physical environmental factors on nature of Chinese material medica. *China journal of Chinese Materia Medica* 35(1): 126–128.

Tang, X. Q., K. C. Wang, and X. A. Chen. 2011. Distribution regulation of indigo, indirubin and polysaccharides of *Isatis tinctoria* at florescence. *Chinese Traditional and Herbal Drugs* 42(7): 1425–1428.

Tang, X. Q., K, C. Wang, and X. Chen. 2011. Effects of waterlogging stress on activity of alcohol dehydrogenase and peroxidase in seedlings of *Isatidis indigotica*. *Acta Agriculturae Jiangxi* 23(2): 70–73.

Tang, Y. M., B. Wang, and X. L. Fan. 2004. Daodi materia medica and the guideline of good agricultural practice (GAP) for Chinese materia medica. *Lishizhen Medicine and Materia Medica Research* 15(6): 361–362.

Tu, Y. Q., J. Sun, and X. H. Ge. 2009. Production and analysis of interinal hybrid calli from protoplast fusion between *Isatis indigotica* Fort. and *Brassicaoleracea* L. var. *alboglabra* Bailey. *Chinese Journal of oil Crop Sciences* 31(4): 522–526.

Wang, H., X. H. Wang, and Y. H. Wang. 2008. Hairy root induction of *Isatis indigotica* Fort. and plantlet regeneration. *Crops* 5: 31–35.

Wang, L. X., and L. L. Xiao. 2000. Significance of medicinal botany to the conservation of endangered species In: Conservation of endangered medicinal wildlife resources in China, Zhang ED & Zheng HC (eds) Second Military Medical University Press, Shanghai, China. pp. 83–86.

Wang, W. B., J. Y. Yu, and J. Z. Xu. 2005. Effect of sowing period on motherwort growth. *Research and practice of Chinese Medicines* 19(3): 13.

Wang, Y., C. Z. Qiao, and Z. R. Wang. 2000. Allozyme analysis of different cultivated populations on *Isatis indigotica*. *Second Military Medical University* 20(3): 209.

Wang, Y., Y. Cha, and C. Z. Qiao. 1999. Difference of five kinds of organic acid content from different cultivated populations leaves of *Isatis indigotica*. *Second Military Medical University* 20(6): 374.

Wu, X. H. 2008. Effect of mineral elements on the growth and accumulation of active ingredient in *Isatis indigotica* Fort. *Hunan Agricultural University: Master's degree thesis*.

Ye, Q. 2006. A research on biological characteristics of *Isatis tinctoria*. *Northwest Agriculture and Forestry University of Science and Technology: Master's degree thesis*.

Zhang, J. H., J. Xie, and C. G. Wang. 2006. Application of orthogonal design in tissue culture of *Isatis tinctoria*. *Journal of Hubei University (Natural Science)* 28(2): 183–186.

Zhang, S. Z., S. Y. Ke, and W. X. Meng. 2009. Study on domestication and transplanting technique of tissue culture plantlets of *Isatis indigotica* Fort. *Northern Horticulture* 2: 237–240.

Medicine Sciences and Bioengineering – Wang (Ed.)
© *2015 Taylor & Francis Group, London, ISBN: 978-1-138-02684-1*

Expression changes of Hes1 of PC12 cells after OGD

Jin-ting He
Department of Neurology, China-Japan Union Hospital, Jilin University, Changchun, Jilin Province, China

Le Yan
People's Hospital of Jilin Province, Changchun, China

Jiao-qi Wang & Yang Cui
Department of Neurology, China-Japan Union Hospital, Jilin University, Changchun, Jilin Province, China

Zong-Shu Li
Department of Neurology, China-Japan Union Hospital, Jilin University, Changchun, Jilin Province, China
People's Hospital of Jilin Province, Changchun, China

Jing Mang*, Yan-Kun Shao* & Zhong-Xin Xu
Department of Neurology, China-Japan Union Hospital, Jilin University, Changchun, Jilin Province, China

ABSTRACT: Ischemic stroke occurs when the blood supply to the brain is obstructed, and it is one of the most common worldwide causes of health problems, disability and death. We investigated the expression of Hes1 of PC12 cells in an Oxygen Glucose Deprivation (OGD) model. In this study, we used nerve growth factor to stimulate PC12 cells and converted them into neuron-like cells, then the OGD of PC12 cells was used to establish a cerebral hypoxia-ischemia model in vitro. Flow cytometry analysis, Western blot, and real-time PCR assays were performed. The results showed that the expression levels of Hes1 mRNA and protein were significantly increased after 3 h of OGD treatment, Our results suggested that OGD can up-regulate the mRNA and protein expression levels of Hes1 cerebral ischemic injury may activate the Notch signaling pathway.

1   INTRODUCTION

The ischemic damage of nerve cells leads to the disruption of a series of complex signaling pathways that affect corresponding biological functions and influence brain function; this terminal differentiated profile of the brain is of particular relevance for cerebral ischemia. We investigated the Notch pathway in regulating proliferation and differentiation of adult neural progenitor cells after stroke. There have been rare reports of expression changes after OGD in the Notch signaling pathway in PC12 cells. The mammalian Hes family includes six members, of which HES1 participate in the Notch signaling pathway (L. Pantoni, F. Pescini & S. Nannucci, 2011). An OGD-damage model is one of the more commonly used models for the study of cerebral ischemia. On the basis of the model of OGD of PC12 cells, we detected the apoptosis ratio of PC12 cells due to different exposure time of OGD and the post-OGD mRNA and protein expression levels of the Notch signaling pathway components Hes1. We used this work to explore whether Hes1 plays a role in the process of cerebral ischemia injury at the gene and protein levels, as well as whether the Notch signaling pathway can be activated as part of cerebral ischemic injury (Shudo, Y. *et al*, 2011).

---

*Corresponding authors

2 RESULTS

2.1 OGD up-regulated Notch1 mRNA expression in PC12 cells

PC12 cells were treated with OGD for 3 h, 6 h, 9 h, 12 h, 16 h or 24 h, respectively. Notch1 mRNA expression levels were measured with real-time PCR (Figure 1). Compared to the control group, Notch1 mRNA expression was significantly increased after 3 h of OGD treatment and then gradually decreased with the extension of OGD exposure. However, the expression of Notch1 mRNA after OGD for 24 h remained somewhat higher than that in the control groups. These results indicated that OGD can up-regulate Notch1 mRNA expression in PC12 cells.

2.2 OGD may activate the Notch signaling pathway

PC12 cells were treated with OGD for 3 h, 6 h, 9 h, 12 h, 16 h and 24 h, respectively. Hes1 protein expression levels were determined using Western blots (Figure 2). Compared to the control groups, Hes1 protein expression levels were significantly increased after 3 h of OGD treatment but then gradually decreased with the extension of OGD exposure. However, the protein expression

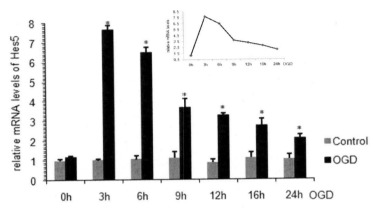

PC12 cells were treated with OGD for 3 h, 6 h, 9 h, 12 h, 16 h and 24 h, respectively. Hes1 mRNA expression level was measured by real-time PCR. Data shown are the mean ± S.E. of relative Hes1 mRNA, measured in three independent experiments and expressed as percentages present compared to the control (untreated) groups, normalized for the cellular expression of ß-actin. *$P < 0.05$.

Figure 1.   The effects of different lengths of OGD treatment on Hes1 mRNA expression in PC12 cells.

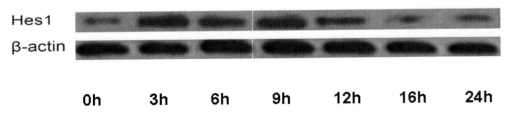

(A) Hes1 protein expression levels at different time points after OGD were measured using western blots. The results shown are representative of three independent experiments. β-actin was used as an internal control. The results indicate that Hes1 protein signal densities increased in OGD groups compared with the control group. (B) Quantitation of the Western blot analysis.

Figure 2.   Western blot analysis. PC12 cells were treated with OGD for 3 h, 6 h, 9 h, 12 h, 16 h and 24 h, respectively.

levels of Hes1 was still slightly higher after OGD for 24 h than in the control groups. These results indicated that OGD may activate the Notch signaling pathway.

3 DISCUSSION

The Notch signaling pathway, a highly conserved system, is under the regulation of the Hes gene family of downstream signal molecules. The Notch pathway has been implicated in the regulation of the fate of several cell types. Notch ligands binding to Notch receptors leads to the cleavage of Notch receptors and the nuclear translocation of Notch intracellular domain (NICD) (N. Sestan, S. Artavanis-Tsakonas, & P. Rakic, 1999)., thereby inducing transcriptional activation of Notch target genes. Hairy/enhancer of split-1 (Hes1) is a well-studied downstream target gene in the Notch signaling pathway (Tara, S *et al*, 2011) Existing animal models are affected by many factors; therefore, a stable cell model of cerebral ischemia was used in this study because of the advantages of the ability to control the experimental conditions, the small amount of sample required and the short experimental period (M. Hayase, *et al*, 2009). In this study, we used NGF to stimulate PC12 cells and converted them into neuron-like cells, which combined with OGD to establish a model of ischemia in nerve cells. We investigated the mRNA and protein expression levels of Notch, Hes1 and Hes5 in an OGD model. Our results showed that the expression levels of Hes1 mRNA and protein increased significantly after 3 h of OGD treatment, and this increase tapered off with the extension of OGD exposure. However, the expression levels of Hes1 remained slightly higher after 24 h of OGD than in the control groups (Chunli Mei *et al*, 2011). The above results indicated that OGD may activate the Notch signaling pathway and that, with OGD, 3 h is the turning point for the activation of the Notch signaling pathway. The above phenomena indicated that the Notch pathway may regulate the apoptosis of cells in the early period of cerebral ischemic injury, but there was no obvious role for Notch signaling after OGD for 12 h. Therefore, further experiments to test the effects of the Notch signaling pathway on the cerebral ischemic injury are needed (S. Oya *et al*, 2009).

4 CONCLUSION

In summary, we have demonstrated for the first time that OGD may up-regulate the mRNA and protein expression levels of Hes1 members of the Notch signaling pathway, and the regulation role changed dynamically with the prolongation of OGD time. We therefore concluded that cerebral ischemic injury may activate the Notch signaling pathway.

5 MATERIALS AND METHODS

5.1 *Cell culture and preparation of the oxygen–glucose deprivation (OGD) model*

PC12 cells were purchased from the Cell Bank of the Chinese Academy of Sciences. PC12 cells were grown at 37°C in 5% CO2. The cells were treated with 100 ng/ml nerve growth factor After 24 h. PC12 cells were treated with NGF (NGF 2.5S; Promega, Madison, WI) for six days. Cells were then washed three times with DMEM, and the cells were cultured with DMEM in the presence of no sugar and 1 mmol/L NaS2O4 in hypoxic conditions (37°C, 5% CO2 and 95% N2) for 16 h (Chunli Mei *et al*, 2011).

5.2 *Flow Cytometry analysis*

To quantitatively assess apoptosis, we used Annexin V-FITC and PI double staining, followed by flow cytometry. The cells were detached using 0.25% trypsin and then harvested, at which point the cells were washed with cold PBS (4°C) three times and floated in195 µL Binding Buffer (1×). The cells were stained with 5 µL Annexin V-FITC (Kaiji Bio Co., Nanjing, China) for 30 min at room temperature in the dark and stained with 5 µL PI staining (Kaiji Bio Co., Nanjing, China) for 5 min. Cells were immediately analyzed using flow cytometry. The signals from apoptotic cells are localized in the lower right quadrant of the resulting dot-plot graph (Han, P; Kang, J.H. & Li, H.L, 2009).

5.3 *Real-Time Polymerase Chain Reaction (RT-PCR)*

Expression levels of the Notch1, Hes1 and Hes5 genes were analyzed using quantitative RT-PCR. Primer sequences were as follows: Hes1, U: 5′-TTC AGC GAG TGC ATG AAC GA-3′ and D: 5′-GTA GGT CAT GGC GTT GAT CT -3′,β-actin, U: 5′-GGT TAC CAG GGC TGC CTT CT-3′ D:5′-ATG GGT TTC CCG TTG ATG AC-3′. Total RNA from cells was extracted using Trizol Plus Columns kit (Invitrogen, USA) according to the manufacturer's specification. cDNA was synthesized with the PrimeScript 1st Strand cDNA Synthesis Kit (TaKaRa, Japan), according to the manufacturer's specification, and then stored at −20°C. Real-time PCR based on SYBR-Green I was performed using the 7500 Fast system (ABI, USA) and SYBR PrimeScript RT-PCR Kit ‖ (TaKaRa, Japan). A 20 µL reaction system was established according to the manufacturer's instructions (Tara, S.; Takagi, G & Mizuno, K, 2011).

5.4 *Western blot analysis*

After the PC12 cells were treated with NGF (100 ng/ml) for 6 days, the samples were treated with OGD for 3 h, 6 h, 9 h, 12 h, 16 h, or 24 h, respectively. Sample cells were washed twice using cold PBS, and 1×10^6 cells were lysed using RIPA buffer [50 mmol/L Tris (pH 8.0), 150 mmol/L NaCl, 0.1% SDS, 1% NP40 and 0.5% sodium deoxycholate] containing protease inhibitors (1% cocktail and 1 mmol/L PMSF). Total protein samples were separated using 15% SDS-PAGE and were transferred to a PVDF membrane. The membrane was blocked using Tris-buffered saline with 0.1% Tween 20 (pH 7.6, TBST) for 1 h at room temperature and was incubated with the primary antibody solution (1:1,000) at 4 °C overnight. After two washes in TBST, the membrane was incubated with the HRP-labeled secondary antibody (Santa Cruz SC-2073) for 1 h at room temperature and was washed three times with TBST (Pieri, A.; Lopes, T.O. & Gabbai, 2011). The final detection was performed using enhanced chemiluminescence (ECL) Western blot reagents (Amersham Biosciences, Piscataway, NJ, USA) and the membrane was exposed to Lumi-Film Chemiluminescent Detection Film (Roche). Loading differences were normalized using a monoclonal ß-actin antibody. The antibodies used in the study included anti-Notch1 (Abcam, rabbit, ab83253) and anti-Hes1 (Abcam, mouse, ab87395) and anti-Hes5 (Abcam, rabbit, ab133424).

6 STATISTICAL ANALYSIS

SPSS software (SPSS10.0, Chicago, IL, USA) was used for statistical analysis, and values were presented as the mean ± S.E. An ANOVA was used to compare the mean values. P-values less than 0.05 were considered statistically significant.

ACKNOWLEDGMENTS

The project is supported by the Youth Research Fund of Jilin Province in China (NO.201205272 and NO. 20130522024JH). Author to whom correspondence should be addressed: Jing Mang, E-Mail: mangjing@jlu.edu.cn, Tel: +8615844031118 and Yan-Kun Shao, E-Mail: yankun-shao@163.com.

REFERENCES

Chunli Mei, Jinting He, Jing Mang, Guihua Xu, Zhongshu Li, Wenzhao Liang, Zhongxin Xu (2011), NGF combined with OGD induces neural ischemia tolerance in PC12 cells. AJBR, 5(10):315–320.

Chunli Mei, Jinting He, JingMang (2011). NGF combined with OGD induces neural ischemia tolerance in PC12 cells. AJBR. 5(10): 315–320.

Han, P.; Kang, J.H. & Li, H.L (2009). Antiproliferation and apoptosis induced by tamoxifen in human bile duct carcinoma QBC939 cells via upregulated p53 expression. Biochem. Biophys. Res. Commun. 385, 251–256.

K. Matsuno, D. Eastman, T. Mitsiades et al. Human deltex is a conserved regulator of Notch signalling. Nat Genet. 1998; 19(1): 74–78.

L. Pantoni, F. Pescini & S. Nannucci (2011). Comparison of clinical, familial, and MRI features of CADASIL and NOTCH3-negative patients. Neurology. 74(1): 57–63.

M. Hayase, M. Kitada, S. Wakao et al (2009). Committed neural progenitor cells derived from genetically modified bone marrow stromal cells ameliorate deficits in a rat model of stroke. J Cereb Blood Flow Metab. 29(8): 1409–1420.

N. Sestan, S. Artavanis-Tsakonas, & P. Rakic (1999). Contact-dependent inhibition of cortical neurite growth mediated by notch signaling. Science. 286(5440): 741–746.

Pieri, A.; Lopes, T.O. & Gabbai (2011) A score is better than CHADS2 score in reducing ischemic stroke risk in patients with atrial fibrillation. Int. J. Stroke. 6, 466.

Shudo, Y.; Miyagawa, S & Sawa, Y. (2011) Establishing new porcine ischemic cardiomyopathy model by transcatheter ischemia-reperfusion of the entire left coronary artery system for preclinical experimental studies. Transplantation. 92, e34–e35.

S. Oya, G. Yoshikawa & K. Taka (2009). Attenuation of Notch signaling promotes the differentiation of neural progenitors into neurons in the hippocampal CA1 region after ischemic injury. Neuroscience. 158(2): 683–692.

Tara, S.; Takagi, G.; & Mizuno, K (2011) Novel approach to ischemic skin ulcer in systemic lupus erythematosus: Therapeutic angiogenesis by controlled-release basic fibroblast growth factor. Geriatr. Gerontol. Int. 11, 527–530.

Medicine Sciences and Bioengineering – Wang (Ed.)
© 2015 Taylor & Francis Group, London, ISBN: 978-1-138-02684-1

Cell immunophenotypic assays more accurately diagnose and classify the different subtypes of acute leukemia

Qing Chi, Yong-zhi Lun & Zeng-guo Yu
Department of Medical Laboratory, College of Medicine, Dalian University, Dalian, Liaoning, China

ABSTRACT: To further explore and objectively evaluate the clinical application of cell immunophenotypic assay in diagnosing immunophenotype and subtype of AL, twelve types of monoclonal antibodies typically used in the clinic were selected for this study. Among 56 patients with newly diagnosed AML, 54 of them were consistent with the results of the immunophenotypic assay. Moreover, all types expressed three or more types of the myeloid antigens, especially CD13 and CD33, and the antigens were expressed at relatively high levels. CD14 antigens were highly expressed in monocytic leukemia cells (M4, M5a, M5b). In M3, there was no positive expression of CD34 antigen, and HLA-DR expression rate was also very low. Except for the 5 AML patients with expression of the lymphoid antigen CD7, about 90% of the patients did not express this particular lymphoid antigen. The results also showed that a misdiagnosis was observed in 2 patients previously categorized by the morphological classification. Hybrid acute leukemia (HAL) expressed at least both the myeloid and lymphoid antigens. Acute megakaryocytic leukemia (M7) mainly expressed CD41 and CD61 antigens. Furthermore, using immunophenotypic assay, 28 patients with ALL were accurately divided into T-ALL, B-ALL and TB-ALL. In addition to the latter, the B-lineage antigens and T-lineage antigens were not mutually expressed and showed strong characteristics of lineage-specific expression, but were also found to express myeloid and lymphoid antigens. T/B-ALL simultaneously expressed both T-lineage and B-lineage antigens. Conclusions Overall, the cell immunophenotypic assay can provide objective and accurate data for diagnosing immunophenotype and subtype of AL, which shows significant improvement over the morphological classification. Immunophenotyping also has improved clinical application that allows differentiation between the AML and ALL subgroups.

1 INTRODUCTION

The identification of leukocyte differentiation antigens and improvements in monoclonal antibodies (McAb) technology has led to the classification of acute leukemia and immunotyping of the MICM leukemia classification. These advances helped characterize unique and novel leukemic cell antigens with high sensitivity and specificity to improve AL diagnosis and prognosis. To further objectively evaluate and investigate the clinical value of using immunophenotypic assay for diagnosing immunophenotype and subtype of AL, twelve types of monoclonal antibodies commonly used in the clinic were selected. The immunophenotypes of 56 patients with acute myeloid leukemia (AML) and 28 patients with acute lymphoblastic leukemia (ALL) that were initially diagnosed by the FAB morphological classification standard were detected and analyzed using flow cytometry (FCM).

2 MATERIALS AND METHODS

2.1 Research subjects

A total of 84 patients with AL were admitted to the Department of Hematology from September 2010 to May 2012 and selected for the study. All patients were initially diagnosed based on the FAB morphological classification standard. The type of leukemia was determined by inspecting the bone marrow cell morphology and the relevant cytochemical staining. Among them, there were 56 cases of AML (7 cases of M1 type, 15 cases of M2a type, 11 cases of M3 type, 6 cases of M4 type, 8 cases of M5a type, 5 cases of M5b type and 4 cases of M6 type) and 28 cases of ALL (11 cases of L1 type, 15 cases of L2 type and 2 cases of L3 type). A total of 53 patients were male and 31 patients were female. The age ranged from 5 years to 68 years, with the average age being 36 years.

2.2 Reagents

Hemolysin (Opti yes C), cell membrane permeability alteration reagent kit (IntraPrp Permeabilization Reagent), fluorescent agent (FTIC, PE, PerCP) and all of the monoclonal antibodies were purchased from Immunotech (France). Twelve kinds of monoclonal antibodies were selected: myeloid monoclonal antibody (CD13, CD14, CD15, CD33), B-cell monoclonal antibody (CD10, CD19), T-cell monoclonal antibody (CD5, CD7), megakaryocytic monoclonal antibody (CD41, CD61) and non-series-specific monoclonal antibody (CD34, HLA-DR).

2.3 Method of immunophenotypic assay and genotyping

The bone marrow was punctured from the anterior superior iliac bone before treatment in all cases and the bone marrow fluid with anticoagulant heparin was prepared. At least 3-5ml of bone marrow fluid with anticoagulant heparin were taken. The conventional separation of mononuclear cell suspension was prepared by lymphocyte separation medium density gradient centrifugation, and the cellular level was sequentially adjusted to 109/L. The monoclonal antibodies were respectively labeled with stain. Twenty microliter (20 μl) of monoclonal antibodies and 50 μl of mononuclear cell suspension were added to each tube and kept in the dark at room temperature for 15 min. The hemolytic agent was added and mixed well. The determination was carried out after 10 min by flow cytometry detection and was analyzed using the three standard method of direct immunofluorescence technique. The instrument was calibrated by standard calibration fluorescent microspheres before the determination. The CD45/SSC dual parameter scatter plot was gated and 104 cells were collected in each measuring tube. Based on the surface antigen positive rate for leukemia cell populations, $\geq 20\%$ is positive for HLA-DR, $\geq 10\%$ is positive for CD34, and the results were analyzed using Cell Quest software. The immunological classification standard was carried out according to the classification method outlined by the European Group for Immunological Characterization of Leukemias (EGIL, 1995) (Bene et al., 1995)

3 RESULTS

3.1 Immuophenotypic assay and genotyping for 56 patients with AML

Among 56 patients with initially diagnosed AML, 54 cases were consistent with the results of the immunophenotypic assay. Among them, myeloid antigens CD13 and CD33 were highly expressed in all types of AML. Myeloid antigen CD14 was highly expressed in monocytic leukemia cells (M4, M5a, M5b). In the M3 type, the non-series-specific antigen CD34 was not detectable and HLA-DR expression levels were low (9%). However, in other types, HLA-DR expression was detected at high levels. There were five cases of AML with lymphoid antigen CD7 expression.

Among two cases of morphological classification error, one was initially diagnosed as leukemic cells of M5a type. The M7 type correlated to cells which expressed megakaryocyte-associated antigens. Other diagnosed cases of M4-type leukemic cells expressed both myeloid antigens (CD13, CD14, CD33) and T-lineage-associated antigens (CD5, CD7), which was diagnosed as hybrid acute leukemia (HAL). Various types of CD antigen expression and immunological classification results are shown in Table 1.

3.2 *Results of immunophenotyping assay and genotyping for 28 cases of ALL*

Using immunophenotypic assay, 28 patients with ALL were classified as following: 9 cases with T-ALL, 18 cases with B-ALL, and 1 case with T/B-hybrid ALL. T-ALL mainly expressed lymphoid antigens CD_5 and CD_7, while B-ALL mainly expressed lymphoid lineage antigens CD_{10} and CD_{19}. Among these antigens, the expression of CD_7 and CD_{19} was highest in T-ALL and B-ALL, respectively, and these two types of antigens were not mutually expressed. T- and B-ALL simultaneously expressed both T-lineage antigens (CD_5, CD_7) and B-lineage antigens (CD_{10}, CD_{19}). There were different degrees of shared expression between myeloid and lymphoid antigens in T-ALL, B-All, and T/B-ALL. Various types of CD antigen expression in ALL and immunological classification results are shown in Table 2.

Table 1. Results of immunophentypic assay and genotyping for 56 cases of AML

| Immunological classification | Cases with antigen positive expression | | | | | | | | | | | | | FAB classification |
	CD 13	CD 14	CD 15	CD 33	CD 41	CD 61	CD 10	CD 19	CD 5	CD 7	HLA-DR	CD 34	*n*	
M1	7	0	5	7	0	0	0	0	0	2	5	6	7	7
M2a	15	0	13	13	0	0	0	0	0	3	14	13	15	15
M3	11	0	8	10	0	0	0	0	0	0	1	0	11	11
M4	5		5	5	0	0	0	0	0	0	2	4	5	6
M5a	7	7	7	7	0	0	0	0	0	0	6	7	7	8
M5b	5	5	4	5	0	0	0	0	0	0	5	1	5	5
M6	4	0	2	3	0	0	0	0	0	0	3	2	4	4
M7	1	0	0	1	1	1	0	0	0	0	0	1	1	0
HAL	1	1	0	1	0	0	0	0	1	1	1	1	1	0

Table 2. Results of immunophenotypic assay and genotypic for 28 cases of ALL

| Immunological classification | *n* | Cases with antigen positive expression | | | | | | | | | | | |
		CD 13	CD 14	CD 15	CD 33	CD 41	CD 61	CD 10	CD 19	CD 5	CD 7	HLA-DR	CD 34
T-ALL	9	2	0	1	3	0	0	0	0	8	9	6	4
B-ALL	18	2	0	0	2	0	0	15	18	0	0	14	9
T/B-ALL	1	0	0	0	1	0	0	1	1	1	1	1	1

4 DISCUSSION

After analyzing the immunophenotypic results derived from 56 patients with AML, the immunophenotypic and morphological characteristics were observed for at least 54 patients expressing three types of myeloid antigens. However, differential expression of a number of myeloid antigens in each subtype were observed, among which 54 patients were CD13 positive (100%), 15 patients were CD14 positive (27.8%), 44 patients were CD15 positive (81.5%), and 50 patients were CD33 positive (92.6%). Apart from a small number of cases (two cases of M1 and three cases of M2a), about 90% of patients with AML did not express any lymphoid antigens. These results indicated there was no specific anti-AML antibodies that can accurately distinguished one leukemic subtype from another. However, the co-expression of a variety of myeloid antigens, such as CD13 and CD33, was able to distinguished AML from ALL. The CD14 antigen is the most specific immune marker of monocytes (Casasnovas *et al.*, 1998 and Krasinskas *et al.*, 1998). The results indicated that immunophenotyping might help morphological classify and identify the M4, M5a and M5b subtypes from all other subtypes (Kaleem & White, 2001). HLA-DR and CD34 are both hematopoietic stem/progenitor cell-associated antigens. Along with cell maturation, their antigen expression are found decreased over during (Testa *et al.*, 2002). In this study, only one patient (1/11) of the M3 type was positive for HLA-DR expression. No other cases showed positive expression for CD34, while other AML subtypes had higher expression. This phenomenon might be related to the derivation of promyelocytic leukemia cells from mature granulocyte progenitor cells and is consistent with previous studies (Paietta, 2003). Therefore, the absent of HLA-DR and CD34 antigen expression is important to help identify atypical M3. In addition, two cases of M1 and M2a showed myeloid-associated antigen expression accompanied with lymphoid antigen (CD7) expression. Moreover, lymphoid antigen expression is associated with acute myeloid leukemia (Ly+-AML), suggesting that AML is poorly differentiated and might be associated with myeloid progenitor cells (Kornblau *et al.*, 1995).

The morphological classification error was found by immunophenotypic assay in two patients. However, among one patient initially diagnosed as M5a type, megakaryocytic antigens (CD41, CD61) expression was observed without the expression of the specific monocytic CD14 antigen. Therefore, it was corrected to the M7 type. The morphology was used to help classify the M4 subtype.. The immunophenotypic assay found co-expression of the myeloid antigens (CD13, CD14, CD33) and the lymphoid antigens (CD5, CD7). No lineage leukemic cell antigen currently exists. HAL leukemic cells expressed at least two types of myeloid and lymphoid antigen rather than the AML-M4 type.

The immunophenotypic assay can accurately classify patients with ALL from those of T-ALL, B-ALL, and T/B-ALL. A number of lymphoid antigens showed high expression in the different types of ALL, among which 8 patients with T-ALL expressed CD5 (88.9%) and 9 patients with T-ALL expressed CD7 (100%). At least 13 patients with B-ALL expressed CD10 (72.2%) and 18 patients with f B-ALL expressed CD19 (100%). The highest rates of CD7 and CD19 were expressed in T-ALL and B-ALL. The lymphoid antigen expression in T-ALL and B-ALL was not mutually expressed. B-lineage antigens (CD10, CD19) and T-lineage antigens (CD5, CD7) had a strong series of specific expression characteristics. This had very high sensitivity and specificity in the classification and identification of ALL. In the present study, there was one patient with T/B-ALL that had co-expression of B-lineage antigens (CD10, CD19) and T-lineage antigens (CD5, CD7), which is essentially similar to the cell clones in pluripotent stem cells or more stages (Paredes-Aguilera *et al.*, 2001). In addition, although CD13, CD33 were relatively specific myeloid antigens, they were found highly expressed in patients (6/9) with T-ALL (66.7%), and in patients (4/18) with T/B-ALL. This indicated that in a significant number of ALL cases, there was co-expression of both myeloid and lymphoid antigens, with one kind of myeloid-associated antigen expressed in acute lymphoblastic leukemia (My+-ALL) and was especially prominent in T-ALL (Kornblau *et al.*, 1995). These observations are consistent with the findings of a previous study (Preti *et al.*, 1995). In addition, 28 patients with ALL were associated with high expression levels of the non-series-specific antigen (HLA-DR and CD34). This suggests that ALL might arise from the malignant transformation of early hematopoietic cells. These results also show a potential benefit for using immunophenotypic assay for the classification of ALL over traditional morphological classification. Immunophenotypic assays can determine the different biological characteristics of ALL in different malignant clones, as well as during cell differentiation.

5 CONCLUSION

The cell immunophenotypic assay could determine the clonogenic source and differentiation stages of myeloid cells and lymphocytes from hematopoietic cells. This study also accurately diagnoses the immunophenotype and subtype of AL to reduce misdiagnosis that might occur using the morphological classification system. The immunophenotypic assay also has unique clinical application by differentiating AML and ALL, and their associated ALL subtypes.

REFERENCES

Bene, M.C., Castoldi, G., Knapp, W., Ludwig, W.D., Matutes, E., Orfao, A., van't Veer, M.B. (1995) Proposals for the immunological classification of acute leukemias. European Group for the Immunological Characterization of Leukemias (EGIL). *Leukemia*, 9(10), 1783–1786.

Casasnovas, R.O., Campos, L., Mugneret, F., Charrin, C., Béné, M.C., Garand, R., Favre, M., Sartiaux, C., Chaumarel, I., Bernier, M., Faure, G., Solary, E. (1998) Immunophenotypic patterns and cytogenetic anomalies in acute non-lymphoblastic leukemia subtypes: a prospective study of 432 patients. *Leukemia*, 12(1), 34–43.

Kaleem, Z. & White, G. (2001) Diagnostic critenria for minimally differentiated acute myeloid leukemia (AML-M0): Evaluation ans a proposal. *Am J Clin Pathol*, 115(6), 876–884.

Kornblau, S.M., Thall, P., Huh, Y.O., Estey, E., Andreeff, M. (1995) Analysis of CD7 expression in acute myelogenous leukemia: martingale residual plots combined with 'optimal' cutpoint analysis reveals absence of prognostic significance. *Leukemia*, 9(10), 1735–1741.

Krasinskas, A.M., Wasik, M.A., Kamoun, M., Schretzenmair, R., Moore, J., Salhany, K.E. (1998) The usefulness of CD64, other monocyte-associated antigens, and CD45 gating in the subclassification of acute myeloid leukemias with monocytic differentiation. *Am J Clin Pathol*, 110(6), 797–805.

Paietta, E. (2003) Expression of cell-surface antigens in acute promyelocyte leukemia. *Best Pract Res Clin Haematol*, 16(3), 369–385.

Paredes-Aguilera, R., Romero-Guzman, L., Lopez-Santiago, N., Burbano-Ceron, L., Camacho-Del Monte, O., Nieto-Martinez, S. (2001) Flow cytometric analysis of cell-surface and intracellular antigens in the diagnosis of acute leukemia. *Am J Hematol*, 68(2), 69–74.

Preti, H.A., Huh, Y.O., O'Brien, S.M., Andreeff, M., Pierce, S.T., Keating, M., Kantarjian, H.M. (1995) Myeloid markers in adult acute lymphocytic leukemia. Correlations with patient and disease characteristics and with prognosis. *Cancer*, 76(9), 1564–1570.

Testa, U., Torelli, G.F., Riccioni, R., Muta, A.O., Militi, S., Annino, L., Mariani, G., Guarini, A., Chiaretti, S., Ritz, J., Mandelli, F., Peschle, C., Foa, R. (2002) Human acute stem cell leukemia with multilineage differentiation potential via cascade activation of growth factor receptors. *Blood*, 99(12), 4634–1637.

Medicine Sciences and Bioengineering – Wang (Ed.)
© *2015 Taylor & Francis Group, London, ISBN: 978-1-138-02684-1*

Conditioned medium mediated immune protection in In Vitro model of endogenous neurotoxin N-methyl-salsolinol in an astrocyte-dependent manner

Fu-li Wang, Xiang-han Wang, Fan Zeng, Hong Qing & Yu-lin Deng
School of Life Science, Beijing Institute of Technology, Haidian District, Beijing, China

ABSTRACT: Parkinson's Disease (PD) is the second largest neurodegeneration disease in the world, and the etiology of PD is unclear now. Enormous studies focus on the neuroinflammation and innate and adaptive immune system in the pathology of PD. In this study, we used endogenous neurotoxin 1(R),2(N)-dimethyl-6,7-dihydroxy-1,2,3,4-tetrahydroisoquinoline-(N-methyl-salsolinol, NMSal)-treated cocultures of dopaminergic neuron SH-SY5Y cells and astrocytomas U87 cells for 24 hours and then reused this 24-hours-old medium to culture human monocyte THP1 cells for another 24 hours and studied the role of this conditioned medium on THP1 cells. We found 24-hours-old medium–protected monocyte THP1 cells from NMSal-mediated apoptosis in an astrocyte U87 cells–dependent manner.

1 INTRODUCTION

Parkinson's Disease (PD) is an age-related and progressive neurodegenerative disease, and the pathology of PD is complex and involves numerous heritable and environmental risk factors (Su and Federoff, 2014). Recent studies establish that innate and adaptive immune system plays an important role in onset and progression in the pathology of PD. One emerging hypothesis is that activation of peripheral immune system exacerbates the progression of neurodegeneration of PD. The evidence for systemic inflammation in PD includes the presence of elevated serum levels of TNF-α and TNF-α receptor in PD patients, increased levels of proinflammatory cytokines including TNF-α, IL-1β, IL-6, and CCL2 in some other tissues, and changes in lymphocytes and monocytes in peripheral blood (Ehses et al., 2007; Funk et al., 2013; Reale et al., 2009; Scalzo et al., 2009; Shoelson et al., 2006).

Endogenous neurotoxin 1(R), 2(N)-dimethyl-6,7-dihydroxy-1,2,3,4-tetrahydroisoquinoline-(N-methyl-salsolinol, NMSal) is a metabolite of 1-methyl-4-phenyl-1,2,3,4-tetrahydroisoquinoline-(Salsolinol, Sal), which is metabolized by N-methyl-transferase in astrocyte, and NMSal is an analog of 1-methyl-4-phenyl-1,2,3,6-tetrahydropyridine (MPTP), which interacts with the mitochondrial respiratory chain and damages mitochondrial complex-1, increasing oxidative stress and leading to cell death (Briggs et al., 2013; Ramsey and Tansey, 2014; Williams and Ramsden, 2005). In the present study, we have used cell–cell coculture system to study the role of human monocyte THP1 cells in endogenous NMSal-treated conditioned medium of cocultures of SH-SY5Y and U87 cells. We found that neuroblastoma SH-SY5Y cells protected THP1 cells from endogenous neurotoxin NMSal-mediated apoptosis along with glioma U87 cells.

2 MATERIALS AND METHODS

2.1 *Cell culture*

Human neuroblastoma cell SH-SY5Y (ATCC, Manassas, VA, USA), human glioma cell line U87 (ATCC, Manassas, VA, USA), and human monocytic cell line THP1 (ATCC, Manassas, VA, USA) were all cultured in Dulbecco's modified Eagle's medium high glucose (Gibco) supplemented with 10% fetal bovine serum (FBS) (Gibco) and 1% penicillin/streptomycin sulfate solution in a humidified incubator at 37°C containing 5% CO_2.

2.2 *Cell–cell coculture*

Cocultured SH-SY5Y and U87 cells were seeded at a ratio of 1:1 in Dulbecco's Modified Eagle's Medium (Gibco) and supplemented with 10% FBS (Gibco) and 1% penicillin/streptomycin; they were then treated by 250 μM NMSal after adhere of cocultures for 24 hours. This 24-hours-old medium was used to culture THP1 cells in a new culture plate for another 24 hours. All cell lines were maintained at 37°C in a humidified incubator with 5% CO_2.

2.3 *Caspase3 activity assay*

Caspase3 activity was measured by Promega caspase3/7 activity kit. THP1 cells were harvested and washed by PBS two times, and cell concentration was regulated to 1×10^5 cells per mL by DMEM medium; add 100 μL (about 1×10^4 cells) cell suspension and 100 μL of caspase3 reaction reagents into the eppendorf 1.5 mL tube at the bottom, incubating for one hour at room temperature without light. The fluorescence of caspase3 activity was observed by Promega Subscription Fluorescence Detector (GLOMAX 20/20 LUMINOMETER).

2.4 *MTS assay*

THP1 cells were seeded into a 96 well plate for 8 hours, and then different concentrations of NMSal (50–1000 μM) were added for 24 hours; then, viability of THP1 cells was measured by MTS (3-(4,5-dimethylthiazol-2-yl)-5-(3-carboxymethoxyphenyl)-2-(4-sulfophenyl)-2H-tetrazolium) assay. The absorbance was measured at 492 nm by THERMO Multiskan ascent (Thermo, Wisconsin-Madison, USA).

2.5 *Data analysis*

All data are presented as mean ± SEM. The differences between groups were analyzed by Student's paired t-test. A $p < 0.05$ was considered significant.

3 RESULTS AND DISCUSSION

3.1 *NMSal-induced apoptosis of human monocyte THP1 cells*

As it is not unclearly whether endogenous neurotoxin NMSal is toxicity to human monocyte THP1 cells, we first check cell viability by MTS assay, and we found NMSal induced toxicity of THP1 cells in an concentration dependent manner, and 250 μM NMSal induced almost 50% percent THP1 cells death at 24 hours (Figure 1a), cell number of THP1 was decreased in NMSal treated medium (Figure 1b), and activity of caspase3 of NMSal treated THP1 cells was strikingly increased compared to THP1 cells not treated by NMSal (Figure 1c). This demonstrated that endogenous neurotoxin NMSal was toxic to human monocyte THP1 cells and 250 μM of NMSal induced the death of almost half of THP1 cells.

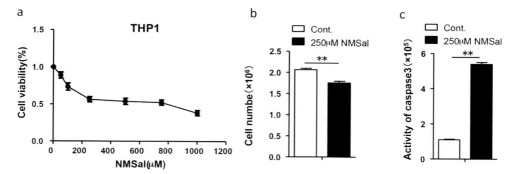

Figure 1. NMSal-induced apoptosis of human monocyte THP1 cells.

a. NMSal-induced toxicity of THP1 cells according to concentration, and 250 μM of NMSal caused apoptosis of almost 50% of THP1 cells. b. 250 μM NMSal induced cell number of THP1 decreased compared to THP1 cells not treated by NMSal. Values are means ± SEM ($n = 3$), **, $P < 0.01$ compared with media controls. c. 250μM NMSal increased caspase3 activity of THP1 cells. Values are means ± SEM ($n = 3$), **, $P < 0.01$ compared with media controls.

3.2 Conditioned medium protected THP1 cells from NMSal-mediated apoptosis in an astrocyte U87 cells–dependent manner

As we wanted to know the role of endogenous neurotoxin NMSal-damaged dopaminergic neuron SH-SY5Y cells on human monocyte THP1 cells, we utilized a cell–cell coculture system to study it. We found that conditioned medium from NMSal-treated cocultures of SH-SY5Y decreased the endogenous neurotoxin NMSal-induced toxicity of THP1 cells in an astrocyte U87 cells–dependent manner (Figure 2a). Meanwhile, we found that conditioned medium decreased the activity of caspase3 in THP1 cells (Figure 2b). All of these indicated that conditioned medium had a protective role in endogenous neurotoxin NMSal–mediated toxicity of human monocyte THP1 cells.

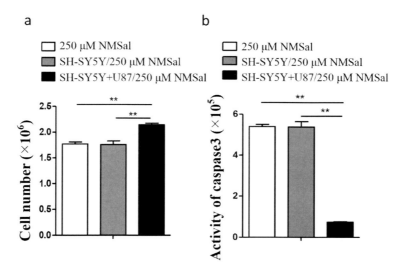

Figure 2. Conditioned medium from NMSal-treated cocultures SH-SY5Y and U87 cells protected THP1 cells form NMSal-mediated apoptosis in an astrocyte-dependent manner.

a. Conditioned medium increased the cell number of THP1. Values are means ± SEM ($n = 3$), **, $P < 0.01$ compared with media controls. b. Conditioned medium decreased caspase3 activity of THP1 cells. Values are means ± SEM ($n = 3$), **, $P < 0.01$ compared with media controls.

SUMMARY

In conclusion, conditioned medium from endogenous neurotoxin NMSal-treated cocultures of SH-SY5Y and U87 cells protects human monocyte THP1 cells from NMSal-mediated apoptosis with decreased caspase3 activity and increased cell number of THP1 cells.

REFERENCES

Briggs, G.D., Nagy, G.M., and Dickson, P.W. (2013). Mechanism of action of salsolinol on tyrosine hydroxylase. *Neurochemistry international* 63, 726–731.

Ehses, J.A., Perren, A., Eppler, E., Ribaux, P., Pospisilik, J.A., Maor-Cahn, R., Gueripel, X., Ellingsgaard, H., Schneider, M.K., Biollaz, G., et al. (2007). Increased number of islet-associated macrophages in type 2 diabetes. *Diabetes* 56, 2356–2370.

Funk, N., Wieghofer, P., Grimm, S., Schaefer, R., Buhring, H.J., Gasser, T., and Biskup, S. (2013). Characterization of peripheral hematopoietic stem cells and monocytes in Parkinson's disease. *Movement disorders: official journal of the Movement Disorder Society* 28, 392–395.

Ramsey, C.P., and Tansey, M.G. (2014). A survey from 2012 of evidence for the role of neuroinflammation in neurotoxin animal models of Parkinson's disease and potential molecular targets. *Experimental neurology* 256, 126–132.

Reale, M., Iarlori, C., Thomas, A., Gambi, D., Perfetti, B., Di Nicola, M., and Onofrj, M. (2009). Peripheral cytokines profile in Parkinson's disease. *Brain, behavior, and immunity* 23, 55–63.

Scalzo, P., Kummer, A., Cardoso, F., and Teixeira, A.L. (2009). Increased serum levels of soluble tumor necrosis factor-alpha receptor-1 in patients with Parkinson's disease. *Journal of neuroimmunology* 216, 122–125.

Shoelson, S.E., Lee, J., and Goldfine, A.B. (2006). Inflammation and insulin resistance. *The Journal of clinical investigation* 116, 1793–1801.

Su, X., and Federoff, H.J. (2014). Immune responses in Parkinson's disease: interplay between central and peripheral immune systems. *BioMed research international* 2014, 275178.

Williams, A.C., and Ramsden, D.B. (2005). Autotoxicity, methylation and a road to the prevention of Parkinson's disease. *Journal of clinical neuroscience: official journal of the Neurosurgical Society of Australasia* 12, 6–11.

Medicine Sciences and Bioengineering – Wang (Ed.)
© 2015 Taylor & Francis Group, London, ISBN: 978-1-138-02684-1

Analyzing couplet medicines in Ma Xiang's treatment of chronic gastritis: Chinese prescription based on association rules

Wen-xue Zhang
School of Sciences, Ningxia Medical University, Yinchuan, China

Hai-hong Zhang
School of Nursing, Ningxia Medical University, Yinchuan, China

Xi-sen Liang
School of Traditional Chinese Medicine, Ningxia Medical University, Yinchuan, China

Liang Bian & Zheng-zhi Li
School of Sciences, Ningxia Medical University, Yinchuan, China

Yong-fu Gu
Department of Information, Ningdong Hospital of Ningxia Hui Autonomous Region, Yinchuan, China

ABSTRACT: Objective: Ma Xiang is Ningxia grassroots famous physician of Traditional Chinese Medicine (TCM). To explore the Chinese medicine compatibility originated from Ma Xiang's treatment of chronic gastritis. Methods: The association rules are discovered using Apriori algorithm. Results: The numbers of couplet medicines, rules consisted of triple herb, and rules consisted of quads herb are 10, 6, and 2, respectively. Conclusions: The experiment demonstrates that couplet medicines, rules consisted of triple herb, and rules consisted of quads herb are based on association rules according to the basic characteristics of TCM.

1 INTRODUCTION

Ma Xiang, a chief physician of Traditional Chinese Medicine (TCM), was honored as a grassroots famous TCM doctor by the Health Department of Ningxia Hui autonomous region in 2010. He was awarded the "Medical Science and Technology Award" by the government of Ningxia Hui autonomous region. Especially, he is good at the treatment of chronic gastritis disease.

The couplet medicines, a particular kind of synergy, consist of relatively fixed two herbals in prescription (FAN *et al.* 2011). It can reflect the theory of Chinese herbs' properties such as nature and flavor, ascending and descending, floating and sinking, and channel tropism (QIN *et al.* 2012). The couplet medicines can closely link with drugs on pathogenesis, and they are composed of simple medicines with specific efficiency and great power. This paper aims to mine couplet medicines from the clinical prescription data of Ma Xiang's treatment of chronic gastritis.

2 MATERIALS AND METHODS

Diagnostic Criteria. The consensus of diagnosis and therapy on chronic gastritis is by using integration of traditional and western medicine (2011 Tianjin) (ZHANG *et al.* 2012).

Cases and Data. The subjects were patients with chronic gastritis who meet the aforementioned diagnostic criteria, and any age and gender. We collected 104 clinical prescriptions from January 2012 to April 2013 Gufang Hospital of Ningxia.

Association Rules. The association rule is a popular and well-researched method for discovering the couplet medicines of TCM clinical data (Wu *et al.* 2013). Apriori is an algorithm for frequent item set mining and association rule learning over transactional databases (Agrawal *et al.* 2012). The parameters sensitivity of Apriori algorithm is analyzed to select a reasonable number of the association rules as shown in Figure 1.

Figure 1 shows that the reasonable minimum support and minimum confidence are 0.3 and 0.8, respectively.

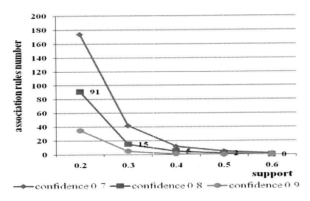

Figure 1. The change trend of association rules number with support and confidence

3 EXPERIMENTAL RESULTS

Mining association rules are shown in Tables 1–3.

Table 1. Couplet medicines

ID	Association rules	Support	Confidence
1	Turmeric root tuber => Chinese thorowax root	0.3	0.95
2	Common yam rhizome => dried tangerine peel	0.3	0.93
3	Zingiber => pinellia tuber	0.3	0.91
4	Pinellia tuber => dried tangerine peel	0.3	0.9
5	Zingiber => dried tangerine peel	0.3	0.89
6	Rhizoma Corydalis => dried tangerine peel	0.3	0.88
7	Chinese thorowax root => turmeric root tuber	0.3	0.86
8	Glabrous greenbrier rhizome => dried tangerine peel	0.3	0.85
9	Liquorice root => dried tangerine peel	0.3	0.82
10	Largehead => dried tangerine peel	0.3	0.81
11	Rhizoma Corydalis => orange fruit	0.3	0.80

Table 2. Rules consisted of triple herb

ID	Association rules	Support	Confidence
1	Common yam rhizome, orange fruit => dried tangerine peel	0.3	0.94
2	Largehead, Rhizoma Corydalis => dried tangerine peel	0.3	0.91
3	Largehead, pinellia tuber => dried tangerine peel	0.3	0.91
4	Rhizoma Corydalis, orange fruit => dried tangerine peel	0.3	0.88
5	Pinellia tuber, orange fruit => dried tangerine peel	0.3	0.87
6	Largehead, pinellia tuber => orange fruit	0.3	0.8

Table 3.   Rules consisted of quads herb

ID	Association rules	Support	Confidence
1	Largehead, pinellia tuber, orange fruit => dried tangerine peel	0.3	0.89
2	Pinellia tuber, dried tangerine peel, orange fruit=> largehead	0.3	0.8

4 DISCUSSIONS

4.1   Couplet medicines

As can be seen clearly from Tables 1–3, the sovereign drugs used for the treatment of chronic gastritis by Ma Xiang are dried tangerine peel, orange fruit, and largehead.

"Turmeric root tuber, Chinese thorowax root." The channel tropism of Chinese thorowax root are heart and abdomen. Clearing heat and purgation and dispersing stagnated liver qi for relieving qi stagnation are its key pharmacological effects. Turmeric root tuber is pungent, bitter, and cold. Nourishing blood and promoting granulation and benefiting qi for activating blood circulation are its key pharmacological effects. "turmeric root tuber, Chinese thorowax root" is clearing stomach and purging heat. They can be used to treat the syndrome of adverse rising of stomach qi.

"common yam rhizome, dried tangerine peel" is harmonizing liver and spleen. They are effective against the syndrome of stagnation of liver qi and spleen deficiency.

"zingiber, pinellia tuber" is the most commonly used couplet medicines by ancient traditional Chinese physicians.

"pinellia tuber, dried tangerine peel" is commonly clinical couplet medicines in favor of regulating qi-flowing for eliminating phlegm. The syndrome of qi stagnation and coagulated phlegm in throat can be treated with them.

"zingiber, dried tangerine peel" is clearing heat and removing food stagnation. It is used in the syndrome of retention of food in stomach.

"Rhizoma Corydalis, dried tangerine peel" with functions of promoting blood circulation for removing blood stasis and regulating qi-flowing for relieving pain, used in the treatment of the syndrome of static blood in stomach collaterals.

"Chinese thorowax root, turmeric root tuber" has the effect of clearing heat and cooling blood and harmonizing qi and blood. It is used in the treatment of the syndrome of stagnation of liver qi and blood stasis, and the syndrome of incoordination between liver and stomach.

"glabrous greenbrier rhizome, dried tangerine peel" is invigorating spleen-stomach and replenishing qi. It is used in the treatment of the syndrome of deficiency of spleen qi and stomach qi. The dried tangerine peel can enhance the efficacy of eliminating dampness and phlegm, and moistening lung for arresting cough of glabrous greenbrier rhizome.

"liquorice root, dried tangerine peel" is invigorating spleen and replenishing qi. Used in the treatment of the syndrome of deficiency of spleen qi.

"largehead, dried tangerine peel" is removing dampness for regulating stomach, and invigorating spleen for dieresis. It is effective against the syndrome of deficient cold of spleen and stomach.

"Rhizoma Corydalis, orange fruit" is relieving oppression and masses. It is used in the treatment of the syndrome of food retention due to spleen deficiency.

4.2   Rules consisting of triple herb

From Table 2, the number of association rules consisted of triple herb is six.

"orange fruit, common yam rhizome, dried tangerine peel" is resolving food stagnation and nourishing spleen and stomach. It is used in the treatment of the syndrome of food retention caused by spleen deficiency.

"largehead, Rhizoma Corydalis, dried tangerine peel" is invigorating spleen-stomach and replenishing qi and benefiting qi for activating blood circulation. It is primarily used to treat the syndrome of blood stasis caused by deficient qi.

"largehead, pinellia tuber, dried tangerine peel" is regulating stomach descending adverse qi and nourishing spleen and stomach. It is used in the treatment of the syndrome of adverse rising of stomach qi, and the syndrome of yin deficiency of spleen and stomach.

"Rhizoma Corydalis, orange fruit, dried tangerine peel" is harmonizing qi and blood and regulating qi-flowing for relieving pain. The syndrome of qi stagnation and blood stasis can be treated using this.

"pinellia tuber, orange fruit, dried tangerine peel" is regulating qi-flowing for harmonizing stomach and resolving food stagnation. It is effective against the deficiency of spleen qi and stomach qi. "largehead, pinellia tuber, orange fruit" is invigorating spleen for benefiting lung and clearing heat-dampness in sanjiao. It can be used to treat the syndrome of qi deficiency of spleen and lung, and the syndrome of phlegm-dampness caused by spleen deficiency.

4.3 Rules consisting of quads herb

From Table 3, the number of association rules consisted of quads herb is two, but it is one in aspect of elements. "largehead, pinellia tuber, orange fruit, dried tangerine peel." The orange fruit works into middle jiao to regulate qi-flowing, and relieve oppression and masses, but it consumes and diffuses qi. Therefore, largehead and dried tangerine peel are used as minister drug to invigorate spleen and replenish qi. The pinellia tuber is a supplementary drug to activate qi for adverse rising of stomach qi.

5 CONCLUSIONS

This paper refined the associated matching models of Ma Xiang's treatment of chronic gastritis on the basis of Chinese prescription including couplet medicines, rules consisted of triple herb, and rules consisted of quads herb. The experiment demonstrates that couplet medicines, rules consisted of triple herb, and rules consisted of quads herb are based on association rules according to the basic characteristics of TCM.

ACKNOWLEDGMENTS

This work is supported by the scientific research foundation of the higher education institution of Ningxia province, China (Grant No. NGY2012053). Thank TCM Ma Xiang to provide the clinical data and interpret the mined patterns.

REFERENCES

Agrawal, R., Imieliński, T. & Swami, A. (1993) Mining association rules between sets of items in large databases. *Proceedings of the 1993 ACM SIGMOD international conference on Management of data – SIGMOD. Washington DC, USA, May 1993.* pp.1–10.

FAN Y., LIANG M.X. & MA J. (2011) Investigation on monarch, minister, adjuvant and dispatcher herbs of Herb Pairs. *China journal of traditional Chinese medicine and pharmacy,* 26(8), 1692–1694.

QIN Z., XU W., XIONG H.Y., et al. (2012) Study on compatibility of depression based on the statistical analysis of drug pairs in ancient and modern prescriptions. *Liaoning Journal of Traditional Chinese Medicine,* 39(10), 1898–1900.

WU, J.R., ZHANG B., YANG B. & CHEN D. (2013) Analysis on YAN Zheng-hua's medication rule in prescriptions on diarrhea based on apriori and clustering algorithm. *China journal of traditional Chinese medicine and pharmacy,* 28(8), 2274–2277.

ZHANG W.D., LI J.X., CHEN Z.S., et al. (2012) The consensus of diagnosis and therapy on chronic gastritis using integration of traditional and western medicine (2011 Tianjin). *Chinese journal of integrated traditional and western medicine,* 32(6), 738–743.

Medicine Sciences and Bioengineering – Wang (Ed.)
© *2015 Taylor & Francis Group, London, ISBN: 978-1-138-02684-1*

Comprehensive rehabilitation treatment and nursing after a surgical repair of hand tendon injuries

Ji-hong Wang
College of Nursing, Beihua University, Jilin, China

Zhong-yan Guo
Affiliated Hospital, Beihua University, Jilin, China

ABSTRACT: The aim of this study was to summarize and analyze methods for the postoperative rehabilitation care of hand tendon injuries. Methods: Twenty-five cases with hand tendon injuries underwent a comprehensive rehabilitation care, including psychological care, postoperative functional exercise, and application of hand function training apparatus according to different circumstances, different degrees, and surgical period. The results showed that the comprehensive postoperative rehabilitation care of tendon injuries with the supervision and guidance of hand function rehabilitation exercise by doctors and nurses could play an important role in the functional rehabilitation after a surgery in patients with hand tendon injuries. In the functional nursing, restoration of the rehabilitation desire of patients is important to enable them to transform from a passive acceptance to an active rehabilitation exercise. The early comprehensive rehabilitation training of patients with hand injuries may be helpful in the prevention of tendon adhesion and ankylosis.

1   INTRODUCTION

The development of society and the increase of accidents in traffic, work, and daily life, resulted in increasing hand tendon injury which had become one of common surgical trauma disorders. It is reported that the incidence of hand injuries has accounted for one-third of total trauma. Although the surgical repair and the surgical methods of hand tendon injuries are reliable currently, different degrees of adhesion of the hand may occur after an operation no matter whether the injured tendon is directly sutured or repaired with a graft because of the elaboration and complexity of hand in anatomy, which may make the clinical efficacy unsatisfactory, even leading to a serious dysfunction of the hand, to lower the daily self-help of the patient. The dysfunction of hand is not only due to the surgery after a tendon injury, but the main factor influencing the functional recovery of hand function is the functional exercise according to the rehabilitation nursing after the surgery. In the last year, a comprehensive functional exercise on the basis of the rehabilitation nursing was conducted in 25 patients with hand injuries, who had undergone a tendon repair surgery. In this paper, the general information, the methods of rehabilitation nursing, especially functional exercise, the rehabilitation results, and the experience on it are discussed.

2   GENERAL INFORMATION

There were 25 patients with hand tendon injuries, 21 cases of fresh injuries, and 4 cases of old injuries, respectively; 18 of them were male and 7 of them were females; they aged from 12 to 50 years with the mean age 32.5 years; the type of injuries included 17 cases of incised injuries and 8 cases of machinery injuries.

3 METHODS

The patients were divided into early-stage (1 to 2 weeks after the operation), medium-stage (3 to 6 weeks after the operation), and late-stage (6 weeks or longer than 6 weeks after the operation) patients (Jing and Miao, 1995) on the basis of the time of operation. Corresponding comprehensive rehabilitation nursing programs were drawn up and the clinical efficacy was evaluated at the 3rd month after the surgery.

3.1 Early-stage rehabilitation nursing

3.1.1 Psychological rehabilitation nursing

Although the rupture of tendon can be surgically repaired, the hand dysfunction caused by the tendon will bring the patient the psychological burden and concerns, such as unwillingness to moving due to the excessive worry about the anastomosis of tendon, the fear of tendon re-rupture after an activity, and the influence of idea of "beating 100 days"; otherwise some of the patients who are particularly sensitive to pain are reluctant to follow the advice of early exercise proposed by doctors and nurses. Aiming at the problems in patients, a psychological counseling was timely given to the patients, including informing the patients regarding the purpose, method, and meaning of rehabilitation exercises, and vigorously promoting the importance of early exercise to the early recovery after injury, so that the patients could understand and accept well the rehabilitation treatment recommendations proposed by doctors and nurses, which lead to the transition from a passive acceptance to an active cooperation with doctors and nurses in treatment to complete the rehabilitation exercise.

3.1.2 Plaster fixation

After the surgery, wrist joints were fixed with plaster at a flexion of 20°–30° and metacarpophalangeal joints were dorsally fixed with plaster at a flexion of 70°. According to the type of injuries, the patients with extension-type injuries could do the functional exercise under the protection of a rubber band traction method. Sports brace could also be used, because the distal joint of each finger or fingernail could make interphalangeal joint naturally extend to prevent the flexion and contracture (Dun and Huang, 1995), in which the color and capillary refill time of nails and each distal fingers should be closely observed.

3.1.3 Functional exercise

The distal and proximal finger joints were gently flexed passively, four times a day, five times each. Generally they were neither flexed actively nor stretched passively, but the fingers could be stretched actively. Once the sutured tendons achieve sufficient tensile strength, an early functional exercise was recommended. The patients could start slowly to move properly under the guidance of a doctor and nurses as soon as the anesthetic effect disappeared, once a day, flexed 2 to 3 times each, and with a magnitude of 1 cm from the fingertip during the first week; then, the amplitude of activities was gradually increased after the first week, and the range and the distance of activities should be increased to about 2 cm by the 3rd week.

3.2 Medium-stage rehabilitation nursing

3.2.1 Rehabilitation nursing from the 3rd to 4th week

The key point was still the systemic functional exercise. At that time, the metacarpophalangeal and interphalangeal joints were in a movable state so that patients were guided actively to flex their fingers gently in the condition without any resistance, passively flex interphalangeal joints with a slightly stronger force, metacarpophalangeal joint flexion, passively stretch gently the interphalangeal joints while metacarpophalangeal joints were in a flexion position, and passively stretch metacarpophalangeal joints when they were in an flexion position. Wrist joints of the patients should be hold at a flexion of 70°.

3.2.2 *Rehabilitation nursing from the 5th to 6th week*

The key point was gradually to increase the mobility and strength of joints. All external fixtures were removed for the transition from a passive movement to an active movement. The patients were taught to flex and stretch actively in a condition without any resistance; the wrist joints could move actively.

3.3 *Early to use the hand function exercise apparatus*

After the tendons were repaired, the joints were continuously moved passively with the hand function exercise apparatus for 2–4 hours daily, which could help to prevent joint contractures. According to the site of injuries, surgery time, and joint flexion contracture, the angle of joints, movement velocity, and movement time were adjusted. When the strength of early tendon healing was not enough, a too large angle of joint movement should be avoided and it should be strictly monitored to ensure the safety of the tendons.

3.4 *Late-stage rehabilitation nursing*

In addition to continuing the functional exercise, the daily living training of the patients should also be enhanced and the patients were asked to do more complex trainings of activities, such as buckling clothing buttons, tying shoes, using chopsticks, cleaning window, and so on. The patients were helped to do exercise in the strength recovery, such as some appropriate household activities and some exercises in works close to each those the patient had been in engaged for before the surgery to lay a foundation for their returning to work. The brace could be used when it was necessary. Meanwhile, the psychological condition of patients should be considered, because the patients had separated themselves from the community and their work for a longer time, which could make them have a psychological burden and prone to low self-esteem, loneliness, and declining in the social adaptability. Nurses should give a psychological support to the patients, help them establish the confidence to return to their homes and the society, and allow patients to achieve the maximum independence.

4 RESULTS

On the basis of the hand surgery function evaluation standards proposed by Hand Surgery Branch, Chinese Medical Society (Tang and She, 1990), the total active activity (TAM), the muscle strength, and the activity of daily living (ADL) of injured hands were measured after the repair. The muscle strength measured on the basis of Lovett rule and ADL recorded on the basis of Bartlel index were used to comprehensively assess the hand functions. The excellent effect indicated the TAM > 75% of the contralateral one, the muscle strength from grade 4 to grade 5, and the ADL > 60; no effect indicated that TAM ≤ 50% of the contralateral one, the muscle strength from grade 0 to grade 2, and ADL ≤ 40. In this study, there were 18 cases with excellent effect, 5 cases with improvement, and 2 cases with no effect; the improvement rate was 92%.

5 SUMMARY

The prognosis of hand tendon injury can be affected by many factors, and the dose depends not only on the surgical technique, and the correct and timely postoperative rehabilitation treatment, but also on the rehabilitation nursing, which is also an important factor (Wang, 2012). The psychological nursing, postoperative functional exercise, hand function training apparatus, and other comprehensive rehabilitation training methods with the supervision and guidance of doctors and nurses to the patients play an important role in the functional rehabilitation after the surgery for hand tendon injuries. After 24–48 h of the surgery, the patients can begin practicing the active movement with full flexion and extension by which local pain and swelling may occur, so the patients have to overcome the pain and persistently do the exercise for a good therapeutic result. The early passive activity under the protection can promote the tendon healing (Sun, 2012), or the adhesion of tendon will often happen if the exercise starts until the surgery reaction disappears and the pain is relieved. It should be noted that in the rehabilitation nursing, the psychological state of patients should be adjusted to a healthy and active state. In the functional nursing, restoration of the rehabilitation desire of patients is very important to enable them to transform from a passive acceptance to an active rehabilitation exercise to restore their hand functions to an optimum degree.

REFERENCES

Duan X.Z. Huang Yongxi. (1995) Modern rehabilitation medicine clinic manual. Beijing: Publishing House of Peking Union Medical College and China Medical University, 76–77.

Jing N.D. & Miao H.S. (1995) *Rehabilitation Medicine.* Beijing: People's Publishing House, 264–72.

Sun H. (2012) Rehabilitation care after distal flexor tendon repair. *Chinese Community Doctors*, 14(4), 323–35.

Tang J.B. & Shi De. (1990) Hand surgery function evaluation. *Journal of Hand Surgery* (6), 75–77.

Wang Z.Q. (2012) Exercise rehabilitation treatment and care of patients after undergoing operation of hand tendon injuries prosthetics. *Chinese Nursing Research*, 26(5), 451–53.

Medicine Sciences and Bioengineering – Wang (Ed.)
© *2015 Taylor & Francis Group, London, ISBN: 978-1-138-02684-1*

An evaluation of the safety and time-saving by the fully automatic ampoule opening device

Ji-hong Wang, Xian-liang Li, Le Zhong & Chang-ping Song*
College of Nursing, Beihua University, Jilin, Jilin, China

ABSTRACT: Needlestick and sharps injuries represent an important workplace issue in contemporary nursing. This study is of a new tool to snap off the neck of sealed ampoule. The idea of the new tool is to reduce injuries to the hands of nurses and save their time for patient care. The tool was evaluated against other methods of snap-off (grinding and slicing and grinding and slicing with gloves) and sizes of ampoule for safety and time saving. We observed that time of snap-off was longer in 10 and 20 ml ampoules by grinding and slicing and grinding and slicing with gloves, and the time of snap-off wase shorter with the new tool. In addition, the degree of satisfaction with the new tool was good. This study provides a novel tool to snap off the neck of ampoules effectively which decreases the time consumed and sharp injuries.

1 INTRODUCTION

Needlestick injuries are an occupational hazard for nurses. The Centers for Disease Control and prevention has estimated that health care professionals suffer 600000 to 1 million injuries caused by conventional needles and sharps annually in the United States, and more than 1000 health care professionals develop serious infection annually from needlestick and sharps injuries (NSI).

In term of statistical analysis from Taiwan, in 527 nursing students under clinical training, the incidences of percutaneous injuries and injuries with blood exposure accidents was 50.1% and 18.2%, respectively. Furthermore, most cases of sharp injuries were from opening ampoules (Guo *et al.*, 1999).

In China, clinical nurses must snap off the neck of sealed ampoules and aspirate the solution with a syringe before administering an injection. However, the glass surface on the neck of the ampoule often cuts the hands of nurses while preparing the drugs; thus, it takes more time to do this work.

For opening glass ampoules in medical care and in other areas, different types of plates and files, usually made of metal, are widely used. Gripping and the use of these openers are troublesome, especially with wet hands. These tools generally have a short life-span, and after a relatively short time, their cutting edge fails. Thus, these tools cannot disrupt the glass surface of the ampoule neck and additional effort by hand may involve the risk of an accident.

This study is of a new tool to snap off the neck of sealed ampoule. The purpose of this study is to evaluate the efficacy and safety of the new tool; an automatic ampoule opener.

2 METHODS

2.1 *Participants*

Eighty nurses were recruited. All were healthy and reported no musculoskeletal problems that might influence performance detrimentally.

---

*Corresponding Author: Song Changping, E-mail: 405693290@qq.com

2.2 Apparatus and materials

Each subject performed 75 combination of snap-off of the neck of sealed ampoule by using three methods (grinding and slicing, grinding and slicing with gloves, and the new tool) and four sizes of ampoule (1, 5, 10, and 20 ml) with five repetition. The automatic opening device has the Chinese Patent ZL 2012 2 0287998.4.

2.3 Evaluation sheet

The automatic opener device evaluation sheet was compiled by our team, and was used to evaluate the quality of the novel tool and degree of satisfaction by 70 users. The scale includes 10 items. The rating criteria include satisfaction, mild satisfaction, and dissatisfaction.

2.4 Data analysis

SPSS13.0 was used to analyze the data that were described as mean ± SD. Statistical significance was defined as $p < 0.05$.

3 RESULTS

3.1 Structure of automatic ampoule opening device

Cutting, disinfecting, breaking off, and collecting ampoule are completed in one step in the machine. Broken ampoules must be discarded quickly to prevent ampoules gathering in the collecting groove. As the rotating speed of the ampoule slot is slow, ampoules can be picked and placed on the rotating slot after being familiar with the machine operation and a set time for ultraviolet disinfection if the machine is not in use, as shown in Figure 1.

3.2 The effects of disinfection

The results showed that the disinfection effects were not significantly different among three snap-off methods ($p > 0.05$, $n = 10$). No bacteria were detected in this test, as shown in Figure 2.

3.3 The time of snap-off ampoule

Results showed that the time of snap-off ampoule were significantly different among the three slice methods ($p < 0.01$, $n = 10$). Mean time of snap-off using the tool was shorter than using grinding and slicing with gloves and grinding and slicing only. In addition, the time to snap-off the ampoule

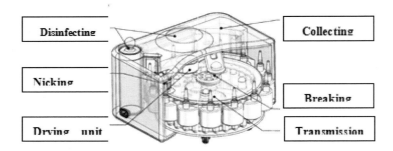

Figure 1. Structure of automatic ampoule opener device.

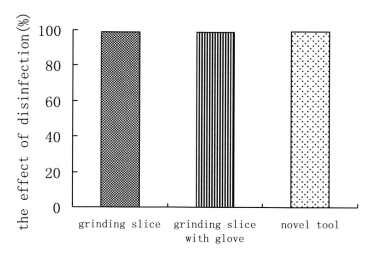

Figure 2. Effect of disinfection among three methods.

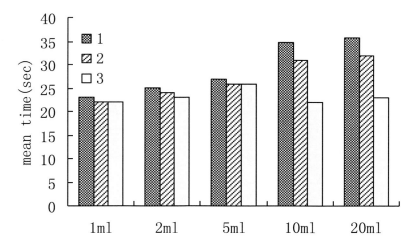

Figure 3. Snap-off time of different sizes of ampoule used by three methods. Grinding and slicing is shown in 1, grinding and slicing with gloves is shown in 2, and the novel tool is shown in 3.

was affected by the size of ampoule. The study indicated that time of snap-off was more longer in 10 and 20 ml of ampoule by grinding and slicing and grinding and slicing with gloves as shown in Figure 3.

3.4 *The evaluation of the degree of the satisfaction with the novel tool-automatic opening device*

The results of this study showed that the novel tool had a positive effect on time saving, safety, and positive attitudes as shown in Figure 4.

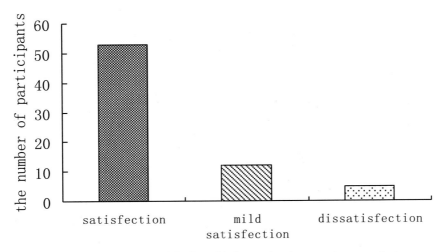

Figure 4.   Evaluation to degree of the satisfaction with the novel tool-automatic opener device.

4   DISCUSSION

It is well known that there are many percutaneous exposure incidents in hospital, of which 38.9% are needle stick injuries, 32.7% were cutaneous exposure, and 28.4% sharps related injuries (Smith *et al.*, 2005). Hagstrom (2006) reported about 54 documented cases of medical personnel in the United States and Canada who were infected with HIV as a result of needle stick injuries.

NSI represent an important cause of injury among nurses. Studies show that Chinese nurses almost all had experienced at least one in their professional lifetime (Smith *et al.*, 2004). Another Japanese study conducted in 2004 also found that ampoules vials, hollow bore needles, and insulin needles were common causes of NSI (Smith *et al.*, 2010).

In China, nurses deal with a large number of ampoules for centralized dispensing on every morning. The risk factor of sharp injuries was opening the glass ampoule. This study was of a novel automatic tool for effective ampoule opening which snaps off the ampoule and improves the efficiency of nurses' work. In addition, sharp injuries caused by snap-off of the ampoules were markedly decreased and satisfaction of nurses was greater with the tool.

We conclude that the automatic ampoule opener is a time-saving, convenient, safe, and efficient device.

REFERENCES

A.M. Hagstrom. (2006) Perceived barriers to implementation of a sucessful sharps safety program. *AORN Journal*, 83, 391–396.

D.R. Smith, P.A. Leggat & K. (2005) Takahashi, Percutaneous exposure incidents among Australian hospital staff. *International Journal of Occupational Safety and Ergonomics*, 11, 323–330.

D.R. Smith, N. Wei & R.S. Wang. (2004) Needlesticks and sharps injuries among chinese hospital nurses. *Advances in Exposure prevention*, 7, 11–12.

D.R. Smith, T. Muto, T. Sairenchi, Y. Ishikawa & S. Sayama, A. (2010) Yoshida and M. Townley-Jones, Hospital safety climate, psychosocial risk factors and needlestick injuries in Japan. *Industrial Health*, 48, 85–95.

Y.H. Guo, J. Shiao, Y.C. Chuang & K.Y. Huang. (1999) Needlestick and sharps injuries among health-care workers in taiwan, *Epidemiology infection*, 122, 256–265.

Medicine Sciences and Bioengineering – Wang (Ed.)
© 2015 Taylor & Francis Group, London, ISBN: 978-1-138-02684-1

Zeta potential of different size of urinary crystallites in lithogenc patients and healthy subjects

Yu-bao Li, Xiao-ling Wen & Jian-ming Ouyang*
Institute of Biomineralization and Lithiasis Research, Jinan University, Guangzhou, Guangdong, China

ABSTRACT: The Zeta potential (ζ) and average particle size ($\bar{d}$) of different sizes of urine crystallites in urine of 15 lithogenic patients and 15 healthy subjects were comparatively investigated by means of nanoparticle size analyzer of Zetasizer Nano-ZS. Different sizes of urine crystallites were obtained after filtration of urine through microporous membrane with different pore sizes (0.22, 0.45, 1.2, 3, and 10 µm), respectively. With the increase of pore size from 0.22 mm to 10 mm, the average value of ζ and $\bar{d}$ in urine of lithogenic patients changed from -4.13 ± 1.33 mV to -8.62 ± 2.11 mV and from 312 ± 134 nm to 3101 ± 781 nm, respectively, however, they changed from -7.61 ± 1.77 mV to -11.9 ± 2.84 mV and from 241 ± 143 nm to 1158 ± 422 nm, respectively, in urine of healthy subjects. Since the greater ζ absolute value indicates greater electrostatic repulsion force between the urine crystallites, thus, the urinary system of lithogenic patients is unstable and the aggregation degree of their urinary crystallites is high. It indicated that the risk of urolithiasis formation of the patients was larger than that of healthy subjects.

1 INTRODUCTION

Urolithiasis is a common disease with high incidence. The occurrence of urolithiasis is still not effectively prevented and its mechanism is still unclear. The first step of calcium oxalate (CaOx) formation is nucleation. The formed nuclei (generally < 10 nm) can grow or/and aggregate to a pathological size (several tens micron). Urinary stones (generally 0.1 cm to several centimeters) are formed after the crystallites are retained in the urinary tract or fixed by the urinary tract organization (He *et al.*, 2010).

In order to clarify the differences of growth and aggregation of different sizes of urine crystallites between stone patients and healthy controls, different pore sizes (0.22, 0.45, 1.2, 3 and 10 µm, respectively) of microporous membrane were used to filtrate the urine of 15 cases of CaOx stone formers and 15 cases of healthy controls, so as to obtain different size ranges of urine crystallites, and the Zeta potential of these crystallites was compared. The results could provide inspiration for clarifying the mechanism of formation of urolithiasis.

2 EXPERIMENTAL SECTION

2.1 *Reagents and apparatus*

All the reagents were analytical purity. Microporous membrane (pore size: 0.22, 0.45, 1.2, 3 and 10 µm, respectively) was purchased from Xinya company (Shanghai, China). The Zeta potential and size distribution of urine crystallites were determined by nanoparticle size analyzer of Zetasizer Nano-ZS (Malvern, England). The experimental conditions were as followings: incident beam of the He-Ne laser, $\lambda = 633.0$ nm, the incident angle of $90°$.

---

* Corresponding authors. E-mail address: toyjm@jnu.edu.cn

2.2 Collection and treatment of urine

The participants in the study included 15 CaOx stones patients and 15 randomly selected healthy persons without prior history of urinary stones. After morning urines were collected, 1% NaN_3 solution was added as antiseptic. The urine samples were centrifuged at 4000 r/m for 15 min and subsequently filtered by microporous membrane with different pore sizes (0.22, 0.45, 1.2, 3, and 10 μm) to remove the cell debris and other distractors in the urines. The filtered urine was stored in clean glassware for detecting.

2.3 Measurement of Zeta potential and size of urine crystallites

After ultrasonication for 3 min, the particle size distribution and ζ of the above filtered urines was immediately detected by nanoparticle size analyzer. All the data were the average values of three parallel tests. The experimental data were expressed as the mean ± standard deviation ($\bar{x} \pm s$).

3 RESULTS AND DISCUSSION

3.1 The Zeta potential of different sizes of urine crystallites

1. The ζ of healthy controls is more negative than that of the patients
As shown in Fig. 1A, the ζ of healthy controls is more negative than that of the patients. ζ can approximate represent for the surface potential of uniform charged spherical particle: $\zeta = 4\pi(\sigma/\varepsilon\kappa)$ (Pawar et al., 2009), where s was the surface charge density of the particles, e was urine dielectric constant, k was Debye–Hückel constant. That is: ζ of urine crystallite is proportional to particle surface charge density (σ), and σ was related to both the concentration of the anionic inhibitors in the urine, and the adsorption ability of the inhibitors on urine crystallites. Since the urine of controls contains more types, more concentrated or more active inhibitory substances than that of CaOx stone patients. Therefore, the ζ of healthy controls was more negative than that of patients. The urine inhibitors include inorganic salts such as citrate and pyrophosphate, and urinary macromolecules such as glycosaminoglycans (GAGs), osteopontin, and prothrombin fragment I (Basavaraj et al., 2007; Boeve et al., 1994).

We have determined the concentrations of GAGs and citrate in the two kinds of the urine by symplectic blue colorimetric method (Whiteman, 1973) and partial ammonium vanadate activation catalytic kinetic spectrophotometry (Ding et al., 2009), respectively. The results showed that urinary GAGs concentration of the patients and controls was 5.18 ± 1.19 and 9.80 ± 2.32 mg/L, respectively, and the urine citrate was 264 ± 118 and 348 ± 108 mg/L, respectively. Since the negative charges of the crystallites in patients' urine were less than those of the controls, the crystallites in patients' urine were easy to aggregate, and thus the possibility of patients to form stones was increased.

2. With the increase of crystallite size, ζ became more negative.
As shown in Fig. 1A, with the increase of filtration membrane aperture from 0.22 μm to 0.45, 1.2, 3 and 10 μm, and the average value of ζ of urine crystallites in 15 cases of controls decreased from −7.61 mV to −8.79, −10.00, −10.70 and −11.90 mV respectively. The rangeability is 4.29 mV. By contrast, ζ of urine crystallites of 15 cases patients decrease from −4.13 mV to −5.34, −6.43, −7.81 and −8.62 mV respectively, and the rangeability is 4.49 mV. This is due to the adsorption capacity of anionic inhibitors on micron-grade urinary crystals were stronger than that of nanoscale crystallites. When urine was filtered through a small size of membrane filter, the large size of the urine crystallites was filtered off, and the small size of urine crystallites was still in the urine. Since the small size of crystallites have many grain boundaries and a large number of lattice defects (Chen et al., 2000), so the ability of these small size of crystallites to adsorb anions was weak (Pawar & Bohidar, 2009), the absolute value of ξ was less, then concentration differences of

the anion inhibitors in the urine was the primary control factor to affect Zeta potential (Sonavane *et al.*, 2008).

However, when urine was filtered through a larger size of membrane filter, both the large size and small size urine crystallites were left in urine. Due to the order of crystal lattice in micron-level crystallite surface, structural integrity, the high degree of crystallization in the crystal surface and more surface charge (such as the surface of COM has positive charge, but it became negative after the adsorption of anionic), and its capacity to adsorb anionic inhibitor was much stronger than that of the small size of nanocrystals. The ability difference of surface adsorption to anions plays a major role to Zeta potential of urine crystallites (Koka *et al.*, 2000). Therefore, with the increase of the membrane pore size, the particle size of urine crystallites increased, their surface charges gradually increased, and their capacity to adsorb anions gradually increased, thereby they could adsorb more anionic inhibitors and thus led to an increase of negative charges density on crystallites' surface, that is, the Zeta potential of urine crystallites become more negative.

ζ reflects directly the electrostatic repulsion force between the crystallites. If the absolute value of ζ was greater (Zeta potential is more negative), the electrostatic repulsion force between the urine crystallites was greater, and the reunion of the crystallites was harder.

3.2 Size distribution of the two types of urine crystallites after filtered by different pore sizes of microporous membrane

The size distribution and average particle diameter ($\bar{d}$) of two types of urine crystallites from 15 cases of CaOx calculi patients and 15 cases of healthy subjects after being filtrated by different pore size microporous membrane were comparatively studied. With the increase of pore size from 0.22 mm to 10 mm, the $\bar{d}$ value in urine of lithogenic patients increased from 312 ± 134 nm to 3101 ± 781 nm (Figure 1B), however, it only increased from 241 ± 143 nm to 1158 ± 422 nm for the crystallites in urine of healthy subjects.

1. Figure 2 shows the size distribution of urinary crystallites of one representative COM stone patients and one healthy control. With the pore size of microporous membrane increasing from 0.22 μm to 0.45, 1.2 and 3 μm, the size of urine crystallites of COM calculus patient grows from 267 nm to 395, 772 and 1718 nm (Figure 2a-d), and that of the control just increase from 184 nm to 384, 499 and 823 nm (Figure 2e-h), respectively.

2. There was less difference of the size between the two types of urine crystallites after filtered through pore size of 0.22 and 0.45 μm filter membrane; while the $\bar{d}$ value of patients was significantly larger than that of controls after filtered through pore size of 3.0 and 10.0 μm filter membrane (Figure 1B). The difference between the two types of urine crystallite size reached 1943 nm when pore size was 10 μm. That is, with the pore size of microporous membrane

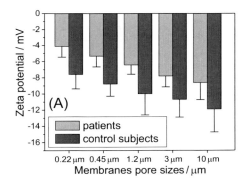
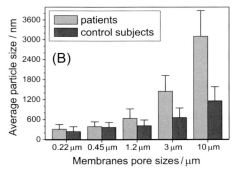

Figure 1. Zeta potential (A) and average particle size (B) of urinary crystallites from 15 calculi patients and 15 healthy controls filtered through membranes with different pore sizes.

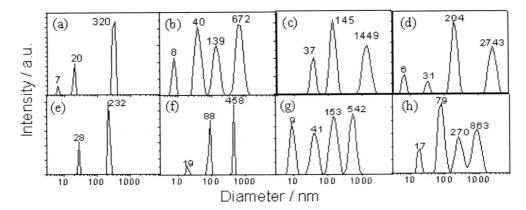

Figure 2. Size distribution of urinary crystallites of one representative COM calculi patient (a–d) and one healthy control (e–h) after filtered through membranes with different pore sizes. Pore size: (a, e): 0.22 μm, (b, f): 0.45 μm, (c, g): 1.2 μm, (d, h): 3 μm.

increasing from 0.22 μm to 10 μm, the average particle size of urine crystallites of calculi patients significantly increased and the increment was 2789 nm; but the increment of controls was only 917 nm. It indicated that the quantity of small size of urine crystallites of the controls was significantly more than that of CaOx calculi patients.

3. The particle size of urine crystallites was much smaller than the corresponding membrane pore size. For instance, the $\bar{d}$ value of lithogenic urine crystallites was 3101 nm, while that of the controls was 1158 nm after filtered through a pore size of 10 μm filter membrane. It showed that the crystallites with a size of more than 4 μm were hard to pass through the filter membrane of 10 μm. This result can help to select an appropriate pore size of the membrane in the future study of the properties of certain size of urine crystallites.

Since the growth of urine crystallites was a very slow process, and the agglomeration of urine crystallites can be completed quickly in a short time (He *et al.*, 2010), the results in this work showed that the urine crystallites of patients were easier to aggregate than that of the controls, and the small size of urine crystallites were easier to aggregate than that of the large one. Therefore, the rapid aggregation of urine crystallites may be one of the key factors of calculi formation.

4   CONCLUSIONS

Different sizes of urine crystallites were obtained after filtration of urine through microporous membrane with different pore sizes (0.22, 0.45, 1.2, 3, and 10 μm), respectively. With the increase of crystallite size, ζ became more negative in both the urines of lithogenic patients and healthy subjects. The Zeta potential (ζ) of healthy controls was more negative than that of the patients. The particle size of urine crystallites was much smaller than the corresponding membrane pore size. Since the greater ζ absolute value indicates greater electrostatic repulsion force between the urine crystallites, thus, the urinary system of lithogenic patients is unstable and the aggregation degree of their urinary crystallites is high. It indicated that the risk of urolithiasis formation of the patients was larger than that of healthy subjects.

ACKNOWLEDGEMENT

This research work was supported by the Natural Science Foundation of China (81170649).

REFERENCES

Basavaraj, D.R., Biyani. C.S., Browing, A.J. & Cartledge, J.J. (2007) The role of urinary kidney stone inhibitors and promoters in the pathogenesis of calcium containing renal stones. *EAU-EBU Update Series*, 5: 126–136.

Boeve, E.R., Cao, L.C., De Bruijn W.C., Robertson, W.G., Romijn, J.C. & Schroder, F.H. (1994) Zeta potential distribution on calcium oxalate crystal and Tamm-Horsfall protein surface analyzed with Doppler electrophoretic light scattering. *The Journal of Urology*, 152: 531–536.

Chen, Q. & Yun, S.R. (2000) Synthesizing nano-sized diamond through explosive detonation and its application. *Journal of Synthetic Crystals*, 29(1): 90–93.

Ding, S.F., Jin, H.M. & Zhu, S.P. (2009) Catalytic activation dynamic determination of citric acid. *Chinese Journal of Health Laboratory Technology*, 19(7): 1520–1521.

He, J.Y., Ouyang J.M. & Yang Y.E. (2010) Agglomeration of urinary nanocrystallites: key factor to formation of urinary stone. *Materials Science & Engineering, C: Materials for Biological Applications*, 30: 878–885.

Koka, R.M., Huang, E. & Lieske, J.C. (2000) Adhesion of uric acid crystals to the surface of renal epithelial cells. *American Journal of Physiology*, 2000, 278: 989–998.

Pawar, N. & Bohidar, H.B. (2009) Surface selective binding of nanoclay particles to polyampholyte protein chains. *Macromolecular Chemistry and Physics*, 131(045103): 1–7.

Sonavane, G., Tomoda, K. & Makino, K. (2008) Biodistribution of colloidal gold nanoparticles after intravenous administration: effect of particle size. *Colloids and Surfaces B*, 66(2): 274–280.

Whiteman P. (1973) The quantitative determination of glycosaminoglycans in urine with Alcian Blue 8GX. *The Biochemical journal*, 131(2): 351–357.

Medicine Sciences and Bioengineering – Wang (Ed.)
© *2015 Taylor & Francis Group, London, ISBN: 978-1-138-02684-1*

Individualized nursing intervention in patients with chronic hepatitis C antiviral treatment adherence

Xiu-li Cheng, Yu-chen Cao, Cheng-jiao Liu & Yan-fu Sun
Gao gan Ward, First Hospital of Jilin University, Changchun, Jilin, China

ABSTRACT: Through individualized interventions, there is an increase in patients with hepatitis C antiviral treatment compliance. Doctor-patient joint efforts are underway in order to obtain longer and more sustained virological response.

1   INTRODUCTION

This paper will take the polyethylene glycol (PEG) 78, restructuring integration interferon variants (PEG IFN-SA) clinical trials of chronic hepatitis C subjects who were randomly divided into intervention group and control group according to their weight. Each group consisted of 39 people. The intervention group was given at 4 weeks, 8 weeks, 12 weeks, and 24 weeks after the treatment the 90 symptom checklist (SCL-90) questionnaire test. In the treatment of patients each with different social, family, physical, and mental health problems, targeted nursing intervention is applied. The control group was provided normal review according to the requirements of the research plan.

The intervention group according to the regulations of the plan had to complete antiviral treatment for 29 cases (29/39, 74.36%). The control group had to complete for 19 cases (19/39, 48.7%). Completion of the intervention group was obviously higher than that of the control group, $p < 0.05$. The intervention group completed an average of $32 + 8$ weeks; the control group completed an average of $26 + 7$ weeks. The intervention group completed longer weeks than the control group on average. The difference was statistically significant ($P < 0.05$). There was no difference between intervention group and control group in influenza-like symptoms, cough, sore throat, and other adverse reactions. Mood changes, irritability, and other mental abnormalities were significantly lesser in the intervention group than the control group, which was statistically significant ($P < 0.05$).

This study provides free treatment; thus, the influence of economic factors is ruled out. Personalized nursing intervention can effectively solve the patient's response to interferon anti-HCV and address the lack of knowledge. It is effective in relieving patients with hepatitis C from adverse reactions caused by negative emotions. To reduce the degree of mental abnormalities, increase the confidence on antiviral treatment, which greatly improves the compliance of HCV patients to improve the sustained response rate.

2   THE OBJECT OF STUDY

Hepatitis C is a global epidemic; it is the biggest cause of end-stage liver disease. In our country, about 42 million people are infected with HCV. The infection rate is 3.2% (Chengjun, 2010). The incidence of HCV infection patients after 20 years, cirrhosis of the liver is about 12.5% (Everson GT, 2005). Due to the height of the hepatitis C virus (HCV), genetic variability and other body tissues surrounding the virus can infect the liver. HCV is very difficult to remove. Interferon (IFN) recurrence rates of 28.6% to 52.9% after treatment; But as the standard antiviral treatment, individualized treatment and direct antiviral drugs, chronic hepatitis C, chronic hepatitis C, CHC) sustained virological response

(SUS - tained virological response, SVR) rate has exceeded 66% in genotype 1 HCV infection, 2, 3, type of HCV infection in more than 80% (Poordad F, 2011). HCV standard antiviral treatment is an important factor, and treatment time must achieve the required course of treatment. *The prevention and treatment of hepatitis* C guide also points out that the patient's compliance is an important factor affecting curative effect. The medical staff in the process of investigate HCV treatment in spiritual, the psychological factors in patients with HCV intervention is important.

This study is polyethylene glycol (PEG) restructuring integration interferon variants (PEG IFN-SA) injection single-center, randomized, positive control, multiple doses, single and multiple dosing in patients with chronic hepatitis C human tolerance and pharmacokinetic study.

Inclusion criteria: (1) Aged 18 to 65 years of age; (2) body mass index (BMI) in the range of 18-26; (3) anti-HCV or HCV RNA positive for more than 6 months; (4) HCV RNA quantitative acuity 2000 iu/mL; (5) the ALT within the upper limit of normal 2.5 times.

Exclusion criteria: (1) malignant tumors, anemia, and other diseases of each system. (2) Received interferon treatment in the past 6 months or always showed no response to interferon treatment. (3) White blood cell count $< 3 \times 10^9/$ L; neutrophil count $< 1.5 \times 10^9$/L; the platelet count $< 90 \times 10^9$/L; hemoglobin is lower than the normal reference value lower limit; serum total bilirubin > 2 times the upper limit of normal reference value. (4) Suspected liver cirrhosis; hepatocellular carcinoma (HCC). When screening, FibroScan values greater than or equal to F3. Of the patients included in this study, 78 met the discharge standard (CHC). According to body mass index (bmi), they were randomly divided into intervention group and control group, with 39 cases in each. The intervention group had 10 female and 29 male cases,2a type of 14 cases, 24 cases of type b, Not parting in 1 case, The average age (48.21 ± 10). The control group had 26 male and 13 female cases. 13 cases of type 2 a, 1 b 23 cases, not parting in 3 patients.The average age was 45.76 ± 11. Between the two groups before the demographic information, genotyping, medication virus quantitative statistical differences ($P > 0.05$) (see table 1).

3 RESEARCH METHODS

3.1 *Treatment and virus detection methods*

PEG IFN-SA mu 1.5 ug/kg to the advantage of warning 0.45 / bid combination therapy. 2 a genotype 24 weeks of treatment, 1 b 48 weeks of treatment. 2 a / 1 b genotypes 48 weeks of treatment. In order to avoid antiviral treatment in patients with chronic hepatitis C by HCV RNA detection, reagent errors result in treatment failure. In the key monitoring point (4, 12, 24, and 48 weeks of treatment, 72 weeks), international standard test is used to detect the contents of HCV RNA (readings minimum 50 IU/mL or less) (Xierao, 2013).

3.2 *Intervention methods*

Intervention group adopt methods such as preparation before intervention, self-management education, process of timely feedback of test results, and psychological nursing of serious adverse events (SAEs). The control group had regular follow-ups and adverse reaction monitoring.

3.2.1 *Medication before intervention*
Medication before propaganda education including told antiviral treatment in patients with the necessity, the possible adverse reaction and response rates reported in the literature. The treatment process must include regular monitoring of content and time and the virus genotype to maximize the SVR must adhere to treatment, guarantee the specification of the dose of drug treatment on the importance of the SVR, etc., should try to avoid unnecessary reduction or withdrawal out (for example, to go out, forgotten, and so on). If during the course of treatment dosage reduction or temporary withdrawal is inevitable for medical factors, you must inform the doctor, perform ShiYanChang treatment at the end of the course, and make up for the reduction or withdrawal and

the loss of the dose (Xieqing, 2013). The prospect of interferon antiviral therapy is introduced to increase confidence on the antiviral treatment. In a timely manner after proper antiviral treatment, quite a proportion (65%) of patients with CHC can achieve SVR; some patients can even be clinically cured (Firpi RJ, 2009). Thus, the CHC antiviral treatment should adopt a more positive attitude. Have a good way of life, learn to self emotion management and self condition monitoring, strict drinking, control of body mass index is not greater than 26 kg/cm squared, and so on. In 2011, the European Association of Liver (EASL) in their guide states that obesity and alcohol affect response rates as "refractory factors" (J Hepatol, 2011).

3.2.2 *Self-management education*

Self-management education can significantly improve a patient's self-management ability. A large number of evidence-based studies have confirmed that effective treatment, self-management support, and regular follow-up are the three important factors of chronic care (Renyuebo, 2012). Through self-management education, the majority of patients can correctly grasp the interferon plus ribavirin treatment during the clinical manifestations of adverse reactions and harmfulness and countermeasures of eliminating patients with the suspicion of adverse reaction and improve the ability of patients to identify incomplete or even wrong information (Huangchangxing, 2006). The curative effect and adverse reaction of the main indicators (such as viruses, white blood cells, neutrophils quantitative absolute value, hemoglobin content, etc.) have a preliminary understanding. They can communicate with follow-up medical staff in time, effectively reduce the complications, and increase the confidence of patients with antiviral treatment. People is the master of the behavior, evaluation and management of their own ability, can through self management to achieve the purpose of stay healthy. Through individualized intervention, help patients to build the health belief model, patients' health belief and the treatment compliance of patients were positively correlated, patients think taking non-compliance behavior will benefit, is the higher compliance (Fenghui, 2005).

3.2.3 *Drug use in the process of timely feedback test results*

Many factors can affect the effect of antiviral treatment of chronic hepatitis C, and the amount of virus in the antiviral treatment changes with SVR to obtain a significant predictive and correlation (Xierao, 2013). Virus ration is the most reliable method of validating antiviral treatment curative effect; Encouraging patients with good effect, strengthen confidence, actively, and looking for the reason of effect of slow and correct in time.

3.2.4 *For Serious Adverse Events (SAEs) of psychological nursing*

Psychological nursing is based on psychotherapy theory and method, through special psychological counseling to eliminate the psychological barrier and restore or improve the patient's physical and mental health (Biaihong, 2006). The intervention group at 4 weeks after the treatment, 8 weeks, 12 weeks and 24 weeks give item symptom checklist 90 (SCL - 90) questionnaire test, understand each patient in the treatment in the process of social, family, physical and mental health problems, such as targeted nursing intervention.

3.3 *Statistical methods*

Age in patients with intervention group and control group by T test, the number of count data such as gender, gene types using chi-square test and the statistical software is SPSS 16.0.

4 RESULTS

4.1 *Adverse reactions of the intervention group compared with the treatment group*

In the intervention group, according to the regulations of the plan it was decided to complete the number of antiviral treatment for 29 (29/39, 74.36%). Compared with 19, 48.7% (19/39), completion intervention group was obviously higher than that of control group ($p < 0.05$). There was no difference between intervention group and control group in influenza-like symptoms, cough, sore throat, and other adverse reactions. Mood changes, irritability, and other mental abnormalities were significantly less in the intervention group than the control group, which was statistically significant (12/39 25/39 intervention group and control group, $P < 0.05$). Adverse reactions to the questionnaire in 5 cases of patients with anxiety and depression symptoms occurred in the observation group, accounting for 6% of the total number of cases.

4.2 Individualized treatment weeks intervention make intervention group was obviously higher than that of control group

According to the plan complete obviously increase the percentage of treatment cycle. Response rates after 12 weeks are shown in table (1). Poor adherence was shown in 22 and 24 weeks. 8 cases suffering from serious adverse reactions, the researchers suggest that exit, accounted for 33% of the number of incomplete treatment. Affect about 60% of the compliance of the reasons for fear of serious adverse reactions. The intervention group showed completion of an average of $32 + 8$ weeks, and the control group showed an average completion of $26 + 7$ weeks; to complete an average week longer than the control group, the intervention group was statistically significant ($P < 0.05$).

5 SUMMARY

The clinical manifestation of chronic hepatitis C is often the specificity; although symptoms are not serious, long-term disease states can lead to effects on patients' health, physiological function, and psychological tolerance and self-health cognition gradually decreases (Wangtingting, 2013). Individual patients after intervention can actively participate in the treatment of diseases, improve the ability of self-management of disease, improve mental and physical health, and develop a good lifestyle, encouraging them to have more confidence to face disease, challenge themselves, and eventually improve their quality of life. Poor adherence are result mainly in failure to finish treatment dose and period of treatment: Some patients do not understand the importance of antiviral treatment, because some adverse reactions often appear with interferon and ribavirin treatment processes. Some poorly compliant patients often do not consult the opinions of clinicians and will perform drug dosage reduction without authorization. Due to insufficient attention to treatment, some patients often forgotten RBV oral or interferon injections. There are also some patients after HCV RNA turn Yin think the virus has disappeared, do not need to continue treatment and drug withdrawal and lost to follow-up on his own. Some patients in the course of treatment cannot continue in the treatment by medical institutions because of work or residence changes and opt for

Table 1. Polyethylene glycol (PEG) resource restructuring integration interferon variation in intervention group compared with control group on the basis of the data and clinical data.

Item	N_1/N	2 a / 1 b/not parting	The number of weeks treatment	Age	Male/female	Response rates
Intervention group	29/39	14/24/1	32 ± 8	45.76 ± 11	29/10	20/39
Control group	19/39	13/23/3	26 ± 7	48.21 ± 10	26/13	11/39
Chi-square value/T	5.41	1.058	3.52	1.02	0.555	4.33
P	<0.05	>0.05	<0.05	>0.05	>0.05	<0.05

N_1: the number in accordance with the scheme rules set to complete resistance drug treatment of people.
N: the number in accordance with the scheme rules set to complete resistance drug treatment of people.

interruption of treatment. Because this group of patients with CHC for free treatment in addition to economic factors Monitoring by medical staff of HCV patients in aspects such as the dosage, course of treatment compliance, and treatment effect is particularly important.

Most of the research hold the standpoint that the mechanism of psychotherapy has two sides. On the one hand, through the direct effect of psychological communication use of certain communication skills affects the human body, to improve the function of circulation and adjust the neuroendocrine system; on the other hand, psychological nursing may improve mood through psychological adjustment, relieve anxiety symptoms, and improve mood stability to avoid damage to human body under various stress states (Zhangwen, 2012). Item symptom checklist 90 (SCL-90) questionnaire test results to give individualized psychological nursing can effectively reduce the degree of abnormal psychology, improve the reliance of medical staff, patients and improve treatment confidence (Renzhen, 2007) adverse events of life had a great influence on negative emotions. This occurs in patients with hepatitis C antivirus during severe adverse reactions. It can cause panic. Medical personnel must use medical and psychological theories. They must make the patients understand that in interferon treatment during the occurrence of serious adverse events (SAEs) there are individual differences. Many basic disease conditions before the occurrence of adverse reactions and drug use, regular review, and timely treatment can avoid the occurrence of SAEs. Seeking good social support can help mobilize the inner psychological process and resources to help patients cope with all kinds of stress and make the patients communicate more with the outside world through the support of family and friends to enhance compliance (Xiaojing, 2012). The intervention group in the study adopts the following methods to intervene: preparation before the intervention, self-management education, process of timely feedback test results, and psychological nursing of serious adverse events (SAEs). The control group is provided regular follow-ups and adverse reaction monitoring. This can significantly improve patient compliance, reduce psychological burden, and improve the curative effect of treatment of HCV patients.

REFERENCES

Biaihong.Zhanglan. Present situation and countermeasure of clinical psychological nursing. The nurse education journal, 2006, 21(9): 814–816.

Chengjun. New progress of chronic hepatitis c treatment. The experiment and the journal of clinical infectious diseases, 2010, 4(1): 1–3.

Everson GT. Management of cirrhosis due to chronic hepatitis C [J]. J Hepatol, 2005, 42(Suppl 1): S65–S74.

European Association for the Study of the Liver. EASL clinical practice guidelines: management of hepatitis C virus infection. J Hepatol, 2011, 55: 245–264.

Fenghui.Heguoping. Self-management education for interferon therapy of chronic hepatitis c patients quality of life. The influence of the people's liberation army nursing journal, 2013, 30(5): 10–13.

Firpi RJ, Clark V, Soldevila Pico C, et al. The natural history of hepatitis C cirrhosis after liver transplantation. Liver Transpl, 2009, 15: 1063–1071.

Huangchangxing.Baixuefan. Chronic viral hepatitis C antiviral treatment of adverse reactions and their processing. Chinese journal of infectious diseases, 2006, 24(3).

Poordad F, McCone J Jr, Bacon BR, et al. Boceprevir for untreated chronic HCV genotype 1 infection[J]. N Engl J Med, 2011, 364(13): 1195–1206.

Renzhen Lihuicong.Baozhiying. Interferon therapy in patients with viral hepatitis c drug compliance of the influencing factors and nursing. The Chinese journal of modern nursing, 2007, 13(35): 3440–3441.

Renyuebo. Zhangyaohui.songxueai, etc. Self-management education for the effect of interferon therapy in patients with hepatitis C. Qilu nursing journal, 2012, 18(18): 19–20.

Shiffm an ML, Suter E Bacon BR, et al. PEG interferon alfa·2a and fibari for 16 or 24 weeks in HCV genotype 2 or 3 . N Engl J Med, 2007, 357: 124–134.

Wangtingting.Xueliming.jinpinpin. Self-management education for interferon therapy of chronic hepatitis C patients quality of life. The influence of the people's liberation army nursing journal, 2013, 30(5): 10–13.

Xiaojing.Chenping.Lixiaoshan, etc. The influence factors of chronic hepatitis b patients quality of life. The liver disease, 2012, 20(9): 649–653.

Xierao Liminghui. How to achieve higher cure rate through standardized antiviral treatment. Chinese journal of liver disease, 2013, 21(6): 408–409.

Xieqing.Guoxinmin. Patients with chronic hepatitis C treatment failure causes and principles of management. Chinese journal of liver disease, 2013, 21(6): 417–419.

Xierao.liminghui. How to achieve higher cure rate through standardized antiviral treatment. Chinese journal of liver disease, 2013, 21(6): 408–409.

Zhangwen.Fangli.niuhaiyan. A-2 a PEG interferon to depressive symptoms in patients with chronic hepatitis b individualized psychological nursing. Journal of college of armed police logistics (medical), 2012, 21(10): 781–783.

Medicine Sciences and Bioengineering – Wang (Ed.)
© *2015 Taylor & Francis Group, London, ISBN: 978-1-138-02684-1*

Unexpected difficult intubation inspired by asymptomatic lingual thyroid

Yang-dong Han, Kai Li* & Peng Chen
Department of Anesthesia, China–Japan Union Hospital of Jilin University, Changchun, China

ABSTRACT: The occurrence of a thyroid gland superficially placed on the pharyngeal portion of the tongue is rare but poses problems to the patient and the anesthetist. This report describes a patient with a lingual thyroid whose only positive sign is a vague tone. The stealthiness during preoperative assessment resulted in an unexpected difficult airway condition in a gynecological case. Comprehensive and programmed anesthetic managements including GlideScope, fiber-optic bronchoscope, LMA, and tracheotomy are utilized in the patient. Indications drawn out from the case are as follows: 1. Ectopic thyroid surrounding airway should be paid great attention in future medical activities, offering particular guidance to clinical treatment. 2. Any trifles and clues associated with airway assessment should be brought to the forefront. 3. Both sufficient oxygen supply and low side injury are the main points in handling the unexpected difficult airway. It is wise to make preliminary preparation and rational choice among the various kinds of auxiliary intubation or ventilation tools based on the actual situation.

1 INTRODUCTION

The anatomical position of the thyroid gland varies considerably. It may cause problems for the anesthetist as a result of compression of the airway, enlargement, or its anatomical position. Ectopic thyroid is a rare developmental anomaly disease, characterized by low incidence rate, and is more often in women (Baldw, 1998 & Rulif, 2000). The lingual thyroid is so called because it lies within, or on the surface of, the pharyngeal portion of the tongue. It is in this latter position that this condition may pose a particular problem to the patient and the anesthetist because of possible hemorrhage during attempts at intubation. It may also completely obscure the laryngeal inlet. Meanwhile, the existence of thyroid neoplasms seldom brings about typical concomitant manifestation due to their peculiar small size. Obvious prefigurative symptoms and signs of difficult airway such as pharyngeal discomfort, dysphagia, expiratory dyspnea, and snoring unusually happened in most of the clinical patients including the following textbook case. The associated experience and tackle procession on the unexpected difficult intubation case caused by rare disease shall be paid more attention in the anesthesia process.

2 CASE REPRESENTATION

The patient presented in this study was a 49-year-old woman (163 cm, 90 kg) with ASA physical status II; she was diagnosed with uterine fibroids and secondary severe anemia and was scheduled for selective laparoscopic total hysterectomy under general anesthesia. The result of conventional preoperative assessment was barely abnormal, and the sole positive sign described as a slurred tone was not taken seriously. Typical symptoms associated with airway neoplasm including pharyngeal discomfort, dysphagia, expiratory dyspnea, and snoring were negative. Airway assessment was

*Corresponding author: Kai Li: likai82@126.com.

normal with a Mallampati score of 2, normal cervical spine extension, a thyromental distance of 6.3 cm, and adequate jaw thrust. In view of her obesity (BMI = 33.87 kg/m²) and higher modified Mallampati scoring, our presupposed plan contained intravenous rapid sequence induction, oral tracheal intubation assisted by GlideScope, and inhalation anesthetics for anesthesia maintenance. In the anesthetic room, full monitoring was applied and intravenous access was established. After premedication with 1.0 mg of penehyclidine hydrochloride intravenously (IV) and preoxygenation with 100% oxygen for three minutes, intravenous induction was performed with midazolam 0.02 mg/kg, propofol 1.5 mg/kg, and sufentanil 0.5 ug/kg. Once adequacy of mask ventilation was confirmed, 0.5 mg/kg of rocuronium was administered intravenously. Mask assist ventilation had been normally processing for 3 minutes. After the patient was placed in the sniffing position, an initial laryngoscopic attempt was performed by an attending anesthesiologist with 15 years of experience. Under the GlideScope (Saturn Biomedical Systems, Burnaby, BC, Canada), there appeared a quasi-circular neuroplasm, 3.0 cm in diameter, with smooth surface beneath the surface of tongue root. Due to the inhibition, tracheal catheter cannot be advanced into the glottis. Subsequently, nasal intubation with flexible fiber-optic bronchoscope guidance failed twice in trials manipulated by an expert. Finally, #4 Supreme laryngeal mask chosen as an emergency instrument was correctly placed. During the mechanical ventilation phase, the patient was under the condition of 35 cmH$_2$O peak airway pressure and 94% S$_p$O$_2$. The operation was canceled. After fully awake extubation, patient was sent back to the ward without any adverse sequelae. Both electronic laryngoscopy (see figure 1) and ^{131}I imaging SPECT/CT (see figure 2) were carried out as further examinations for the cause of obstruction on the next day. The result is described as radioactivity increased shadow considered as ectopicthyroidgland Three days later, the patient was scheduled for the gynecological operation once again. She and her relatives rejected conscious nasal intubation with the assistance of fiber bronchoscope based on misgiving regarding the high incidence of failure and complication associated with the plan. After tracheotomy under local anesthesia, general anesthesia and operation proceeded uneventfully. The patient was discharged from the hospital after recovery 11 days later.

3   DISCUSSION

It is found in this asymptomatic case that the unexpected difficult intubation during general anesthesia is related to ectopic thyroid located in the superficial layer of tongue root. As a rare developmental anomaly disease, ectopic thyroid neoplasms are unnoticeable because they seldom bring about typical concomitant manifestation that points to difficult airway due to their peculiar small size. Close attention has not been paid to vague tone as the only positive sign. The stealthiness gives rise to the risk of unexpected difficult airway. Anesthetic managements with regard to urgent difficult airway are closely related to the safety and quality of anesthesia. Experience based on the case has the following important enlightenments.

3.1   *Scrupulous presurgical evaluation plays an indispensable role in the safety and quality of anesthesia*

This patient presented with very limited physical features indicative of the possibility of difficult intubation, which is extremely challenging. Provided that slurred tone as the only positive sign

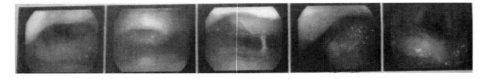

Figure 1.   View of electronic laryngoscopy displaying neoplasm at the foramen cecum of the tongue.

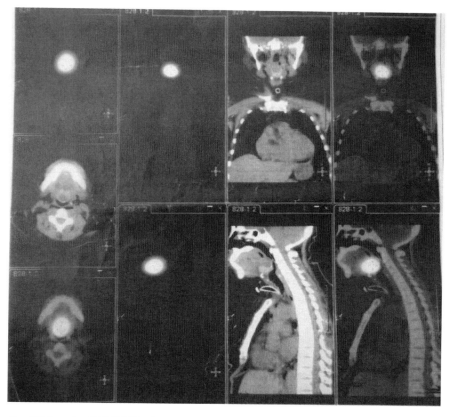

Figure 2. [131]I imaging SPECT/CT picture confirms the radioactivity-increased shadow as ectopic thyroid benign tumor.

was taken seriously, an additional electronic laryngoscopy examination should have been strongly recommended to the suspected case besides routine airway assessment. The emergency condition of unexpected difficult intubation in the operation theater and primary intubation failure would have been avoided. Any subtle symptom should have been paid adequate attention. Full-scale evaluation and comprehensive plane provide effective safeguards for the anesthetic procedure including airway management.

3.2 Strategy for the unexpected difficult airway

It is a disaster to come across with unexpected difficult airway after induction without spontaneous breathing. In a case of difficult airway management, it is clear that a "can't ventilate" situation is more critical than a "can't intubate" one. The American Society of Anesthesiologists Task Force on Management of the Difficult Airway recommends establishing emergency invasive airway for the "can't ventilation" situation (American Society of Anesthesiologists Task Force on Management of the Difficult Airway, 2003). Both cricothyroid membrane puncture or incision and tracheotomy are imperative strategies (Goon & Green, 2009) in order to ensure the oxygen supply. However, it is very lucky for us that the adequacy of mask ventilation was confirmed. Repeated blind and violent attempts should be averted in this kind of simple unexpected difficult intubation case caused by local lesion. Associated iatrogenic injury such as pharyngolaryngeal edema, trauma, and subsequent hemorrhage will lead to more serious intubation complications and deteriorate the situation into the "can't ventilate" condition. Various kinds of auxiliary video intubation systems may be definitely useful in improving the view of glottic structures in case of poor laryngoscopic vision. Laryngeal mask airway (LMA) considered as a supraglottic device is strongly recommended for the failure intubation condition after temperate attempts even with advanced auxiliary equipments.

3.3 *Both primary and secondary strategies should be scheduled for difficult airway management*

In the representative case, a sufficient and handy assistant kit such as video laryngoscope, fiber-optic bronchoscope, and LMA makes the whole process sleek. GlideScope (Saturn Biomedical Systems, Burnaby, BC, Canada) and McGrath laryngoscopes (Aircraft Medical Ltd., Edinburgh, UK) are useful in the improvement of glottic views. Besides fiber bronchoscope, special tubes such as Parker flex tip (Parker Medical, Englewood, CO) and styles such as Gliderite (Verathon Medical, Bothell, WA), Trachlight (Laerdal Medical Corp, Long Beach, CA), and Seeing Optical Stylet System (SOS, Clarus Medical, Minneapolis, MN) may be used to aid glottic entry. Abundant clinical studies and case reports reveal the significant role of the esophageal tracheal double-lumen airway (Combitube™, Kendall–Sheridan, Argyll, USA) and laryngeal mask airway (LMA) in emergency medicine and in difficult airway management. The original difficult airway algorithm devised in 1991 by the ASA stated that "if there is a good possibility that intubation and/or ventilation by mask will be difficult, then the airway should be secured while the patient is still awake." Because of its safety and its effectiveness, awake fiber-optic intubation (AFOI) has become the "gold standard scheme" in difficult airway situations, especially in expected cases. It is wise to make preliminary preparation and rational choice among various kinds of auxiliary intubation or ventilation tools based on the actual situation.

4 SUMMARY

Operaion process should been carried out in a well-organized pattern according to recommended guidelines in the situation of unexpected difficult airway. All these sensible strategies should be based on principles combined with sufficient oxygen supply and less side injury. It is wise to make preliminary preparation and rational choice among various kinds of auxiliary intubation or ventilation tools based on the actual situation. Sufficient accumulation on relevant experience and operation skills plays an important role on the emergency condition.

REFERENCES

American Society of Anesthesiologists Task Force on Management of the Difficult Airway. (2003) Practice guidelines for management of the difficult airway: an updated report by the American Society of Anesthesiologists Task Force on Management of the Difficult Airway. Anesthesiology, 98, 1269–1277.
Baldwin RL, Copeeland SK. (1998) Lingual thyroid and associated epiglottitis. S Med J, 81, 1538.
Goon SS, Stephens RC, Smith H. (2009) The emergency airway. Br J Hosp Med (Lond), 70(12), M186–M188.
Green L. (2009) Can't intubate, can't ventilate! A survey of knowledge and skills in a large teaching hospital. Eur J Anaesthesiol, 6(6), 480–483.
Rulif TG. (2000) Follicular carcinoma in ectopic thyroid gland. G Chir, 18(3), 97.

Medicine Sciences and Bioengineering – Wang (Ed.)

Development and validation of bioactive components of *Xiao xianggou (Ficus)*

Hui-qing Lv
Zhejiang Chinese Medical University, Hangzhou, China

Xue-zhi Chen
People Hospital of Jingning, Lishui, China

Zhi-jun Xie & Cheng-ping Wen*
Zhejiang Chinese Medical University, Hangzhou, China

ABSTRACT: *Xiao xianggou (Ficus)*, was widely used as traditional "She" medicine in Zhejiang Province, China. In this work, a Reversed-Phase High-Performance Liquid Chromatography (RP-HPLC) coupled with Diode Array Detection (DAD) and electrospray ionization mass spectrometry (ESI-MS) method was developed and validated for the simultaneous identification and determination of bioactive components from *Xiao xianggou*. The separation of the six compounds was accomplished through a C18 column, with good specificity and satisfactory resolution. The chromatographic peaks of the four investigated compounds were identified by comparing their retention time, UV and MS spectrum with the corresponding reference compounds. The method showed a good linearity ($r^2 > 0.999$), high precision (RSD < 5.0%), and recoveries (ranged from 87.9 to 95.3%) were acceptable. The developed method exhibited good sensitivity for the determination of such bioactive compounds, and that it constructed a basis for the comprehensive evaluation of the quality of *Xiao xianggou*.

1 INTRODUCTION

Ficus, Moraceae family, constitutes one of the largest species of the flowering plants with approximately 800 genera (Phan *et al.*, 2011). As natural sources of antioxidant agents (Singh *et al.*, 2011), many *Ficus* species are used in Traditional Chinese Medicine (TCM), and their uses originated from the Middle East (Bankeu *et al.*, 2010). *Ficus pandurata* H., commonly known as *Xiao xianggou* in Lishui district (Zhejiang, China), is widely used as food condiment and "She" medicine in Traditional Chinese Medicine to treat arthritis, rheumatism, indigestion, edema, etc (Lei *et al.*, 2007, Lv *et al.*, 2013).

Recently, the chromatographic fingerprint technique has been internationally accepted as an efficient tool for the integral quality control of herbal medicines (Niu *et al.*, 2013, Tang *et al.*, 2014, Peng *et al.*, 2013). Following the general research trend devoted to the development of analytical methods, our current investigation describes a RP-HPLC coupled with DAD and ESI-MS method for both separation and determination of major constitutes in "*Xiao xianggou*". To the best of our knowledge, little information has been reported regarding the phytochemistry of *Xiao xianggou*. Therefore, the objective of the present work, is to provide preliminary data for a comprehensive HPLC-DAD-MS analysis of chemical constitutes present in this traditional "She" medicine, and to lay a scientific and technical basis for the utilization and development of the plant resources.

*Correspondence: Dr. Cheng-Ping Wen, Zhejiang Chinese Medical University
E-mail: wenchengping@126.com

2 EXPERIMENTAL

2.1 *Reagents, materials and instrumentation*

Text HPLC-grade acetonitrile and methanol; HPLC-grade formic acid; Other analytical grade reagents. Reference compounds (> 99.0%). Aerial parts of *Xiao xianggou (XXG)*. were collected from Lishui district (Zhejiang, China) and identified. HPLC analysis was performed with a Surveyor HPLC system consisting of binary pumps and a diode array detector. HPLC-ESI-MS peak identification was performed using the above described HPLC system coupled with a LCQ mass spectrometer equipped with an electrospray interface. Instrument control and data acquisition were performed using Xcalibur 2.0 software.

2.2 *Preparation of sample and standards solution*

The aerial parts of *XXG* were dried, pulverized and extracted with 65% ethanol for 2 hours under reflux. The extracts were combined together and concentrated to dryness. The dried extract was weighed and dissolved to prepare sample solution. The standards were accurately weighed and dissolved to prepare the stock solutions. The standards solutions were diluted from the stock solutions, filtered through a 0.45 μm membrane and stored in a refrigerator (4°C) for the subsequent HPLC analysis.

2.3 *HPLC and MS conditions*

HPLC-DAD quantification was performed on a reversed-phase Dionex C18 column (4.6 mm × 250 mm, 5.0 μm) maintained at 25°C. The compounds were monitored at 320 nm for peak characterization. The mobile phase was composed of methanol (A) and 0.1% acetic acid aqueous solution (B) with the gradient elution (0 min to 5 min, 25% A; 5 min to 40 min, 25% to 70% A; and 40 min to 45 min, 70% A). The flow rate used was set at 0.80 mL/min throughout the gradient. The injection volume was 10 μL.

HPLC-ESI-MS analysis was operated in ESI full scan mode. The sheath gas (N_2, 99.99%) in the ESI source was set at 25 arbitrary units. The spray voltage was set at 4.5 kV for the positive mode and −3.5 kV for the negative mode. The heated ion transfer tube (350°C) was set at +55 V for ion introduction. Pure helium (99.999%) was used for the trapping and collision activation of the selected ions. Each mass spectrum was the average of over 10 scans.

2.4 *Validation of method*

The developed method was validated in terms of specificity, stability, linearity, limit of detection (LOD), precision, and accuracy (Leonardo *et al.*, 2013, Wu *et al.*, 2014). Linearity was determined using the square correlation coefficients of the calibration curves generated by three repeated injections of standard solutions at six concentration levels. The LOD was determined at a signal-to-noise ratio of 3 for standard solutions. Intra- and inter-day variations precisions were investigated on a single day and three successive days, respectively. The relative standard deviation (RSD) was taken as a measure of precision. The method accuracy was evaluated in terms of recovery test. Three replicates were measured at three concentration levels to determine the recovery.

3 RESULTS AND DISCUSSION

3.1 *Optimization of the chromatographic conditions and identification by HPLC-MS*

Chromatographic conditions such as mobile phase gradient, flow rate, column temperature and injection volume were optimized in order to limit run time while obtaining the best possible peak symmetry and resolution. Formic acid, acetic acid, and ammonium formate were tested as a mobile phase to enhance the resolution. Among them, only acetic acid effectively improved the peak resolution. As a result, gradient elution of the mobile phases consisting of methanol and 0.1% acetic acid buffer solution at a flow rate of 0.8 mL.min^{-1} was optimized as RP-HPLC conditions. It can be seen from Figure 1 that good separation and detectability of target compounds were obtained with minimal interference from the herb. Hence, it is relatively easy to estimate the peak area with acceptable accuracy. A representative DAD (320 nm) chromatograms for the standard solution of target components and the solution of herbal extract of *XXG* are shown in Figure 1, respectively. HPLC–ESI-MS experiments were employed for online identification in this study. Positive and negative ion modes were utilized for the targets, respectively. The detailed information are listed in Table 1, including their retention time, UV absorption, and ESI-MS signal of target six components.

3.2 *Validation of the method*

Specificity was determined by the calculation of peak purity facilitated by DAD. The results showed that the migration time and peak area of each analyte remained almost unchanged, and that no significant degradation is observed within the given period, indicating the solutions are stable for at least 1 week without the results being affected. A series of standard samples were prepared to study the relationships between the peak area and the concentrations of the targets under selected

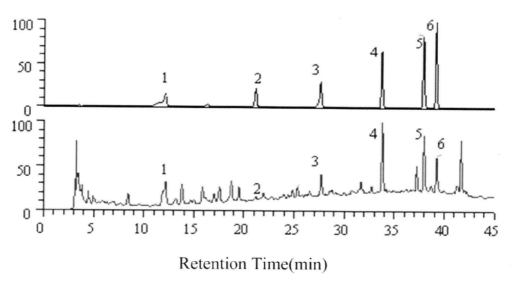

Figure 1.   Typical chromatograms of reference compounds and *XXG* extract from jingnan

Table 1.   HPLC-ESI/MS results of the six constituents

NO.	Retention time (min)	UV absorption (nm)	[M+H]+	[M–H]-	Constituents
1	13.27	240, 325	355	353	Chlorogenic acid
2	22.29	325	163	161	7-hydroxycoumarin
3	29.00	255, 320, 355	611	609	Rutin
4	35.11	245, 295	187		Psoralen
5	39.42	255,320, 350	287	285	Luteolin
6	40.66	265, 315	217		Bergapaten

Table 2. Calibration curves, linear range and LOD of the six constituents

Constituents	Calibration curve	r^2	Linear range (ug/mL)	LOD (ug/mL)
Chlorogenic acid	y = 49297x − 14250	0.9995	0.2−100	0.20
7-hydroxycoumarin	y = 68282x − 4241	0.9991	0.32−53.3	0.32
Rutin	y = 140000x + 2886.2	0.9998	0.24−40	0.24
Psoralen	y = 170000x + 6172.6	0.9994	0.34−58.3	0.34
Luteolin	y = 250000x − 69128	0.9997	0.29−48.3	0.29
Bergapaten	y = 270000x + 50378	0.9994	0.3−50	0.30

Table 3. Contents of the six constituents

Cultivar	Contents (%)					
	Chlorogenic acid	7-hydroxycoumarin	Rutin	Psoralen	Luteolin	Bergapaten
Jingnan	14.8	1.0	3.0	6.9	3.8	2.5
Shawan	14.2	0.9	2.6	4.9	3.4	2.3
Bohai	11.7	0.8	1.8	3.3	2.7	1.7
Dajun	10.2	0.6	1.2	2.9	2.0	1.6

conditions. Table 2 showed the results of the calibration curves and the LOD of target compounds. The correlation coefficients were higher than 0.9990 for all of the analytes studied. The precision test was carried out by the intra-day and inter-day variability for relative compound at three concentrations. The RSD of intra-day and inter-day variability was less than 5.0% and recoveries ranged from 87.9 to 95.3%, which demonstrated good precision and satisfactory average recovery of this method.

3.3 Sample analysis

The established method was applied to determine the six constituents of XXG. extracts from various geographic cultivars without any apparent interference from the other constituents. Under the analytical conditions, the results are shown in Table 3. The results demonstrated the successful application of HPLC-MS for the quantification of both coumarins and flavonoids with a wide dynamic range in various ethanol extracts of XXG. The findings also showed that different extracts differ in their quantities of coumarins and flavonoids, resulting in different qualities and efficacies. Jingnan contained the richest amounts of bioactive components, whereas Dajun had the least amount of six constituents.

4 CONCLUSION

An accurate and reliable HPLC-MS method was developed for the qualitative and quantitative analyses of bioactive constituents of *Xiao xianggou* ethanol extracts. This method was validated for its specificity, linearity, precision, accuracy, and extraction recovery. It was successfully applied to compare the six constituents. Among the four cultivars studied, Jingnan showed the highest phenolic contents and antioxidant activities. Thus, Jingnan is an excellent source of natural antioxidants for food condiments and medical uses. The results of the present study provide important information for the development of "She" medicine.

ACKNOWLEDGMENTS

This work was supported by Zhejiang Provincial Public Technology Research and social development project of China (Grant No. 2013C33114); Zhejiang traditional Chinese medicine scientific research Foundation (Grant No. 2013ZA030); Zhejiang Provincial Program for the Cultivation of High-level Innovative Health talents.

REFERENCES

Bankeu J.J., Mustafa S.A., Gojayev A.S., Lenta B.D., Tchamo Noungoué D., Ngouela S.A., Asaad K., Choudhary M.I., Prigge S., Guliyev A.A., Nkengfack A.E., Tsamo E., Shaiq Ali M.(2010) Ceramide and Cerebroside from the stem bark of Ficus mucuso (Moraceae). *Chem Pharm Bull* (Tokyo). 58(12):1661–1665.

Lei H.X., Li S.F. (2007) *The Chinese "She" medicine*. Beijing: China Press of traditional Chinese medicine. pp. 307.

Leonardo P. Landim, George S. Feitoza, José G.M. da Costa. (2013) Development and validation of a HPLC method for the quantification of three flavonoids in a crude extract of Dimorphandra gardneriana. *Revista Brasileira de Farmacognosia*, 23(1), 58–64.

Lv H.Q., Zhang X.P., Chen X.Z., Xie Z.J., Hu C.F., Wen C.P., and Jiang K.Z. (2013) Phytochemical Compositions and Antioxidant and Anti-Inflammatory Activities of Crude Extracts from *Ficus pandurata* H. (Moraceae). *Evid Based Complement Alternat Med*. 215036, 1–8.

Niu T.Z., Zhang Y.W., Bao Y.L, Wu Y., Yu C.L., Sun L.G., Yi J.W., Huang Y.X., Li Y.X. (2013) A validated high-performance liquid chromatography method with diode array detection for simultaneous determination of nine flavonoids in Senecio cannabifolius Less. *Journal of Pharmaceutical and Biomedical Analysis*, 76(25), 44–48.

Peng R., Ma P., Mo R.Y., Sun N.X. (2013) Analysis of the bioactive components from different growth stages of Fritillaria taipaiensis P. Y. Li. *Acta Pharmaceutica Sinica B*, 3(3),167–173.

Phan V.K., Nguyen X.C., Nguyen X.N., Vu K.T., Ninh K.B., Chau V.M., Bui H.T, Truong N.H., Lee S.H., Jang H.D., Kim Y.H. (2011) Antioxidant activity of a new C-glycosylflavone from the leaves of Ficus microcarpa. *Bioorg Med Chem Lett,* 21(2), 633–637.

Singh D., Singh B., Goel R.K. (2011) Traditional uses, phytochemistry and pharmacology of Ficus religiosa: a review. *J Ethnopharmacol*, 134(3), 565–583.

Tang D.Q., Zheng, X.X., Chen X., Yang D.Z., Du Q. (2014) Quantitative and qualitative analysis of common peaks in chemical fingerprint of Yuanhu Zhitong tablet by HPLC-DAD–MS/MS. *Journal of Pharmaceutical Analysis*, 4(2), 96–106.

Wu X.Y., Zhou Y., Yin F.Z., Mao C.Q., Li L., Cai B.C., Lu T.L. (2014) Quality control and producing areas differentiation of Gardeniae Fructus for eight bioactive constituents by HPLC–DAD–ESI/MS. *Phytomedicine*, 21(4), 551–559.

Medicine Sciences and Bioengineering – Wang (Ed.)
© 2015 Taylor & Francis Group, London, ISBN: 978-1-138-02684-1

Active constituents' determination in *Schisandra chinensis* by HPLC and evaluation of the uncertainty

Jane yu-xia Qin, Xiong Ye, Chen Yan & Dian-shuai Gao
Department of Neurobiology, Xuzhou Medical College, Jiangsu Province, China

ABSTRACT: *Schisandra chinensis* contains schisandrin, deoxyschisandrin, r-schisandrin, and other active substances, which have many medical functions such as neuroprotective effects, anti-cancer function, etc. This study, using High-Performance Liquid Chromatography (HPLC) method, determined the contents of three active ingredients, established an Evaluation of Uncertainty factor mathematical model for HPLC method detecting these three active contents in *Schisandra*, and fully analyzed the uncertainty sources in the measurement process. Then, uncertainty was evaluated and calculated. The results showed that when the sample amount was 2.00 mg the determination of schisandrin and deoxyshisandrin in *Schisandra* shows a good linear relationship. In conclusion, the method developed using high-performance liquid chromatography in this study is suitable for uncertainty factors' assessment in the determination of schisandrin, deoxyshisandrin, and r-schisandrin in *Schisandra*. This study lays the foundation to testify the quality of *Schisandra chinensis* using an international union standard.

1 INTRODUCTION

This experiment established the RP-HPLC simultaneous determination method of schisandrin (S), deoxyshisandrin (D), and r-schisandrin (R) contents in *Schisandra* and uncertainty assessment for the test results, the analysis of the error sources, and the confidence interval determination of the measurement results. Pharmacological studies on animals have shown that Schisandra increases physical working capacity and affords a stress-protective effect against a broad spectrum of harmful factors including heat shock, skin burn, cooling, frostbite, immobilization, swimming under load in an atmosphere of decreased air pressure, aseptic inflammation, irradiation, and heavy metal intoxication. The phytoadaptogen exerts an effect on the central nervous, sympathetic, endocrine, immune, respiratory, cardiovascular, and gastrointestinal systems, on the development of experimental atherosclerosis, on blood sugar and acid-base balance, and on uterus myotonic activity (Panossian A & Wikman G, 2012).

2 INSTRUMENT AND REAGENT

Agilent 1200 high-performance liquid chromatography with quaternary pump, autosampler, MWD detector, and ChemSation workstation; electronic analytical balance: 1712 mp8 type, Germany Sartorius Company; KQ-500TDE high-frequency digital ultrasonic cleaner from Kunshan Ultrasonic Instrument Ltd. Schisandrin, Lot: 110857-200,507; deoxyschizandrin Lot: 110764-200,408; r-schisandrin, batch 110765-200508. Reference substances were purchased from China Drug Biological Products; methanol, analytical grade, Beijing Chemical Plant; Wahaha water as pure water, HPLC grade, U.S. Dumas companies. Samples, S 0.0012 g, D 0.0026 g, and R 0.0018 g, were placed in a 25-mL volumetric flask, dissolved in methanol by the ultrasonic, and incubated at room temperature; methanol was added to the mark, and the working solution was obtained.

About 2 g of *Schisandra* powder was weighed with a 0.1-mg precision balance and placed in a 25-mL volumetric flask, which was dissolved in methanol by the 30 min ultrasonic incubated at room temperature; a constant volume was made with methanol, and the mixture was shook and filtered with a 0.22-µm nylon membrane before loading onto the machine.

Chromatographic conditions: Agilent XDB-C18 column (250 mm × 4.6 mm, 5 um), In sheath fluid, methanol: water = 70:30, flow rate 1.0 mL/min, column temperature 26°C, and detection wavelength 254 nm. S, D, R, and other components were separated well.

3   RESULTS AND DISCUSSION

3.1   *Preparation of standard curve*

With a 1-mL single drawing precision pipette, 0.1, 0.2, 0.3, 0.4, 0.5, 1, and 1.5 mL schisandrin, deoxyschizandrin, and r-schisandrin reference substances were placed automatically into the sample bottles, according to 2.2.1, and the peak areas were measured according to chromatographic conditions. Peak area and *Schisandra* A standard solution concentration C (mg/mL) were linearly fit with the least-squares method; the obtained values were as follows: S.A = 14684C-6.422, D.A = 12435C-11.851, R.A = 11364C-7.033, and correlation coefficient r = 0.9998.

3.2   *Mathematical model and main source of uncertainty evaluation*

The mathematical calculation formula is as follows:

$$R = \frac{C_{standard} \times A_{sample} \times V_{metered}}{A_{standard} \times m \times 10^3} \times 100 \tag{1}$$

Note: R is the percentage of schisandrin, deoxyschizandrin, r-schisandrin in *Schisandra chinensis*; $C_{standard}$: the reference substance concentration, mg/mL; $V_{metered}$: the constant volume of sample, mL; A_{sample}: the sample peak area, mAu; $A_{standard}$: the peak area of the reference substance, mAu; and m: the sample weight, g.

The content-determining uncertainty sources are mainly from the following aspects: ① the uncertainty introduced by sample weighing; ② uncertainty introduced by the sample's metered volume; ③ uncertainty introduced by sample-handling processes; ④ uncertainty introduced by the sample peak area measurement; ⑤ uncertainty introduced by sample repeated measurements; and ⑥ uncertainty introduced by the nonlinearity of the standard curve.

The sample solution was filtered with a 0.22-um nylon membrane and then uploaded onto the machine for measurement according to "Chromatographic conditions." The results mean value (%) (n = 6). Schisandrin, 0.4671; D-schizandrin, 0.1466; and r-schisandrin, 0.3421.

The uncertainty introduced by balance calibration: The given error limit of analytical balance was 0.1 mg; according to a rectangular distribution ($k = \sqrt{3}$), the uncertainty caused by the balance calibration component is $u_1(m) = 0.1mg/\sqrt{3} = 0.00005g$.

The uncertainty introduced by weighing variability: Based on the "uncertainty evaluation guide in the chemical analysis," the obtained analytical balance variation is about 0.5 times the last significant figure, and the balance was 0.1 mg. Therefore, the uncertainty components was caused by weighing variability: $u_2(m) = 0.5 \times 0.1mg = 0.00005g$; using the minus weighing method, 2× uncertainty should be calculated for twice weighing, so it is $u(m) = \sqrt{2[(0.00005)^2 + (0.00005)^2]} = 0.0001g$. Weighing the sample, m = 2.0737 g; then, the relative standard uncertainty introduced by weighing is $u_{rel}(m) = 0.0001g / 2.0737g = 0.0000482$.

The uncertainty introduced by 25-mL volumetric flask [u(V)]: This includes four sources, calibration error: 25-mL A Grade volumetric flask, permit error: ±0.03 mL (Zhao Min, 2006), error according to a rectangular distribution ($k = \sqrt{3}$), and the uncertainty introduced by the calibration of

25-mL volumetric flask: $u_1(V_{volume25}) = 0.03mL / \sqrt{3} = 0.0173mL$. The 25 mL volumetric flask was filled 10 times in one experiment, and the obtained standard deviation is 0.02 mL, $u_2(V_{capacity}25)$ = 0.02 mL. Temperature range is $\pm 5°C$, water expansion coefficient is 2.1×10^{-4} at room temperature, so the volume change of 25 mL volumetric flask is $\Delta(V_{volume25}) = 25 \times 2.1 \times 10^{-4} \times 5 = 0.0262mL$. When the confidence level is 0.95, coverage factor K = 1.96 and the uncertainty introduced by the temperature change is $u_3(V_{volume25}) = 0.0262mL / 1.96 = 0.0133mL$.

The uncertainty components introduced by reading were as follows: 1% error for the actual volume of container allowed: $u_4(V_{volume25}) = 0.01 \times 25mL / \sqrt{6} = 0.0102mL$; relative standard uncertainty introduced by the 25-mL volumetric flask: $u_{rel}(V_{volume25}) = \sqrt{0.0173^2 + 0.02^2 + 0.0133^2 + 0.102^2} / 25mL = 0.00424$; uncertainty caused by repeatable measurement, which belong to class A; and the entire procedures refer to GB/T 5009.1-2003 (Zhao Min, 1990). The measured data are shown in Table 1.

The standard deviation was obtained by the Bessel formula: $S_x = \sqrt{\dfrac{\sum_{n=1}^{i}(x_i - \bar{x})^2}{n-1}}$ Repeatability uncertainty:

$$u_{(rep)} = S_x / \sqrt{n}\,; \quad u_{rel}(rep) = u_{(rep)} / R \tag{2}$$

Schisandrin $u_{rel}(rep) = u_{(rep)} / R = 0.00412$; deoxyschizandrin $u_{rel}(rep) = u_{(rep)} / R = 0.0137$; and r-schisandrin $u_{rel}(rep) = u_{(rep)} / R = 0.00204$. The uncertainties introduced by repeated measurements of the peak are shown in Table 2. The range method was used for assessment.

Based on "Evaluation and Expression of Uncertainty in Measurement" (Zhao Min, 1990),

$u_A = \dfrac{R_{range}}{A_{rangecoefficent}}$; S. $u_{rel} = \dfrac{u_A}{A} = 0.0167$; D. $u_{rel} = \dfrac{u_A}{A} = 0.0503$; R. $u_{rel} = \dfrac{u_A}{A} = 0.0134$.

Uncertainty introduced by the instrument data processing system: According to the instrument manual and the general performance of the integrator, so far, the maximum error of peak area convolution procedure by liquid chromatography is 0.2% to 1%, and then the peak area relative uncertainty components is $u_A = \dfrac{0.01}{\sqrt{3}} = 0.00577$. Liquid chromatography used a microinjector for measurement, and the injection uncertainty was 1%; then the relative uncertainty components

Table 1. The repeatable measurement results of *Schisandra* (n = 10).

No.	1	2	3	4	5	6	7	8	9	10
Schisandrin	0.479	0.482	0.467	0.462	0.473	0.475	0.478	0.468	0.471	0.469
D-schizandrin	0.147	0.148	0.14	0.159	0.158	0.142	0.156	0.148	0.151	0.145
R-schisandrin	0.338	0.339	0.342	0.347	0.35	0.348	0.356	0.337	0.352	0.349

Table 2. The peak area measurement results of *Schisandra* (n = 6) [u (AS)], C = 2.53.

Sample	1	2	3	4	5	6	Mean value
S	8753.81543	8799.83741	8525.98355	8434.69893	8635.52509	8672.03894	8636.983225
D	2272.70763	2291.1676	2167.48784	2461.22728	2442.67531	2198.40778	2305.61224
R	4780.14941	4789.28149	4831.65202	4902.26955	4946.05243	4917.80541	4861.201718

were $u\,u_{injection} = \dfrac{0.01}{\sqrt{3}} = 0.00577$. The uncertainty introduced by the instrument data processing system was $u_{machine} = \sqrt{u_A^2 + u_{load}^2} = 0.0082$. So, the uncertainty caused by the sample peak area measurement was as follows: $u_{rel}(A_S) = \sqrt{u_{machine} + u_{rel}}$. S: $u_{rel}(A_s) = \sqrt{0.0167^2 + 0.0082^2} = 0.0186$; D: $u_{rel}(A_s) = \sqrt{0.0503^2 + 0.0082^2} = 0.0509$; and R: $u_{rel}(A_S) = \sqrt{0.0134^2 + 0.0082^2} = 0.0157$. The standard deviation was obtained by the Bessel formula: $S_x = \sqrt{\dfrac{\sum_{n=1}^{i}(x_i - \overline{x})^2}{n-1}}$. The repeatability uncertainty was as follows: $u_{(rep)} = S_x/\sqrt{n}$, $u_{rel}(rep) = u_{(rep)}/R\,[u\,(rep)]$. S: $u_{rel}(rep) = 0.00899$; D: $u_{rel}(rep) = 0.00716$; R: $u_{rel}(rep) = 0.00543$.

The uncertainty introduced by the nonlinear standard curve [u (line)]: Precise concentrations of 0.1, 0.2, 0.3, 0.4, 0.5, 1.0, and 1.5 mL standard *Schisandra* solution were taken, and each concentration was measured twice. The standard curve equation was prepared using the least-squares method: S.A = 14684C−6.422, D.A = 12435C−11.851, R.A = 11364C−7.033, and correlation coefficient r = 0.9998. The standard deviation of the standard curve equation was calculated, which is the standard deviation of the residuals. The absorbance values by apparatus measurement or calculation according to the linear equation are shown in Table 3.

The residual standard deviation of the standard curve and the uncertainty caused by standard curve fitting are as follows:

$$S_R = \sqrt{\dfrac{\sum_{j=1}^{n}[A_{0j} - (a + bC_{oj})]^2}{n-2}}\;;\quad u_{(line)} = \dfrac{S_R}{b}\sqrt{\dfrac{1}{p} + \dfrac{1}{n} + \dfrac{(\overline{C} - \overline{C}_0)^2}{\sum_{j=1}^{n}(C_{0j} - \overline{C}_0)^2}} \tag{4}$$

Notes: S_R: residual standard deviation of the standard curve (residual standard deviation); b: slope; p: repeated measurement numbers of the samples tested; n: standard curve points; $\overline{C}$: C average concentration of the sample; $\overline{C}_0$: mean concentration for the standard curve points; C_{0j}: standard concentration value; the relative standard uncertainty caused by the standard curve: S

$$S_R = 13.003\ mg/ml; b = 14684; \overline{C} = 0.3833; \overline{C}_0 = 0.02742; urel(line) = \dfrac{0.4098}{0.4671} = 0.0114;$$

$$S_R = 24.042 mg/ml; b = 12435; C = 0.1205; C_0 = 0.05942;$$

$$D: urel(line) = \dfrac{0.01320}{0.1466} = 0.0900 \tag{5}$$

$$R: S_R = 17.375\ mg/ml; b = 11364; \overline{C} = 0.2808; \overline{C}_0 = 0.04114; urel\ (line) = \dfrac{0.004142}{0.3421} = 0.0121$$

Table 3. Residual calculation results of the standard curve.

Concentration C0j (mg/mL)			Response value A0j			[A0j - (a + bC0j)]2		
S	D	R	S	D	R	S	D	R
$\overline{C}_0$ 0.02742	0.05942	0.04114				Σ 845.462	Σ2890.143	Σ1509.49

S = schisandrin; D = D-schizandrin; R = R-schisandrin.

3.3 Combined standard uncertainty and expanded uncertainty

The above uncertainty components are unrelated, and the synthetic relative uncertainty is as follows:

$$u_{rel}(R) = \sqrt{[u_{rel}(m)]^2 \ [u_{rel}(V_{volume25})]^2 + [u_{rel}(rep)]^2 + [u_{rel}(A_S)]^2 + [u_{rel}(rep)]^2 + [u_{rel}(line)]^2}$$

The synthetic uncertainty is $u(R) = u_{rel}(R) \times R = 0.01984 \times 4.60\% = 0.0912\%$. If the coverage factor is K = 2, then the expanded uncertainty is $U = ku(R) = 2 \times 0.0912\% = 0.18\%$. The *Schisandra* content results are expressed as $R = (4.60 \pm 0.18)\%$, $k = 2$.

4   SUMMARY

Currently, the quality of *Schisandra* varies widely, so an effective, steady, and repeated method to measure its active components is needed. Then, we can formulate a quality standard for this product. From the uncertainty of the assessment process, we can see that for determining the functional factors' content of *Schisandra* by high-performance liquid chromatography the uncertainty mainly comes from sample peak area measurement uncertainty, so the uncertainty component can be reduced by the control precision of the liquid system. So, reduction of the sample peak area measurement uncertainty has the most obvious effect on the total uncertainty reduction of using the High-Performance Liquid Chromatography method.

REFERENCES

Lee TH, Jung CH, Lee DH. (2012) Neuroprotective effects of Schisandrin B against transient focal cerebral ischemia in Sprague-Dawley rats. Food Chem Toxicol. 50(12): 4239–45.

Liu Z, Zhang B, Liu K, Ding Z, Hu X. (2012) Schisandrin B attenuates cancer invasion and metastasis via inhibiting epithelial-mesenchymal transition. PLoS One. 7(7): e40480.

Panossian A. Wikman G. (2008) Pharmacology of *Schisandra chinensis* Bail.: an overview of Russian research and uses in medicine. Journal of Ethnopharmacology. 118(2): 183–212.

Zhao Min, JJG 196-2006. (2006) Metrology Verification Regulation of the People's Republic of China Working Glass Container [S]. 6–9.

Zheng S, Aves SJ, Laraia L, Galloway WR, Pike KG, Wu W, Spring DR. (2012) A concise total synthesis of deoxyschizandrin and exploration of its antiproliferative effects and those of structurally related derivatives. Chemistry. 18(11): 3193–8.

Zhao Min JJ. G705-1990 liquid chromatograph test procedures. (1990) China National Accreditation board for laboratories. Guide to the evaluation of uncertainty in chemistry analysis [M].

Medicine Sciences and Bioengineering – Wang (Ed.)
© 2015 Taylor & Francis Group, London, ISBN: 978-1-138-02684-1

Reconstruction of central aortic pressure using continuous peripheral arterial blood pressure at two separate sites on lower arms

Chao Ma
Guangdong Provincial Key Laboratory of Robotics and Intelligent System, Shenzhen Institutes of Advanced Technology, Chinese Academy of Sciences, Shenzhen, China
Harbin Institute of Technology Shenzhen Graduate School, Shenzhen, China

Jia Liu* & Pan-deng Zhang
Guangdong Provincial Key Laboratory of Robotics and Intelligent System, Shenzhen Institutes of Advanced Technology, Chinese Academy of Sciences, Shenzhen, China

Xiao-ping Yang*
Harbin Institute of Technology Shenzhen Graduate School, Shenzhen, China

ABSTRACT: We proposed a new mathematical model to reconstruct the waveform of the Central Aortic Pressure (CAP) using continuous peripheral arterial blood pressure measured from the radial artery and finger artery separately. First, we formulated mathematical relations between Blood Pressure (BP) waveforms at the radial artery and finger artery. The radial blood flow waveforms are estimated via linear least-square and multichannel linear least-square deconvolution algorithm. Then combine with the measured radial BP waveforms to derive the CAP. To demonstrate the feasibility of this technique, we use three interventional surgery patients conducting human trials. The estimated CAP waveforms are very close to it's measured (selected 10s segments, the RMSE is 2.74 mmHg). In conclusion, this new technology will be wider application in clinical trials and clinical practice.

1 INTRODUCTION

Central aortic pressure and waveforms convey important information of cardiovascular condi-tions, it plays an important role in evaluation of occurrence and development of cardiovascular disease (Safar *et al*., 2009). Clinically, invasive CAP measurement, however, is still the "gold standard", which imposes significant clinical risk as well as high cost. Though the non-invasive peripheral arterial pressure (PAP) measurement is much easier and widely used, it is different from CAP (Morgan *et al*., 2004). Therefore, recently, the measurement of the CAP using non-invasive approach has attracted great attention.

Substantial research efforts have been made to develop non-invasive methods in estimating CAP from peripheral circulatory measurements. These methods can be divided into two types: 1) General Transfer Function (GTF); 2) Pulse Wave Separation (PWS). Based on a "black box" model, the GTF can be derived from clinical data between CAP and PAP (Chen *et al*., 1997), However, clinical studies indicate that the GTF can be affected by age and disease (Bos *et al*., 1996), the use of GTF can result in errors in the prediction of CAP. The PWS derives the CAP from the sum of the forward and backward traveling waves at the corresponding position. It was proposed by Westerhof *et al*. (1972) earlier, then Stergiopulos *et al*. (1998) used a BP and blood flow velocity measured at a single peripheral location to derive CAP. However, blood flow waves can not be readily acquired.

This paper presents a new technique to derive the CAP by two continuous peripheral arterial blood pressure signals. Unlike most single-vessel model, which used a single peripheral location measured, we added a measurement site after radial artery to estimate the unknown flow (Swamy *et al*., 2010). Subsequently, combine with the measured radial waveforms to derive the CAP.

We test the method on three interventional surgery patients by simultaneous recording the CAP/FBP/RBP waveforms. Finally, We conclude this technique.

2 METHODS

2.1 Physics-based model analysis technique

The physics-based model is divided into two parts [see Figure 1.(a)], one from central condition to radial arterial line, is still used to classical model (Swamy et al., 2010). The characteristic impedance is Z_{RC}. From the measured pressure and flow waves [$P_R(t)$ and $Q_R(t)$] at the radial artery. The forward and backward waves can be separated as follows:

$$p_{fc}(t) = [Q_R(t) \bullet Z_{FC} + P_R(t)]/2$$
$$p_{bc}(t) = [P_R(t) - Q_R(t) \bullet Z_{FC}]/2 \tag{1}$$

These pressure waves are then time shifted by Δt_0, forward and backward, respectively, to calculate the CAP as follows:

$$P_C(t) = p_{fc}(t + \Delta t_0) + p_{bc}(t - \Delta t_0) \tag{2}$$

Where $P_C(t)$ is the CAP waveform, Δt_0 is the time delay between central aorta and radial artery. Another one from the radial artery to finger artery [see Figure 1.(a)] has independent characteristic impedance Z_{RF}. At the terminal load, the impedance mismatch causes wave reflection, the relationship of backward and forward wave at the terminal can be expressed as:

$$p_{br}(t) = \Gamma_R(t) \otimes p_{fr}(t) \tag{3}$$

Where $\otimes$ is the convolution operation, Γ_R is the unknow reflection coefficient $\Gamma_R = (Z(w) - Z_{RF})/(Z(w) + Z_{RF})$. $Z(w)$ is a frequency-dependent impedance arising from the resistance, compliance and inertance of the arteries. After time shifting and ignoring the terminal transit time, the measured finger and radial pressure waves ($P_F(t)$ and $P_R(t)$) can be expressed as the sum of $p_{br}(t)$ and $p_{fr}(t)$ as follows:

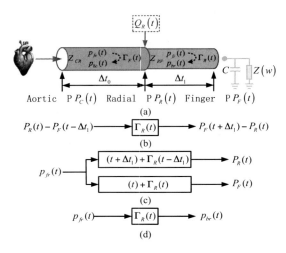

Figure 1. Physics-based model for reconstructing CAP $P_C(t)$ using two continuous peripheral pressure signals measured from raidal and finger artery ($P_F(t)$ and $P_R(t)$).

$$P_F(t) = p_{fr}(t) + \Gamma_R(t) \otimes p_{fr}(t) \tag{4}$$

$$P_R(t) = p_{fr}(t + \Delta t_1) + \Gamma_R(t) \otimes p_{fr}(t - \Delta t_1) \tag{5}$$

Where Δt_1 is the recorded time delay for wave travels between radial artery and finger artery. Combining (4) with (5), the relationship between $P_F(t)$ and $P_R(t)$ can be re-written in discrete-time domain as follows:

$$y(n) = \Gamma_R(n) \otimes x(n) \tag{6}$$

Where $y(n) = P_F(n + \Delta n_1) - P_R(n)$, $x(n) = P_R(n) - P_F(n - \Delta n_1)$, are the measured SISO time-varying model, $\Gamma_R(n)$ is causal filter impulse response [see Figure 1.(b)]. Noting the Poiseuille's law, mean blood pressure is the same along the tube. We extended our time-varying univariate model identified by an least-squsres estimation to minimizing the prediction error energy effectively.

Once the reflection coefficient $\Gamma_R(n)$ for a tube is determined by system identification, the $p_{fr}(n)$ then can be estimated by measured discrete-time sequences $P_F(n)$ and $P_R(n)$ using multi-channel linear least-squares deconvolution (Abed-Meriam et al., 1997) [see Figure 1.(c)]. $\delta(n)$ is the unit impulse response. Finally, the corresponding backward $p_{br}(n)$ is readily computed via (4) [see Figure 1.(d)]. It is noted that the flow waveforms ($Q_R(t)$) at radial artery can be expressed as the difference of $p_{br}(t)$ and $p_{fr}(t)$ as:

$$Q_R(t) = \left[p_{fr}(t + \Delta t_1) - p_{br}(t - \Delta t_1) \right] / Z_{RC} \tag{7}$$

The corresponding instantaneous CAP $P_C(n)$ then can be estimated via (1) (2).

2.2 Experimental protocol

We verified the new model using the collected hemodynamic data from the patients in inter-ven-tional surgery. It was approved by The Second Affiliated Hospital of Guangzhou University of Medical Health Research Ethics Board and informed consent from the patients. Before disin-fect-ing patients, a servo-controlled finger plethysmograph (finapres-1000, Ohmeda, USA) was in-stalled on the left hand positioned at the horizontal level with the heart, and a tonometric device (CBM-7000, Colin Medical Instruments, Japan) was installed on the same hand wrist artery, the instrumentation was properly calibrated before the beginning of surgical case to ensure that ac-curate BP data were collected. After local anesthesia, the reference CAP in the ascending aorta was recorded from indwelling catheters via rigid fluid-filled tubing to external BP transducers (DPT-248, China) connects to a patient monitor (PM-9000, China). All the subjects resting time of 10 minutes, the analog output BP signals were recorded simultaneously in computer using an interface cable (BNC, USA) and a transducer connector interface by connect a data acquisition equipment (USB2811, China) with a sampling rate of 500 Hz for the duration of 1min.

3 STATISTICAL ANALYSIS AND RESULTS

The physics-based model analysis was applied to 10s continuous BP segments extracted from simultaneously recorded CAP/RBP/FBP resample to 250 HZ. A fifth-order butterworth low-pass filter with cut off frequency at 0.1 Hz was applied to obtain transfer function coefficient of the zero-phase digital filter. All BP signals were then filtered by zero-phase digital filter, respectively. Noting that the analogue waveforms were essentially discrete-time sequences, the validity of physics-based model could be assessed by comparing the estimated CAP sequences against collected reference data in the ascending aorta. For further comparsion, the accuracy of estimated CAP was quantified by the root-mean-squared error (RMSE) versus the actual CAP in the corresponding data segment.

Table I summarizes the physiologic paremeter and the results of the experimental evaluation. It indicates that the subjects are in diverse physiologic states. The RMSE between the estimated and measured reference CAP waveforms are 2.74 mmHg. Figure 2 shows the recorded radial and finger artery as well as the reference central aortic blood pressure waveforms segments. It is obvious that the different arterial tree sites have diverse blood pressure waveforms. The upper left panel of Figure 3 shows the comparison of reference and estimated CAP, center and right panels show corresponding prediction results of the raw radial artery and finger artery pressure waveforms. And the corresponding correlation is illustrated in the lower panel of Figure 3. Obviously, the CAP can be reconstructed very accurately, and the estimated CAP is close in morphology to its reference counterpart.

Table 1   Physiologic condition of the human subject. PTT is shown the time delay between aortic-radial/ radial-finger paths.

Subject	HR[bpm]	MAP[mmHg]	SP[mmHg]	PP[mmHg]	PTT[ms]	RMSE[mmHg]
1	63.9	96.4	137.3	61.2	32/28	2.23
2	73.5	100.8	141.4	40.6	44/92	3.09
3	91.2	89.5	100.5	32.4	56/48	2.91
ALL	77.5	92.9	118.9	46.8	44/56	2.74

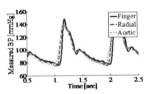

Figure 2.   Measured BP: Invasive central aortic, non-invasive radial and finger BP measurement.

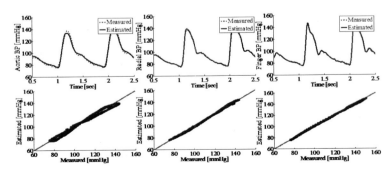

Figure 3.   Model validation: comparison of measured versus estimated aortic, radial and finger artery pressure waveforms.

4 SUMMARY

In this paper, we proposed a new mathematical model which allows us to estimate the CAP us-ing peripheral arterial blood pressure waves collected from two separate sites (wrist and finger from radial and finger arteries) on lower arms. As peripheral arterial blood pressure waves can be relatively easy be measured (when comparing with blood flow), our method is more practical than the original method of pulse wave separation which requires both waves of blood pressure and blood flow simultaneously.

ACKNOWLEDGMENTS

This work was supported by a grant from Shenzhen Science and Technology Project [ReferenceNo. ZDSY20120617113312191], the work described in this paper was partially supported by Sh-enzhen Fundamental Research Program (JC201005280481A), Guangdong Innovative Research Team Program (201001D0104648280) and The Project of Chinese Academy of Sciences and Foshan City Collaborative Platform (2013HT100051).

REFERENCES

Abed-Meriam, K., Qiu, W. & Hua, Y. (1997) Blind system identification. Proc. IEEE. [Online] 85, 1310–1332.

Bos, W. J et al. (1996) Reconstruction of brachial artery pressure from noninvasive finger pressure measure-ments. Circulation. [Online] 94, 1870–1875.

Chen, C. H. & E. Nevo. et al. (1997) Estimation of central aortic pressure waveform by mathematical trans-formation of radial tonometry pressure: validation of generalized transfer function. Circulation. [Online] 95, 1827–1836.

Morgan, T. et al. (2004) Effect of different antihypertensive drug classes on central aortic pressure. American journal of hypertension. [Online] 17 (2), 118–123.

Safar, M. & Jankowski, P. (2009) Central blood pressure and hypertension: Role in cardiovascular risk assess-ment. Clin. Sci. [Online] 116 (4), 273–282.

Stergiopulos, N. et al. (1998) Physical basis of pressure transfer from periphery to aorta: a model-based study. American Journal of Physiology-Heart and Circulatory Physiology. [Online] 274 (4), H1386–H1392.

Swamy, G. et al. (2010) Calculation of Forward and Backward Arterial Waves by Analysis of Two Pressure Waveforms. Biomedical Engineering, IEEE Transactions. [Online] 57, 2833–2839.

Westerhof, N. et al. (1972) Forward and backward waves in the arterial system. Cardiovascular Research. [Online] 6, 648–656.

Medicine Sciences and Bioengineering – Wang (Ed.)
© 2015 Taylor & Francis Group, London, ISBN: 978-1-138-02684-1

Experimental study on reduction of Aβ by berberine in serum and brain of diabetic rats

You Zhou, Ying Tan, Lun Li, Dong-xue Wang & Ying Zhao[*]
School of Pharmacy, Harbin University of Commerce, Harbin, China

ABSTRACT: Objective: Study the influence of berberine on β amyloid protein in brain and serum of diabetic rats. Method: Male Wistar rats were fed a high-fat diet for 8 weeks and were induced with diabetes by the intraperitoneal injection of streptozotocin (STZ). The model rats were randomly divided into five groups by blood glucose levels and body weights: negative control group, model control group, high dose group of berberine (H, 129.45 mg/kg·d), low dose group of berberine (L, 64.72 mg/kg·d), and positive control group (Pioglitazone, 2.72 mg/kg·d). Rats were sacrificed after being administered for 8 weeks continuously, and serum and brain tissue were separated. Fasting glucose, insulin levels, and Aβ levels in serum and brain were observed. Results: Compared with the negative control group, there was a significant increase in weight of the model rats ($P < 0.01$) and there was a significant ($P < 0.05$) decline in FPG, INS, and insulin sensitivity index of the model rats. We measured the Aβ content levels in brain and serum of the model rats after 8 weeks. Compared with the negative control group, there was a significant increase in the Aβ content levels in brain and serum of the model rats ($P < 0.01$), and after administration for 8 weeks compared with the model group there was a significant decline in the Aβ content levels in brain and serum of high dose groups of berberine ($P < 0.01$). Conclusions: High-fat diet for 8 weeks combined with intraperitoneal injection of 1% STZ 35 mg/kg can be successfully replicated in diabetic rat model with insulin resistance; there was a significant decline in Aβ content levels in brain and serum of high dose groups of berberine. High doses of berberine could significantly reduce the Aβ content levels in brain and serum of diabetic rats.

1   INTRODUCTION

Diabetes as a systemic disease can cause a variety of tissue, organ, structural, and functional changes with lesions involving the whole body (Gilberto, 2009). Cognitive dysfunction is a chronic complication of diabetes; it is mainly shown as damage in learning and memory function decline (BoddaertJ *et al.* , 2008). Berberine have good effects to intervene metabolism syndrome. Therefore, this paper aims to explore the intervention effect of diabetes on Aβ levels in brain and blood of rats and the effect of berberine on it.

2   MATERIALS

2.1   *Animals*

A total of 50 healthy adult Wistar male rats weighing 180–220 g for this study were provided by the Bethune Medical University. Normal diet (53% cornmeal, 24% soybean meal, 16% wheat bran, 5% fish powder, 1% bone powder, and 1% salt) and high-fat diet (10% lard, 10% egg yolk powder, 1% cholesterol, 0.5% sodium cholate, and 78.5% basic diet) were obtained from the Heilongjiang University of Chinese Medicine.

---

[*]correspondence

2.2 Drugs and reagents

Glucose Oxidase Method was obtained from Changchun HuiLi Biotech Co.; insulin radioimmunoassay kit was obtained from 3V Biological Engineering Group Co. Streptozotocin was obtained from Sigma; pioglitazone was obtained from Zhinuo Biotech Co. Berberine was obtained from Zhinuo Biotech Co.

2.3 Instrument

Ultraviolet–visible light detector was obtained from UNICO Instruments Co.; low-speed refrigerated centrifuge was obtained from Beijing Medical Centrifuge Factory, and GC-2010γ RIA counter was obtained from USTC ZONKIA Co.

3 METHODS

3.1 Model replication

A total of 70 male Wistar rats were given adaptive feeding with normal diet and water for 1 week, and then they were randomly divided into two groups. Whereas the normal control group was given normal diet, the model groups were given high-fat diet after 8 weeks. The diabetic model was established by intraperitoneal injection of 1% STZ 35 mg/kg. Rats in the normal control group were injected with the same dose of citric acid-sodium citrate buffer. Fasting blood glucose values were detected after 72 h. Animals with fasting blood glucose levels greater than 16.7 mmol/L were included in the experiment.

3.2 Grouping and administration

According to blood glucose, rats were randomly divided into four groups: The negative control group (ig, same volume of saline), high-dose group (ig, berberine 129.45 mg/kg·d), low-dose group (ig, berberine 64.72 mg/kg·d), and positive control group (ig, pioglitazone 2.72 mg/kg·d). All drug groups were given high-fat diet, and each group was given intragastric administration once daily; the animals were sacrificed after being administered for 8 weeks.

3.3 Preparation of plasma samples and brain tissue samples

Collected ocular fundus venous plexus for blood after model group were high-fat diet for 8 weeks, intraperitoneal injection of 1% STZ for 72 h, administered for 8 weeks, collect blood 1 to 2 mL, the samples were centrifuged at 3000 rpm for 10 min. The supernatant was cryopreserved at −80°C for measurement. The animals were sacrificed after administration for 8 weeks. Rats were decapitated, and the brain tissues were stripped quickly. Take the side of the half-the brain tissue and then adding 8 times amount of physiological saline after weighing, and mashed with a tissue homogenizer, 3000 r/min, centrifugal 10 min, the supernatant cryopreserved were stored in the refrigerator at 80°C until analysis.

3.4 Observed indicators and detection methods

3.4.1 General observation
Animal spirits, activity, coat color, eating conditions, etc., were observed during the experiment.

3.4.2 Determination of blood glucose concentration (FBG), plasma insulin concentration (FINS), and insulin sensitivity index (IAI)
FBG and FINS were measured by using glucose oxidase method and radioimmunoassay. Concrete operation was performed according to kit instructions. Insulin sensitivity index (IAI) was calculated by the following formula: insulin sensitivity index (IAI) = Ln[1/(FPG × FINS)].

3.4.3 Determination of Aβ 42 and Aβ 40 levels in blood and brain

Determination of double-antibody sandwich ELISA and Aβ levels was performed in order to calculate the sum of the two. Concrete operation was performed according to kit instructions.

3.5 Statistical analysis

All the data were processed by variance analysis in SPSS 17.0 for Windows statistical software. A P-value less than 0.05 was considered statistically significant. A P-value less than 0.01 was considered extremely statistically significant.

4 RESULT

4.1 All indexes change in diabetic rats

4.1.1 The general situation in rats

Compared with the negative control group, model group rats showed listlessness, depression, hair scattering, loose stools, and other states and their polydipsia, polyphagia, and polyuria were consistent with the clinical symptoms of diabetes manifestations. In this way diabetic rat mode was induced successfully.

4.1.2 Changes of body weight in rats fed a high-fat diet

Compared with the negative control group, there was a significant ($P < 0.01$) increase in weight in the model groups after administration for 8 weeks. There was a significant ($P < 0.05$) decline in weight of the model groups after intraperitoneal injection of 1% STZ for 72 h, the result are listed in Table 1.

4.2 Glucose metabolic markers in diabetic rats

Compared with the negative control group, there was a significant ($P < 0.05$) increase in blood glucose of model groups. There was also a significant ($P < 0.01$) increase in insulin levels of the model groups, the result are listed in Table 2.

Table 1. The influence of high-fat diet on body weights of rats.

Group	N	1 week (g)	6 weeks (g)	8 weeks (g)	STZ 72 h (g)
Control	10	227.79 ± 21.94	284.89 ± 33.37	304.76 ± 37.45	312.89 ± 34.23
Model	60	231.72 ± 11.63	$317.85 \pm 40.86**$	$342.89 \pm 42.32**$	$324.34 \pm 26.77*$

Compared with control, $*P < 0.05$, $**P < 0.01$.

Table 2. Effects of high-fat diet on blood glucose, insulin, and insulin sensitivity index.

Group	N	FPG (mmol/L)	INS (μIU/L)	IAI
Control	10	4.73 ± 1.58	21.19 ± 6.14	-4.57 ± 0.46
Model	60	$5.81 \pm 1.18*$	$34.79 \pm 6.74**$	$-5.26 \pm 0.58*$

Compared with control, $*P < 0.05$, $**P < 0.01$.

Table 3. Improving the effect of berberine on the Aβ content levels in brain and serum of diabetic rats.

Group	N	Aβ of serum (pg/mL)	Aβ of brain (pg/mL)
Control	13	116.92 ± 5.61	200.99 ± 5.59
Model	5	125.61 ± 7.12**	999.22 ± 85.08**
BerH	6	113.28 ± 4.71△△	201.29 ± 19.11△△
BerL	5	122.47 ± 2.78	691.33 ± 73.53
PIO	5	116.98 ± 3.39△	653.69 ± 58.63△

Compared with control, △ $P < 0.05$, △△ $P < 0.01$.
Compared with model, *$P < 0.05$, **$P < 0.01$.

4.3 Improving the effect of berberine on the Aβ content levels in brain and serum of diabetic rats

Compared with the negative control group, there was a significant ($P < 0.01$) increase in Aβ content levels of the model groups. Compared with the model group, there was a significant ($P < 0.01$) decrease in Aβ content levels of the high-dose group and there was a significant ($P < 0.05$) decrease in Aβ content levels of the positive control group, the result are listed in Table 3.

5 DISCUSSION

In this study, we adopted a high-fat diet for 8 weeks for rats, after which the diabetic rat model was induced by the intraperitoneal injection of 1% STZ. Compared with the negative control group, insulin sensitivity index significantly decreased in the model group by high-fat diet after 8 weeks. Fasting blood glucose was significantly increased but did not reach the diagnostic criteria for diabetes. The results instructions that islet function was normal. This case of induced rats with insulin resistance is the early defect of diabetes. But at this stage insulin levels in the blood of rats were higher than those in normal rats. But the ability of blood insulin levels combined with insulin receptors and post receptor are reduced. In order to overcome this case, insulin secretion rate is increased, but it still cannot make blood sugar levels return to normal basis. Destruction β-cell function of pancreatic slightly by intraperitoneal injection of 1% STZ (35 mg/kg), and leading to β-cell function cannot be fully compensated, blood glucose was increased significantly.

Compared with the negative control group, model group rats showed listlessness, depression, hair scattering, loose stools, and other states and their polydipsia, polyphagia, and polyuria were consistent with the clinical symptoms of diabetes manifestations, which can induce diabetic model successfully. The results suggest that there was a significant increase in Aβ content levels of the model groups compared with those of the negative control group. Diabetes can promote the formation of Aβ in brain and serum, and berberine can reduce the Aβ levels of serum and brain in diabetic rats.

ACKNOWLEDGMENT

The work was supported by the 2013 National Natural Science Foundation of China Project (81373548).

REFERENCES

Boddaert J, Barrou Z, Lemaire A, et al. Diabetes mellitus and cognition: 15 there a link? Psychol Neuropsychiatr Vieil, 2008, 6(3):189–198

Gilberto. Exercise and cognitive function: a hypothesis for the association of type II diabetes mellitus and Alzheimer's disease from an evolutionary perspective, Diabetology & Metabolic Syndrome 2009, 1:7.

Medicine Sciences and Bioengineering – Wang (Ed.)
© 2015 Taylor & Francis Group, London, ISBN: 978-1-138-02684-1

Metabonomic characterization of aging rats by means of RRLC-Q-TOF-MS-based techniques

Jing-hui Sun[1], Chun-mei Wang, Hao Jia, Hong-xia Sun, Cheng-yi Zhang,
Jian-guang Chen & He Li[*]
Country College of Pharmacy, Beihua University, Jilin, China

ABSTRACT: A metabonomics approach based on Rapid Resolution Liquid Chromatography coupled with Quadruple-Time-Of-Flight mass spectrometry (RRLC-Q-TOF-MS) method was applied to analyze the characteristics of plasma samples of Wistar rats from four ages (4, 12, 18 and 24 month-old). 14 potential biomarkers were identified by MS/MS analysis. The analysis of metabolic pathways indicated the decrease of fatty acid, phospholipids metabolism and energy metabolism, disorder of lipid metabolism were the main features of aging.

1 INTRODUCTION

Aging, as a complex physiological process involving numerous endogenous metabolites, is difficult to be fully characterized only by single or limited metabolites. Metabonomics is a discipline based on NMR spectroscopy and Mass spectrometry to describe the nontargeted 'global' analysis of tissues and biofluids for small molecular mass organic endogenous metabolites (Yin *et al.*, 2005). In the present study, a RRLC-Q-TOF-MS-based metabonomic approach was applied to analyze the characteristic of plasma samples of rats at different ages.

2 EXPERIMENTAL

2.1 *Chemicals and materials*

HPLC-grade methanol and acetonitrile were purchased from TEDIA (USA). All the reference standards were purchased from Sigma Corporation (St. Louis, Mo, USA). The water used in the experiments was collected from a Milli-Q Ultra-pure water system (Millipore, Billerica, USA). Other chemicals were of analytical grade.

2.2 *Animals and sample preparation*

Sixty male Wistar rats (190 $\pm$ 15 g; 8 weeks old) were purchased from Experimental Animal Center of Jilin University (Changchun, China). The rats were randomly divided into four groups (15 per group). The blood samples of each group of rats were collected in respective ages (4, 12, 18 and 24 month-age). The blood samples were then centrifuged at 3000 × g for 10 min to get 100 µL plasma and then stored at −20°C until analysis. 400 µL methanol were added into each plasma sample and vortex for 30 s, and then the sample was centrifuged at 13000 × g for 5 min. The aliquot of 5 µL was injected into the LC/MS.

---

[1] E-mail: sunjinghui2008@126.com
[*] Corresponding Author E-mail: yitonglh@126.com

2.3 *RRLC/MS analysis*

Agilent 1200 RRLC (Santa Clara, CA, USA); Agilent 6520 Q-TOF MS, (Santa Clara, CA, USA).

The liquid chromatography separation was performed on an Agilent SB-C18 column (100 mm × 3.0 mm, 1.8 μm, 600 bar) at a temperature of 25°C. 0.1% formic acid (v/v) and acetonitrile were used as the mobile phases A and B, respectively. The initial elution was 95% A and 5% B, and the gradient elution was programmed as followed: 0–15 min (5%–61% B), 15–16 min (61%–95% B). The flow rate was 0.3 mL/min. The injected sample volume was 5 μL. This RRLC system was connected to Q-TOF mass spectrometer.

The Q-TOF-MS scan range was set at m/z 50–1000 in negative modes. The conditions of the ESI source were as follows: drying gas (N2) flow rate was 8.0 L/min, drying gas temperature was set at 350°C, nebulizer was set as 30 psig, capillary voltage was 3500 V, fragmentor was 175 V, skimmer was 65 V.

2.4 *Data analysis*

The analysis of RRLC/MS data was performed on Agilent software Masshunter (version B 03.01) and Mass Profiler Professional (version B 02.02). To compare the metabolite profiles of the four groups of each age and TGRG treatment of each group, statistical methods including t-test and principal component analysis (PCA) were used. For the identification of potential biomarkers, the following databases were used: HMDB (http://www.hmdb.ca/), LIPID MAPS (http://www.lipidmaps.org/), METLIN (http://metlin.scripps.edu/), MassBank (http://www.massbank.jp/) and KEGG (http://www.genome.jp/kegg/).

3 RESULTS AND DISCUSSION

3.1 *Analysis of plasma metabolite profiles*

In this study, RRLC-Q-TOF-MS analysis was performed to acquire plasma metabolic profiles in negative ion mode. The principle component analysis (PCA) was performed to discover the potential age-related metabolites of plasma samples from 4, 12, 18, 24 month-old rats. PCA, as a common method for multivariate data analysis, can be used to reduce the dimensionality with minimal information loss while retaining the characteristics that contribute most to the variance. Figure 1a shows the 3D-PCA score plots, in which the scattered points of various samples exhibit

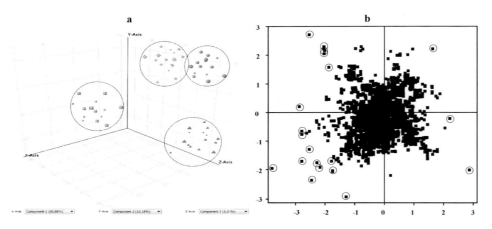

Figure 1. (a) 3D-PCA score plots of 4, 12, 18, 24 month-old rats. (■: 4 month-old rats; ▲: 12 month-old rats; ◆: 18 month-old rats; ●: 24 month-old rats); (b) loading plots from the result of PCA of 4, 12, 18, 24 month-old rats.

an obvious separation and are classified into four groups according the age of the rats. Figure 1b shows the loading plots from the result of PCA. The spots further from the center were more likely to be the potential biomarkers for the analysis of aging process. There were total 14 potential age-related metabolites which showed significant differences according to the T test ($p < 0.01$). To identify these potential biomarkers, the retention time, accurate molecular ion mass and characteristic fragment ions with MS/MS were compared with those from authentic standards and database resources. The related information of potential biomarkers is list in Table 1.

3.2 Characterization of aging based on plasma metabolites

To observe the trends of these metabolites in each group, the extracted ion chromatogram (EIC) and the average peak area of every biomarker of respective groups were analyzed to achieve the specific peak information for the relative intensity. Every average peak area of all the metabolites in each group was presented as the mean ± standard deviation (SD). The statistical analysis was performed by ANOVA and the differences between the means were assessed by Turkey's test. The statistical significance was considered as the value of $p < 0.05$ and $p < 0.01$. Figure 2 showed the change of biomarkers in each group and most of them were displayed based on age-related trend.

As Figure 2 shows, all the metabolites were decreased clearly with the increase of aging. The decreasing of metabolites related fatty acid and phospholipids metabolism such as phytosphingosine indicated that the phospholipids on the cell membrane were consumed for excessive free radicals attack with the growth of age (Liu et al., 2002). The decreasing of citric acid (intermediate in the tricarboxylic acid cycle, TAC) indicates the mitochondria function of liver cell was reduced with aging (Schieke & Finkel, 2006). Taurocholic acid as physiological detergents that facilitate excretion, absorption, and transport of fats and sterols in the intestine and liver, the decreasing of its level with aging indicates the disorder of lipid metabolism balance (Williamson, et al., 2001). Phenylalanine is the precursor of tyrosine or catecholamines in the body, the decreasing of

Table 1. Data of identified metabolites.

No.	mass	Metabolite	Element composition	Related metabolic pathway
1	610.9066	DG(14:1(9Z)/22:6(4Z,7Z,10Z,13Z,16Z,19Z)/0:0)	$C_{39}H_{62}O_5$	Saturated and unsaturated fatty acid
2	810.1348	PC(18:2(9Z,12Z)/20:2(11Z,14Z))	$C_{46}H_{84}NO_8P$	Phospholipids metabolism
3	784.013	PE(20:5(5Z,8Z,11Z,14Z,17Z)/20:5(5Z,8Z,11Z,14Z,17Z))	$C_{45}H_{70}NO_8P$	Phospholipids metabolism
4	515.6197	LysoPC(18:4(6Z,9Z,12Z,15Z))	$C_{26}H_{46}NO_7P$	Saturated and unsaturated fatty acid
5	495.6301	LysoPC(16:0)	$C_{24}H_{50}NO_7P$	Palmitic acid metabolism
6	317.5072	Phytosphingosine	$C_{18}H_{39}NO_3$	Phospholipids metabolism
7	392.4672	cPA(16:0/0:0)	$C_{19}H_{37}O_6P$	Phospholipids metabolism
8	436.5198	LPA(18:1(9Z)/0:0)	$C_{21}H_{41}O_7P$	Phospholipids metabolism
9	499.5772	LysoPE(20:5(5Z,8Z,11Z,14Z,17Z)/0:0)	$C_{25}H_{42}NO_7P$	Phospholipids metabolism
10	515.703	Taurocholic acid	$C_{26}H_{45}NO_7S$	Taurine metabolism
11	192.1235	Citric acid	$C_6H_8O_7$	Tricarboxylic acid cycle
12	304.4669	Arachidonic acid	$C_{20}H_{32}O_2$	Mediates inflammation and the functioning of several organs and systems
13	165.1891	Phenylalanine	$C_9H_{11}NO_2$	Catecholamine or energy metabolism
14	278.4296	Linolenic acid	$C_{18}H_{30}O_2$	Phospholipids metabolism

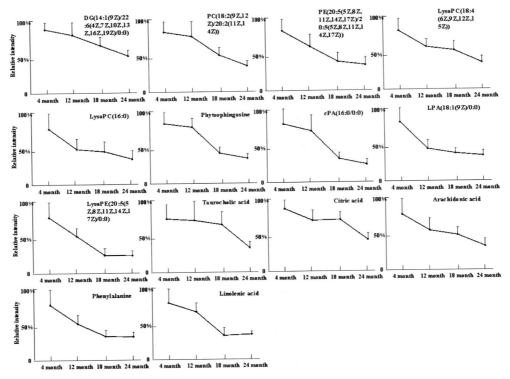

Figure 2.   Age-associated changes in the relative intensity of metabolites in plasma sample from 4, 12, 18 and 24 month-old group of rats.

phenylalanine in aging rats maybe caused by inhibition of catecholamines metabolism or reducing of energy metabolism with aging (Simpkins, *et al.*, 1997; McIntosh & Westfall, 1987).

4   CONCLUSIONS

In this study, a metabonomics method based on RRLC-Q-TOF-MS has been developed to study the characteristics of aging process of rats. After multivariate statistical analysis, a clear separation between the four different aging rats was achieved. 14 age-related potential biomarkers have been found and identified. The results showed that the decrease of fatty acid, phospholipids metabolism and energy metabolism, disorder of lipid metabolism were the main characteristics of the aging.

ACKNOWLEDGEMENTS

This research work was supported by project of Jilin province education department (No. 2013-200, No. 2014-191) and Health department of Jilin Province (No. 2013-Q017).

REFERENCES

Liu, H.M. Luo, Z.S. & Li, X.F, (2002) Relationship of aging and the metabolism of saturated fatty acid in rats. *Chin J Gerontol*, 22(2): 42–43.

Mclntosh, H.H. & Westfall, T.C. (1987) Influence of aging on catecholamine levels, accumulation, and release in F-344 rats. Neurobiol Aging, 8: 233–239.

Schieke, S.M. & Finkel, T. (2006) Mitochondrial signaling, TOR and life span. *Biol Chem*, 387(10–11): 1357–1361.

Simpkins, J.W. Mueller, G.P. Huang, H.H. & Meites, J. (1977) Evidence for depressed catecholamine and enhanced serotonin metabolism in aging male rats: possible relation to gonadotropin secretion. Endocrinology, 100: 1672–1678.

Williamson, C. Gorelik, J. Eaton, B.M. Lab, M. de Swiet, M. & Korchev, Y. (2001) The bile acid taurocholate impairs rat cardiomyocyte function: a proposed mechanism for intra-uterine fetal death in obstetric cholestasis. *Clin Sci (Lond)*. Apr, 100 (4): 363–369.

World Health Organization's Ageing & Health. http://www.who.int/ageing/en/; accessed Jan 3, 2012.

Yin, D.Z. & Chen, K.J. (2005) The essential mechanisms of aging: Irreparable damage accumulation of biochemical side-reactions. *Experimental gerontology*. 40(6): 455–465.

Medicine Sciences and Bioengineering – Wang (Ed.)

Precision analysis of the Nintendo Balance Board for assessment of wheelchair stability

Xian-zhi Jiang* & Liang-liang Yang
Faculty of Mechanical Engineering & Automation, Zhejiang Sci-Tech University, Hangzhou, China

Chao Zhang
Department of Internal Neurology of the First Affiliated Hospital of Zhejiang Chinese Medicine University, Hangzhou, China

ABSTRACT: This paper studies the validity and reliability of the Nintendo Wii Balance Board by analyzing the precisions on measurement of weight and coordination. Results showed that smaller load resulted in worse precision. Without filters, the minimum error of weight measurement was about 0.4 kg and that of the center of position was 16.8 mm. The results showed that the WBB can work as an effective measuring tool for the low-precision system.

1 INTRODUCTION

Every year, there are many wheelchair-related injuries in the world and most of which are caused by the loss of stability of the wheelchairs (Louise *et al.*, 2012; Kirby *et al.*, 1995). The wheelchair stability assessment aims to enhance wheelchair prescription to improve the stability of the wheelchair which can be helpful in selecting and reconfiguring the wheelchair to reduce the injuries caused by tips and falls of the wheelchair. On the basis of these data, all the other important parameters of the wheelchair can be calculated such as center of gravity (COG) and distances between the wheels of the wheelchair as shown in Figure 1.

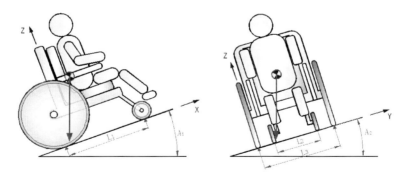

Figure 1. Center of gravity of the wheelchair.

To measure the vertical ground reaction force and center of position (COP) of the wheel, the simplest solution is using a scale with four load cells on its corners. Four such scales can measure the four vertical ground reaction forces and COPs of the wheelchair's four wheels. With these data, the COP of the wheelchair and the distances between the wheels can be calculated. When inclined

---

*Corresponding author Xianzhi Jiang can be contacted at: xianzhi@zstu.edu.cn

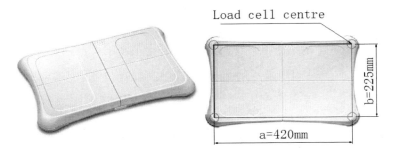

Figure 2.   The Nintendo Wii Balance Board (WBB).

to a fixed angle, the COG of the wheelchair can be worked out too. These parameters are essential to the wheelchair stability assessment system. Therefore, the selection of the scale is quite important and the precision of the scale as well.

The Nintendo Wii Balance Board (WBB) is considered as a suitable measuring device to the health care measuring tool as shown in Figure 2 (Erik, 2012).

Lucio and Giovanni (2011) focused on an application of navigation and interaction in a virtual environment by using a WBB. Their purpose was to simulate the use of a mouse and a keyboard starting from the properly interpreted and translated inputs received from the WBB. Michael et al (2011) developed the WeHab system, a low-cost rehabilitation instrument, by using two WBBs to enhance rehabilitation for patients with balance disorders.

The WBBs were also introduced in some other studies as the input or testing devices (Emily et al., 2011; Barbara *et al.*, 2011; Ross *et al.*, 2011), in which, some claimed that the WBB had a high precision but some not. But none of these articles gave the detailed precision analysis of the WBB. Therefore, the aim of our study is to analyze the precision of the WBB and to verify whether it is a valid and reliable tool in assessment of wheelchair stability system.

2   METHOD

2.1   *Noise of the load cell*

Figure 3(a) shows the voltage of the top-left load cell of the WBB that works without any load. Figure 3(b) shows the same load cell with a load of about 10 kg.

In Figure 3(a), without any load on the WBB, the original voltage of the top-left load cell is 0.154 V and the noise is about 0.04 V. In addition, the voltages and noises are not always the same to the four load cells. In Figure 3(b), with a load of 10 kg on the top-left load cell, the voltage increases to 0.244 V but the noise is the same. The voltages show that the noise of the load cell is about 0.04 V. The experimental data showed that the noise was about 0.04 V and smaller load will result in poorer measuring precision.

2.2   *Data capture*

In our study, the WBB is synchronized with a laptop via Bluetooth as shown in Figure 4. The WBB is covered by a graph paper to read the real COP. A 5.4 kg calibrated weight is also used to verify the precision of force measurement.

After synchronization, the WBB will report 7 kinds of data, such as X_{raw}, X of the COP; Y_{raw}, Y of the COP; M_{raw}, mass of the load; M_{TL}, value of the top-left load cell; M_{TR}, value of the top-right load cell; M_{BL}, value of the bottom-left load cell; and M_{BR}, value of the bottom-right load cell.

We developed the software to access the data of the WBB in Labview by loading the library of WiimoteLib, which can access the reported data of the WBB when paired via Bluetooth. The sample rate was set to 10 Hz.

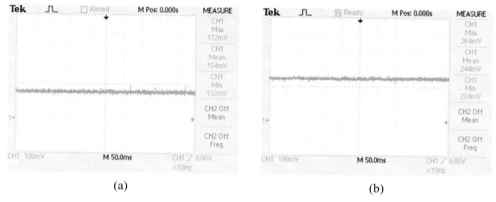

(a)   (b)

Figure 3.   Amplified voltage of the top-left load cell of the WBB.

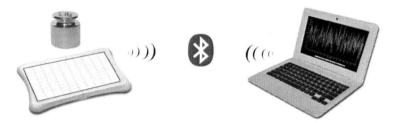

Figure 4.   WBB is synchronized with a laptop via Bluetooth.

2.3   *Precision of the raw data*

Figure 5 shows the values of the four load cells with the WBB working without any load. From Figure 5, we can find out that the values of the four load cells are quite different and the maximum error is about 0.8 kg, but the noises are nearly the same, so the reported data should be calibrated.

These parameters are reported directly by the WBB, while X, Y, and M can be calculated by MTL, MTR, MBL, and MBR:

$$M_{cal} = M_{TL} + M_{TR} + M_{BL} + M_{BR} \tag{1}$$

$$X_{cal} = \frac{a(M_{TR} + M_{BR} - M_{TL} - M_{BL})}{2(M_{TL} + M_{TR} + M_{BL} + M_{BR})} \tag{2}$$

$$Y_{cal} = \frac{b(M_{TL} + M_{TR} - M_{BL} - M_{BR})}{2(M_{TL} + M_{TR} + M_{BL} + M_{BR})} \tag{3}$$

where $a = 420$ mm is the length of the working area and $b = 225$ mm is the width.

Theoretically, X_{cal} should be equal to X_{raw}, Y_{cal} should be equal to Y_{raw}, and M_{cal} should be equal to M_{raw}, but the experimental data and curves indicate that it was not so. One of the recorded data shows that the error range of M_{raw} is −2.35 to −2 kg but that of M_{cal} is −9.3 to −8 which indicate that the precision of M_{raw} is better than M_{cal}.

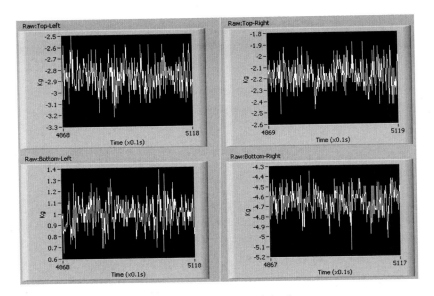

Figure 5. Curves of the four load cells of the WBB without any load.

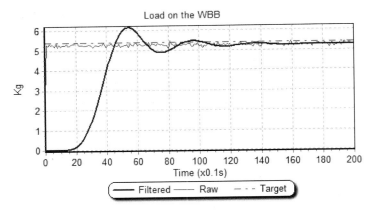

Figure 6. The curves of M_{raw} and filtered M_{raw}.

2.4 *Precision of the filtered data*

As studied in the preceding section, there are serious noises in the raw data which will make the precision of the assessment of wheelchair stability very poor. To improve the precision of the WBB, the raw data was filtered by an eight-order low-pass Butterworth filter with a cut-off frequency of 10 Hz. Figure 6 shows the results after the Butterworth filter.

In Figure 6, the applied load is 5.4 kg. The calibrated raw load ranges from 5.10 to 5.46 kg. After filteration, the rise time increase to 4.6 s, the maximum overshoot is 0.74 kg, and the setting time is about 15 s. The filtered data ranges from 5.23 to 5.29 kg after stable. These results indicate that although the precision is improved by filter, the response is very slow.

3 SUMMARY

The noise of the load cell in the WBB is about 0.04 V which means the error is about 20% when applied a load of 5.4 kg on it. Although the COP and the load can be calculated by the data of the four load cells, the calculated values are not as precise as the reported data. The experimental data showed that the precision of the WBB was not as good as claimed in some other studies. However, because the WBB has so many advantages such as low cost, portability, and wireless communication, it is quite suitable for the low-level, low-precision product for the wheelchair stability assessment system.

ACKNOWLEDGMENTS

This work was supported by the Science Foundation of Zhejiang Sci-Tech University (ZSTU) under Grant 13022152-Y, the Key Projects of the National Science & Technology Pillar Program under Grant 2013BAF05B01, and the Zhejiang Scientific Research Foundation of Chinese Medicine Program under Grant 2012ZB053. The authors would like to thank the Health Design Technology Institute (HDTI, Coventry University, UK,) and Dr. Dimitar Stefanov.

REFERENCES

Barbara Williams, Nicole L. Doherty, Andrew Bender, Holly Mattox, & Jesse R. Tibbs. (2011) The Effect of Nintendo Wii on Balance: A Pilot Study Supporting the Use of the Wii in Occupational Therapy for the Well Elderly. *Occupational Therapy in Health Care*, 25, 131–139.

Emily Bainbridge, Sarah Bevans, Brynne Keeley, & Kathryn Oriel. (2011) The Effects of the Nintendo Wii Fit on Community-Dwelling Older Adults with Perceived Balance Deficits: A Pilot Study. *Physical & Occupational Therapy in Geriatrics*, 29(2), 126–135.

Erik A. Wikstrom. (2012) Validity and Reliability of Nintendo Wii Fit Balance Scores. *Journal of Athletic Training*, 47(3), 306–313.

Lucio Tommaso De Paolis, Giovanni Aloisio. (2011) Walking in a Virtual Town Using Nintendo Wii Mote And Balance Board, *Scientific Research and Information Technology*, 1(2), 21–32.

Michael W. Kennedy, James P. Schmiedeler, Aaron D. Striegel, Charles R. Crowell, Michael Villano, and Johan Kuitse. (2011) Enhanced Feedback in Balance Rehabilitation using the Nintendo Wii Balance Board. *IEEE International Conference on e-Health Networking Applications and Services*, pp.162–168.

Lee Kirby R. Maria T. Sampson, Fredrik A.V. Thoren, Donald A. MacLeod. (1995) Wheelchair stability: Effect of body position. *Journal of Rehabilitation Research and Development*, 32(4), 367–372.

Ross Allan Clark, Rian McGough, Kade Paterson. (2011) Reliability of an inexpensive and portable dynamic weight bearing asymmetry assessment system incorporating dual Nintendo Wii Balance Boards. *Gait & Posture*, 34, 288–291.

William Young, Stuart Ferguson, Sebastien Brault, Cathy Craig. (2011) Assessing and training standing balance in older adults: A novel approach using the 'Nintendo Wii' Balance Board. *Gait & Posture*, 33, 303–305.

Medicine Sciences and Bioengineering – Wang (Ed.)
© *2015 Taylor & Francis Group, London, ISBN: 978-1-138-02684-1*

Blood lipid components in functional tradeoffs and risk of coronary heart disease due to type 2 diabetes mellitus

Qian Guo*, Rui Gong, Guang-hao Xia, Li-min Tian, Shu-hong Zhou,
Lu-yan Zhang & Hui-qin Niu
Department of endocrinopathy, Gansu Provincial Hospital, Lanzhou, China

ABSTRACT: **Objective:** Exploring the effects of ABCA1R219K polymorphism on changes in blood lipid profiles and the contribution of ratios of blood lipid components to Type 2 Diabetes Mellitus (T2DM) complications with Coronary Heart Disease (CHD) risk. **Method:** Analyzing effects of ABCA1R219K polymorphism on the T2DM complications with CHD risk by changing blood lipid components ratios. **Results:** (1) The significant difference in frequency of KK genotype appeared between T2DM with CHD and T2DM or control ($p < 0.05$). (2) The levels of Triglyceride (TG) and Low-Density Lipoprotein Cholesterol (LDL-C) decreased obviously, whereas high-density lipoprotein cholesterol (HDL-C) increased in KK genotype ($p < 0.05$). The difference in ratios of LDL-C/HDL-C, TG/HDL-C, and total cholesterol (TC)/HDL-C was greater than the individual components between groups. Only LDL-C/HDL-C was significantly higher in T2DM with CHD than that in T2DM and control, but there was no difference between T2DM and control. **Conclusion:** KK homozygous genotypes have some contribution to improve the blood profile to prevent from the risk of CHD in patient with T2DM. Maybe the risk of CHD in patients with T2DM complications depends mainly on the relative levels of LDL-C, HDL-C, and their functional tradeoffs, rather than the alteration in absolute concentrations of individual components.

1 INTRODUCTION

Coronary Heart Disease (CHD), which is closely related to disorder of blood lipid metabolism, is the most common chronic complication in patients with diabetes mellitus (DM). Abnormality of lipid metabolism would result in the process of atherosclerosis (AS) and CHD in patients with DM (Smaoui *et al* 2004, Murase *et al* 2008). HDL-C would give a great contribution to prevent from the pathogenesis of AS (Goldbourt *et al* 1997). Some studies further manifest that there is a close contact between the ratio of low-density lipoprotein cholesterol (LDL-C)/ high-density lipoprotein cholesterol (HDL-C) and CHD pathogenesis (Manninen *et al* 1992, Kannel 2005, Mohan 2005). Scholars believe that the ratio of LDL-C/HDL-C is a more available clinical marker for determining risk of pathogenesis of cardiovascular disease (Packard *et al* 2005, Fernandez et al 2008).

The ATP-binding cassette transporter (*ABCA1*) gene as an important genetic factor involves in lipid metabolism and its polymorphism might play an important role to result in pathogenesis of CHD in patients with T2DM (Brousseau *et al* 2001, Hong *et al* 2002). The common SNPs polymorphism of *ABCA1R219K* gene would affect the transfer of cholesterol, that is, reversely from periphery cellular to liver by changing the level of blood lipid components (Fielding et al 1995).

We hypothesize that T2DM complications of CHD might be certainly related to the functional tradeoffs of blood lipid components. This study examines the contribution of *ABCA1R219K* polymorphism to improve the blood profile ratio of blood lipid components, and analyzes the effects of functional tradeoffs of blood lipid components on the risk of CHD pathogenesis in T2DM patients.

---

*Corresponding author: Guo Qian.

2 MATERIAL AND METHOD

2.1 Subjects

All cases in the study were recruited from inpatients in Gansu Provincial Hospital from 2005 to 2006 and categorized as follows:

Group of T2DM: 73 cases, male/female: 39/34, 57 years old in average. The diagnosis of T2DM is based on the criteria of diagnosis and classification of DM approved by WHO in 1998, and all patients had no family history of CHD.

Group of T2DM complications with CHD risk: 71 cases, male/female: 37/34, 58 years old in average. The diagnosis of T2DM is the same as aforementioned. The group included patients with myocardial infarction, acute myocardial infarction, angina, and CHD were confirmed using coronary arteriography.

Group of control was recruited from healthy people simultaneously. Eighty-three healthy volunteers, male/female: 47/36, 57 years old in average, without family history of DM and CHD.

The study was approved by the ethical committee of hospital. Written informed consent was obtained from all patients and healthy volunteers enrolled.

2.2 Method

2.2.1 Sample collection

Five milliliters fasting peripheral blood was collected from each object and put into the tube with EDTA.

2.2.2 Genotype assay

Genomic DNA was extracted from peripheral blood according to Montgomery and Sise (1990). Briefly, the target fragment of 177 bp in 7th exon of *ABCA1* gene was amplified by PCR by using the following primers according to Clee *et al* (2001): Forward primer: 5'-GTATTTTTGCAAGGCTACCAGTTACATTTGACAA-3'; and reverse primer: 5'-ATTGGC TTCAGGATGTCCATGTTGGAA-3'. Ten microliters of PCR product was digested with 10 U of the restriction enzyme *Xag*I at 37°C for more than three hours. The digested fragments were analyzed by electrophoresis on 2% agarose gel. The bands were visualized by staining with ethidium bromide. Three Genotypes RR, RK, and KK were performed according to Cenarro *et al* (2003).

2.2.3 Blood lipid components determination

Peripheral fasting blood was collected from all subjects who had not used lipid-lowering drugs at least 15 days. Total cholesterol (TC), triglyceride (TG), LDL-C, and HDL-C levels were determined using automatic biochemistry analyzer (Express Plus, Bayer Health Care, Germany).

2.2.4 Statistical analysis

Statistical analyses were performed by SPSS v.11.5 program for Windows.

3 RESULTS

3.1 The genotypes analysis

The results of genotypes analysis for 227 subjects confirmed the presence of three genotypes: homozygous RR (177 bp), heterozygous RK (177, 107, and 70 bp), and homozygous KK (107 and 70 bp) (Figure 1).

The genotype frequency distribution of R219K polymorphism is shown in Table 1. The frequency of the KK in group of patients with T2DM complications at a risk of CHD was significantly lower than that in control and T2DM groups ($p < 0.05$); though the KK in T2DM group was also lower than that in control group, but the difference was not significant in statistics between them. Moreover, there was no significant difference in frequencies of the RR and RK between any two groups (Table 1).

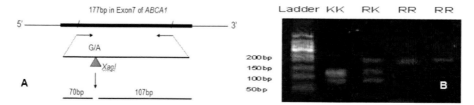

Figure 1. Determination of the R219K genotype by PCR amplification and restriction analysis. Upper part: the G/A polymorphism position is indicated by a triangle. When the nucleotide A is present, a *Xag*I restriction site is created. Lower part: 2% agarose gel electrophoresis of *Xag*I-digested PCR products is shown. After cleavage with *Xag*I, either a 177 bp fragment (homozygous GG, lane RR) or 177, 107, and 70 bp fragments (heterozygous GA, lane RK) or 107 and 70 bp fragments (homozygous AA, lane KK) are produced.

Table 1. Distribution in frequency of ABCA1 R219K genotypes in three groups.

| Groups | Cases | Genotype (frequency) (%) | | | Chi-square Test | | |
		RR	RK	KK	df	X^2	p
T2DM + CHD	71	30 (42.3)	37 (52.1)	4 (5.6)*,$^{\triangle}$	1	2.94408	>0.05
T2DM	73	27 (37.0)	34 (46.6)	12 (16.4)	1	0.05499	>0.05
Control	83	29 (34.9)	38 (45.8)	16 (19.3)	1	0.31193	>0.05

*Compared with control, $p < 0.05$; $^{\triangle}$Compared with group of T2DM, $p < 0.05$. X^2 test, the distribution of genotype frequency comply with Hardy–Weinberg genetic equilibrium ($p > 0.05$).

Table 2. Concentration of blood lipid components in the three genotypes.

| Components of blood lipids (mmol/L) | Genotype | | |
	RR ($n = 57$)	RK ($n = 71$)	KK ($n = 16$)
HDL-C	1.27 ± 0.20	1.28 ± 0.17	1.38 ± 0.15*
LDL-C	2.92 ± 0.77	2.97 ± 0.68	2.84 ± 0.31
TG	2.09 ± 1.02	1.96 ± 0.93	1.76 ± 0.58*
TC	4.88 ± 0.80	4.98 ± 0.82	4.92 ± 0.64

Compared with RR genotype: *$p < 0.05$.

3.2 *R219K polymorphism, blood lipid profile, and ratio of lipid components between genotypes*

Blood lipids profile was in association with the R219K polymorphism. The TG and LDL-C levels were obviously lower in subject with KK, and especially the TG was lower 15.8% than that in subject with RR ($p < 0.05$). On the contrary, the HDL-C was higher 8.7% (p < 0.05) in subject with KK than RR. LDL-C and TC in subject with KK increased by 2.74% and decreased by 0.82% only, respectively, in comparison with RR. Moreover, the levels of four kinds of blood lipid components had insignificant difference between RK and RR genotypes (Table 2).

However, the difference in ratio of blood lipid components was much greater than that of individual lipid components among genotypes. The ratios of LDL-C/HDL-C, TG/HDL-C, and TC/HDL-C in the subject with KK were lower 13.0%, 22.4%, and 7.3%, respectively, than those in subjects with RR. The ratios had more obvious difference in comparison with individual lipid components between genotypes, but there was no significant difference between RK and RR (Figure 2).

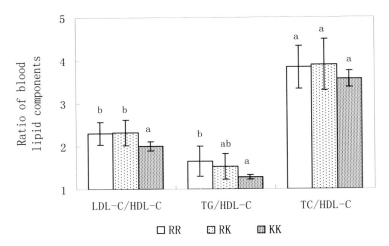

Figure 2. Ratios of blood lipid components in three genotypes. The three kinds of ratio value in genotype KK are lower than those in genotype RR and RK. Different letters indicate significant differences between genotypes.

Table 3. Concentration of blood lipid components in three groups.

Components of blood lipid (mmol/L)	Control ($n = 83$)	T2DM ($n = 73$)	T2DM+CHD ($n = 71$)
HDL-C	1.43 ± 0.13	1.32 ± 0.11	1.25 ± 0.14*
LDL-C	2.74 ± 0.30	2.91 ± 0.46	2.97 ± 0.31*
TG	1.72 ± 0.39	1.93 ± 0.43*	2.04 ± 0.41**
TC	4.65 ± 0.36	4.94 ± 0.41*	4.93 ± 0.54*

Compared with control group: * $p < 0.05$; ** $p < 0.01$.

3.3 The ratio of lipid components between groups

TG and LDL-C levels of T2DM were higher 12.2% and 6.2%, respectively, than those of control, and their levels in group of T2DM complications with CHD risk were, respectively, up to 18.6% and 8.4% higher ($p < 0.05$) than those of control. Especially, TG was more significantly raising ($p < 0.01$) in patients with T2DM complications. On the other hand, the HDL-C in two patient groups were lower 7.7% and 12.6% ($p < 0.05$), respectively, than those of control. However, the TG and HDL-C levels increased by 5.7% and decreased, respectively, by 5.3% in patient with complication, in comparison to those of T2DM, which suggested that TG and HDL-C had a more close connection with T2DM complications with CHD risk (Table 3).

Similarly, the difference in ratio of blood lipid components between groups was greater than that of individual lipid components. The ratios of LDL-C/HDL-C, TG/HDL-C, and TC/HDL-C in group of complication were higher 25.0%, 35.8%, and 21.2%, respectively, than those in control. The changes were more obvious in ratios than in individual lipid components, especially the value of LDL-C/HDL-C in patient with complication was significant higher than that in control and T2DM.

The ratios of LDL-C/HDL-C and TG/HDL-C in patient of T2DM with CHD were also higher 17.8% and 11.6%, respectively, than those in T2DM. But among three ratios, only LDL-C/HDL-C in patient with complication was significantly higher than that in both T2DM and control, and that in T2DM and control have no difference (Figure 3).

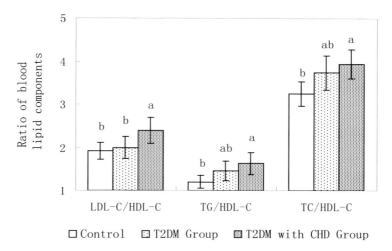

Figure 3. Ratios of blood lipid components in three groups. Three kinds of ratio value in complication group increased significantly, LDL-C/HDL-C in group of T2DM with CHD was significantly higher than that in groups of control and T2DM. Different letters indicate significant differences between groups.

4 DISCUSSIONS

The HDL-C level was the strong inversely correlated with CHD incidence. Low level of HDL-C was the most common lipid abnormality in patients with early and familial CHD, which is generally accepted as an independent risk factor in the development of CHD (Genest *et al* 1992). T2DM was also associated with dyslipidemia defined as increased TC, TG, LDL-C and decreased HDL-C (Zimmet *et al* 2005, Pladevall *et al* 2006). However, the decrease in HDL-C level in T2DM plays an important role in liability of CHD (Laakso *et al* 1997).

Clee *et al* (2001) reported that common *ABCA1* cSNPs are associated with altered blood lipids level and severity of AS and, importantly, may decrease the risk of coronary events. It was found that HDL-C level in T2DM was increasing along with RR, RK, KK, and the difference of HDL-C level was also significant between the RR and KK genotypes ($p < 0.05$) (Table 2), which suggested that the allele *k* might lead to increase in HDL-C level and reduce risk of CHD in patient of T2DM with KK genotype (Xiang *et al* 2007).

This study has shown that the frequency of the KK genotype was lower 2.9% and HDL-C concentration was also lower 7.7% in T2DM than that in control, and the KK frequency was up to 13.7% lower and HDL-C was also up to 12.6% lower in T2DM with CHD than those in control. Meanwhile, increase in other blood lipid components have led to a great increase in ratios of LDL-C/HDL-C and TG/HDL-C. Epidemiological and clinical studies have also shown that increase in ratios of LDL-C/HDL-C and TG/HDL-C was more commonly associated with dyslipidemia in patient of coronary syndrome (Kannel 2005, Mohan *et al* 2005). Therefore, the changes in ratio of blood lipid components caused by the decrease in frequency of KK genotype might greatly increase risk of CHD in patient of T2DM.

The ratios of LDL-C/HDL-C, TG/HDL-C, and TC/HDL-C in two patient groups were significant higher than those in control. However, only LDL-C/HDL-C among them was still significantly higher in complication group than that in T2DM as well as control groups (Figure 3). Therefore, it revealed that the ratio of LDL-C/HDL-C might be more closely connected to complicate CHD in T2DM, and thus it could be used as a more reliable factor to judge the risk of CHD due to complications in patient of T2DM.

The ratio of LDL-C/HDL-C was significantly lower in subject with KK than that in subject with the RK and RR genotypes. However, the lowest frequency (5.6%) of the KK genotype appeared only in patients with T2DM complications, which suggested that the KK genotype might be available for preventing from T2DM complications with CHD risk by improving efficiently the blood lipids profile in T2DM patients. Inversely, the patients with T2DM complication possessed higher frequency (16.4% and 19.3%) of RK and RR genotypes and higher value of ratio of LDL-C/HDL-C, and there was no difference in statistics in the ratio of LDL-C/HDL-C between the RK and RR genotypes (Figure 1). It might suggest that the risk of CHD was greater in T2DM patients with RK or RR genotypes than with the KK genotype. These results illustrated a notable effects of the homozygote KK genotype on the blood lipids profile and also shown that the ratio of LDL-C/HDL-C could be more efficient to reflect the risk of CHD pathogenesis; Natarajan *et al* (2003), Kannel (2005), and Fernandez *et al* (2008) reported the similar results. Manninen *et al* (1992) reported that LDL-C/HDL-C ratio had more prognostic value than LDL-C or HDL-C. Some epidemiological and clinical studies have also found that the LDL-C/HDL-C ratio to be an excellent predictor of CHD risk (Manninen *et al* 1992, Kannel 2005). On the basis of our results, we considered that the ratio of LDL-C/HDL-C could reflect the more comprehensive conditions and influence of changes in blood lipids metabolism. Because of diverse functions of HDL and LDL during AS process, their influence was antagonistic to each other (Manninen *et al* 1992, Oram 2002). Therefore, we concluded that the risk of AS process and T2DM complications with CHD risk in T2DM patients was dependent on relative levels of both of HDL and LDL and their functional tradeoffs, rather than the changes in the absolute concentration of individual blood lipid component.

ACKNOWLEDGMENTS

This work was supported by the Lanzhou Scientific and Technological program Projects under Grant 2013-3-32 and the Natural Science Fund of Gansu Province under Grant 3YS061-A25-027.

REFERENCES

Brousseau ME, Bodzioch M, Schaefer EJ, Goldkamp AL, Kielar D, Probst M, Ordovas JM, Aslanidis C, Lackner KJ, Bloomfield Rubins H, Collins D, Robins SJ, Wilson PW and Schmitz G (2001) Common variants in the gene encoding ATP binding cassette transporter 1 in man with low HDL cholesterol levels and coronary heart disease. *Atherosclerosis,* 154(3), 607–611.

Cenarro A, Artieda M, Castillo S, Mozas P, Reyes G, Tejedor D, Alonso R, Mata P, Pocoví M, Civeira F (2003) A common variant in the ABCA1 gene is associated with a lower risk for premature coronary heart disease in familial hypercholesterolaemia. *Journal of Meddicial Genetics*, 40(3),163–168.

Clee SM, Zwinderman AH, Engert JC, Zwarts KY, Molhuizen HOF, Roomp K, Jukema JW, van Wijland M, van Dam M, Hudson TJ, Brooks- Wilson A, Genest J, Kastelein JPK and Hayden MR (2001) Common genetic variation in ABCA1 is associated with altered lipoprotein levels and a modified risk for coronary artery disease. *Circulation*, 103(9), 1198–1205.

Fernandez ML. and Webb D (2008) The LDL to HDL cholesterol ratio as a valuable tool to evaluate coronary heart disease risk. *Journal of American College Nutrition,* 27(1), 1–5.

Genest JJ Jr, Martin-Munley SS, McNamara JR, Ordovas JM, Jenner J, Myers RH, Silberman SR, Wilson PW, Salem DN and Schaefer EJ (1992) Familial lipoprotein disorders in patients with premature coronary artery disease. *Circulation*, 85(6), 2025–2033.

Goldbourt U, Yaari S, Medalie JH (1997) Isolated low HDL cholesterol as a risk factor for coronary heart disease mortality: A 21 year follow-up of 8000 men. *Arteriosclerosis Thrombosis, and Vascular Biology,* 17(1),107–113.

Hong SH, Riley W, Rhyne J, Friel G and Miller M (2002) Lack of association between increased carotid intima-media thickening and decreased HDL-Cholesterol in a family with a novel ABCA1 variant, G2265T. *Clinical Chemistry*, 48(11), 2066–2070.

Kannel WB (2005) Risk stratification of dyslipidemia: Insights from the Framingham Study. *Current Medicinal Chemistry Cardiovascular Hematology Agents*, 3(3), 187–193.

Laakso M. and Letho S (1997) Epidemiology of microvascular disease in diabetes. *Diabetes Reviews*, 5: 294–315.

Manninen V, Tenkanen L, Koskinen P, Huttunen JK, Manttari M, Heinonen OP, Frick MH (1992) Joint effects of serum triglyceride and LDL cholesterol and HDL cholesterol concentrations on coronary heart disease risk in the Helsinki Heart Study. Implications for treatment. *Circulation*, 85(1), 37–45.

Mohan V, Deepa R, Velmurugan K, Gokulakrishnan K (2005) Association of small dense LDL with a coronary artery disease and diabetes in urban Asian Indians - the Chennai Urban Rural Epidemiology Study (CURES-8). *The Journal of the Association of Physicians India*, 53, 95–100.

Montgomery GW and Sise JA (1990) Extraction of DNA from sheep white plasma cells. *N.Z.J. Agriculture Research,* 33: 437–441.

Murase T, Okubo M, Amemiya-Kudo M, Ebara T, Mori Y (2008) Impact of elevated serum lipoprotein (a) concentrations on the risk of coronary heart disease in patients with type 2 diabetes mellitus. *Metabolism: Clinical and Experimental,* 57(6), 791–795.

Natarajan S, Glick H, Criqui M, Horowitz D, Lipsitz SR, Kinosian B (2003) Cholesterol measures to identify and treat individuals at risk for coronary heart disease. *American Journal of Preventive Medicine,* 25(1), 50–57.

Oram JF (2002) ATP-binding cassette transporter ABCA1 and cholesterol trafficking. *Current Opinion Lipidology,* 13(4), 373–381.

Packard CJ, Ford I, Robertson M, Shepherd J, Blauw GJ, Murphy MB, Bollen ELEM, Buckley BM, Cobbe SM, Gaw A, Hyland M, Jukema W, Kampe AM, Macfarlane PW, Perry IJ, Stott DJ, Sweeney BJ, Twomey C and Westendorp RGJ (2005) Plasma lipoproteins and apolipoproteins as predictors of cardiovascular risk and treatment benefit in the PROspective Study of Pravastatin in the Elderly at Risk (PROSPER). *Circulation*, 112(20), 3058–3065.

Pladevall M, Singal B, Williams LK, Bortons C, Guyer H, Sadurni J, Falces C, Serrano-Rios M, Gabriel R, Shaw JE, Zimmet PZ and Haffner S (2006) A single factor underlies the metabolic syndrome: A confirmatory factor analysis. *Diabetes Care*, 29(1), 113–122.

Smaoui M, Hammami S, Chaaba R, Attia N, Hamda KB, Masmoudi S, Mahjoub S, Bousslama A, Farhat MB, Hammami M (2004) Lipids and lipoprotein(a) concentrations in Tunisian type 2 diabetic patients; Relationship to glycemic control and coronary heart disease. *Journal of Diabetes and its Complications,* 18(5), 258–263.

Xiang GD, He YS, Zao SL, Hou J, Le L (2007) The association between high-density lipoprotein cholesterol and endothelium-dependent arterial dilation in type 2 diabetes mellitus with dyslipidemia. *Chinese Journal of Diabetes*, 15(4): 474–477. (IN CHINESE)

Zimmet P, Magliano D, Matsuzawa Y, Alberti G, Shaw J (2005) The metabolic syndrome: a global public health problem and a new definition. *Journal of Atherosclerosis Thrombosis*, 12(6): 295–300.

Medicine Sciences and Bioengineering – Wang (Ed.)
© *2015 Taylor & Francis Group, London, ISBN: 978-1-138-02684-1*

Application of problem-based learning in the clinical practice teaching of neurology

Wei Sun[1]
Affiliated Hospital of Beihua University, Jilin, Jilin, China

Jia-le Liu[*]
JiLin Central General Hospital Jilin, Jilin, China

ABSTRACT: In this study, Problem-Based Learning (PBL) teaching was applied in the teaching of neurology probation class, and its methods and results were explored. Sixty 5-year clinical undergraduate students were randomly divided into two groups, a PBL group and a traditional teaching group, with 30 students in each group. The students' behaviors and test scores were observed and compared statistically. The results showed that the students' learning enthusiasm, self-evaluation, and interest in neurology practice in the PBL group were significantly higher than those in the traditional teaching group; 98% of the students were satisfied with PBL method; test scores of the students in the PBL group were significantly higher than those in the traditional teaching group ($P < 0.05$). PBL teaching method should be better than the traditional method in improving students' flexible use of knowledge and overall levels. The method is beneficial to the training of students in their learning enthusiasm and interest, self-evaluation, clinical thinking, problem-solving skills, and innovative abilities.

1 INTRODUCTION

Problem-Based Learning (PBL), proposed by Professor Barrow of the American Academy of Neurology, McMaster University in 1969, Canada, is a teaching method in which a problem-centered research study is conducted (Norman GR & Schmidt HC, 2000). Its advantages are to create opportunities for students to think and solve problems, and guide students to combine theoretical knowledge with clinical practice, focusing on students' clinical thinking and applied capabilities to overcome the drawback of the separation of basic medical theory from the clinical medical practice in the traditional medicine education (Yang Di *et al.*, 2008). In this study, PBL was applied in the teaching of neurology probation class and its practical methods were explored.

2 SUBJECTS AND METHODS

Sixty clinical internships from five-year medical undergraduates at Beihua University were divided into PBL and traditional teaching groups, 30 in each group. The PBL group includes 21 males and 9 females, aged 22–27 years with a mean age of 25.1 ± 1.2 years. There were 30 students in the traditional teaching group, 19 males and 11 females, aged 24–26 years with a mean age of 25.2 ± 1.4 years. There was no statistically significant difference in the general information (age, gender, etc.) between the two groups ($P > 0.05$).

---

[1] First Author: Sun Wei (1979),
[*] Corresponding Author: Liu Jiale (1979), E-mail: 6172279@qq.com

2.1 *Teaching methods in the traditional teaching group*

In the traditional teaching group, the teachers mainly led the students to review the theoretical knowledge first, and then led the students to make the rounds of the wards and check patients, in which the students were required to ask questions and the teachers explained those.

2.2 *Teaching methods in the PBL group*

2.2.1 *Selection of problems*
The teachers responsible for the practical teaching were required to prepare case materials and carefully conceive series of "problems." The designed problems should be scientific, with certain level, depth, and difficulty, some artistic and rhythmic, and paid more attention to the contact with the relevant disciplines.

2.2.2 *Students' preparation*
On the basis of the problems, some reference books were recommended to the students, such as Cerebrovascular Disease Prevention and Treatment Guidelines, neurology, 700 Questions for Neurology Physician and Neuroanatomy; the students were encouraged to consult more related reference materials as possible, write a speech outline, ask new questions, and prepare for the class discussion.

2.2.3 *Classroom discussion*
Focusing on the problems raised by the students, the discussion was organized. Students in each group recommended their representative to give the speech. According to the personal volunteer, 8–10 students were in one discussion group to explain and debate their views, and record the problems. The teachers recorded the problems that were not clear or needed to be corrected. Finally, the discussion was briefly summarized by the group leader.

2.2.4 *Summary by the teachers*
Aiming the problems found by the students, the teacher commented on them and explained them in detail, answered students' questions, and pointed out common problems in the practice and the key knowledge that should be grasped. The teachers should mainly play an inspiration and guidance role in the process to control the discussion.

2.2.5 *Clinical application*
With reference to patient diagnosis and treatment information, the answers to questions were verified and adjusted, to stimulate the students' interest in learning and enhance their memory.

2.3 *Unified assessment*

2.3.1 *Questionnaire survey*
The questionnaire survey focused on the learning enthusiasm, initiative, independent analysis, problem-solving skills, self-evaluation, satisfaction of teaching, and the interest in the neurology internship and the pathway of access to knowledge.

2.3.2 *Theoretical examination*
The theoretical examination was conducted using unified examination papers. The examination time, paper content, and assessment standard of papers were exactly the same in the two groups. The results in the two groups were compared and the data were processed with SPSS19.0 statistical software.

3 RESULTS

The learning enthusiasm, self-evaluation, and interest in neurology practice of students in the PBL group were significantly higher than those in the traditional teaching group; 98% of the students were satisfied with PBL method; there were 10–14 accesses to knowledge in the PBL group, but only 5–7 in the traditional teaching group; as shown in Table 1, the average score of theoretical examination in the PBL group was 92.5 ± 6.5 points, whereas that in the traditional group was 80.2 ± 5.3 points, and the difference was statistically significant ($P < 0.05$).

4 DISCUSSION

The traditional medical education focuses on imparting knowledge, but the PBL medical education emphasizes on "problem-centered" learning. The "problem-centered" approach can break the separation of basic medical education from clinical education in a staging way and the traditional boundary among disciplines, which emphasizes on placing the study in a complex, meaningful, relatively real environment, allowing the learners to try to solve problems with authenticity in an exploration and cooperation process, and focus on the problems to learn the scientific knowledge hiding in the question (Chen Ning & Zhang Qinglin, 2006). It aims at enabling learners to build up a broad and flexible knowledge base, efficiently understand, analyze, and solve problems, and at the same time, focuses on the cultivation of students in the self-learning and cooperative learning ability, which can play a positive role in making up for deficiencies of the past teaching mode in the practice (Li Hongwei et al., 2008; Yu Zhengmiao & Chen Jing, 2008; Liu Zhongxiu, 2008).

The problem is both the start point and the focus of PBL. It is of vital importance to create some problems closely linked with the content of teaching materials and practical cases. The teachers should not directly tell students how to solve the problems faced, but provide references for them, encourage them to find the answer through Internet, and consult relevant experts to solve the problems, through which the students can develop their self-learning ability. Through the group discussion and academic exchange, the students can deepen the understanding of the current issues and share the information obtained by the different perspectives clash, supplement, and modification, which can train both their "collaborative learning" capability and their teamwork spirits, thus improving their comprehensive quality.

As the teacher, they must have the necessary professional knowledge, change the traditional image of authority, focus on the organization and guidance in the learning process, and rethink, study and improve their own teaching practice to enhance their ability and quality. Neurology, as an important part of clinical medicine, is a subject with a strong practicality, and the knowledge of it is abstract and difficult to understand, so that the students' initiative should be given full play in the teaching process to achieve the desired goal of teaching. For the students, if they can combine the problems to learn by thinking and discussing them, their initiatives and thinking abilities can be greatly stimulated (Eshach H. et al., 2003; Dochy F. et al., 2003; Ehrenberg Ac & Haggblom M, 2007). With PBL teaching method, an effective integration of clinical practice and basic medical knowledge can be achieved, so that this teaching method is considered to be a bridge link between the theory and the practice (Lycke KH et al., 2006) to help the students understand diseases well, broaden the students' horizons and open up a new path for the training of more qualified medical personnel.

Table 1. Comparison on the results of theoretical examination between the two groups (points, X ± s)

Groups	n	Results
PBL	30	92.5 ± 6.5
Traditional teaching	30	80.2 ± 5.3

REFERENCES

Chen Ning, Zhang Qinglin. (2006) Implementation of problem-based learning and challenge of it to teachers [J].*Basic Education Research,*1(1):27–29.

Dochy F, Segers M, Van den Bossche P, et al .(2003)Effects of problem-based learning: am eta ana lysis[J]. *Learn Instruct,* 13: 533.

Ehrenberg Ac, Haggblom M. (2007)Problem-based learning in clinical education: integrating theory and practice [J]. *Nurse Edu Pract,* (2): 67.

Eshach H, B itterm an H. (2003)From case based reasoning to problem-based learning[J]. *A cad Med,*78(5): 4916.

Li Hongwei, Liu Liyi, Zheng Yu, et al. (2008) Application of PBL teaching in the teaching of coronary heart diseases[J]. *Journal of Clinical and Experimental Medicine,* 7 (8): 196–197.

Liu Zhongxiu. (2008)Discussion on the application PBL teaching model in medical education[J]. *China High Medical Education.* 1 (1) 1–2.

Lycke KH, Grttum P, Strms HI.(2006) Student learning strategies, mental models and learning outcomes in problem-based and traditional curricula in medicine [J]. *Med Teach,* 28(8): 717–22.

Norman GR, Schmidt HC. (2000) The effect of the PBL courses [J]. *Medical Education,* 34 (9) : 721–728.

Yang Di, Qiu Lihong, Li Zimu, Wang Xuemei. (2008) Application and reflection of PBL teaching model in oral medicine [J].*China High Medical Education,* (12);117–118.

Yu Zhengmiao, Chen Jing. (2005) Problems PBL teaching in single courses[J]. *Journal of Shanxi Medical University(Preclinical Medical Education Edition),* 7 (5): 501–503.

Medicine Sciences and Bioengineering – Wang (Ed.)
© *2015 Taylor & Francis Group, London, ISBN: 978-1-138-02684-1*

Neuroprotective effects of Breviscapine against oxidative-stress-induced cell death in PC12 cells:Involvement of Nrf2/HO-1 pathway

Gui-lan Jin
China Three Gorges University people's Hospital & Yichang First People's Hospital, Yichang, China

Hui-lin Qin, Hai-bo He*, Fan Cheng & Da-chun Gong
Biological and Pharmaceutical College of China Three Gorges University, Yichang, China

Bang Xu, Liang-liang Jia & Wei Xi
China Three Gorges University people's Hospital & Yichang First People's Hospital, Yichang, China

Hong-wu Wang
Tongji Hospital of Huazhong University of Science and Technology, Wuhan, China

Xiang-fei Xing
China Three Gorges University people's Hospital & Yichang First People's Hospital, Yichang, China

ABSTRACT: The present study was designed to explore the protective effects of Breviscapine (Bre) against 6-hydroxydopamine (6-OHDA)-induced neurotoxicity with cultured PC12 cells and the possible mechanisms involved. The PC12 cells were cultured and exposed to 6-OHDA in the absence or presence of Bre. Its neuroprotective effects in PC12 cells were evaluated by cell viablity, ROS, LDH release assay, intracellular antioxidant enzyme and caspase activities, Nrf2), HO-1 and Bcl-2 family expressions. In the study, we found that Bre might significantly inhibit 6-OHDA-induced oxidative stress in PC12 cells, as indicated by its ability to increase cell viability and inhibit LDH release. The effectiveness of Bre against 6-OHDA-induced oxidative stress may due to restore the intracellular antioxidant defense, thereby reduce ROS production, prevent the development of apoptosis through activating the Nrf2/HO-1 pathways, and reverseing the abnormal expression of Bcl-2 family and caspase, and then alleviating 6-OHDA-induced PC12 cell injury and cell death.

1 INTRODUCTION

Breviscapine (Bre) is the flavonoid constituent isolated from a traditional Chinese herb *Erigerin breviscapus* (Vant.) Hand-Mazz, which contains two main flavonoids: scutellarin-7-O-glucuronide and a small amount of apigenin-7-O-glucuronide, the former makes up more than 90% of the extract and the latter is only about 4% of the extract. Bre has several commercially produced preparations like tablets and injections available in the market and has been extensively used in the clinic to treat acute cerebral infarction and paralysis induced by cerebrovascular diseases (Liu *et al.*, 2014). Our previous studies and literatures had demonstrated that Bre had protective effects for cerebral injury (Guo *et al.*, 2014). However, the underlying mechanisms remain poorly understood especially for antioxidant and apoptosis. Recent evidence has showed that nuclear factor erythroid 2-related factor 2 (Nrf2)/heme oxygenase-1(HO-1) pathway is considered as a new therapeutic target for the treatment of many oxidative stress-associated diseases such as cerebrovascular disease. Therefore, the purpose of the present study was to investigate the

---

* Correspondence to: Hai-bo He, Biological and Pharmaceutical College of China Three Gorges University, University Avenue, Yichang, China. E-mail: hjy219@126.com

effects of Bre on 6-hydroxydopamine (6-OHDA)-induced cell death and to explore the roles of the Nrf2/HO-1 pathways in PC12 cells.

2 MATERIALS AND METHODS

Drugs and Reagents Bre injection was provided by Longjin pharmaceutical Co. Ltd. (China). 6-OHDA, dimethyl sulfoxide (DMSO) and 2′,7′-dichlorodihydrofluo- rescein diacetate (DCFH-DA) were purchased from Sigma-Aldrich (USA). Lactate dehydrogenase (LDH), superoxide dismutase (SOD), Glutathione peroxidase (GSH-Px) and malondialdehyde (MDA) were purchased from Nanjing Jianchen Bioengineering Institute (China). Caspase activity assay kit was purchased from Millipore (USA). RNA PCR kit was obtained from TaKaRa (Japan). Antibodies to Nrf2, HO-1 and β-actin were obtained from Santa Cruz Biotechnology (USA). All other reagents and solvents were of analytical grade.

Cell culture and drug treatment PC12 cells were purchased from the Center of Basic Medical Cell of Chinese Institute of Basic Medical Sciences (China), and was cultured as previously described (Wang *et al.*, 2014). In the study, cells were pretreated with various concentrations of Bre for 2 h without other description, and followed by treatment of 6-OHDA (200μM) for 24 h. Control group was treated with 0.1% DMSO.

MTT assay and LDH release assay The cell viability was determined by MTT assay, and the release of LDH in the culture medium was measured according to the directions of the reagent kit.

Intracellular ROS measurement The intracellular ROS content was determined by oxidative conversion of cell-permeable DCFH-DA to fluorescent dichlorofluorescein (DCF) according to literature report (Wang *et al.*, 2014).

Intracellular antioxidant assay After different treatments, whole-cell lysate was prepared according to manufacturer's instructions, and the contents of GSH-Px, SOD and MDA were examined according to the directions of the reagent kits.

Caspase-3 and Caspase-9 activities measurement Treated PC12 cells were resuspended in 500 μL of cell lysis buffer, and then centrifugated, the supernatant was collected. Caspase-3 and caspase-9 activities were determined by the caspase activity assay kits (USA).

Bcl-2 and Bax mRNA expression analysis by real-time PCR Total RNA was extracted from the PC12 cells using Trizol Reagent according to manufacturer instructions. Real-time PCR for cardiomyocyte Bcl-2, Bax and HO-1 were undertaken as described previously description (Wang *et al.*, 2014).

Western Blotting Total protein and nuclear protein of ischemic cortex were extracted using Protein Extraction Kits (USA) following the manufacturer's protocol. Nrf2 western blotting analysis was performed as previously described (Wang *et al.*, 2014).

Statistical analyses Data were expressed as mean±standard deviation (SD), and differences among groups were analyzed by one-way analysis of variance (ANOVA). Resulting P values of less than 0.05 was regarded as statistically significant.

3 RESULTS AND DISCUSSION

Effects of Bre on cell viability of PC12 cells Our results showed that Bre (12.5~200 μg/mL) alone exhibited no apparent cytotoxicity. Next, the protective effects of Bre on 6-OHDA-induced PC12 cell were examined. In the 6-OHDA alneo group, the survival was only $43.33 \pm 2.10\%$ of cells compared with control group, pretreatment with Bre (12.5, 25 and 50 μg/mL) significantly increased cell viability to $50.67 \pm 2.91\%$, $57.07 \pm 3.36\%$ and $71.23 \pm 1.99\%$ that of the control ($P < 0.05$, $P < 0.01$, respectively).

Effects of Bre on LDH release Usually, cytosolic enzyme of LDH, which serve as the diagnostic markers of cerebrovascular injury, releases into the cell culture following damage of membrane integrity. So, its release is the main indicators of the extent of cerebrovascular injury (Wang *et al.*, 20014). In the study, the results showed 6-OHDA alone induced significantly LDH release, and was markedly reversed by Bre ($P < 0.05$, $P < 0.01$, respectively) (Table 1).

Effects of Bre on intracellular ROS content Increasing evidence suggests a critical role of oxidative stress in cerebrovascular disease. elevated reactive oxygen species (ROS) produced in cerebral ischemia could directly disrupt the structures of lipids, proteins and DNA, and induce cell death in various ways. Accordingly, cleaveing excess of ROS is an important means for the prevention and treatment of cerebrovascular disease. In the present study, exposure of the cells to 6-OHDA increased intracellular ROS generation to $256.12 \pm 7.46\%$ of the control, but this was significantly reduced to $167.97 \pm 8.06\%$, $143.17 \pm 4.78\%$ and $107.67 \pm 6.30\%$ of the control by Bre ($P < 0.05$, $P < 0.01$, respectively) (Figure 1).

Effects of Bre on intracellular antioxidant enzyme activity Under physiological conditions, intracellular ROS levels are tightly controlled by a sophisticated cellular antioxidant system, including SOD and enzymes of the GSH-dependent families. Our present study indicated that SOD, GSH-Px activities of whole-cell lysate remarkably decreased, MDA content significantly increased in the 6-OHDA group compared with the control group ($P < 0.01$, respectively). These aforementioned abnormal changes might significantly be reversed by Bre ($P < 0.05$, $P < 0.01$, respectively) (Table 1).

Effects of Bre on Nrf2/HO-1 pathways It is clear that Nrf2 is an attractive target for prevention of cerebrovascular disease and neurodegeneration induced by multifaceted response. When oxidative stress is increased, Nrf2 is released from Keap1 and quickly translocated to the nucleus, and results in transcriptional activation of antioxidant genes such as HO-1 and so forth (Wang *et al.*, 2014). In the study, we found that breviscapine activated the Nrf2 pathway and induced Nrf2 nuclear translocation, increased the level of HO-1, which suggested that the Nrf2/HO-1 pathway might be involved in the antioxidative capability of Bre (Table2, Figure 2).

Table 1.   Effects of Bre LDH release and intracellular antioxidant enzyme activity

Group	LDH (% of control)	GSH-Px(mU/mg)	SOD (U/mg)	MDA (nmol/mg)
Control	6.40 ± 1.45	150.2 ± 7.6	15.22 ± 0.99	6.02 ± 0.12
6-OHDA	$52.23 \pm 0.57^{\#\#}$	$79.8 \pm 6.2^{\#\#}$	$5.61 \pm 0.55^{\#\#}$	$22.04 \pm 2.50^{\#\#}$
Bre (12.5 μg/mL)	$41.78 \pm 4.63^{*}$	$97.0 \pm 2.1^{**}$	$6.78 \pm 0.41^{*}$	$16.99 \pm 0.47^{*}$
Bre (25 μg/mL)	$32.13 \pm 2.91^{**}$	$112.7 \pm 2.7^{**}$	$8.46 \pm 0.83^{**}$	$15.07 \pm 0.40^{**}$
Bre (50 μg/mL)	$25.64 \pm 1.67^{**}$	$121.0 \pm 3.3^{**}$	$10.71 \pm 0.76^{**}$	$11.06 \pm 0.61^{**}$

Note: Data are shown as the mean $\pm$ SD ($n = 5$). $^{\#\#}P < 0.01$ compared with control group; $^{*}P < 0.05$, $^{**}P < 0.01$ compared with 6-OHDA group.

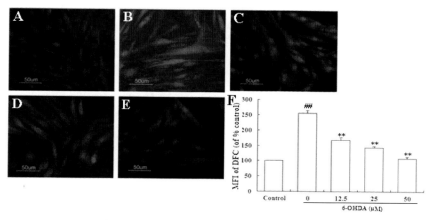

Figure 1.   Effect of Bre on ROS concentration. (A) Control group; (B) 6-OHDA group; (C-E) Bre (12.5, 25 and 50 μg/mL); (F) Quantitative analysis of the mean fluorescence intensity (MFI) of DCF. Data are shown as the mean $\pm$ SD ($n = 5$). $^{\#\#}P < 0.01$ compared with the control group; $^{**}P < 0.01$ compared with the 6-OHDA group.

Table 2. Effects of Bre on Bcl-2 family mRNA levels and caspase activity

Group	HO-1/ β-actin	Bcl-2/ β-actin	Bax/ β-actin	Bcl-2/ Bax ratio	Caspase-3 (nm/μgpro)	Caspase-9 (nm/μgpro)
Control	0.41 ± 0.02	1.72 ± 0.13	0.45 ± 0.08	3.91 ± 0.55	524.4 ± 77.1	401.7 ± 43.2
6-OHDA	$0.47 \pm 0.03^{\#\#}$	$0.81 \pm 0.19^{\#\#}$	$1.22 \pm 0.09^{\#\#}$	$0.66 \pm 0.13^{\#\#}$	$1236.8 \pm 105.5^{\#\#}$	$820.4 \pm 38.4^{\#\#}$
Bre (12.5μg/mL)	$0.58 \pm 0.04^{*}$	$1.28 \pm 0.17^{*}$	$0.88 \pm 0.13^{*}$	$1.46 \pm 0.04^{**}$	$970.4 \pm 113.5^{*}$	$722.9 \pm 44.3^{*}$
Bre (25.0μg/mL)	$0.63 \pm 0.03^{**}$	$1.46 \pm 0.11^{**}$	$0.74 \pm 0.11^{**}$	$2.02 \pm 0.39^{**}$	$836.7 \pm 99.8^{**}$	$614.1 \pm 67.5^{**}$
Bre (50.0μg/mL)	$0.70 \pm 0.04^{**}$	$1.55 \pm 0.12^{**}$	$0.64 \pm 0.12^{**}$	$2.47 \pm 0.27^{**}$	$819.4 \pm 94.6^{**}$	$548.1 \pm 71.6^{**}$

Note: Data are shown as the mean $\pm$ SD ($n = 4$). $^{\#}P < 0.05$, $^{\#\#}P < 0.01$ compared with control group; $^{*}P < 0.05$, $^{**}P < 0.01$ compared with 6-OHDA group.

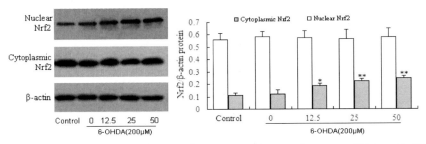

Figure 2. Effects of Bre on Nrf2 protein expresion. Data are shown as the mean $\pm$ SD ($n = 4$). $^{*}P < 0.05$, $^{**}P < 0.01$ compared with the 6-OHDA group.

Effects of Bre on Bcl-2 family mRNA levels It is well known that the balance in mitochondrial homeostasis is tightly regulated by the equilibrium between anti-apoptotic Bcl-2 and pro-apoptotic Bax. Bax and Bcl-2 determine whether a cell survives or undergoes apoptosis (Wang *et al.*, 2014). Our results showed that the mRNA expression of Bcl-2 was significantly reduced in the 6-OHDA group, whereas the mRNA expression of Bax was increased compared with that in the control group ($P<0.01$). As a result, Bcl-2/Bax ratio remarkably decreased ($P < 0.01$). By contrast, Bre might significantly increase Bcl-2 expression and decreased Bax expression ($P < 0.05$, $P < 0.01$, respectively), thus elevating Bcl-2/Bax ratio (Table 2).

Effect of Bre on caspase-3 and caspase-9 levels Several studies show that that activated caspase-3 and caspase-9 were considered to be a hallmark of apoptosis process. To verify this, we analyzed caspase-3 and caspase-9 activities. As Table 2 indicated, the caspase-3 and capase-9 activities of the 6-OHDA group were significantly increased compared with the control group ($P < 0.01$). Bre resulted in a significant reduction compared with the 6-OHDA group ($P < 0.05$, $P < 0.01$, respectively).

4 CONCLUSIONS

In this study, our study indicated that Bre inhibited 6-OHDA-induced oxidative stress in PC12 cells, as indicated by its ability to increase cell viability and inhibit LDH release. The effectiveness of Bre against 6-OHDA-induced oxidative stress may due to restore the intracellular antioxidant defense, thereby reduce ROS production, and prevent the development of apoptosis through activating the Nrf2/HO-1 pathways, and reverseing the abnormal expression of Bcl-2 family and caspase, and then alleviating 6-OHDA-induced PC12 cell injury and cell death.

ACKNOWLEDGEMENT

This study was supported by the Natural Science Fund Project of Hubei province (No: 2012FFB03705).

REFERENCES

Liu, Z. Okeke, C.I. Zhang, L. Zhao, H. Li, J. Aggrey, M.O. Li, N. Guo, X. Pang, X. Fan, L. Guo.L (2014). Mixed polyethylene glycol-modified breviscapine-loaded solid lipid nanoparticles for improved brain bio-availability: preparation, characterization, and in vivo cerebral microdialysis evaluation in adult Sprague Dawley rats. AAPS PharmSciTech.15(2): 483–496.

Guo, C. Zhu, Y. Weng, Y. Wang, S. Guan, Y. Wei, G. Yin, Y. Xi, M. Wen, A. (2014). Therapeutic time window and underlying therapeutic mechanism of breviscapine injection against cerebral ischemia/reperfusion injury in rats. J Ethnopharmacol. 151 (1): 660–666.

Wang, L. Wang, R. Jin, M. J. Huang, Y. J. Liu, A.M. Qin, J. Chen, M.H. Wen, S.J. Pi, R.B. Shen,W (2014). Carvedilol attenuates 6-hydroxydopamine-induced cell death in PC12 cells: involvement of akt and Nrf2/ARE pathways. Neurochem Res. DOI 10.1007/s11064-014- 1367–2.

Medicine Sciences and Bioengineering – Wang (Ed.)
© 2015 Taylor & Francis Group, London, ISBN: 978-1-138-02684-1

Oxidative stress injury caused by 1800-MHz electromagnetic radiation

Huan Liu, Ming-lian Wang*, Ru-gang Zhong, Xue-mei Ma, Qiao-li Liu, Yan Li, Fei Xie & Qing-xia Hou
College of Life Sciences and Bioengineering, Beijing University of Technology, Beijing, China

ABSTRACT: Objective: To investigate the potential adverse effect of 1800-MHz intermittent Electromagnetic Fields (EMF). Method: Cells were exposed to 1800-MHz GSM signals in GSM-Talk mode (5 min on/10 min off) at a Specific Absorption Rates (SAR) of 4 W/kg for 2 h. ROS and MDA were detected every 20 min. A DCFH-DA fluorescence probe was used to detect ROS levels and thiobarbituric acid (TBA) was used to detect the MDA. Result: The ROS levels of the 20 min and 80 min exposure groups were significantly higher than respective sham groups. No difference was found of MDA in the experiment group except 120 min group. The MDA level of the 120 min exposure group was the highest. Conclusion: 1800-MHz EMF exposure at 4 W/kg could induce ROS-mediated oxidative stress injury.

1   INTRODUCTION

Nowadays, the worldwide use of mobile phones has rapidly increased. Public concern about the potential effects of mobile phone use has been growing. Radiofrequency electromagnetic fields (RF-EMF) emitted from cellular phones ranging from 800 to 2,000 MHz (Hardell L *et al.*, 2008; Health Protection Agency 2013) fall in the microwave spectrum. Several recent epidemiological studies have investigated the effects of RF-EMR from mobile phones on the organism (Hardell, L *et al.*, 2013; Aitken, R.J *et al.* 2005; Ahlers M.T *et al.* 2013; Lantow, M *et al.* 2006), but results to date have been contradictory and inconclusive.

The current guideline in Europe reports that microwave exposure from mobile phones is 2 W/kg for the brain. While using cell phones, some parts of tissue or some cells in the brain might be exposed to the radiation much higher than 2 W/kg. Several studies reported DNA damage at an intensity of lower than 4 W/kg (Lennart Hardel *et al.*, 2008). And the reactive oxygen species (ROS) could induce DNA damage. Oxidative stress is a state where increased formation of ROS overwhelms body antioxidant protection and subsequently induces DNA damage, lipid peroxidation, protein modification, and other effects. All the effects are the symptoms for numerous diseases including cancer, cardiovascular disease, etc. Lipid peroxidation leads to the formation of MDA, which is worthwhile to note in many pathophysiological processes. The by-products of lipid peroxidation could mediate, at least in part, many chronic diseases involving oxidative stress (Manjeet Singh *et al.*, 2010). The reduction of lipid peroxidation or the regulation of different pathways activated by downstream products of lipid peroxidation could be a potential alarm in preventing or decelerating disease progression (Pamela D *et al.*, 2010).

---

*Minglian Wang is the corresponding author for the study (E-mail: mlw@bjut.edu.cn).

2 MATERIALS AND METHODS

2.1 Cell culture

The mouse epidermic cell line (JB6-C41) were diluted with 10 mL of RPMI 1640 culture medium (Gibco, USA), supplemented with 10% fetal bovine serum (FBS; Gibco, USA) and 1% strepto-mycin and penicillin (Gibco, USA). Cells were incubated at 37°C in a 5% CO_2 incubator (Thermo Scientific, USA), and cells grown to 75–85% confluence were washed with phosphate buffer saline (PBS), trypsinized with 0.5 mL of 0.25% (v) trypsin (Gibco, USA), diluted with fresh medium, and counted using a hemacytometer before seeding into 35-mm culture dishes (Thermo NUNC, USA).

2.2 Exposure procedure

At 24 h after cell seeding, the cells were subjected to an exposure to 1800-MHz GSM-Talk signals with an intermittent cycle of 5 min on/10 min off for 2 h. An sXc-1800-MHz exposure system (IT'IS, Zurich, Switzerland) was used. To explore the role of oxidative stress in RF-EMR-induced effects, the following groups were examined: (1) RF exposure; (2) sham exposure, the presence or absence of the electromagnetic field was the only difference. After exposure, cells were simulta-neously subjected to the measurement of ROS and MDA every 20 minutes. Cells were washed in phosphate-buffered saline solution (PBS) twice. The pellet was resuspended in PBS for the ROS or fixed with the lysis buffer for MDA detection (see below).

2.3 ROS detection

ROS were measured with the 2′,7′-dichlorofluorescein diacetate (DCFH-DA) (Beyotime Company, China). After exposure to RF-EMR, the culture medium was removed and cells were washed with PBS, then incubated to 10 μM DCFH-DA for 30 min. After incubation, the cells were detached by trypsin and washed with PBS three times, and finally, the cells were resuspended in 300 μL PBS and analyzed using flow cytometry (Merck Millipore, Germany) for fluorescence. The increase in sample's fluorescence values relative to control fluorescence values was regarded as representative of the increase in intracellular ROS.

2.4 MDA detection

All samples were collected into 15 mL tubes and centrifuged at 1600 rpm for 10 min. The cell pel-lets were resuspended with ice-cold lysis buffer. 200 μL aliquot of the sample was assayed for MDA according to the lipid peroxidation assay kit protocol (Beyotime Company, China). Cells were homog-enized in ice-cold lysis buffer and centrifuged. The resulting supernatant was mixed with trichloro-acetic acid (TBA) and 100°C heated for 15 min. The lysate was cooled and centrifuged to remove the flocculent precipitate. The absorbance of the sample was monitored at 570 nm with 1420 Multilabel Counter (Perkin Elmer, USA), and the concentration of MDA was determined from a standard curve.

2.5 Data analyses

The results were analyzed using the SPSS17.0 program (SPSS). The data were analyzed for statistical significance between the control and experimental groups with an analysis of variance (one-way ANOVA) and paired t test, p-Values < 0.05 were considered statistically significant.

3 RESULTS

The statistical data of intracellular ROS and the data of endogenous MDA are shown in Table 1 and Table 2, respectively. As the results showed that the level of ROS in the exposed groups are higher than sham groups, the 80 min exposure group is the highest, and it increased at 20 min and 80 min significantly ($p < 0.05$) (Figure 1). In the EMF-exposed groups, the MDA level of 120 min exposure group reached the highest. And compared with the sham groups, there were no distinctions in MDA levels except the 120 min group ($p < 0.05$) (Figure 2).

4 DISCUSSION

The data showed that exposure to 1800-MHz EMF for different times promotes ROS and MDA increase in the cells. Hou has come to the conclusion that a significant increase in intracellular ROS levels after EMR exposure and it reached the highest level at an exposure time of 1 h(Qingxia Hou, 2014), we have slightly different with her maybe because the different of cells. The increases of MDA can most likely be ascribed to an excessive production of ROS, which could be related to antioxidant enzyme leakage (Sudheesh, N. P. et al., 2013).

Table 1. The ROS level for the control and experimental groups ($\bar{x} \pm 2S_E$).

Time	20 min*	40 min	60 min	80 min*	100 min	120 min
Exposure	18.3 ± 3.0	25.7 ± 4.6	25.3 ± 5.5	26.1 ± 6.6	21.4 ± 4.6	27.3 ± 9.0
Sham	14.5 ± 3.7	23.1 ± 4.7	21.5 ± 5.2	19.2 ± 3.1	18.4 ± 4.6	23.2 ± 7.3

*$p < 0.05$

Table 2. The MDA level for the control and experimental groups ($\bar{x} \pm 2S_E$).

Time	20 min	40 min	60 min	80 min	100 min	120 min*
Exposure	20.0 ± 1.9	17.9 ± 1.2	17.9 ± 1.0	22.6 ± 3.1	17.8 ± 2.1	40.8 ± 11.6
Sham	18.3 ± 1.1	18.4 ± 1.6	18.3 ± 1.0	23.0 ± 3.1	19.7 ± 1.3	20.9 ± 3.4

*$p < 0.05$

There are multiple defenses against the ubiquitous MDA adducts, for example, complement factor H (CFH), which is an innate defense protein against MDA (Charbel Issa et al., 2011). MDA is a major ligand for CFH on apoptotic/necrotic cells. MDA binding on CFH demonstrates that the organism could resident the oxidation-specific injuries. So we can infer that the level of MDA did not escalate until 120 min, whereas ROS escalated immediately at 20 min due to the contribution of the defense mechanisms.

EMF exposure induced ROS-mediated oxidative stress injury. We can infer that DNA base damage with no detectable DNA strand breakage occurs subsequently. Further research will be required to understand the long-term effects of mobile phone use.

ACKNOWLEDGMENTS

This work was funded by the grants from Beijing Municipal Education Commission Science and Technology Project (KM201310005029) and National Key Basic Research Project (2011CB503705).

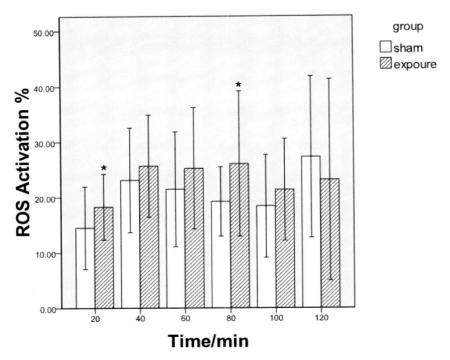

Figure 1.   Intracellular ROS in JB6-C41 cells after exposure to an 1800-MHz EMR.

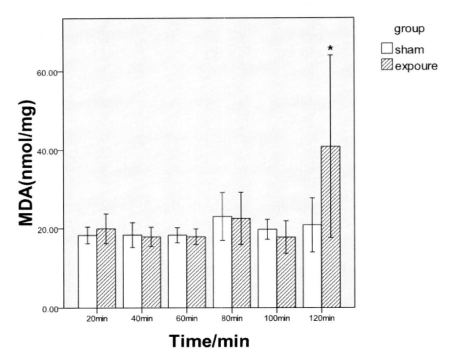

Figure 2.   Endogenous MDA data in JB6-C41 cells after exposure to an 1800-MHz EMR.

REFERENCES

Aitken, R.J., Bennetts, L.E., Sawyer, D., et al. (2005). Impact of radio frequency electromagnetic radiation on DNA integrity in the male germline. Int J Androl 28:171–9.

Ahlers M.T., Ammermüller, J. (2013). No influence of acute RF exposure (GSM-900, GSM-1800, and UMTS) on mouse retinal ganglion cell responses under constant temperature conditions. Bioelectromagnetics, doi: 10.1002/bem.21811. [Epub ahead of print].

Charbel Issa, Marisol Cano, Hubert Brandstatter, Sotirios Tsimikas, Christine Skerka, Giulio Superti-Furga, James T. Handa, Peter F. Zipfe, Joseph L. Witztum3 & Christoph J. Binder. (2011) Complement factor H binds malondialdehyde epitopes and protects from oxidative stress. Nature 478:76–81

Hardell L, Sage C. (2008) Biological effects from electromagnetic field exposure and public exposure standards. Biomed Pharmacother, 62: 104–109.

Health Protection Agency. (2013)Radiation: Mobile telephony and health background information. [Online] Available from: http://www.hpa.org.uk/webw/HPAweb&HPAwebStandard/HPAweb_C52558? p115893460778.

Hardell, L., Carlberg, M., Söderqvist, F., et al. (2013) Pooled analysis of case-control studies on acoustic neuroma diagnosed 1997–2003 and 2007–2009 and use of mobile and cordless phones. Int J Oncol.43:1036–1044.

Kumar S. (2004) Occupational exposure associated with reproductive dysfunction. J Occup Health; 46:1–19.

Lantow, M., Lupke, M., Frahm, J.,et al. (2006a). ROS release and Hsp70 expression after exposure to 1,800 MHz radiofrequency electromagnetic fields in primary human monocytes and lymphocytes. Radiat Environ Biophys 45: 55–62.

Lennart Hardell, Cindy Sage. (2008) Biological effects from electromagnetic field exposure and public exposure standards. Biomedicine & Pharmacotherapy 62: 104–109.

Meltz ML. (2003)Radiofrequency exposure and mammalian cell toxicity, genotoxicity, and transformation. Bioelectromagnetics ; 24:S196–213.

Manjeet Singh, Dang Thanh Nam, Madeleine Arseneault and Charles Ramassamy. (2010) Role of ByProducts of Lipid Oxidation in Alzheimer's Disease Brain: A Focus on Acrolein. Journal of Alzheimer's Disease 21: 741–756

Pamela D. Moore, Clement G. Yedjou, Paul B. Tchounwou. (2010) Malathion-Induced Oxidative Stress, Cytotoxicity, and Genotoxicity in Human Liver Carcinoma (HepG2) Cells.Toxicol 25: 221–226.

Qingxia Hou, Minglian Wang, Shuicai Wu, Xuemei Ma, Guangzhou An, Huan Liu, and Fei Xie, (2014) Oxidative changes and apoptosis induced by 1800-MHz electromagnetic radiation in NIH/3T3 cells. Electromagnetic Biology and Medicine Posted online 1–8.

Seung-Kwon Myung, Woong Ju, Diana D. McDonnell, Yeon Ji Lee, Gene Kazinets, Chih-Tao Cheng, and Joel M. Moskowitz. (2009) Mobile Phone Use and Risk of Tumors: A Meta-Analysis. American Society of Clinical Oncology. 27:5565–5572.

Sheiner EK, Sheiner E, Hammel RD, Potashnik G, Carel R. (2003) Effect of occupational exposures on male fertility: literature review. Ind Health. 41:55–62.

Sudheesh, N. P.; Ajith, T. A.; Janardhanan, K. K.(2013)Hepatoprotective effects of DL-alpha-lipoic acid and alpha-Tocopherol through amelioration of the mitochondrial oxidative stress in acetaminophen challenged rats. TOXICOLOGY MECHANISMS AND METHODS. 23: 368–376.

Medicine Sciences and Bioengineering – Wang (Ed.)
© *2015 Taylor & Francis Group, London, ISBN: 978-1-138-02684-1*

Clinical analysis of Baoxinbao film for elderly patients with unstable angina pectoris

Li-juan Guo

Jilin Beihua University hospital, Jilin, Jilin, China

ABSTRACT: The purpose is to observe the clinical curative effect of Baoxinbao film for elderly patients with unstable angina pectoris and to carry on the analysis. The method is that 161 patients with unstable angina were randomly divided into treatment group and control group, in which 105 cases belong to the treatment group and 56 cases belong to the control group. Two groups are given conventional treatment, including nitrates, aspirin, beta blockers, calcium channel blockers, angiotensin-converting enzyme inhibitors or angiotensin II receptor blockers, and so on. Based on the above treatment, the treatment group is added with Baoxinbao film, which is added one for every 4 days but two for the first time. Treatment course for the two groups is 20 days. After treatment, angina pectoris clinical symptoms relieved, electrocardiogram improved, and blood rheology indexes in the treatment group raised than those in the control group ($P < 0.05$). The curative effect of Baoxinbao film for the treatment of unstable angina pectoris is good and no obvious side effects observed.

1 OBJECT AND METHOD

1.1 Object

From September 2006 to September 2007, selected 161 cases of elderly patients with coronary artery disease are in line with the "diagnostic criteria of diagnosis and treatment of unstable angina pectoris," (The Chinese Medical Association cardiovascular Association, 2002) including 82 male cases and 79 female cases. The treatment group includes cases with ages 40–70 year old, average 60 ± 6 years old; 26 with hypertension; 14 with diabetes; and 28 with hyperlipidemia. One-hundred and sixty-one patients were randomly divided into two groups, where treatment group comprised 105 cases and control group comprised 56 cases; the two groups in age, gender, comorbidity, symptoms, ECG, and blood rheology indexes were not significantly different ($P < 0.05$).

1.2 Treatment method

Two groups of patients are given conventional treatment, including oxygen, bed rest, low salt, low-fat diet (diabetic patients were given diabetic diet), drugs including nitrates, aspirin, beta blockers, calcium channel blockers, angiotensin-converting enzyme inhibitors, angiotensin II receptor blockers. The treatment group is added with Baoxinbao film on the basis of basic treatment (Beijing Huaheng Hanfang Pharmaceutical Co Ltd provides), in the area before the heart, once every 4 days, twice for the first time, and the two groups were treated for 20 days to assess the curative effect.

1.3 Curative effect evaluation

Curative effect evaluation is according to the "guidelines for clinical research on new drugs of TCM (The Ministry of health of the People's Republic of China, 1993)." Angina pectoris curative effect judgment standard: significant reduction in angina attacks and nitroglycerin consumption reduced by more than 80%; effective: reduction in angina attacks and nitroglycerin consumption reduced by more than 50–79%; reduce the number of invalid: angina and nitroglycerin consumption less than 50%. Electrocardiogram curative effect judgment standard: excellence: resting ECG returned to normal or nearly normal; effective: resting ECG ST segment recovery above 0.05 mV, or the main lead T-wave inversion of shallow ≥50% or T waves by a flat to erect. Invalid: changes before and after treatment without resting electrocardiogram.

1.4 Statistical methods

Measurement data with the X + S, the data of the two groups are compared with t test.

2 RESULTS

After treatment, clinical symptoms of angina pectoris relieved and ECG improved than those in the control group (shown in Table 1, Table 2), and a significant difference is noted (P < 0.05). The indexes of blood rheology in treatment group is superior to the control group (shown in Table 3), and the difference is significant.

Table 1. Comparison of coronary heart disease in two groups with angina pectoris [cases (%)].

Groups	Number of cases	Markedly effective	Effective	Ineffective	Overall efficiency
Treatment group	105	58 (55.24)	37 (35.24)	10 (9.52)	95 (90.48)
Control group	56	20 (35.71)	25 (44.64)	11 (19.64)	45 (80.36)

Note: Comparison of curative effect of two groups of Ridit, $u = 2.3237$, $P < 0.05$. There is an improving rate of angina pectoris in the treatment group than the control group.

Table 2. Comparison of ECG improvement in two groups [cases (%)].

Groups	Number of cases	Markedly effective	Effective	Ineffective	Overall efficiency
Treatment group	105	26 (24.76)	44 (41.91)	35 (33.33)	70 (66.67)
Control group	56	8 (14.29)	23 (41.07)	25 (44.64)	31 (55.36)

Note: After treatment, total ECG effective was for 70 cases (66.67%), and the control group was 31 cases (55.36%); compared with two groups curative effect analysis of Ridit, $u = 0.1622$, $P < 0.05$. The treatment group was better than control group.

Table 3. Blood flow changes before and after treatment in two groups (x ± S).

Groups	Number of cases		High-shear whole blood viscosity	Low-shear whole blood viscosity	Plasma viscosity	Hematocrit	Erythrocyte electrophoresis rate	Fibrinogen
Treatment group	57	Before	62.1 ± 1.83	9.06 ± 2.11	2.54 ± 0.67	45.16 ± 4.35	10.09 ± 1.24	482.96 ± 80.11
		After	4.09 ± 1.27	7.01 ± 1.52	1.91 ± 0.03	45.21 ± 3.20	0.88 ± 2.13	313.45 ± 99.63
			**ΔΔ	*Δ	*		**Δ	**Δ
Control group	50	Before	6.6 ± 1.60	9.36 ± 1.68	2.75 ± 0.44	46.07 ± 5.81	10.24 ± 1.32	504.28 ± 68.11
		After	5.69 ± 1.71	8.47 ± 1.24	2.15 ± 0.19	43.93 ± 0.19	11.01 ± 1.66	415.36 ± 83.24
			□	□	□	□	□	□

Note: □ The comparison between the two groups before treatment P < 0.05, *, ** The comparison before treatment P < 0.05, Δ, ΔΔ Compared with control group P < 0.05.

3 DISCUSSION

Refers to unstable angina pectoris and acute myocardial infarction and sudden cardiac death are among the clinical status, its pathological basis of atherosclerotic lesions in the original coronary arteries occurs on the basis of internal capsule hemorrhage, plaque rupture and damaged platelets and fibrin forms blood clots, coronary artery spasm, causing incomplete stenosis or occlusion of coronary artery based on block (Chen Haozhu, 2001).

The important factors like blood vessels, nerve, endocrine factors, and abnormal blood rheology also contribute to the occurrence of coronary heart disease unstable angina pectoris. In elderly patients, often hypertension, high blood sugar, blood lipid abnormalities, obesity, and other metabolic syndrome merge with coronary heart disease unstable angina pectoris. Increased vascular endothelial damage prompted the formation of thrombus, and causes coronary artery spasm and narrow, incomplete occlusion leads to myocardial microcirculation, tissue hypoperfusion ischemia, and hypoxia. It is often to expand blood vessels and anticoagulation as the main treatment method. Through the clinical observation, application of pericardium lamination treatment of elderly unstable angina pectoris, no matter in alleviating clinical symptoms, ECG ischemia change state, blood rheology indexes are significantly better than the control group.

Topical application of Baoxinbao film is the first treatment of cardiovascular disease, injury pathway through tissue penetration against inflammatory injury of myocardial ischemia, and ischemia reperfusion. Animal experiments and clinical trials have confirmed that Baoxinbao film with antiplatelet aggregation, decreasing blood viscosity role, can adjust the release of various vasoactive substances, dilating blood vessel, and improve the microcirculation; with inflammatory damage after hypoxia ischemia, the effective protection of vascular endothelial function in the role of the heart. The main pharmacological mechanisms of Baoxinbao film are as follows: inhibit macrophage production of prostaglandin E (PGE2) and thromboxane B2 (TXB2); inhibit vascular endothelial cell adhesion molecule-1 (ICAM-1) and could reduce the myocardial infarct size; improve ECG S-T segment to decrease the occurrence of abnormal rhythm of the heart; inhibit serum lactate dehydrogenase (LDH), creatine kinase (CPK), and malondialdehyde (MDA) increased; the hemodynamics test has certain protective effect on damaged diastolic and systolic function after myocardial ischemia.

In short, Baoxinbao film has better clinical value in elderly coronary heart disease unstable angina pectoris prevention. Even though it has small side effect, it is simple, safe, effective, and convenient to use.

REFERENCES

Chen Haozhu. (2001) *Practical Department of internal medicine*. 11nd edition. Beijing: People's Medical Publishing House. pp. 1376.
Shen Luhua. (2001) Strengthen the diagnosis and treatment of unstable angina pectoris. *China Medical Journal*, 39(11), 39.
The Chinese Medical Association cardiovascular Association. (2002) Diagnosis and treatment of unstable angina pectoris. *Chinese Journal of cardiovascular disease*, 28, 409.
The Ministry of health of the People's Republic of China (1991) Guidelines for new drug clinical medicine. 1nd edition. pp. 141.

Medicine Sciences and Bioengineering – Wang (Ed.)
© 2015 Taylor & Francis Group, London, ISBN: 978-1-138-02684-1

A preliminary study of high-pressure CO_2 on the crystal transformation of heat-sensitive drugs

De-dong Hu*
College of Electromechanical Engineering, Qingdao University of Science & Technology, Qingdao, China
State Key Laboratory of Generic Manufacture Technology of Chinese Traditional Medicine, LuNan Pharmaceutical Group, Linyi, China

Shou-zhong Zhang, Qi Wang, He Zhang & Wei-qiang Wang
College of Electromechanical Engineering, Qingdao University of Science & Technology, Qingdao, China

ABSTRACT: The research of the crystal structure of solid drug has great significance due to the influence of the crystal structure of solid drug on clinical efficacy, safety, and the drug quality stability. In this paper, spironolactone, atorvastatin calcium, orlistat, and dexibuprofen were treated using the high-pressure CO_2 and characterized by the X-ray diffractometer. The spec-trograms of XRD characterization show that the crystal structure of drugs have changed after being treated using the high pressure CO_2. The results indicate that it is feasible using the high-pressure CO_2 to transfer the crystal of heat-sensitive drugs.

1 INTRODUCTION

The traditional solid chemical drug crystal preparation methods such as solvent crystallization, melting method, and salting out method have great limitations in the preparation of drug crystal. Solvent crystallization method has a lot of requirements in operation condition with appropriate boiling point. Peng Ying et al (Y. Huang, Z.D. Song & F.Z. Liu, 2008) mentioned that crystal character is easy to change in the purification of stigmasterol process conditions using solvent crystallization method. Melting method is not applicable to the heat-sensitive drug (J. Huang, R.Y. Zhang & B. Wu, 2006). The biggest drawback of salting out method is mother liquor treating and the solvent and diluents separating (D.A. Roston, M.C. Walters & R.R. Rhinebarger, 1998).

Recently, the high-pressure CO_2 is applied in the transformation of drug crystal structure. The advantages of high-pressure CO_2, i.e., moderate physical property, security, no pollution and no residue after decompression, the easily controlled process parameters, and the simple technological process, ensure the stability of effective components and product quality (Y.G. Lei, 2008). Ruggero et al (R. Bettini, L. Bonassi & V. Castoro, 2001) successfully obtained pure stable crystalline phase of carbamazepine using high-pressure CO_2 to treat carbamazepine polymorphs.

The aim of this paper is indicating that the high-pressure CO_2 method is favorable to transfer the crystal of heat-sensitive drugs through investigating the crystal of spironolactone, atorvastatin calcium, orlistat, and dexibuprofen.

2 EXPERIMENTAL INSTRUMENTS AND MEDICINES

The experimental instruments: extraction experiment device type of CLJ-2*1L/320P (the highest extraction pressure: 30 MPa, single cylinder extraction volume: 1 L, the extraction temperature: the room temperature to 100°C, and maximum flow: 50 L/h), electronic balance (Model: FA2004B), and DMAX-2500PC X-ray diffractometer (XRD).

The experimental drug: spironolactone, atorvastatin calcium, orlistat, and dexibuprofen.

3 EXPERIMENTAL METHOD

3.1 *Method of dealing with drugs*

Weigh the required amount of untreated medicines, wrap it with a multilayer filter cloth, and then place into the processing vessel. Using high-pressure CO_2 process the drugs under 30 MPa, 288 K, and 20 L/h. After 5 h, remove the powdered medicine from the filter cloth wrapping, then allow to stand for some time for the sublimation of dry ice so that the collecting drugs can be saved.

3.2 *Detection method of drug crystal shape*

After preheating X-ray diffraction instrument for 20 to 30 minutes, start the XRD commands. Set the working conditions under KV = 40, MA = 100 and use copper target as the radiation source. Double-click the DIFFRACplus Measurement Part icon to open testing software, set the step size, scan time, scan range and other parameters in the appropriate column, and start to begin testing the X-ray detector to obtain diffraction patterns.

4 EXPERIMENTAL RESULTS AND DISCUSSION

The chromatogram analysis of the four drugs was shown in the Figures 1–8.

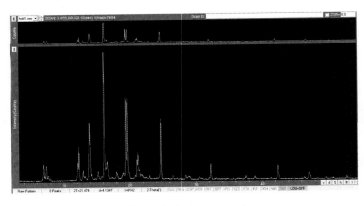

Figure 1.   Chromatogram analysis of dexibuprofen before processing.

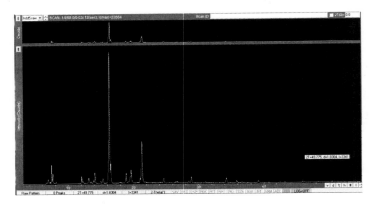

Figure 2.   Chromatogram analysis of dexibuprofen after processing.

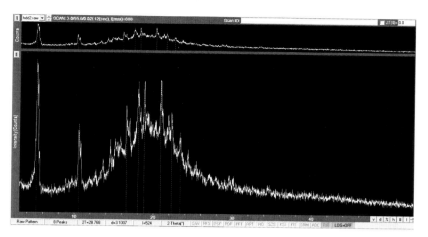

Figure 3.   Chromatogram analysis of orlistat before processing.

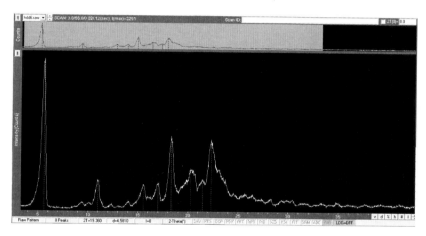

Figure 4.   Chromatogram analysis of orlistat after processing.

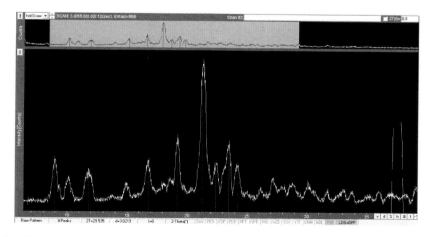

Figure 5.   Chromatogram analysis of atorvastatin calcium before processing.

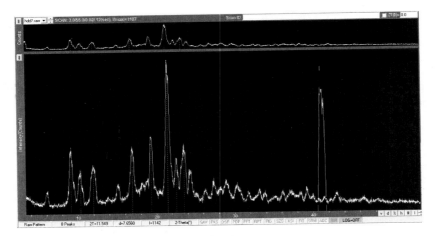

Figure 6.   Chromatogram analysis of atorvastatin calcium after processing.

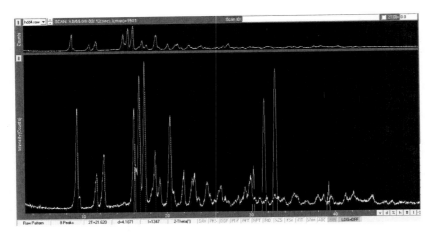

Figure 7.   Chromatogram analysis of spironolactone before processing.

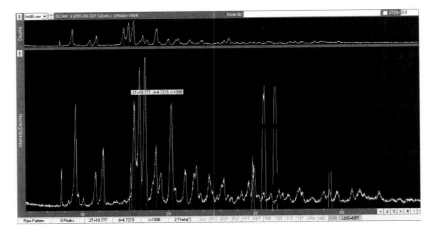

Figure 8.   Chromatogram analysis of spironolactone after processing.

The two theta angles of eight strong peaks located at 12.260°, 13.898°, 16.079°, 19.342°, 19.601°, 21.218°, 24.716°, and 32.257° before processing of dexibuprofen are shown in Figure 1. The two theta angles of eight strong peaks located at 7.406°, 7.622°, 12.060°, 14.080°, 16.339°, 18.880°, 19.623°, and 21.320° after processing of dexibuprofen are shown in Figure 2. The two theta angles of eight strong peaks located at 8.920°, 11.762°, 16.796°, 19.182°, 21.261°, 22.421°, 23.499°, and 24.221° before processing of atorvastatin calcium are shown in Figure 5. The two theta angles of eight strong peaks located at 9.100°, 10.280°, 11.920°, 16.881°, 19.282°, 21.440°, 22.541,° and 23.541° after processing of atorvastatin calcium are shown in Figure 6. By comparing the changes of the two theta angles between Figure 1 and Figure 2, and Figure 5 and Figure 6, it can be found that the positions of the eight strong peaks of dexibuprofen and atorvastatin calcium have greatly changed, indicating that there is a change in the crystal structures before and after processing.

The two theta angles of eight strong peakslocated at 5.144°, 10.519°, 16.541°, 18.020°, 18.784°, 20.811°, 22.240°, and 23.359° before processing of orlistat are shown in Figure 3. The two theta angles of eight strong peaks located at 5.599°, 10.980°, 15.540°, 17.021°, 18.301°, 20.221°, 21.479°, and 22.300° after processing of orlistat are shown in Figure 4. By comparing the changes of the two theta angles between Figure 3 and Figure 4, it can be found that the positions of the eight strong peaks of orlistat almost have no change. The peaks shown in Figure 3 are dispersion peaks with larger FWHM, whereas in Figure 4, the peaks transfer to sharp-pointed peaks with narrow FWHM. It could be concluded that the crystal structures have not changed, but the crystallinity of the drug has improved after processing.

The two theta angles of eight strong peaks located at 9.320°, 11.582°, 12.481°, 16.119°, 16.760°, 17.339°, 18.600°, and 20.439° before processing of spironolactone are shown in Figure 7. The two theta angles of eight strong peaks located at 7.641°, 9.318°, 12.518°, 16.100°, 16.759°, 17.398°, 18.581°, and 20.439° after processing of spironolactone are shown in Figure 8. From Figure 7 and Figure 8, it can be concluded the positions of the first two peaks have greatly changed, but another six peaks have no change. The chromatograms proved that a part of the crystal structure has changed, but it is unobvious.

5 CONCLUSION

From the above analyses and relevant data, it can be concluded that high-pressure CO_2 is a good method for the crystal transformation of heat-sensitive drugs.

ACKNOWLEDGMENTS

This research was financially supported by Science and Technology Project of Shandong Province Colleges and Universities (J13LM08) and Shandong Province Postdoctoral Innovation special funds (201203011).

REFERENCES

Bettini, R., Bonassi, L. & Castoro, V. (2001) Solubility and conversion of carbamazepine polymorphs in supercritical carbon dioxide. *Pharmaceutical Sciences*. [Online] 13, Available from: http://www.sciencedirect.com/science/article/pii/S0928098701001154 [Accessed 7th June 2014].
Huang, Y., Song, Z.D. & Liu, F.Z. (2008) Study on crystallization conditions for separation of stigmasterol. *Modern Chemical Industry*. [Online] 28 (2), Available from: http://www.cqvip.com/qk/95539x/2008s2/1000556381.html [Accessed 21th June 2014].
Huang, J., Zhang, R.Y. & Wu, B. (2006) Crystal forms transformation and thermal expansion property of polycrystalline Na2SO4/SiO2 composite phase-change energy storage materials. *Materials Engineering*. [Online] (12), Available from: http://d.wanfangdata.com.cn/Periodical_clgc200612004.aspx [Accessed 18th June 2014].

Lei, Y.G. (2008) Study on extract technique by the CO2 supercritical and subcritical fluid extraction and analysis components of star anise oil. *Guangxi University.* [academic dissertation], Available from: http://cdmd.cnki.com.cn/Article/CDMD-10593-2008135220.htm [Accessed 10th June 2014].

Roston, D.A., Walters, M.C. & Rhinebarger, R.R. (1998) Characterization of polymorphs of a new anti-inflammatory drug. *Journal of Pharmaceutical and Biomedical Analysis.* [Online] 16 (322), Available from: http://www.sciencedirect.com/science/article/pii/0731708593800202 [Accessed 16th June 2014].

Medicine Sciences and Bioengineering – Wang (Ed.)
© *2015 Taylor & Francis Group, London, ISBN: 978-1-138-02684-1*

Effect of external use of fresh aloe juice on the scald model of rats

Ming-san Miao & Lin Guo
Henan University of Traditional Chinese Medicine, Zhengzhou, Henan, China

ABSTRACT: Objective: To verify the external use of fresh aloe juice for the treatment of scald. Methods: To evaluate the scald, to observe pathological changes of scald skin tissue in rats, and to observe the effect of external use of fresh aloe juice for the treatment of scald. Results: Compared to the model group, for large, medium, and small doses of aloe juice group, scald area deviations between before and after treatment increased significantly, and all rats in the aloe juice group significantly improved the pathological changes of scald. Conclusion: Aloe juice has a good curative effect on scald.

1 INTRODUCTION

Aloe can be used as an astringent for sores, eliminates stasis to activate blood circulation, maintains hemostasis, and so on and from the records of "collection of Chinese herbal medicines" it is applied externally for the treatment of scald. Fresh aloe juice contains enzymes (Wang, 2013), which is rich in amino acids (Li, 2012) and has pharmacological effects on anti-inflammatory, antibacterial, and wound healing. This paper will report the use of fresh aloe juice for the treatment of scald and provide experimental basis for the clinical use of aloe.

2 MATERIALS

2.1 *Animal and instruments*

Whistar rats (certificate number: 804122) weighing 180–220 g, half male and half female, provided by medical experimental animal center of Hebei Province; electronic balance of FA (N)/JA(N) series (Shanghai Minqiao Precision Instrument Co., Ltd); HWS12 type electric thermostatic water bath (Shanghai Heng Scientific Instrument Co) were used in the experiment.

2.2 *Drugs and reagents*

Liliaceae aloe Kuraso (scientific name: Aloe barbadensis Mill.) purchased from Henan Zhang Zhongjing large pharmacy Co Ltd, identified by the teacher from the Department of Pharmacognosy of Henan Traditional Chinese Medicine University, was used for the experiment.

Fresh aloe juice preparation: clean the leaf of fresh aloe and cut into small pieces of 3 cm–5 cm. Pare off leaf thorn on both sides firstly with a ripped blade, scrape transparent collagen with a knife, and stir evenly to obtain fresh aloe juice; Jing Wan Hong ointment for the application on scalded wound (Tianjin Darentang Jing Wan Hong Pharmaceutical Co Ltd, batch number 211646); and sodium chloride injection (Zhengzhou Yonghe Pharmaceutical Factory Co Ltd, batch number: 070302221) were also used for the experiment.

3 METHOD

The experimental procedure includes the following steps: removal of back hair in 70 mice of 180–220 g 1 day before the experiment. On the next day, give anesthesia to 60 rats by intraperitoneal injection of pentobarbital sodium (45 mg/kg) and make scald in the back hair removed area of 5 cm × 8 cm, approximately 10% of body surface area (for light-degree scald) by immersing in a water bath for 10 seconds at a constant temperature of 80°C. Then immediately give 5 mL of ip sterilized saline to all rats for bromogeramine disinfection. According to the scald area, divide evenly large, medium, and small doses of aloe juice group (these groups can also be called as LG, MG, SG for short), Jing Wan Hong group, ice water group, model group, with 10 rats in each group and another 10 as the blank group. Immediately after modeling, rats in the LG, MG, SG group were treated with fresh aloe vera juice on the scalded area in the thickness of 3 mm, 2 mm, and 1.5 mm, respectively (diluted to 50% original liquid with physiological saline); at the same time, rats in the Jing Wan Hong group were treated with Jing Wan Hong ointment on scalded wound in the thickness of 1.5 mm, and rats in the model group and blank group were treated with saline. After administration, the wound is covered with cling film and adhesive tape is fixed. In the rats of ice water group, gauze soaked in ice water was kept over the wound with cling film to maintain moisture, it be an ice pack to keep the temperature. To maintain contact with the skin, the drugs were administered continuously for every 6 h; from the second day onwards, only the ice group received the drugs. Other groups administered drugs every 2 h and 4 times one day, continuously 15 days. Every 5 days with the transparent sulfuric acid paper painted skin scald area graph once, weight the scalded skin area of paper, the weight change show the change in skin scald area. The weight loss percentage can be calculated by dividing the weight deviations of the scald area between before and after treatment from the weight of scald area before treatment; it means that the tested drug effect can be evaluated on the basis of weight loss percentage in the scalded skin area (for results see Table 1). The next day after the last administration, every group of scald rats were sacrificed by cervical mortar, scald skin was cut, fixed in 4% formaldehyde solution, embedded in paraffin, stained using HE and viewed under the microscope to observe the level of skin healing (results shown in Table 2).

4 STATISTICAL METHODS

Statistical analysis was done with the Windows software package SPSS Statistics 13, measurement data with the mean ± standard deviation ($\bar{x} \pm s$), and count data using rank analysis.

Table 1. Effect of fresh aloe juice on rats scald model ($\bar{x} \pm s$).

| Group | N | At different times after scald with paper weight difference before treatment (mg) | | |
		5d	10d	15d
Blank	10	0.00 ± 0.00	0.00 ± 0.00	0.00 ± 0.00
Model	10	10.33 ± 6.78	35.27 ± 7.24	104.17 ± 13.37
Ice water	10	13.31 ± 6.14	35.17 ± 6.20	110.47 ± 12.76
Jing Wan Hong	10	33.71 ± 7.22	84.97 ± 6.27*	146.46 ± 8.05*
LG	10	31.09 ± 6.74	94.19 ± 11.04*	147.46 ± 6.07*
MG	10	20.57 ± 6.69	84.58 ± 11.93*	134.94 ± 12.86*
SG	10	19.60 ± 7.15	47.52 ± 8.55**	117.11 ± 11.49**

Note: compared with model group, *$P < 0.01$, **$P < 0.05$.

Table 2. Effect of fresh aloe juice on the change of pathological tissue on rats scald model.

Group	N	−	+	++	+++
Blank	10	10	0	0	0*
Model	10	0	0	1	9
Ice water	10	0	1	2	5
Jing Wan Hong	10	0	7	3	0*
LG	10	0	2	8	0*
MG	10	0	4	6	0*
SG	10	0	3	7	0*

Note: compared with model group, $*P < 0.01$

"−" the experimental animal skin epithelial cells, subcutaneous tissue, and accessory glands were normal; "+" experimental animal skin epithelial cells and subcutaneous tissue are replaced by new granulation tissue; "+ +" experimental animal skin epithelial cells, subcutaneous tissue, and accessory glands were replaced by granulation tissue and scar tissue; "+ + +" skin epithelial cells, subcutaneous tissue, and accessory glands were completely replaced by large areas of necrosis tissue.

5 RESULT

5.1 *Effect of fresh aloe juice on rats scald model*

Table 1 shows that compared with the model group, before treatment scald area in other groups had no significant difference ($P > 0.05$), but after fifth day of treatment, scald area deviations in large, medium, and small doses of aloe juice group and Jing Wan Hong group increased significantly ($P < 0.01$), and ice water group showed no significant increase ($P > 0.05$); in the tenth day of treatment scald area deviations in large, medium, and small doses of aloe juice group and Jing Wan Hong group increased significantly ($P < 0.01$), and ice water group has no significant increase ($P > 0.05$); in fifteenth day of treatment scald area deviations in large and medium doses of aloe juice group and Jing Wan Hong group increased significantly ($P < 0.01$), but small doses of aloe juice group have slight increase ($P < 0.05$) and ice water group has no significant increase ($P > 0.05$).

5.2 *Effect of fresh aloe juice on the change of pathological tissue in rats scald model*

Results of histopathological observation in scald skin of each group were as follows: in blank group, epithelial cell, subcutaneous tissue, and accessory glands of skin are normal (Figure 1); in model group, epithelial cell disappeared for skin lesions, and subcutaneous tissue and accessory glands are large areas of necrosis (Figure 2); in Jin Wan Hong group, epithelial cell, subcutaneous tissue, and accessory glands of skin are replaced by granulation tissue (Figure 3); in large doses of aloe juice group, epithelial cell, subcutaneous tissue, and accessory glands of skin are replaced by granulation tissue (Figure 4); in medium doses of aloe juice group epithelial cell, subcutaneous tissue and accessory glands of skin are replaced by granulation tissue (Figure 5); in small doses of aloe juice group, epithelial cell, subcutaneous tissue, and accessory glands of skin are replaced by granulation tissue and scar tissue (Figure 6); in ice water group, epithelial cell disappeared, subcutaneous tissue are large areas of necrosis, and accessory glands appear as a little gland (Figure 7).

Table 2 shows that compared with blank group, there is a significant pathological damage of scald in model group ($P < 0.01$), and compared with the model group, Jin Wan Hong group, large, medium, and small doses of aloe juice group can significantly improve the scald pathological changes ($P < 0.01$); pathological changes of scald in ice water group cannot improve obviously ($P > 0.05$).

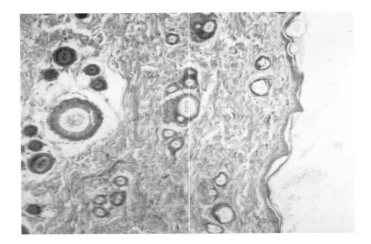

Figure 1.   Blank Group HE × 100.

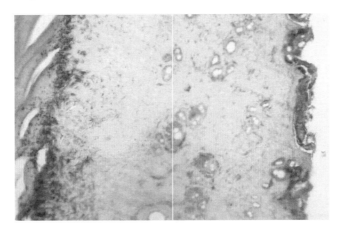

Figure 2.   Model Group HE × 100.

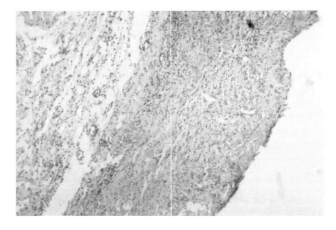

Figure 3.   Jing Wan Hong Group HE × 100.

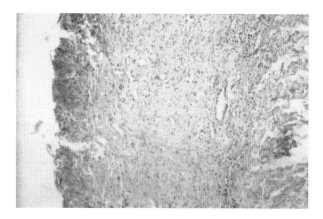

Figure 4.   Large doses of aloe juice group HE × 100.

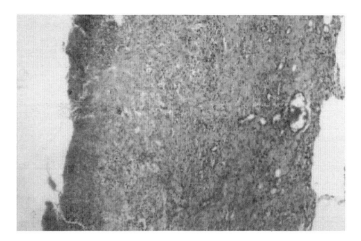

Figure 5.   Medium doses of aloe juice group HE × 100.

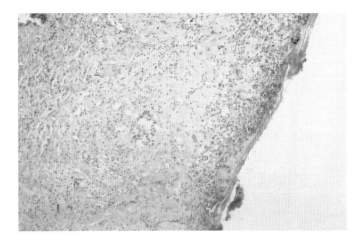

Figure 6.   Small doses of aloe juice group HE × 100.

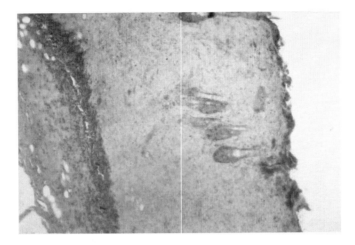

Figure 7.   Ice water group HE × 100.

"-" the experimental animal skin epithelial cells, subcutaneous tissue, and accessory glands were normal; "+" experimental animal skin epithelial cells and subcutaneous tissue are replaced by new granulation tissue; "+ +" experimental animal skin epithelial cells, subcutaneous tissue, and accessory glands were replaced by granulation tissue and scar tissue; "+ + +" skin epithelial cells, subcutaneous tissue, and accessory glands were completely replaced by large areas of necrosis tissue.

6   SUMMARY

According to medical statistics, at present our country scald incidence rate is about 2%, and the number of annual incidence is in the above of tens of millions of people [Ma, H. M et al., 2014]. For better study of fresh aloe juice effect on scald, the experiment evaluates the scald area and scald skin tissue pathological changes of rats. Scald area can reflect the effect of aloe on scald treatment from the macroscopic point of view. Histopathological changes of scald skin can reflect the skin inflammatory cell infiltration and healing in each degree of damaged tissue, from the microscopic point of view.

Modern research thinks, wound repair is affected by many factors, the early stage is mainly inflammatory response, and late stage are mainly associated with connective tissue and epithelium proliferation. In the early stage of scald, wounds microcirculation disorder and inflammatory react excessively. Poor blood flow causes local inflammation and accumulate metabolin. Inflammatory factor aggravate local inflammation response and tissue edema, compress local blood vessels, and aggravate the ischemia and hypoxia. These two are cause - and - effect, vicious circle.

Aloe has pharmacological effects on anti-inflammatory, antibacterial, and wound healing, suggesting a role for treatment of scald.

The experimental results show that the different doses of aloe could significantly increase the scald area difference, can significantly improve the pathological changes of scalded tissues, suggesting that fresh aloe juice has a good curative effect on scald. The experiment provides the basis for external efficacy of aloe on treating scald, provides scientific support for the clinical use of aloe, and offers a new method for traditional Chinese medicine an external treatment of scald.

REFERENCES

Li, Y. K. (2012) Study on the main chemical components and pharmacological action of aloe. Youth, 10, 374.
Ma, H. M & He, G. H. (2014) The curative effect of Shao Shang ointment on wound healing of deep second-degree scald in rabbits. *JOURNAL OF GANNAN MEDICAL UNIVER SITY*, 34(1):8–10.
Wang, S. (2013)Separation, extraction, purification of active components in Aloe. Guide of China medicine, 11(5):66–67.

Medicine Sciences and Bioengineering – Wang (Ed.)
© *2015 Taylor & Francis Group, London, ISBN: 978-1-138-02684-1*

A detection method of lung cancer–characteristic expired gases based on a cross-responsive sensor array

Jin-can Lei

Postdoctoral Station of Science and Technology of Instrumentation, College of Optoelectronic Engineering, Chongqing University, Chongqing, China

Chang-jun Hou*, Dan-qun Huo, Xiao-gang Luo, Mei Yang, Yan-jie Li & Ming-ze Bao

Key Laboratory of Biorheology Science and Technology, Ministry of Education, College of Bioengineering, Chongqing University, Chongqing, China

ABSTRACT: A simple and rapid discrimination method of four lung cancer-related Volatile Organic Compounds (VOCs) with a colorimetric sensor array was presented. The sensor system showed high sensitivity to selected lung cancer biomarkers with concentrations of 50-500 ppb. By means of Fisher Linear Discriminant (FLD), it exhibited good selectivity and fine discrimination of selected gases via extracting array pattern information. And different concentrations of selected VOCs were discriminated by the employment of Back Propagation Neural Network (BPNN). It is also suggested that the proposed method could not only distinguish different kinds of lung cancer–related VOCs but also perform quantitative determination of some VOC concentrations with the correct rate almost up to 100%. It is expected that this method will have potential application for clinical and commercial value in the near future.

1   INTRODUCTION

It was shown that lung cancer accounts for 1.3 million deaths per year worldwide by the statistics of the World Health Organization in 2009 (G. Liu *et al.*, 2013). If lung cancer can be detected in the early stage, the five-year survival rate can be remarkably increased (K. H. Kim *et al.*, 2012). However, the existing methods of early diagnosis of lung cancer are not satisfactory because of low accuracy rate or being very expensive.

A method for the detection of volatile organic compounds (VOCs) in the breath proposed by Pauling in 1971 seems promising in the early diagnosis of lung cancer. Some studies showed that some VOCs that originate from the oxidation of unsaturated fatty acids caused by excessive oxidation in cell membrane in lung cancer patients can be used as specific biomarkers in the early detection of lung cancer. Compared with other detection methods, these VOCs can be used as a potential easy-to-use diagnostic tool with the advantages of being noninvasive, simple, and inexpensive (X. Chen *et al.*, 2007). Recently, the design and revision of gas sensors for detection of VOCs of lung cancer has become an important field of development.

A colorimetric sensor array designed by our laboratory succeeded in not only discriminating proteins but also detecting and classifying toxic gases (C. J. Hou *et al.*, 2011; C. J. Hou *et al.*, 2012), and the latter showed that the sensor array had high specificity and sensitivity for VOCs, so it will attempt to discriminate lung cancer-characteristic expired gases with concentrations from 50 to 500 ppb. The four VOC biomarkers (decane, benzene, styrene, and heptanal) selected by us have been confirmed as biomarker candidates in former studies (M. Phillips *et al.*, 2003).

---

*Corresponding author: Changjun Hou. Tel. no.: +862365112673; e-mail: houcj@cqu.edu.cn.

In this study, the discrimination of the four selected VOCs was on the basis of data analysis methods including fisher linear discriminant (FLD) and back propagation neural network (BPNN). And it intended to allow fine discrimination of the four VOCs with high selectivity. Thus, maybe it will become a new test method in the early diagnosis of lung cancer.

2 EXPERIMENT MATERIALS AND METHODS

2.1 *The cross-responsive sensor array system*

A cross-responsive sensor array consists of chemically responsive dyes, porphyrin, and porphyrin derivatives. The preparation of the cross-responsive sensor array and system is described in our previous work (C. J. Hou *et al.*, 2011; C. J. Hou *et al.*, 2012). The size of the array is 25 mm × 25 mm, and there are 36 (6 × 6) chemically responsive spots whose color can be changed on interacting with different gases or different concentrations. After exposure of the array to the as-prepared VOCs, the sensor array images were automatically collected by a camera every 1 min. A colorful RGB (red-green-blue) difference map was acquired by a series of image processing by means of the control and data processing system.

2.2 *Methods of data analysis*

Figure 1 (a) shows the original image gained from the camera. Figure 1(b) shows the image grayed and the local threshold segmented. And the edge could be extracted (as shown in Figure 1(c)). With a target image, the image processing software locates each spot; samples pixels within a radius of 70% of each spot (as shown in Figure 1(d)); and determines the average red, green, and blue values to be fetched as the coloring information for each spot. When the coloring information of each spot is collected, the standardization image is completed (as shown in Figure 1(e)). Then, the difference maps are obtained through the RGB change of "initial" image and "final" image (as shown in Figure 1(f)). The color change of each certain spot (Xi, Yj) with some time exposures is given by Equation 1.

$$\Delta R_{t1\ (Xi,\ Yj)} = R_{t1\ (Xi,\ Yj)} - R_{t0\ (Xi,\ Yj)}$$

$$\Delta G_{t1\ (Xi,\ Yj)} = G_{t1\ (Xi,\ Yj)} - G_{t0\ (Xi,\ Yj)} \tag{1}$$

$$\Delta B_{t1\ (Xi,\ Yj)} = B_{t1\ (Xi,\ Yj)} - B_{t0\ (Xi,\ Yj)}$$

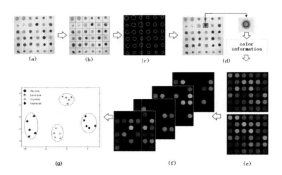

Figure 1.   The methods of data analysis.

Nevertheless, the value of RGB is closely related to the spectrum, which cannot be described by the signal color component. Thus, the change values as characteristics of sensitive spots within the cross-responsive sensor array image can be described as ΔS given by Equation 2.

$$\Delta S = [_{\varepsilon}(\Delta R^2 + \Delta G^2 + \Delta B^2)/3_{\sigma}]^{1/2} \qquad (2)$$

3 RESULTS AND DISCUSSION

3.1 *Dynamic response of cross-responsive sensor array to selected VOCs*

Take decane at the lowest concentration of 50 ppb at room temperature for example, and the different maps of the cross-responsive sensor array exposed every three minutes are shown in Figure 2. Visibly, within the array some sensitive points change the color, whereas some do not.

The trend of the color change could be visualized in a time-dependent graph. Taking the points (3, 3), (3, 5), and (4, 2) for example, the trend is shown in Figure 3. Each line represents the color change for a spot. The trends of every point are almost the same and reach a maximum at the approximate exposure time of 12 min. All the color changes for spots gradually increase as the exposure time is increased before 12 min, and after that time there is no obvious change. It shows that the reaction has reached equilibrium at 12 min. Similarly, we also found that the chemical reactions between sensor array and each of the other three VOCs can reach equilibrium within 12 min. So, it is suggested that 12 min is suitable for the test of the VOCs we selected.

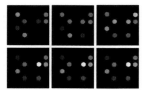

Figure 2.   Difference maps of decane (50 ppb) at specified time values, 3, 6, 9, 12, 15, and 18 min.

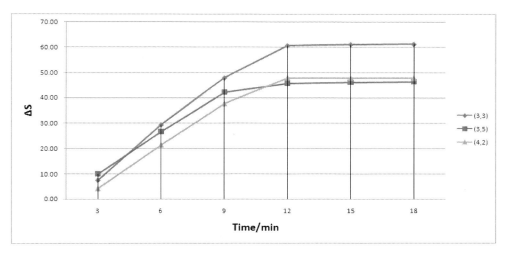

Figure 3.   Typical cross-responsive sensor array response to decane (50 ppb).

3.2 *Response of cross-responsive sensor array with various selected VOCs of lung cancer*

Four kinds of gases were selected to react with the cross-responsive sensor array in the same conditions, at a concentration range of 50–500 ppb and 12 min, including decane, benzene, styrene, and heptanal. Figure 4 shows the difference maps obtained from the system and aforementioned methods of data analysis mentioned. Obviously, for each VOC, although the concentrations are different, there are certain fixed color-changed sensitive points. It means that different target gases have different peculiar difference maps. Under the same conditions, the typical difference maps of different concentrations of all four VOCs at 12 min were also obtained (Figure 4). With the change in concentration, the changes of absorption spectral reaction were different; so the changes of RGB were different, but the points of obvious change in color were at the similar position. It suggested that concentration and difference map had some corresponding relationships.

The response values of the sensor array reacted with the four VOCs at four different concentrations were analyzed by FLD. Figure 5 shows the results. The response of the sensor array to benzene and heptanal were not distinguished completely at the concentration of 50 ppb. However, there was just a little confusion. And it shows that each of the four analytes can be separated well from others at 200 ppb and the analytical results of the response at 500 ppb were better than those at other concentrations. The best rate of classification by using FLD could reach 100%. The results were satisfactory and showed that the sensor array could quickly detect various characteristic VOCs of lung cancer at low concentrations in a short time.

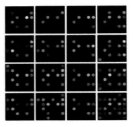

Figure 4. Difference maps of decane, benzene, styrene, and heptanal (from left to right) at 12 min and concentrations of 50 ppb, 200 ppb, 350 ppb, and 500 ppb (from top to bottom).

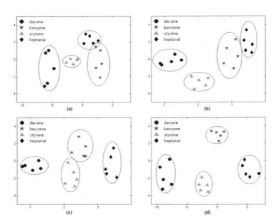

Figure 5. Fisher linear discriminant (FLD) of response patterns for four VOCs at 12 min with different concentrations: (a) 50 ppb; (b) 200 ppb; (c) 350 ppb; and (d) 500 ppb.

3.3 *Pattern recognition with Back Propagation Neural Network (BPNN)*

In this study, BPNN was applied to quantitative analysis of styrene with various concentrations, which are shown in Figure 4. There are 160 samples (40 specimens for each of the four concentrations) randomly divided into two parts for each test. One part contains 96 samples (24 specimens of each concentration) used for training. The other contains 64 samples (16 specimens of each concentration) for the test. The input is a 21- dimensional vector, which comprises ΔR, ΔG, and ΔB of the seven points of which colors are changed. The output layer has two neurons, and (0, 0), (0, 1), (1, 0), and (1, 1) represent the four concentrations. Table 1 shows the test results of the rest. The correct rate is almost 100%.

Table 1. Results of TSFNN analysis.

	Actual value (ppb)	Correct number	Error (%)
Test 1	50	16	0
	200	16	0
	350	16	0
	500	16	0
Test 2	50	15	6.67
	200	17	0
	350	16	0
	500	16	0
Test 3	50	14	12.5
	200	17	0
	350	17	0
	500	16	0
Test 4	50	16	0
	200	16	0
	350	16	0
	500	16	0

4 SUMMARY

A simple and rapid lung cancer–characteristic expired gas detection method is presented in this paper. It exhibited high sensitivity to four lung cancer–characteristic expired gases (decane, benzene, styrene, and heptanal) at the ppb level, based on cross–responsive sensor arrays and data analysis methods. The results show a good selectivity. Through further research, low–cost and fast detection devices of various lung cancer–characteristic expired gases can be expected to be used in the clinical detection of lung cancer. We believe that this method has potential for further clinical application in early diagnosis of lung cancer.

ACKNOWLEDGMENTS

The authors would like to acknowledge the financial support extended by NSFC (81271930, 81171414), Key Technologies R&D Program of China (2012BAI19B03), and Sharing Fund of Chongqing University's Large Equipment.

REFERENCES

Chen, X., Xu, F., Wang, Y., Pan, Y., Lu, D., Wang, P., Ying, K., Chen E. & Zhang W. (2007) A study of the volatile organic compounds exhaled by lung cancer cells in vitro for breath diagnosis. *Cancer*, 110(4); 835–844.

Hou, C. J., Dong, J. L., Zhang, G. P., Lei, Y., Yang, M., Zhang, Y. C., Liu, Z., Zhang S. Y. & Huo D. Q. (2011) Colorimetric artificial tongue for protein identification. *Biosensors & Bioelectronics*, 26(10), 3981–3986.

Hou, C. J., Li, J. J., Huo, D. Q., Luo, X. G., Dong, J. L., Yang, M. & Shi. X. J. (2012) A portable embedded toxic gas detection device based on a cross-responsive sensor array. *Sensors and Actuators B-Chemical*, 161(1); 244–250.

Kim, K. H., Jahan, S. A. & Kabir, E. (2012) A review of breath analysis for diagnosis of human health. *Trac-Trends in Analytical Chemistry*, 33, 1–8.

Liu, G., Cheresh, P. & Kamp, D. W. (2013) Molecular basis of asbestos-induced lung disease. *Annual Review of Pathology-Mechanisms of Disease*, 8, 161–187.

Medicine Sciences and Bioengineering – Wang (Ed.)
© 2015 Taylor & Francis Group, London, ISBN: 978-1-138-02684-1

Detection of follicle stimulating hormone expressed in CHO cell

Rong-mao Hua, Lu Jiang & Bin Zeng[*]

School of Life Science, Jiangxi Science & Technology Normal University, Nanchang, China

ABSTRACT: Follicle Stimulating Hormone (FSH) is a glycoprotein hormone which is secreted by animal anterior pituitary basophils. It is mainly used to treat human infertility disorders in the medical field. FSH is currently used in clinical urine mainly derived urin FSH (uFSH) containing traces of LH and needs to be further processed. FSH expressed by eukaryotic genetic engineering is an effective and low cost method. The paper focuses on CHO cells which were transfered by recombinant vector plasmids and selected by G418 and hygromycin B later, then the expressed FSH was detected by ELISA. So we established eukaryotic systems to express FSH and used ELISA to detect it.

1 INTRODUCTION

Follicle Stimulating Hormone (FSH) is a glycoprotein hormone which is secreted by animal anterior pituitary basophils. FSH is a heterodimer which consisted of alpha subunit and beta subunits composed by non-covalently bound. It plays an important role in the hypothalamus - pituitary - gonad reproductive axis. In the same species, the amino acid sequences of alpha subunit in various glycoprotein hormones (e.g. luteinizing hormone, thyroid stimulating hormone, human chorionic gonadotropin, pregnant mare serum gonadotropin) are the same. There are 92–96 amino acids (the type composed of different mammals)in alpha subunit gene and 109–115 amino acids in beta subunit gene (He, T.P., 2011). The biological specificity of FSH was determined by beta subunit. Alpha subunits and beta subunits alone are not biologically active but they combinated together (Wang, J.W., 2005). Glycoprotein hormone synthesized in cells gets the biological activity after glycosylation subject (Fu, W.Z., 2012). At present, the recombinant glycoprotein hormone drugs in the international markets were mainly expressed by animal cells (Liu, X., 2013, p.382–384). Therefore this is a meaningful research of FSH to be expressed by genetic engineering which aims to obtain CHO cells expressing FSH selected by G418 and hygromicineB and establish the ELISA system to detect FSH. This paper provides some experiences of FSH eukaryotic expression by genetic engineering and methods to detect FSH.

2 MATERIALS AND METHODS

2.1 *Plasmid and cell strains*

The plasmid was transfered into the human FSH alpha gene and FSH beta gene by gene synthesis methods, then purified to get the target plasmid (Recombinant plasmids completed by Nanjing GenScript companies). CHO cells were presented by Shuai Liang from South China Agricultural University.

---

*Correspondence should be addressed to Bin Zeng: zengtx001@aliyun.com.

2.2 Main reagents and instruments

Reagents: cell culture medium RPMI-1640 (Heclone), fetal bovine serum (Wuhan Sanli), lipofectamine 2000 (Invitrogen), G418 (Solarbio), hygromycin B (Amresco), FSH alpha antibody (1.4 mg/mL, Abcam), FSH beta antibody (2.0 mg/mL, Abcam), HRP antibody (1mg/mL, Kangwei Century), zFSH positive control (From animal hospital).

Main Instruments: Microplate reader (Thermo), Carbon dioxide incubator (Thermo), Inverted microscope (Thermo).

2.3 Cell culture

Cells were cultured in complete medium containing RPMI 1640 and 15% fetal bovine serum at 37°C and 5% CO_2 incubator and passaged three generations before transfection.

2.4 Cell transfection

CHO cells were seeded into each well at a density 6×10^5 in 6-well culture plate. After 24 hours, the CHO cells grew to 90%–95% in the well were prepared to be transfected (Liu, Z., 2002). 2 ug FSH alpha plasmid and 2 ug FSH beta plasmid were diluted in 250 ul serum-free medium, then mixed gently. 10 ul lipofectamine 2000 were diluted by 250 ul serum-free medium, and incubated at room temperature. After five minutes, the plasmid and the liposomes were mixed together, incubated at room temperature for 20 minutes. Then the cells were washed twice with serum-free medium. At last, each well was added to 500 ul compound. After the cells were incubated in carbon dioxide incubator for 4-6 hours, the serum-free medium was replaced with serum-containing medium (Liu, X., 2013, p. 4–6).

2.5 Screening and expressing cells

After 24 hours of transfection, the cells were digested and seeded in 96 cell culture plate with the density of 1 cell/well, 5 cell/well in 10 cell/well, 20 cell/well, 50 cell/well, 100 cell/well, 200 cell/well, 500 cell/well, 1000 cell/well, 2000 cell/ well, which were numbered as 1, 2, 3, 4, 5, 6, 7, 8, 9 and 10. Until the cells density reached 60%, a certain concentration of G418 and hygromycinB in medium were added into every well. After 3–4 days, the old complete medium containing antibiotics was replaced into new one. Two weeks later, the stable survived cell lines which could express FSH were initially selected out (Kim, D.J., 2010).

2.6 ELISA test FSH

The supernatant of transfected cells after 24 hours was taken to detect by indirect ELISA. Firstly, preliminary experiment was done to determine the optimal antibody concentration. Indirect ELISA specific methods: Antigen were coated overnight under 4°C and washed three times. Each well added 5% skim milk and incubated under 37°C, washed four times. Then each well added FSH alpha antibody dilution 100 ul, incubated in 37°C for 1 hour, washed four times. Later each well was added 100 ul HRP secondary antibody dilutions, incubated under 37°C for 45 minutes. Then TMB solution 100 ul was used in each well, incubated for 8-10 minutes at 37°C and dark. At last each well was added 50 ul 2M H_2SO_4 to stop the reaction and test the OD values by microplate reader. Experimental methods of blank, negative control and positive control were the same methods.

3 RESULTS

3.1 Cell culture

Cells recovered were passaged for three generations and in good condition. The following photos were cells before transfection.

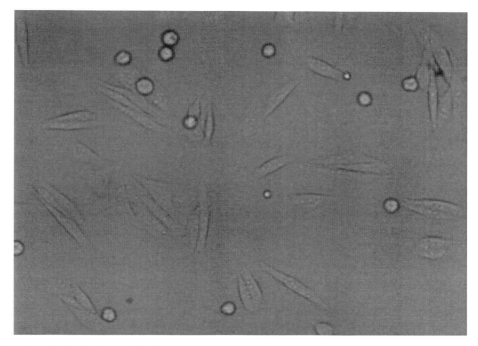

Figure 1. CHO cells in magnification microscope.

3.2 *Cell transfection results*

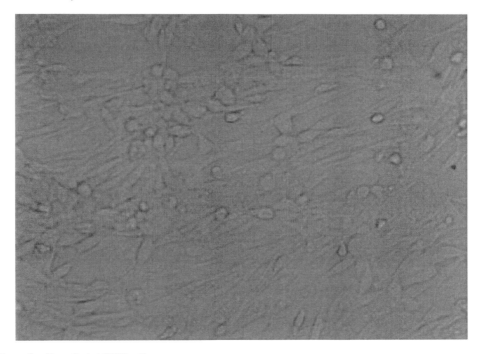

Figure 2. Transfected CHO cells.

3.3 *Filter cell line*

After screened by G418 and hygromycinB concentration, the optimal G418 screening concentration was found to be 100 ug/mL, the optimal hygromycinB screening concentration was 50 ug/mL. Cells were stable survival after screened by antibiotics for two weeks which indicated that FSH was expressed in this cells.

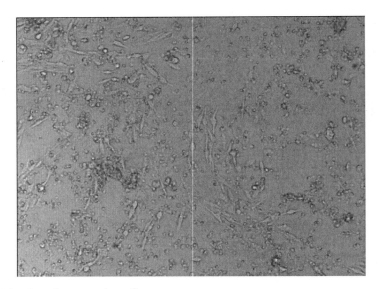

Figure 3. After three days screening cells.

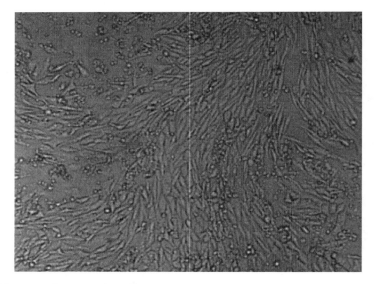

Figure 4. After seven days screening cells.

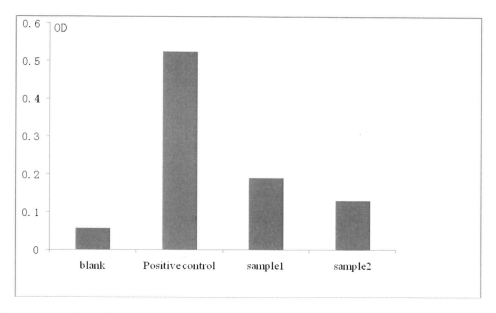

Figure 5.　Blank, positive control, sample1, sample2 OD.

3.4　*ELISA results*

Through preliminary experiments to determine the optimal coating concentration of antibody (1.2 ug/mL), antigen was diluted into 200 and 400 times (sample1 and sample2). Then indirect ELISA was applied to test sample, the positive control, negative control and blank control. The following were OD values of sample, positive control and blank in Figure 5.

4　SUMMARY

1. CHO cells were successfully recovered and cultured in good condition.
2. FSHα plasmid and FSHβ plasmid were successfully transferred into CHO cells, the transfected cells were in good condition.
3. After CHO cells were screened by G418 and hygromycin B for two weeks, the stable survival CHO cells were obtained.
4. Cell culture supernatants were detected by ELISA, it indicated that the supernatant contain the FSH.

ACKNOWLEDGMENTS

This work was financially supported by National Natural Science Foundation of China (No. 31171731), project 3000035402, project 00001384, project 30000389, project 3000039703 and project 30000402.

315

REFERENCES

Fu, W.Z, Chen, Y.J., Wang, Q.Z., Zhang, X.K., Ma, Y., Zhang, X.G.(2012) Construction of eukaryotic express-ing vector of mouse PD- L1 and establishment of stable transfectant CHO cell line. *Journal of Soochow University (Medical Science Edition)*, 02:80–83.

He, T.P., Tang, Y.J., Xu, L., Song, C.L., Tan, X.J., Nie, Y.T., Yang, B., Lei, T. (2011) Expression of recombinant human follicle-stimulating hormone in CHO cell. *Chinese Journal of Biologicals,* 12:1409–1412.

Kim, D.J., Seok, S.H., Baek, M.W., et al. (2010) Highly expressed recombinant human follicle-stimulating hormone from Chinese hamster o-vary cells grown in serum-free medium and its effect on induction of folliculogenesis and ovulation. *Fertility and Sterility*, 08:120–129.

Liu, X., Liu, F., Liu, S.Y., Zhu, X.Q., Ling, P.X. (2013) Construction of recombinant human thrombin eukar-yotic expression vector and its stable expression in CHO cells. *Food and Drug*, 06:381–384.

Liu, X., Liu, F., Liu, S.Y., Zhu, X.Q., Ling, P.X. (2013) Construction of eukaryotic expression vector of human hyaluronidase and establishment of its stable transfected CHO cell line. *Food and Drug,* 02:80–83.

Liu, Z.G., Qu, S. (2002) Research of DNA transfected CHO cell efficiently. *Journal of Wuhan Polylechnic University*, 01:4–6.

Wang, J.W., Chen, X.P., Yan, Z.J., Ding, J.T. (2005) Construction of eukaryotic expressing vector Goat FSH pVITRO-FSHαβ and establishment of stable transfectant CHO cell line. *Chinese Journal of Animal and Veterinary Sciences*, 36(11):1130–1136.

Medicine Sciences and Bioengineering – Wang (Ed.)
© 2015 Taylor & Francis Group, London, ISBN: 978-1-138-02684-1

The protective potential of fasudil hydrochloride in liver injury induced by intestinal ischemia reperfusion in rats

Xiaowei Hu
Department of Pharmacology Dalian Medical University, Dalian, China

Xiao-feng Tian & Zhe Fan
Department of General Surgery, Second Affiliated Hospital of Dalian Medical University, Dalian, China

Liang Chu
Department of Pharmacology Dalian Medical University, Dalian, China

Yang Li
Department of General Surgery, Second Affiliated Hospital of Dalian Medical University, Dalian, China

Li Lv, Dong-yan Gao* & Ji-hong Yao*
Department of Pharmacology Dalian Medical University, Dalian, China

ABSTRACT: Background/Aims: To investigate the protective effects of fasudil hydrochloride, a Rho-kinase inhibitor, on liver and intestine injury induced by intestinal ischemia/reperfusion in rats. Methods: The intestinal I/R model were established by blocking the superior mesenteric artery with clap in rats. Fasudil (7.5 mg/kg and 15 mg/kg) was administered intraperitoneally 1h before the operation. Results: Administration of fasudil markedly ameliorated tissue injury demonstrated as the decreasing levels of serum AST, ALT, CK-B, cytokines and MPO and SOD activity increased. The expressions of Rho-kinase in liver tissue markedly attenuated and the expression of eNOS in liver enhanced markedly compared with I/R group. Conclusions: Fasudil can alleviate liver and intestine injury induced by intestinal I/R, which may be attributed to the inhibition of neutrophil infiltration through inhibiting the activity of Rho-ROCK.

1 INTRODUCTION

The obstacle of intestinal Ischemia-Reperfusion (IR) is one of the most serious injuries which not only occurs in acute abdomen diseases such as intestinal obstruction, mesentery arterial embolism but also in shock after serious hurt and burn. Intestinal IR injury induces a systemic inflammatory response, the release of harmful substances like ROS causes the death of intestine mucous cell, the barricade of intestine mucous is destroyed. Then, the permeability of blood vessel increases, endotoxin is absorbed into blood and systemic circulation. Finally, it may affect the function and integrity of distant organs such as respiratory system, liver, heart, and kidney, cause the systemic inflammatory response syndrome and multiple organ dysfunction syndrome occurs (Pierro & Eaton, 2004). The precise mechanism of organ injuries induced by intestinal I/R is complicated and unclear yet.

Rho kinase is a downstream target molecule of small GTP-binding proteins. It was originally identified as a regulator of actin cytoskeleton organization and thereby mediates cell adhesion, motility and contractility. The previous studies have demonstrated that Rho kinase regulates the production of ROS in neutrophils and mediates other cellular functions such as proliferation or

---
*Correspondence to: Jihong Yao and Dongyan Gao,Tel: 86-411-8611-0412, Fax: +86-411-8611-0410 E-mail: yaojihong65@hotmail.com, gaody1975@163.com This work was supported by the grants of the Dalian Scientific Research Foundation, No. 2008E13SF217.

apoptosis. In addition, Rho-kinase inhibition is known to be useful for the treatment of ischemic disease, including cerebral vasospasm, renal and liver ischemia reperfusion.

Hence, we conducted this study to find out if the Rho/Rho-kinase pathway is involved in the liver injury induced by intestinal I/R and the inhibition of Rho-kinase by hydrochloride fasudil is effective to alleviate the disorder.

2 MATERIALS AND METHODS

2.1 *Experimental design*

Male Sprague-Dawley rats weighing 200–240 grams (the Animal Center of Dalian Medical University, Dalian, China) were given a standard pellet diet and water in accordance with institutional animal care policies. The rats were randomly divided into four experimental groups (n = 6 in each): (1) control group: the rats underwent full surgical preparation including the superior mesenteric artery (SMA) without occlusion; (2) intestinal IR group: the rats were subjected to 1 h intestinal ischemia and 2 h reperfusion after SMA was isolated and ischemia was occluded; (3) and (4) fasudil pretreatment group: the rats underwent surgery as in the II/R group with intraperitoneal administration of fasudil (7.5 mg/kg, 15 mg/kg) 1 h before the operation. The rats in the control and II/R groups were treated with an equal volume of normal saline solution. All animals were killed after 2 h of reperfusion, and the blood samples, intestine and liver tissues were obtained for further study.

2.2 *Histopathologic evaluation of intestine and liver*

Tissue samples were fixed in 10% formalin, then embedded in paraffin and cut into 4μm sections. Slides were stained with hematoxylin and eosin (H.E.) and examined with a light microscopy (Olympus BX 51, Olympus Instruments Service, Tokyo, Japan). Each slide was evaluated by two separate investigators blinded to the data.

2.3 *Determination of ALT, AST, CK and TNF-α in serum and MPO, SOD in intestinal and liver*

The serum levels of ALT, AST and creatine kinase B (CK-B) were determined using an automated analyzer (Olympus au 1000). The serum level of TNF-α was determined using a RIA kit (Radioimmunity Institute of PLA General Hospital, Beijing, China) according to the manufacturer's instructions and expressed as ng/L. Proximal Intestine 15 cm away from ileocecal valve and the left lobe of liver tissues were collected, weighed, and immediately homogenized on ice in 5 volumes of normal saline separately. MPO and SOD activity in the supernatants were measured using assay kit (Nanjing Jincheng Corp., China) following the manufacturer's instructions and expressed as U/g or U/mg prot.

2.4 *Determination of Rho-kinase activity (P-Moesin) and eNOS by Western blot*

P-Moesin, as the substrate of Rho kinase, the activity of P-Moesin could identify with the activity of Rho kinase. Cellular plasma protein were extracted from the frozen intestine and liver tissues with a protein extraction kit (Pierce, Meridian Road, Rockford, IL, USA). The proteins were separated by 10% SDS-PAGE gel electrophoresis and were electrophoretically transferred to a PVDF membranes (Millipore, Bedford, MA, USA) at 9 V. The transferred membranes were incubated overnight at 4°C with rabbit polyclonal antibodies against rat (p-Moesin and eNOS both at 1:1000 dilution, Santa Cruz Corp.) in PBS-T containing 5% skim milk. The membranes were incubated with anti-rabbit IgG conjugated to horseradish peroxidase in PBS-T containing 5 % skim milk for 1 h at 37°C. After three additional washes with PBS-T, the signals were visualized by DAB assay kit and analyzed with a gel imaging system (Kodak system EDAS120).

2.5 Statistical analysis

Statistical analyses were carried out with SPSS statistical software (SPSS for Windows, Version 13.0, SPSS Inc., Chicago, IL). All data were expressed as the mean ± SD. Statistical analysis was performed using F test. P values less than 0.05 was considered statistically significant.

3 RESULTS

3.1 Fasudil alleviates intestinal injury induced by intestinal I/R in rats

After the administration of fasudil, a significant improvement in edema and inflammatory infiltrate was seen in intestinal villi, and tissue damage was alleviated (Figure 1). The serum CK-B level (a sensitive diagnostic marker of intestinal injury) in intestinal IR group were significant rising as compared to the control group(P < 0.01). Administration of fasudil markedly ameliorated the increase of serum CK-B level(P < 0.01). In comparison to the control group, serum TNF-α level significantly increased in intestinal I/R group (P < 0.01), while fasudil pretreatment markedly decreased serum level of TNF-α in comparison to the intestinal I/R group (P < 0.01).

3.2 Fasudil alleviates acute liver injury induced by intestinal I/R in rats

Serum levels of AST and ALT, marker of hepatocellular injury, were measured 2h after intestinal I/R. Fasudil pretreatment markedly suppressed the concentrations of AST and ALT (P < 0.01, figure 2A and B), suggesting that fasudil markedly ameliorates liver injury induced by intestinal I/R. This was consistent with the liver histopathologic evaluation (figure 2 right).

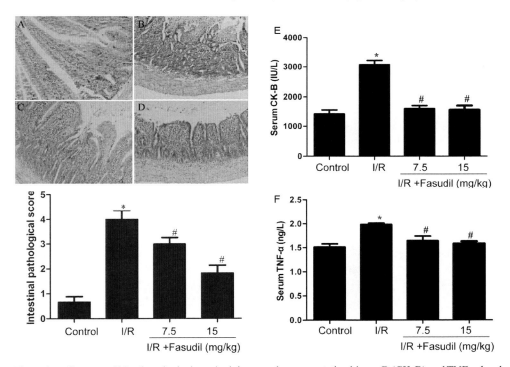

Figure 1. Changes of histology in the intestinal tissue and serum creatine kinase B (CK-B) and TNF-α levels after 60 min ischemia and 120 min reperfusion in rats ($\times$ 200). n = 6. A: Control; B: I/R; C: I/R + Fasudil (7.5mg/kg); D: I/R + Fasudil (15mg/kg). CK-B (E) and TNF-α (F) *p < 0.01 vs control; #p < 0.01 vs I/R.

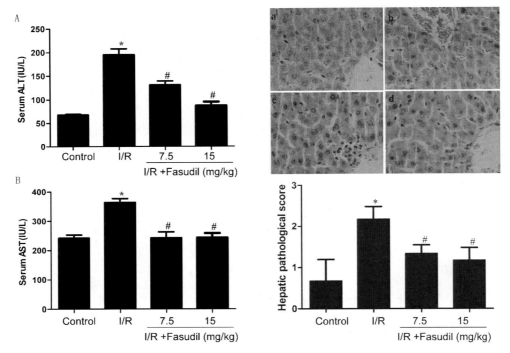

Figure 2.   Serum ALT (A), AST (B) levels and pathological score in the liver tissue on acute liver injury after intestinal ischaemia-reperfusion (I/R). a: Control; b: I/R; c: I/R + Fasudil (7.5 mg/kg); d: I/R + Fasudil (15mg/kg).*p < 0.01 vs control; #p < 0.01 vs I/R.

3.3   *Effect of fasudil on intestine and liver neutrophil infiltration and SOD activity*

MPO activity was assayed for estimating the tissue leukocyte recruitment. The tissue MPO activity decreased significantly after fasudil pretreatment in comparison to the intestinal I/R group (P < 0.01, P < 0.01, figure 3 A and B). SOD is the major enzyme for scavenging oxygen radicals. The SOD increased significantly after fasudil pretreatment in comparison to the intestinal I/R group (P < 0.01, P < 0.01, figure 3 C and D).

3.4   *Effects of fasudil on Rho-kinase activity and eNOS Expression*

To quantify Rho-kinase activity, the extent of phosphorylation of the ezrin, radixin, and moesin (P-ERM) family, substrates of Rho-kinase, was determined by Western blot by rabbit anti-rat moesin polyclonal antibody. The result showed that significant increase of P-Moesin protein and decrease of eNOS protein expression were found in intestinal I/R group. Fasudil Pretreatment markedly decrease P-Moesin and increase eNOS protein expression separately (figure 4).

4   DISCUSSION

The liver is known to be vulnerable to injury in intestinal I/R. The present study is the first report to provide evidence of the protective effect of hydrochloride fasudil against intestine and liver injury induced by intestinal I/R in an experimental model. Our findings showed that intestinal I/R upregulated Rho-kinase activity in the intestine and liver tissues, pharmacologic inhibition of Rho-kinase by fasudil effectively alleviates liver injury caused by intestinal I/R.

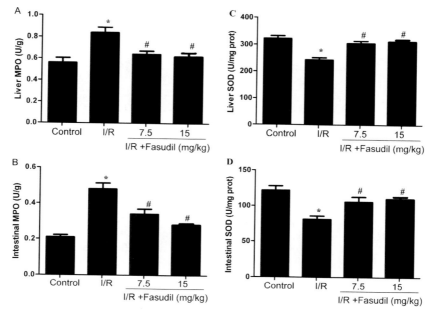

Figure 3.   Activity of myeloperoxidase (MPO) and activity of superoxide dismutase (SOD) in the liver and intestinal tissue in different groups (mean ± SD). MPO contents in the tissue were analyzed with an MPO assay kit as the index of neutrophil recruitment. A: Activity of MPO in the liver tissue; B: Activity of MPO in the intestinal tissue. C: Activity of SOD in the liver tissue; D: Activity of SOD in the intestinal tissue. *$P < 0.01$ vs control; #$P < 0.01$ vs I/R.

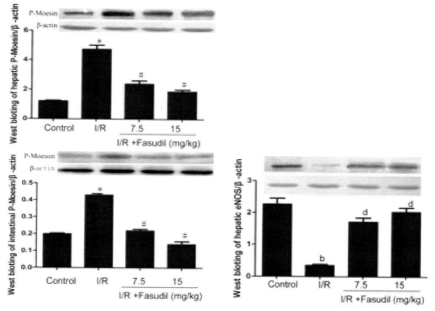

Figure 4.   Effects of fasudil on Rho-kinase activity in liver and intestine and eNOS expression in the liver. The data were normalized to endogenous protein expression in different groups (mean±SD). *$p < 0.01$ vs control; #$p < 0.01$ vs I/R.

It has been demonstrated that ROS generated during tissue reperfusion contribute to the organ injury in intestinal I/R and Rho kinase enhances the production of ROS by neutrophils. In this study a decrease of SOD was observed in the intestinal I/R, however, SOD level was elevated markedly after 7.5 and 15 mg/kg fasudil pretreatment, suggesting that Rho kinase inhibition by fasudil suppress superoxide production during intestinal I/R. Proinflammatory cytokines and activated polymer-phonuclear neutrophils (PMNs) play pivotal role in the liver injury caused by intestinal I/R (Yao et al, 2009). In the early stage of intestinal I/R, the gut barrier function is damaged and the activated cytokines and neutrophils are released into the circulation, interacting with the vascular endothelium of distant organs such as liver and inducing a systemic inflammatory reactions. Thus, we examined whether the cytokine production could be suppressed by Rho-kinase inhibition. In our study inhibition of Rho-kinase by fasudil resulted in a down-regulation of proinflammatory cytokine TNF-α, which in turn limited activation of circulation leukocytes in the microcirculation of liver and other organs, leading to reduced inflammatory mediated intestine and liver injury. The liver and intestine MPO activity which reflects the level of accumulation of PMNs in tissues were markedly reduced with fasudil in this study.

Recent study reported that a selective ROCK inhibitor fasudil decreased neurologic deficit by augmenting eNOS and NO production after ischemia reperfusion (Li et al, 2009). The present study showed a decrease in eNOS expression in the liver tissue after intestinal I/R, while fasudil Pretreatment up-regulated the eNOS protein expression. The augmentation of eNOS expression by fasudil could lead to beneficial anti-inflammatory effects in the vascular wall, which may involved in the protection of liver injury after intestinal I/R. Intestinal I/R is complex and multifactorial pathophysiological process that involves many mediators such as ROS, cytokines and eNOS. These mediators can be regulated by Rho kinase. Rho kinase may directly catalyze MLC phosphorylation, or act indirectly via inactivation of myosin light chain phosphatase by phosphorylation at Thr695, Ser894, and Thr850. These mechanisms cause activation of actin polymerization, stress fiber formation, MLC phosphorylation and actomyosin-driven cell contraction resulting in endothelial cell barrier disruption. Previous Studies have demonstrated that Rho kinase or increased Rho kinase activity is involved in the pathogenesis of various vascular lesions through the downregulation of endothelial nitric oxide synthase (eNOS) activity and production of O2- in neutrophils and vessels (Baba et al, 2010). In our present experiment, 1 h of intestinal ischemia followed by 2 h of reperfusion induced liver injury manifested as a significant increase of pathological injury score as well as PMN infiltration. These changes were parallel to the increased level of liver Rho kinase activity (P-Moesin), suggesting that the activation of Rho kinase activity is involved in the pathogenesis of liver injury induced by intestinal I/R. While Fasudil can prevent this disorder by inhibiting the activity of Rho kinase, downregulating the neutrophil infiltration, and upregulating liver eNOS expression.

In summary, this study demonstrated a pivotal role of Rho-kinase in the pathogenesis of liver injury induced by intestinal I/R. The results confirm the potential therapeutic importance of Rho-kinase and the feasible implication of Rho-kinase inhibitor fasudil in intestinal I/R.

REFERENCES

Baba, H., Tanoue, Y., Maeda, T., et al. (2010). Protective effects of cold spinoplegia with fasudil against ischemic spinal cord injury in rabbits. *J. Vasc. Surg.*, 51(2) : 445–452.

Li, Q., Huang, X.J., He, W. et al. (2009). Neuroprotective potential of fasudil mesylate in brain ischemia-reperfusion injury of rats. *Cell Mol. Neurobiol.*, 29(2) : 169–180.

Pierro, A., Eaton, S.. Intestinal ischemia reperfusion injury and multisystem organ failure. Semin Pediatr Surg. 2004 Feb; 13(1) : 11–17 [PMID: 14765366].

Yao, J.H., Zhang, X.S., Zheng, S.S., et al. (2009) Prophylaxis with carnosol attenuates liver injury induced by intestinal ischemia/reperfusion. *World J. Gastroenterol.*, 14; 15(26) : 3240–3245.

Medicine Sciences and Bioengineering – Wang (Ed.)
© 2015 Taylor & Francis Group, London, ISBN: 978-1-138-02684-1

Simulation and prediction of the material foundation of Rhubarb based on molecular docking

Yue-ying Rong & Li Lu
Department of Traditional Chinese Medicine, Guangdong Pharmaceutical University, Guangzhou, China

Yuan-xin Tian
Department of Pharmaceutical Analysis, School of Pharmaceutical Sciences, Southern Medical University, Guangzhou, China

Jie-xin Lin, Qin-xiao Guan, Sheng-wang Liang, Lu Zhao & Shu-mei Wang*
Department of Traditional Chinese Medicine, Guangdong Pharmaceutical University, Guangzhou, China

ABSTRACT: Rhubarb is a widely used Traditional Chinese Medicine (TCM) which has been extensively applied in the clinical treatment of ischemic stroke. However, the underlying mechanism of clinical administrating Rhubarb on ischemic stroke is not clear. In this study, by using the molecular docking, virtual screening of the active molecules of Rhubarb was performed. We obtained a group of compounds from Rhubarb, and identified 21 targets that are related to the mechanism of cerebral ischemia. The results show that a number of components have good binding activity after docking with the above targets. The action mechanism of Rhubarb is most probably due to the active compounds target at multiple proteins in the biological network. This study not only made a contribution to a better understanding of the mechanisms of Rhubarb on the treatment of cerebral ischemia-reperfusion injury, but also proposed a strategy to develop novel TCM candidates at a network pharmacology level.

1 INTRODUCTION

The clinical curative effect of traditional Chinese medicine, essentially via a plurality of small molecule drugs combined with biological target protein, plays the synergistic effect of the biological process. Modern research results show that the chemical nature of the combination of drug and target is actually that drugs interacting with receptors and forming drug-receptor complexes. In addition to the electrostatic interactions include covalent and non-covalent bond, such as the ionic bond, hydrogen bond, van der Waals force, etc. (Duan *et al.*, 2009). Molecular docking technology (Zhang *et al.*, 2010), as an important means of computer-aided drug design, is mainly used between protein receptor and small drug molecules and mutual recognition process to realize the computer-aided drug screening by geometric matching and energy matching. A study found that the positive rate of the active compounds using the molecular docking virtual screening than using high throughput screening increases seven times (Liu & Du, 2003).

Rhubarb is one of the common traditional Chinese medicine, with wide effects. Rhubarb, rhubarb extracts and rhubarb aglycone have been confirmed to play a remarkable curative effect on ischemic stroke. Rhubarb aglycone could clear a large number of free radicals caused by brain ischemia-reperfusion (Li *et al.*, 2004), effectively reduce NO-mediated cytotoxicity (Li *et al.*, 2003), inhibit inflammatory cascade reaction with cerebral ischemia-reperfusion injury (Li *et al.*, 2005a; Li *et al.*, 2007), inhibit the thrombosis, the aggregation and adhesion of platelet (Li *et al.*, 2005b), and

---

*The corresponding author of this study is Prof. Shumei Wang. Her basic information are: Tel: 86-(0)20-3935-2559, Fax: 86-(0)20-3935-2174 and E-mail: shmwang@sina.com.

have protective effects on rats with cerebral ischemia (Liu *et al.*, 2004). However, the mechanism of Rhubarb in treatment of stroke is not clear. Therefore, in this experiment, we apply molecular docking technology to study the effective substances of Rhubarb. Study on current literature contained compounds of Rhubarb, preferably select with the effective chemical compositions on the treatment of cerebral ischemia.

2 MATERIALS AND METHODS

2.1 *Materials*

The docking studies were carried out with Surflex-Dock program of Sybyl-7.3 version software installed on Microsoft Windows XP system. This research was conducted in the School of Pharmaceutical Sciences, Southern Medical University. And the Compound-Target Networks were generated by Cytoscapse 2.8.1. All chemical compounds of Rhubarb were retrieved from Chinese Academy of Sciences Chemistry Database and Chinese Herbal Drug Database. Finally, to the most extent 52 compounds were collected. The structures of these molecules were produced by ChemBioDraw (MDL Information Systems, Inc.).

2.2 *Targets collecting*

Through scanning, a large number of patents and references on ischemic cerebral apoplexy, and according to the clinical pharmacology experiments, we selected 21 targets that play a significant role in the pathological mechanism of cerebral ischemia as research objects, namely VEGFR, Bcl-2, ICAM-1, IL-1β and so on. The three-dimensional molecular structures and bioactive ligand complexes' structures of above 21 targets which were obtained by searching the PDB. The protein targets were shown in Table 1.

2.3 *Molecular docking*

Molecular docking was performed with Surflex-Dock program that is interfaced with Sybyl 7.3 (Jain, 2007; Sun *et al.*, 2010). The programs adapted an empirical scoring function and a patented searching engine. Two-dimensional structure of all the compounds was constructed by ChemBioOffice2008 and transformed into 3D structure. Hydrogen and Gasteiger-Hückel charges were added to every molecule. Then, the receptor structure was minimized in 1000 cycles with the Powell method in Sybyl 7.3. And then their geometries are optimized by the Powell energy

Table 1. Cerebral ischemia-associated protein targets.

Protein	PDB code	Protein	PDB code
Vascular endothelial growth factor (VEGFR)	1VR2	Caspase-3	2CNK
Tumor necrosis factor-a (TNF-α)	2AZ5	B-cell lymphoma-2(Bcl-2)	1YSW
Intercellular adhesion molecule- 1 (ICAM-1)	1P53	B-cell lymphoma(Bcl-XL)	2YXJ
Vascular cell adhesion molecule-1 (VCAM-1)	1VSC	Interleukin-1B(IL-1β)	1RWN
Nuclear transcription factor-KB (NF-KB)	4G3D	Angiopoietin receptor (Tie-2)	3L8P
Transforming growth factor-B (TGF-β)	1PY5	Superoxide dismutase (SOD)	2VOA
Matrix metalloproteinase-9 (MMP-9)	1GKC	Prostacyclin synthase (PGIS)	3B6H
Matrix metalloproteinase-2 (MMP-2)	1QIB	Cycloxygenase-1 (COX-1)	3N8X
Inducible nitric oxide synthase (iNOS)	2Y37	Cycloxygenase-2 (COX-2)	3NT1
Insulin-like growth factor-2 (IGF-2)	1GPO	Interleukin-6 (IL-6)	1ALU
Heat shock protein 70 (HSP70)	3D2F		

gradient method in the TRIPOS force field. The energy convergence criterion is 0.05 kcal/mol. The purpose of energy optimization is to find the lowest energy conformation of ligand molecular structure to simulate the molecular stable conformation of natural systems.

2.4 *Network construction*

The Candidate Targets and Potential Targets were respectively used to build the Compound-Target Networks with the Candidate compounds. The Compound-Target Networks were generated by Cytoscapse 2.8.1 (Smoot *et al.*, 2011), a standard tool for integrated analysis and visualization of biological networks. The Compound-Pathway Network was produced by linking the Candidate compounds and the signal pathways in which they participated.

3 RESULTS

3.1 *Docking accuracy*

Got the Total Score, Crash and Polar parameter values for docking success, with the Total Score parameters as evaluation index. To compare the Total Score values of the successful docking compounds and the original ligand, the result is that the former is higher than the latter, or similar. Surflex is a fully automatic flexible molecular docking and assessment show that more than 80% of the forecast and actual model the RMSD are within the 2.5 Å, and can significantly reduce false-positive ratio, the true positive rate is greater than 80% (Jain, 2003).

3.2 *Molecular-docking results*

The study will deal with 52 active small molecules docking to the 21 protein targets respectively. We count the screening results, the score value is more than 5.0 indicating that molecules and target have good binding activity, more than 7.0 showing the combination of molecules and target configuration has strong activity. The results are shown in Table 2. It reveals that there are 23 components with 10 or more than 10 targets which have a strong interaction. Molecular docking results reveal the comprehensive effects of multiple components and multiple target of Rhubarb in the treatment of cerebral ischemia.

3.3 *Study of multi-target effects of Rhubarb 23 active ingredients*

We applied Cytoscape software to establish the multiple Compounds-targets network, the relationship between the 23 active components and multiple targets visually presented in Fig. 1. By the network analysis, we found that the 23 active ingredients can control 21 genes associated with cerebral ischemia.

4 DISCUSSION

Comprehensive analysis of lots of literature domestic and foreign (Durukan & Tatlisumak, 2007; Mazumdar *et al.*, 2008), at present, the main pathology and pathogenesis of ischemic stroke are: ①glutamate neurotoxicity, ②free radicals generated, ③intracellular calcium overload, ④inflammatory reactions, ⑤changes in neurotransmitters and neuroactive substances, ⑥the blood-brain barrier damage, ⑦energy failure, etc.

TGF-β is mainly expressed after cerebral ischemia. A large number of TGF-β will promote to generate capillaries and activate vascular endothelial cells, etc (Liu *et al.*, 2010). In the process of cerebral ischemia, angiogenin (ANG) mainly through combination with its receptor (Tie-2) induces the formation of blood vessels (Li *et al.*, 2013). In this study, after docking 52 compounds

Table 2. The results of 23 compounds of Rhubarb with more than 10 targets docking.

Compounds	VEGFR	Caspase-3	Bcl-2	Bcl-XL	TNF-A	IL-1B	ICAM-1	VCAM-1	NF-KB	Tie-2
Rhaponticin	6.44	—	5.02	7.49	5.34	5.69	5.79	5.49	5.00	7.22
Aloe-emodin-o-O-β-D-glucopyranoside	5.62	5.23	5.01	5.39	—	5.61	7.31	5.51	5.04	7.66
Toraehrysone-8-O-β-D-glucoside	5.82	—	5.33	5.77	5.58	5.51	7.55	5.61	—	7.61
Phenylbutanone-glucoside	5.28	—	—	5.28	—	6.93	5.04	5.24	5.80	7.69
Emodin-1-O-β-D-glucopyranoside	5.32	—	6.08	5.12	6.01	—	7.25	—	5.49	7.81
Isorhapontigenin	5.02	—	—	6.13	—	5.15	5.88	5.05	6.19	5.68
Emodin-8-O-β-D-gentiobioside	7.18	—	—	5.22	6.46	5.89	7.52	—	6.71	6.62
5-carboxyl-7-glucose based oxygen-2-methyl benzopyran-y-ketone	6.12	5.00	—	—	—	5.25	7.82	5.02	5.52	5.05
1,2,6-Tri-O-galloyl-glucose	7.63	5.84	5.36	—	—	6.36	7.32	—	8.25	7.65
3,5,4'-Trihydroxystilene-4'-glucoside	5.99	—	—	7.01	—	5.54	5.18	—	6.05	6.53
1,6-Di-0-galloyl-β-D-glucose	7.43	—	6.20	5.37	—	—	—	—	6.43	5.53
Rheidin A	6.60	—	—	6.05	5.50	—	7.54	6.68	6.17	5.86
GaUoyl-4-O-(6'-O-galloyl)glucoside	5.65	—	—	—	—	—	5.88	—	8.26	8.84
1-O-galloyl-β-D-glucose	5.36	—	—	—	—	—	—	—	6.05	5.94
Musizin-8-O-β-D-glucoside	5.34	—	—	—	—	—	5.13	7.14	—	6.21
(+)-Catechin-5-O-glucoside	5.21	—	—	—	—	—	5.15	5.66	7.02	8.60
6-Hydroxy-inusizin-8-O-β-D-glucoside	—	—	5.06	5.17	5.05	6.00	6.62	—	5.84	6.36
Chrysophanol-8-O-β-D-glucopyranoside	—	5.25	5.45	—	—	—	6.92	—	—	8.61
Emodin-8-O-β-D-(6'-oxalyl)glucopyranoside	—	—	7.30	—	5.47	—	5.39	—	6.57	7.46
Rhein-8-O-β-D-glucopyranoside	—	—	6.07	5.68	—	5.11	5.69	—	—	9.72
Physcion-8-O-β-D-glucopyranoside	—	6.21	—	—	—	—	7.61	—	5.76	7.27
Rheidin C	7.86	—	5.74	—	5.72	5.70	7.43	7.96	5.84	6.39
GaUoyl-3-O-(6'-O-galloyl)glucoside	—	—	5.59	—	—	—	5.67	5.67	6.46	—

Table 2.   The results of 23 compounds of Rhubarb with more than 10 targets docking (*Continued*).

Compounds	TGF-β	SOD	HSP70	MMP-9	MMP-2	iNOS	IL-6	IGF-2	PGIS	COX-1	COX-2
Rhaponticin	7.85	6.64	9.15	6.38	5.10	6.47	—	—	6.59	—	—
Aloe-emodin-ω-O-β-D-glucopyranoside	7.74	5.12	9.58	7.02	6.57	8.95	—	—	5.99	—	—
Toraehrysone-8-O-β-D-glucoside	7.40	6.45	9.76	7.50	5.83	8.44	—	5.17	7.17	—	—
Phenylbutanone-glucoside	7.81	6.24	7.50	6.02	6.41	6.51	—	—	6.68	5.30	—
Emodin-1-O-β-D-glucopyranoside	10.07	5.86	8.97	6.55	6.15	6.26	—	—	6.98	—	—
Isorhapontigenin	7.66	—	6.11	5.60	5.58	5.73	—	—	—	7.01	6.38
Emodin-8-O-β-D-gentiobioside	6.18	5.82	—	6.39	5.82	5.71	—	—	6.79	—	—
5-carboxyl-7-glucose based oxygen-2-methyl benzopyran-y-ketone	7.51	6.04	8.01	7.15	—	7.22	—	—	7.36	—	—
1,2,6-Tri-O-galloyl-glucose	7.56	—	8.23	5.70	—	9.21	5.97	—	7.33	—	—
3,5,4'-Trihydroxystilene-4'-glucoside	7.66	6.57	9.37	6.12	7.12	7.01	—	—	8.09	—	—
1,6-Di-0-galloyl-β-D-glucose	7.68	5.29	5.87	6.81	6.99	7.56	—	—	—	—	—
Rheidin A	6.86	—	—	—	—	7.47	5.05	—	5.44	—	—
GaUoyl-4-O-(6'-O-galloyl)glucoside	5.74	—	5.93	6.06	6.51	6.20	6.16	—	5.45	—	—
1-O-galloyl-β-D-glucose	6.98	5.63	9.93	7.17	—	5.37	—	—	5.98	6.34	6.95
Musizin-8-O-β-D-glucoside	5.90	5.44	7.34	5.19	5.01	7.02	—	—	5.23	—	—
(+)-Catechin-5-O-glucoside	7.07	—	8.50	7.52	7.08	7.05	—	—	5.12	—	—
6-Hydroxy-inusizin-8-O-β-D-glucoside	—	5.45	8.34	8.02	—	—	—	—	6.39	—	—
Chrysophanol-8-O-β-D-glucopyranoside	6.96	6.15	7.27	—	—	6.85	5.74	—	7.10	—	—
Emodin-8-O-β-D-(6'-oxalyl)glucopyranoside	6.35	6.91	8.12	5.88	—	—	—	—	5.76	—	—
Rhein-8-O-β-D-glucopyranoside	9.40	—	6.96	6.22	—	7.43	—	—	6.78	—	—
Physcion-8-O-β-D-glucopyranoside	7.84	5.53	7.86	5.93	—	7.90	—	—	5.49	—	—
Rheidin C	9.43	—	—	—	—	6.60	—	—	—	—	—
GaUoyl-3-O-(6'-O-galloyl)glucoside	6.14	—	10.29	8.30	5.17	7.32	—	—	8.32	—	—

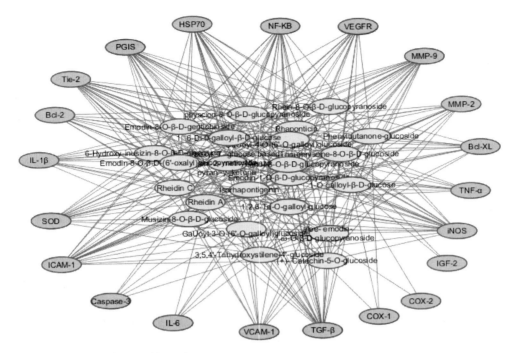

Figure 1.   Compound-Target Network.

of Rhubarb with TGF-β and Tie-2, respectively, the result is that there are 22 compounds combined with these two proteins, respectively, and their docking scores are more than 5.0. According to Table 2, a total of 20 compounds, both with two kinds of protein targets have good binding activity, of which there are nine compounds and their docking score are more than 7.0. Analysis of the above nine kinds of compounds with TGF-β and Tie-2 targets have strong binding activity, speculating that may be the effective substances of Rhubarb in the treatment of cerebral ischemia, via affecting the expressing of TGF-β and Tie-2 targets. However, the pharmacodynamics research needs further verification.

The Bcl-2 protein is one of the important inhibiting apoptosis protein that are known. Over expression of Bcl-2 can inhibit the apoptosis of nerve cells caused by oxygen-free radical, calcium overload, excitatory amino acid, etc. (Gustavsson *et al.*, 2007). The Caspase family is a kind of cytokine in the regulation of apoptosis, and is also the initiator and executor during the cell apoptosis. Caspase-3 plays the pivotal role in the apoptotic process (Rosell *et al.*, 2008). According to the results of Table 2, there are 12, 12, and 5 kinds of compounds, respectively, combined with Bcl-2, Bcl-XL, and Caspase-3, and their docking scores are more than 5.0. In which, there are seven compounds, both with Bcl-2 and Bcl-XL having good binding activity. We speculate that the above seven kinds of compounds may be the effective substances of Rhubarb for the treatment of cerebral ischemia, via affecting the expressing of Bcl-2 and Bcl-XL targets. Analysis of the results, finding that aloe-emodin-ω-O-β-D-glucopyranoside can combine with Bcl-2, Bcl-XL and Caspase-3, and has good binding activity. It may be the effective substance of Rhubarb in the treatment of cerebral ischemia, via influencing the main targets of cerebral ischemia.

The characteristics of TCM are multi-components, multi-channel, multi-target, and multi-effect, making the material foundation of traditional Chinese medicine, the process in vivo, biological effects and mutual relations are quite complex. In general, the more compositions of TCM, the more targets applied to the body in different ways (Wu *et al.*, 2012). According to the results of Table 2, there are 11 compounds, both with the 21 targets having good binding activity. From this, we speculate that these molecules are likely to be very important roles on the expression of the regulation of protein targets related to cerebral ischemia of Rhubarb or with the interaction of these proteins. In addition, these molecules simultaneously targeting multiple protein, as those shown on Fig.1, it demonstrates the characteristics of TCM of synergistic effect of multi-target and multi-effect.

5 SUMMARY

Virtual screening via molecular docking method can be used not only to find the active components of Rhubarb in the treatment of cerebral ischemia, but also to the traditional Chinese medicine compound provide a new reference to the research on multiple targets. Molecular docking simulation is applied to predict the effective substance group of Chinese medicine, improve the efficiency of active component screening, construct the interaction relations between effective material group and target protein interaction, explain the multi-component and multi-target synergy of traditional Chinese medicine composition, and provide a demonstration for studies of the pharmacodynamic material basis of traditional Chinese medicine.

ACKNOWLEDGMENTS

The corresponding author of this study is Prof. Shumei Wang. Her basic information are: Tel: 86-(0)20-3935-2559, Fax: 86-(0)20-3935-2174 and E-mail: shmwang@sina.com.

This study was financially supported by the National Natural Science Foundation of China (Nos. 81073024 and 81274060).

REFERENCES

Duan, A.X., Chen, J., Liu, H.D., Liu, X.H., & Lu, X.Q. (2009) Application and development of molecular-docking method. *Journal of Analytical Science*, 25(4), 473–476.

Durukan, A., & Tatlisumak, T. (2007) Acute ischemic stroke: Overview of major experimental rodent models, pathophysiology, and therapy of focal cerebral ischemia. *Pharmacology, Biochemistry and Behavior*, 87(1), 179–197.

Gustavsson, M., Wilson, M.A., Mallard, C., Rousset, C., Johnston, M.V., & Hagberg, H. (2007) Global gene expression in the developing rat brain after hypoxic preconditioning:involvement of apoptotic mechanisms? *Pediatric Research*, 61(4), 444–450.

Jain, A.N. (2007) Surflex-Dock2.1: Robust performance from ligand energetic modeling,ring flexibility,and knowledge-based search. *Journal of Computer-Aided Molecular Design*, 21(5), 281–306.

Jain, A.N. (2003) Surflex: Fully Automatic Flexible Molecular Docking Using a Molecular Similarity-Based Search Engine. *Journal of Medicinal Chemistry*, 46(4), 499–511.

Li, J.S., Hou, X.J., Zheng, X.K., Li, X.L., Wang, Z.W., & Zhou, Q.A. (2003) Effect of Rhubarb and it's abstract on nitric oxide and tumor necrosis factor of cerebral ischemia rats. *Chinese Journal of Gerontology*, 23(11), 769–771.

Li, J.S., Liu, J.X., Fang, J., Liang, S.W., Wang, D., & Zhang, W.Y. (2005a) Effects of Rhubarb aglycone antagonising cerebral ischemic injury and influence on inflammatory factors in rats with cerebral ischemia. *Journal of Integrated Traditional and Western Medicine in Intentire Critical Care*, 12(5), 275–278.

Li, J.S., Liu, J.X., Liang, S.W., Zhao, J.M., Liu, K., & Wang, M.H. (2004) Effects of glucoside and aglycone parts of Rhubarb on the metabolism of free radicals in rats with ischemic brain injury. *Chinese Journal of Clinical Rehabilitation*, 8(34), 7748–7750.

Li, J.S., Liu, K., Song, Z.J., Gao, L.X., Yang, X.K., Liu, J.X., Zhou, Y.L., Liu, Z.G., & Han X.H. (2013) Effect of Naomaitong on expression of Ang and Tie after cerebral ischemia/reperfusion in aged rats. *China Journal of Traditional Chinese Medicine and Pharmacy*, 28(1), 200–203.

Li, J.S., Liu, J.X., Wang, D., Liang, S.W., Zhang, W.Y., & Fang, J. (2007) Rhubarb aglycone injection antagonism to inflammatory cascade reaction of rats with cerebral ischemia injury. *Chinese Pharmacological Bulletin*, 23(1), 114–118.

Li, J.S., Wang, D., Fang, J., Zhang, W.Y., Liu, J.X., & Zhou, H.X., (2005b) Effect of different-dose Rhubarb aglycone on thrombosis, platelet aggregation and adhesion, and blood coagulation in rats with cerebral ischemia: comparison with aspirin and Nimodipine. *Chinese journal of clinical rehabilitation*, 9(21), 142–144.

Liu, A.L., & Du, G.H. (2003) Method research on virtual screening of acetylcholinesterase inhibitors. *Computers and Applied Chemistry*, 20(5), 547–550.

Liu, J.X., Li, J.S., Liang, S.W., Gao, J.F., Zhao, J.M., Zhang, W.H., (2004). Protective effects of Rhubarb aglycone and its monomers on rats with cerebral ischemia. *Journal of Henan College of Traditional Chinese Medicine*, 19(115), 23–25.

Liu, K., Li, J.S., Zhou, Y.L., Gao, J.F., Yang, X.K., Zhao, Y.W., Liu, Z.G., & Liu, J.X. (2010) Effect of Naomaitong on cerebral angiogenesis and expressions of TGF, bFGF after cerebral ischemia/reperfusion in aged rats. *China Journal of Traditional Chinese Medicine and Pharmacy*, 25(8), 1188–1192.

Mazumdar P.A., Kumaran D., Swaminathan S., & Das, A.K. (2008) A novel acetate-bound complex of human carbonic anhydrase. *Acta Crystallographica Section F, Structural Biology and Crystallization Communications*, 64(3), 163–166.

Rosell, A., Cuadrado, E., Alvarez-Sabín, J., Hernández-Guillamon, M., Delgado, P., Penalba, A., Mendioroz, M., Rovira, A., Fernández-Cadenas, I., Ribó, M., Molina, C.A., & Montaner, J. (2008) Caspase-3 is related to infarct growth after human ischemic stroke. *Neuroscience Letters*, 430(1), 1–6.

Smoot, M.E., Ono, K., Ruscheinski, J., Wang, P.L., & Ideker, T. (2011) Cytoscape 2.8:new features for data integration and network visualization. *Bioinformatics*, 27(3), 431–432.

Sun, J.Y., Cai, S.X., Yan, N., & Mei, H. (2010) Docking and 3D-QSAR studies of influenza neuraminidase inhibitors using three dimensional holographic vector of atomic interaction field analysi. *European Journal of Medicinal Chemistry*, 45(3), 1008–1014.

Wu, K.Z., Zuo, Y., & Li, A.X. (2012) The study of Traditional Chinese Medicine-target using computer-aided drug design. *Journal of Logistics University of CAPF(Medical Sciences)*, 21(6), 479–483.

Zhang, Jin-liang,Guo Y.H., & Gao, C.H. (2010) Design,Synthesis and Molecular Docking of a Novel Small-molecule Inhibitor of Caspase-3.*Chemical Research in Chinese Universities*, 26(2), 256–258.

Medicine Sciences and Bioengineering – Wang (Ed.)
© 2015 Taylor & Francis Group, London, ISBN: 978-1-138-02684-1

Analysis of effect of Pueraria lobata flavone in the cerebral ischemia-reperfusion rats using ^{1}H-NMR-based metabonomics

Chun-wei Wu, Qin-xiao Guan, Shu-mei Wang*, Fan Yang, Lu Zhao, Li Lu &
Yue-ying Rong
Department of Traditional Chinese Medicine, Guangdong Pharmaceutical University, Guangzhou, China

ABSTRACT: Puerariae radix, the dried root of *Pueraria lobata* (Willd.) Ohwi, is one of the most important edible crude herbs used for various medical purposes. Pueraria lobata flavone, a kind of major active components, has been confirmed to play a remarkable curative effect on cerebral ischemia, but the mechanism is not clear. Therefore, in this study, ^{1}H-NMR-based metabonomics approach has been used to investigate the protective effect of PLF on rats of cerebral ischemia-reperfusion. Through principal component analysis, it was observed that metabolic alterations induced by ischemic cerebral-reperfusion were restored after treatment with PLF. Metabolites with significant changes induced by ischemic cerebral-reperfusion, including lactate, taurine, glutamate, choline, glucose, lipids, creatine, which were characterized as potential biomarkers involved in the pathogenesis of ischemic cerebral-reperfusion. All those biomarkers can be regulated by Pueraria lobata flavone treatment, which suggested that the therapeutic effect of PLF on ischemic cerebral-reperfusion may involve in regulating the dysfunctions of energy metabolism, amino acid metabolism, energy metabolism. This study indicated that the Pueraria lobata flavone had protective effect on rats of cerebral ischemia-reperfusion and explored the metabolic regulation mechanism and the NMR-based metabonomics approach might be a promising approach to study mechanisms of traditional Chinese medicines.

1 INTRODUCTION

Stroke, as a cerebrovascular disease, with high incidence and mortality rate, is serious to the public health worldwide every year (Strong *et al*., 2007). Almost, most of the strokes are ischemic cerebral events in both developed and developing countries (Palm *et al*., 2010).

Puerariae radix, the dried root of *Pueraria lobata* (Willd.) Ohwi, is an important crude herb used for various medical purposes. The effective ingredient for treatment of stroke is Pueraria lobata flavone (PLF), which can anti-oxidant (Guerra *et al*., 2000), anti-inflammatory (Lim *et al*., 2013), hypoglycemic (Chung *et al*., 2008), as well as protective effects of nerve cells (Wang *et al*., 2014). But the mechanism of the PLF on stroke is not clear.

Metabonomics is a new scientific techniques for the investigation of the metabolic response of living systems to physiological, disease and drugs stimuli (Nicholson et al., 1999). The application of metabonomics was widely used in the study of Chinese medicine. These include mechanism of new drugs (Zheng *et al*., 2014), evaluation drug toxicity (Xue *et al*., 2014), diagnosis and treatment of disease (Zhang *et al*., 2011). NMR spectroscopy is a powerful tool for generating multivariate metabolic data by measuring hundreds of compounds. ^{1}H-NMR spectroscopic analysis of biofluids has successfully showed lots of novel metabolic biomarkers for drug development and disease diagnosis (Lindon *et al*., 2004). A strategy of data reduction followed by multivariate analysis

---

*Prof. Shumei Wang, department of Traditional Chinese Medicine, Guangdong Pharmaceutical University, is the corresponding author of this research. (Tel:020-39352559; E-mail:shmwang@sina.com)

techniques, such as principal components analysis (PCA), is typically employed. Therefore, we investigated the treatment effect of PLF on cerebral ischemia-reperfusion rat model and explored the metabolic regulation mechanism by using ^{1}H-NMR spectroscopy combined with PCA.

2 MATERIALS AND METHODS

2.1 Reagents and chemicals

The *Pueraria lobata* (Willd.) Ohwi was purchased from Guangzhou Zhixin Chinese medicine Pieces Co. Ltd. and identified by Prof. Shu-yuan Li, Guangdong Phaemacutical university, Guangzhou. The purity of PLF reached 81.8%, which was laboratory-made. Nimodipine (20120508) was purchased from Zhengzhou Ruikang Pharmaceutical Co.Ltd. 2,3,5-Triphenyltetrazolium chloride (TTC) was purchased from Shanghai Shanpu Chemical Industry Co. Ltd. D_2O containing 0.05% sodium 3-trimethylsilyl-(2, 2, 3, 3-$^2H_4$)-1-propionate (TSP) were purchased from Beijing Dimma Technology Co.Ltd.

2.2 Animal grouping and drug administration

42 male Wistar rats (270 $\pm$ 20 g) were purchased from Shandong Lukang Pharmaceutical Co., Ltd. The animals were kept at a temperature of 24$\pm$1° with a humidity of 50$\pm$10% on a 12-h light/dark cycle. This study was approved by the Ethics Committee of Guangdong Pharmaceutical University (No. SPF20120001). 42 rats were randomly divided into six groups, i.e. control group, model group, Nimodipine group and PLF groups (in high, middle and low dose). Rats in the control group and model group were daily given 0.5% CMC-Na suspension. Nimodipine group Rats were daily given nimodipine (6 mg/kg) 0.5% CMC-Na suspension, and rats in PLF group were daily given PLF (200 mg/kg, 100 mg/kg, 50 mg/kg). After 4 days administration, they were administered an hour before surgery on the fifth day.

2.3 Model preparation

The model of focal cerebral ischemia reperfusion is established with the suture-occluded method by Longa (Longa *et al.*, 1989). The rats were injected intraperitoneally with 10% chloral hydrate (0.3 ml/100g) to be anesthetized. After a midline incision was made at the ventral surface of the neck skin, the right common carotid artery (CCA), external carotid artery (ECA), and internal carotid artery (ICA) were isolated. The CCA and ECA were clamped, leaving a small cutting in the crotch of the CCA and ECA. A 4-0 monofilament nylon surgical suture with a rounded tip (Beijing Sunbio Biotech Co. Ltd, Beijing, China) was introduced through the right CCA to the ICA until resistance was felt. After occlusion for 2 hours, the suture was withdrawn, allowing reperfusion. The rats in the control group conduct the same surgical procedures, but without arterial occlusion.

2.4 Observation and evaluation of neurologic impairment

According to the method described by Longa (Longa *et al.*, 1989), the neurologic assessments were scored on a five-point scale: a score of 0 indicated no neurologic deficit; a score of 1 (failure to extend left forepaw fully) indicated a mild focal neurologic deficit; a score of 2 (circling to the left) indicated a moderate focal neurologic deficit, and a score of 3 (falling to the left) indicated a severe focal deficit; rats with a score of 4 did not walk spontaneously and had a depressed level of consciousness.

2.5 Serum collection and sample processing

After 24 h reperfusion, 2 ml blood was acquired via Orbital cavity into EP tube, centrifuged for 10 min (4000 r/min, 4°C). The supernatant was pipetted into EP tube and refrigerated at –80°C.

130 µL of phosphate buffer (0.2 M, Na_2HPO_4/NaH_2PO_4, pH7.4) and 300 µL serum were mixed, After, centrifugation at 4°C and 4000 r/pm) for 5 min, the supernatant was transferred to the 5 mm NMR tube with 150 µL of D_2O containing 0.05% sodium 3-trimethylsilyl-(2, 2, 3, 3-$^2H_4$)-1-propionate (TSP) for ^1H-NMR analysis.

2.6   Brain tissue TTC staining and measurement of infarction area

The brain was rapidly removed and placed in a refrigerator at –20°C for 15 min. The brain was sliced coronally into four pieces beginning from optic chiasma. The second piece of brain slices incubated for 20 minutes in a 2% solution of 2,3,5-triphenyltetrazolium chloride (TTC) at 37°C for vital staining (Bederson et al., 1986). The stained brain slices were washed by saline three times and fixed in 10% formaldehyde solution for being photographed after 24 h. The infarct volumes of brain slices were measured by the computer image processing system.

2.7   Pathological examination of brain tissue

The third piece of brain slices was fixed with 10% formaldehyde solution overnight at 4°C. The thickness of paraffin-embedded sections stained with HE was 4 µm. Brain tissue was observed under a light microscope ($\times$ 400). A slice of each rat was observed in 10 horizons, and calculated the number of normal neuronal cell under each view.

2.8   Data acquisition and processing

All ^1H-NMR experiments were carried out at 298 K on a Bruker Avance 500 MHz spectrometer. The NMR spectrum was recorded using the water-presaturated standard one-dimensional Carr-Purcell-Meiboom-Gill (CPMG) pulse sequence (recycle delay-90°-(τ-180°-τ) $_n$-acquisition). 128 transients were collected into 32k data points using a spectral width of 10 kHz with a relaxation delay of 3 s, and total echo time ($2n\tau$) of 100 ms.

Following phase and baseline correction, each spectrum was automatically segmented into 0.04 ppm width using the software package XWINNMR across the chemical shift 0.50–5.50. Regions containing resonance from residual water (δ4.6–5.5) was excluded. The data of each sample was normalized to the total area to compensate for the effects of variation in concentration. The data were submitted to Simca-P$^+$ 12.0 (Umetrics, Sweden) software for PCA. This was effected by converting each metabolite peak into a coordinate in N-dimensional space and calculating the factors which contribute to the greatest variation across a group of samples. The normalized integral areas of the selected metabolites form PCA results were further statistically analyzed using SPSS17.0 using One-Way ANOVA analysis.

3   RESULTS

3.1   Evaluation of neurologic impairment

After 2 h occlusion, model rats showed piloerection, sluggish, irritability. Neurological score results are shown in Table 1. It is shown that the neurological symptoms have been alleviated in PLF group rats compared with model rats, showing the curative effects of PLF.

3.2   Brain tissue TTC staining and measurement of infarct area

The results of TTC staining are shown in Figure 1 and Table 1. The ischemic tissue was white and the normal brain tissue looked reddish. The brain slice of the control group showed no infarction. In model group, the left half of brain slice was of most infarction. Compared to the model group, infarction areas of brain slices of the PLF group reduced, especially in a middle dose group. It is shown that PLF had a protective effect on cerebral ischemia brain tissue.

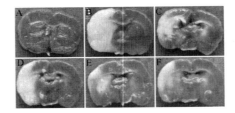

Figure 1. The TTC colorable graphs of cerebral tissue from A. Control group; B. Model group; C. Nimodipine group; D. Low-dose group (50 mg/kg) of PLF; E. Middle-dose group (100 mg/kg) of PLF; F. High-dose group (100 mg/kg) of PLF.

Table 1. The results of nervous symptom score and cerebral infarction area (n = 7).

	Evaluation of neurologic impairment(score)	Infarct area (%)
Control group	0.00 ± 0.00**	0.00 ± 0.00
Model group	$2.53 \pm 0.26^{\Delta\Delta}$	35.88 ± 1.8
Nimodipine group	1.50 ± 0.31*	24.44 ± 3.7
Low-dose group of PLF group	2.00 ± 0.29*	20.17 ± 4.4
Middle-dose group of PLF group	2.00 ± 0.32*	19.27 ± 2.7
High-dose group of PLF group	1.83 ± 0.32*	23.73 ± 3.8

Note: *as compared with model group, **$p < 0.01$*, $p < 0.05$; $^{\Delta}$as compared with control group, $^{\Delta\Delta}p < 0.01$, $^{\Delta}p < 0.05$.

3.3 Brain pathological examination

As shown in Figure 2 and Table 2, compared to control rats, the number of normal cells reduced in model rats. However, the number of normal cells in PLF group were more than model group, showing that PLF, especially a middle dose, could reduce neuronal apoptosis.

3.4 ¹H-NMR analysis of serum

3.4.1 Metabolites Identification of 1H CPMG Spectra of serum

Figure 3 shows representative 500 MHz ¹H-NMR CPMG spectra of serum from all groups. Assignments of endogenous metabolites were based on the literature (Shi et al., 2013; Chen et al., 2011; Peng et al., 2011) and confirmed by 2D spectroscopy. The serum NMR spectra were dominated by lipid (δ0.86, δ1.26), leucine (δ0.95, 0.97), valine(δ1.03), 3-hydroxybutyrate (δ1.18), lactate (δ1.33, δ4.12), alanine (δ1.48), N-acetyl aspartate (NAA) (δ2.02), glutamate (δ2.14), acetoacetate (δ2.24), pyruvate (δ2.38), citrate (δ2.54, δ2.68), dimethylamine (δ2.72), creatine (δ3.02), choline (δ3.22), taurine (δ3.26, δ3.42), glycine (δ3.54), Glycerol (δ3.64), citrulline (δ3.71), tyrosine (δ3.94) and glucose (δ3.4-4.0).

3.4.2 PCA and statistical analysis of plasma spectra data

A PCA model was performed for model group and the control group (Figure 4A) and revealed a satisfactory discrimination. The loading plots (Figure 4B) revealed that the resonances responsible

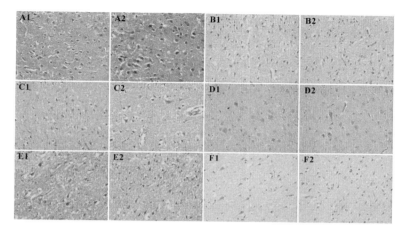

Figure 2. HE colorable graphs of cerebral tissue (×400) A1: Cells of cerebral cortex in control group; A2: Cells of hippocampus in control group; B1: Cells of cerebral cortex in model group; B2: Cells of hippocampus in model group; C1: Cells of cerebral cortex in nimodipine group; C2: Cells of hippocampus in nimodipine group; D1, E1, F1: Cells of cerebral cortex in 200, 100, 50 mg/kg of PLF group; D2, E2, F2: Cells of hippocampus in 200, 100, 50 mg/kg of PLF group.

Table 2. The semi-quantitative results of the pathological sections of cerebral issue ($n = 7$).

Group	–	+	++	+++	Group	–	+	++	+++
Control group	7	0	0	0	Low-dose group of PLF group	1	2	1	3
Model group	0	0	0	7	Middle-dose group of PLF	3	2	1	1
Nimodipine group	2	2	2	1	High-dose group of PLF group	2	3	1	1

Note: "–" Neuronal cells and glial cells were normal; "+" A small number of neurons were edema or atrophy, glial cells were normal; "+ +" Neuronal cells were edema or atrophy, glial cells were disappeared; "+ + +" Neuronal cells were clear edema or partial atrophy, glial cells were disappeared.

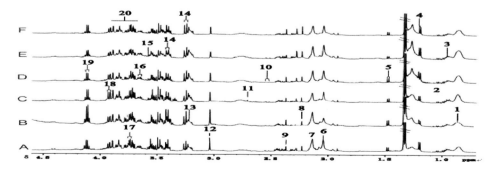

Figure 3. Typical ^{1}H NMR cpmg spectra of plasma from four groups: (A) Control group; (B) Model group; (C) Nimodipine group; (D) Low-dose group of PLF group; (E) Middle-dose group of PLF group; (F) High-dose group of PLF group. Main metabolites: 1. Lipid; 2.Leucine; 3.Valine; 4. 3-Hydroxybutyrate; 5.Alanine; 6.N-Acetyl Aspartate; 7.Glutamate; 8.Acetoacetate; 9.Pyruvate; 10.Citrate; 11.Dimethylamine; 12.Creatine; 13.Choline; 14.Taurine; 15.Glycine; 16.Glycerol; 17.Citrulline; 18.Tyrosine; 19.Lactate; 20.Glucose.

for the discrimination were lactate, glutamate, glycine, taurine, choline, glucose, 3-hydroxybutyrate, lipids, creatinine. Meanwhile, PCA plot was obtained when the analysis was performed for model group and PLF groups (Figure 4C), which showed clear clustered separation. Last, a PCA model was performed for model group and middle-dose of PLF group. The loading plots (Figure 4D) revealed that the discrimination attributed to the same variables as mentioned above.

Table 3 listed the results of the statistical analysis for comparison. The resonances assigned to lactate, taurine, glutamate, choline, glucose were significantly increased, but the level of lipids, creatine was statistically decreased in model group compared to control group. Middle-dose PLF group had higher levels of lipids and creatine, but lower levels of lactate, taurine, glutamate, choline and glucose. However, the levels of glycine and 3-Hydroxybutyrate did not present significant alterations in middle-dose PLF group compared to model group.

4 DISCUSSION

In our study, we conducted experiments of neurologic impairment evaluation, brain tissue TTC, and HE staining, showing that the PLF could reduce the neurologic impairment, brain infarct area and cell apoptosis. Consequently, a ^{1}H-NMR-based metabonomics method combined with PCA

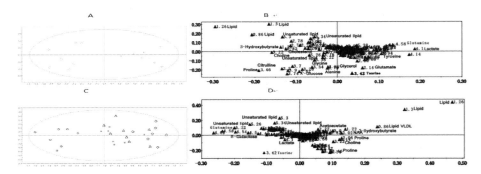

Figure 4. PCA results of plasma ^{1}H-NMR spectra A: score plots of model group vs control group; B: loading score plots of model group vs control group; C: score plot of model group vs PLF groups; D: loading plots of model group vs middle-dose group of PLF group; + Control group; ○ Model group; △ High-dose group of PLF group; *Middle-dose group of PLF group; ◇ Low-dose group of PLF group.

Table 3. Main metabolite changes of serum by statistical analysis ($n = 7$).

Main metabolite	Model vs Control group	PLF vs Model group	Main metabolite	Model vs Control group	PLF vs Model group
Lactate	↑$^{\Delta\Delta}$	↓**	Glucose	↑$^{\Delta\Delta\Delta}$	↓***
Taurine	↑$^{\Delta}$	↓	Lipids	↓$^{\Delta\Delta}$	↑**
Glutamate	↑$^{\Delta\Delta}$	↓**	3-Hydroxybutyrate	↓	↑
Glycine	↑	↓	Creatine	↓$^{\Delta\Delta\Delta}$	↑***
Choline	↑$^{\Delta\Delta}$	↓**			

Note: $^{\Delta}$as compared with control group, $^{\Delta\Delta\Delta}p < 0.001$, $^{\Delta\Delta}p < 0.01$, $^{\Delta}p < 0.05$; * as compared with model group, ***$p < 0.01$, **$p < 0.01$, *$p < 0.05$.

was employed to study the serum metabolite changes of cerebral ischemia-reperfusion and the effect of PLF. PCA scores plots demonstrated that the cluster of model rats was separated from control rats; rats of PLF group were classified from model rats.

4.1 *Energy metabolism*

Normally, there is sufficient supply of oxygen and glucose. While in the cerebral ischemia, glucose is difficult to through the blood brain barrier, which becomes the rate limiting step of its utilization (Li *et al.*, 2005). The level of glucose in the serum decreased in the PLF group in comparison with those in the model group, indicating that the PLF had a regulatory effect of the glucose metabolism in cerebral ischemia rats.

Creatine (Cr) can reflect the changes of energy metabolism in the brain (Ross & Michaelis, 1994). Balestrino found Cr can effectively restrain the injury of hypoxia ischemia caused by depolarization, which speculated that Cr could protect brain tissue of ischemia hypoxia (Balestrino *et al.*, 2002). Our research showed that the PLF can effectively improve the concentration of Cr in order to increase the energy supply.

Once cerebral ischemia, ATP rapidly depletes and anaerobic glycolysis strengthens in brain tissue, which will produce large quantities of lactate. With the accumulation of lactate H+, it may cause lactic acidosis, which further aggravates the injury of nerve cells. The research showed that the level of lactate in serum decreased in the PLF group in comparison with the model group, indicating that the PLF avoid lactic acidosis to protect the nerve cells.

4.2 *Amino acids metabolism*

Glutamate is released in superphysiological amounts during cerebral ischemia. This excitotoxicity is mediated by several glutamate receptor subtypes (Akins & Atkinson, 2002), consequently, causing the ion imbalance and calcium overload. The level of glutamate in serum decreased obviously in PLF group compared with the model group, indicating that the PLF could significantly reduce the level of glutamate by possibly reducing the influx of Ca^{2+}.

Taurine possesses antioxidant properties and Wang found that PLF could improve the activity of SOD and reduce the level of MDA in the brain (Wang *et al.*, 2006). It is key for osmoregulation, membrane stabilization (Wang *et al.*, 1996), Ca^{2+} flux regulation (Condron *et al.*, 2003). This study showed that compared with control rats, the level of taurine increased significantly in model rats, while the level of taurine decreased in PLF group compared with the model group, indicating that the PLF continued to maintain the moderate level of taurine.

4.3 *Lipid metabolism*

Choline is a constituent of cell membranes. The increase of choline served as a biomarker of cerebral ischemia, which probably came from the products of membrane breakdown (Yang *et al.*, 2013). Decreased choline was found in the serum of PLF rats compared with model rats. It indicated that the PLF may keep the balance of lipid metabolism in cerebral ischemia.

5 SUMMARY

In our study, a ^{1}H-NMR-based metabonomics method combined with PCA was employed to study the protective effect of the PLF. The PLF regulated the metabolic disorders and promoted the regression of the metabolic phenotype close to the normal range. This study could provide evidence that ^{1}H-NMR-based metabonomics method is a useful tool in the investigation of metabolic regulation mechanisms of traditional Chinese medicine.

ACKNOWLEDGMENTS

This work was supported by the National Natural Science Foundation of China (81073024 and 81274060).

REFERENCES

Akins, P.T. & Atkinson, R.P. (2002) Glutamate AMPA receptor antagonist treatment for ischaemic stroke. *Current Medical Research and Opinion*, 18(suppl 2), S9–S13.

Balestrino, M., Lensman, M., Parodi, M., Perasso, L., Rebaudo, R., Melani, R., Polenov, S. & Cupello, A. (2002) Role of creatine and phosphocreatine in neuronal protection from anoxic and ischemic damage. *Amino Acids*, 23(1–3), 221–229.

Bederson, J.B., Pitts, L.H., Germano, S.M., Nishimura, M.C., Davis, R.L. & Bartkowski, H.M. (1986) Evaluation of 2,3,5-triphenyltetrazolium chloride as a stain for detection and quantification of experimental cerebral infarction in rats. *Stroke*, 17(6), 1304–1308.

Chen, F., Zhang, J., Song, X., Yang, J., Li, H., Tang, H. & Liao, Y.C. (2011) Combined metabonomic and quantitative real-time PCR analyses reveal systems metabolic changes of Fusarium graminearum induced by Tri5 gene deletion. *Journal of Proteome Research*, 10(5), 2273–2285.

Chung, M.J.; Sung, N.J.; Park, C.S.; Kweon, D.K.; Mantovani, A.; Moon, T.W.; Lee, S.J. & Park, K.H (2008) Antioxidative and hypocholesterolemic activities of water-soluble puerarin glycosides in HepG2 cells and in C57 BL/6J mice. *European Journal of Pharmacology*, 578(2-3), 159–170.

Condron, C.; Neary, P.; Toomey, D.; Redmond, H. P. & Bouchier-Hayes, D. (2003) Taurine attenuates calcium-dependent, Fas-mediated neutrophil apoptosis. *Shock*, 19 (6), 564–569.

Guerra, M.C.; Speroni, E.; Broccoli, M.; Cangini, M.; Pasini, P.; Minghett, A.; Crespi-Perellino, N.; Mirasoli, M.; Cantelli-Forti, G. & Paolini, M. (2000) Comparison between chinese medical herb Pueraria lobata crude extract and its main isoflavone puerarin antioxidant properties and effects on rat liver CYP-catalysed drug metabolism. *Life Sciences*, 67(24), 2997–3006.

Li, X.Y., Li, X.Z. & Zhang, A.M. (2005) The expression of glucose transporter1(GLUT1) in blood-brain barrier following cerebralischemia in rats. Shandong Medicine, 45(7), 10–11.

Lim, D.W., Lee, C., Kim, I.H. & Kim, Y.T. (2013) Anti-Inflammatory Effects of Total Isoflavones from Pueraria lobata on Cerebral Ischemia in Rats. *Molecules*, 18(9), 10404–10412.

Lindon, J.C., Holmes, E. & Nicholson, J.K. (2004) Metabonomics and its role in drug development and disease diagnosis. *Expert Review of Molecular Diagnostics*, 4(2), 189–199.

Longa, E.Z., Weinstein, P.R., Carlson, S. & Cummins, R. (1989) Reversible middle cerebralatery occlusion without craniectomy in rats. *Stroke*, 20(1), 84–91.

Palm, F., Urbanek, C., Rose, S., Buggle, F., Bode, B., Hennerici, M.G., Schmieder, K., Inselmann, G., Reiter, R., Fleischer, R., Piplack, K.O., Safer, A., Becher, H. & Grau, A.J. (2010) Stroke Incidence and Survival in Ludwigshafenam Rhein, Germany: the Ludwigshafen Stroke Study (LuSSt). *Stroke*, 41(9), 1865–1870.

Peng, J.B., Jia, H.M., Xu, T., Liu, Y.T., Zhang, H.W., Yu, L.L. & Cai, D.Y. (2011) A 1H-NMR based metabonomics approach to progress of coronary atherosclerosis in a rabbit model. *Process Biochemistry*, 46(12), 2240–2247.

Ross, B. & Michaelis, T. (1994) Clinical application of magnetic resonance spectroscopy. *Magn Reson Q*, 10, 191–247.

Shi, B., Tian, J., Xiang, H., Guo, X., Zhang, L., Du, G. & Qin, X. (2013) A ^{1}H-NMR plasma metabonomic study of acute and chronic stress models of depression in rats. *Behavioural Brain Research*,241, 86–91.

Strong, K., Mathers, C. & Bonita, R. (2007) Preventing stroke: saving lives around the world. *Lancet Neurology*, 6(2), 182–187.

Wang, J. H.; Redmond, H. P.; Watson, R. W.; Condron, C. & Bouchier-Hayes, D. (1996) The beneficial effect of taurine on the prevention of human endothelial cell death. *Shock*, 6 (5), 331–338.

Wang, N., Zhang, Y., Wu, L., Wang, Y., Cao, Y., He, L., Li, X. & Zhao, J. (2014) Puerarin protected the brain from cerebral ischemia injury via astrocyte apoptosis inhibition. *Neuropharmacology*, 79, 282–289.

Wang, P.Y., Wang, H.P. & Li, G.W. (2006) The protective effects of Pueraria lobata flavone on cerebral ischemia reperfusion rats. *China Journal of Chinese Materia Medica*, 31(7), 577–579.

Xue, L.M., Zhang, Q.Y., Han, P., Jiang, Y.P., Yan, R.D., Wang, Y., Rahman, K., Jia, M., Han, T. & Qin, L.P. (2014) Hepatotoxic constituents and toxicological mechanism of Xanthium strumarium L. Fruits. *Journal of Ethnopharmacology*, 152(2), 272–282.

Yang, Y., Wang, L., Wang, S., Liang, S., Chen, A., Tang, H., Chen, L. & Deng, F.Study of metabonomic profiles of human esophageal carcinoma by use of high-resolution magic-angle spinning ¹H-NMR spectroscopy and multivariate data analysis. Analytical and Bioanalytical Chemistry, 405(10), 3381–3389.

Zhang, B., Halouska, S., Schiaffo, C.E., Sadykov, M.R., Somerville, G.A. & Powers, R. (2011) NMR analysis of a stress response metabolic signaling network. *Journal of Proteome Research*,10(8), 3743–3754.

Zheng, X.F., Tian J.S., Liu, P., Xing, J. & Qin, X.M. (2014) Analysis of the restorative effect of Bu-zhong-yi-qi-tang in the spleen-qi deficiency rat model using ¹H-NMR-based metabonomics. *Journal of Ethnopharmacology*, 151(2), 912–920.

Medicine Sciences and Bioengineering – Wang (Ed.)
© *2015 Taylor & Francis Group, London, ISBN: 978-1-138-02684-1*

Solid-phase synthesis of octapeptide GHGKHKNK

Xiao Han, Meng-chuan Zhang, Shuang Jiang, Li-ping An, Guang-yv Xv,
Guang-hong Wang & Pei-ge Du*
*Department of Microbial and Biochemical Pharmacy, College of Pharmaceutical Science, Beihua
University, Jilin, Jilin Province, China*

ABSTRACT: This work introduces the solid-phase synthesis process of octapeptide GHGKHKNK.
2-Chlorotrityl resin, trityl resin, 4-methyl trityl resin, or 4-methoxy trityl resin was used as the starting
materials; by the method of solid-phase synthesis, amino acids having a protecting group were
connected sequentially, to acquire protected octapeptide resin. The process has the advantages of
simple operation and high yield. In addition, the antitumor drugs having GHGKHKNK as the main
active ingredient can inhibit tumor metastasis.

1 INTRODUCTION

In recent years, increasing attention has been paid to synthetic antitumor peptides. Modern
chemotherapy based on synthetic peptides has the potential to provide an effective anti-metastasis
treatment for cancer patients while minimizing severe side effects (Oyston *et al.*, 2009).

GHGKHKNK, an octapeptide derived from domain 5 (D5) of human high-molecular weight
kininogen (HKa), was initially found to inhibit the invasion and migration of melanoma cells
(Kawasaki *et al.*, 2003). In recent years, our group members are researching the effect and mechanism of the GHGKHKNK peptide in anti-metastasis. In our previous study (Xiao *et al.*, 2012),
we measured the effect of the octapeptide on tumor metastasis of a HCCLM3 human hepatocarcinoma cell line and in a nude mouse model of hepatocellular carcinoma and to detect the underlying mechanisms of any inhibitory effects. The results showed that, GHGKHKNK, an octapeptide
derived from HKa D5, showed a significant inhibitory effect on the metastatasis by the HCCLM3
cell line in vitro and in vivo. This effect appeared to occur, at least in part, through regulation of
MMP-2 expression. Our study will provide fundamental basis for R&D of this drug.

Currently, chemical synthesis becomes the main method of obtain small-molecule peptides.
But we all know that the raw material for synthesis is very expensive, and the yield is low. Also,
it is difficult to purify and brought many difficulties to the researchers (Ariamala *et al.*, 2000).
Therefore, solid-phase synthesis technology was used in this study to simplify and improve the
process of GHGKHKNK synthesis.

2 MATERIALS AND METHODS

2.1 *Materials*

2-Chlorotritylresin, ethanol, methyl alcohol, ether, ethylene, mercaptan, thioanisole, acetonitrile,
ethyldiisopropylamine, N,N-Dimethylformamide, 2,2-dimethylolbutanoicacid, piperidine,
O-(Benzotriazol1yl)-N,N,N',N'-tetramethyluronium tetrafluoroborate, O-(7-Azabenzotriazol1yl)-
NNN'N'-tetramethyluronium hexafluophosphate, N-hydroxybenzotrizole, ammonium acetate,

---

*Pei-ge Du is the corresponding author of this article; e-Mail: dupeige2001@126.com.

tallow fatty acid, trityl chloride resin, and various amino acids were bought from Beijing Dingguo Changshengh Biotechnologh Co. Ltd . The above reagents were of analytical grade. Hat reagent: PIP:DMF = 1:5 (v/v); Coupling reagent: NMM:DMF = 1:9 (v/v); Cut peptide reagent: TFA:H$_2$O:Ethanedithio:Thioanisole = 650:17:17:4 (v/v).

2.2   Methods

2.2.1   *Preparation of Fmoc-Lys (Boc)-resins*
Fifty grams of 4- methyl trityl resin (2-chlorotrityl resin, trityl resin, 4-methoxy trityl resin) was soaked with DMF (Mian *et al.*,2005) for 30 minutes until the resin is fully swollen. A volume of 44 mL DIPEA (or DMPA) was added to 46.9 g Fmoc-Lys (Boc)-OH, and kept at 10°C-15°C for 3 hours. A volume of 50 mL methanol was added in, and again kept for 3 hours. Nitrogen dried, washed with DMF for three times, and Fmoc-Lys (Boc)-resin was obtained.

2.2.2   *Removal of amino protection group*
A volume of 500 mL Hat reagent was added to the Fmoc-Lys (Boc)-resin , kept at 25°C for 30 minutes, filtered with nitrogen; washed with DMF, methanol, and again with DMF, and finally dried with nitrogen.

2.2.3   *Coupling reaction*
Fmoc-Asn(Trt)-OH (MV: 596.7,200 mmol) 119.9 g, TBTU (MW: 321,200 mmol) 64.2 g, HOBT (MW: 153,200 mmol) 30.6g, and coupling reagent 440 mL were added into the above reaction, then the mixture reacts for 1 hour at 25°C. Nitrogen dried, then washed with DMF, anhydrous methanol, and DMF. Dried by nitrogen to obtain Fmoc-Asn (Trt)-Lys (Boc) - resins. According to the above method, Fmoc-Lys (Boc)-OH, Fmoc-His (Trt)-OH, Fmoc-Lys (Boc)-OH, Fmoc -Gly-OH, Fmoc-His (Trt)-OH, and Boc-Gly-OH were added to the reaction separately in accordance with the amino acid sequence of the peptide chain.Then repeat the coupling reaction process to receive the desired peptide chain. The feeding amount of each amino acid, coupling reaction time, and deprotection reaction time was presented in Table 1.

2.2.4   *Peptide cutting*
The octapeptide resin obtained was precisely weighed, transferred into an eggplant-shaped bottle, and chopped peptide reagent: (TFA/water/ethanedithiol/thioanisole = 650 mL/17 mL/17 mL/34 mL) was added under cooling condition and 25°C and stirred for 2 hours. Filtered, drained, and the filtrate was precipitated by anhydrous ether. Then filtered and collected the sediment, dried by P$_2$O$_5$ in vacuum, receiving crude octapeptide.

Table 1.   The feeding amount of each amino acid, coupling reaction time and deprotection reaction time.

Amino acid	Feeding amount of amino acids(g)	Coupling reaction time (min)	Deprotection reaction time (min)
Fmoc-Lys(Boc)-OH	93.7	60	30
Fmoc-His(Trt)-OH	123.9	60	30
Fmoc-Lys(Boc)-OH	93.7	60	30
Fmoc-Gly-OH	59.5	60	30
Fmoc-His(Trt)-OH	123.9	60	30
Boc-Gly-OH	35.4	60	30

2.2.5 Purification of peptide

The crude peptide was dissolved in NH₄AC, filtered, separated and purified by HPLC. The filtrate was purified in batches through C18.The mobile phase was 0.1M NH₄AC:acetonitrile (7.5:2.5); the flow speed was 380 mL/min; detection wavelength: 280 nm; the effluent was collected by liquid chromatography. The sample peak was desalted after combination, and then lyophilized to obtain a massive white loose product. The purity of the peptide was tested by Agilent HPLC 1100. The column was sepaxGp-C18 reverse phase column (5 um, 4.6 mm × 150 mm, 120 A), and eluent was 0.1M; NH₄AC: acetonitrile (v/v) = 7.5:2.5; flow speed 380 mL/min; detection wavelength: 280 nm. Flight mass spectrometer (Agilent, LC/MSD TOF) was used to detect the relative molecular mass of the target product.

3 RESULTS

In this study, 4-methyl trityl resin was used as raw material for the synthesis of octapeptide, the amount of other materials are shown in Table 1, and the resin feeding amount, product yield, and product purity are shown in Table 2.

This research, through the method of solid-phase to synthetise GHGKHKNK peptide, using flight mass spectrometer to detect the relative molecular mass of the synthesized product, proved the correctness of the experimental results , as shown in Figure 1. The sample molecular ion peak M + 1 is 905.124, so the measured molecular mass of the sample is 904.124. The difference between the theoretical and measured values of the relative molecular mass of octapeptide compounds in the range of ±1.0 is allowed.

Table 2. Resin feeding amount,yield, purity and yield.

Resin species	resin amount(g)	crude peptide yield (mg)	refined peptide yield (mg)	purity %	peptide yield %	pure product yield %
4-Methyl trityl resin	50	37	14.5	98.3	88	32.0

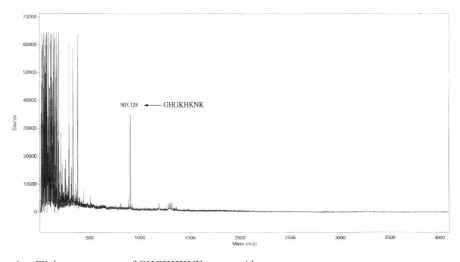

Figure 1. Flight mass spectra of GHGKHKNK octapeptide.

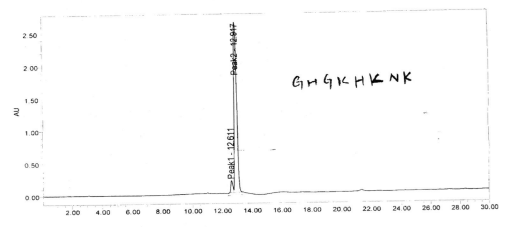

Figure 2.   HPLC spectrum of GHGKHKNK octapeptides.

The crude octapeptide was purified by HPLC, with a purity up to 98%, and it has stable physical and chemical properties, as shown in Figure 2. The retention time tR of GHGKHKNK octapeptide compound is 12.917 min.

4   SUMMARY

In 1963, Merrifield proposed the solid-phase synthesis of peptide for the first time (Merrifield, 1986).This method is an iterative process of adding amino acids. First, the C-terminal of amino acid is fixed to the insoluble resin, followed by the condensation of the amino acid on the resin to extend peptide chain. Solid-phase synthesis methods can greatly reduce the difficulty of purification of the product in each step (Pantarotto *et al.* 2002). To prevent side reactions, the side chains of amino acids are protected, but the carboxyl terminal is free. So the amino acids must be activated before the reaction. In this study, the first protected amino acid Fmoc-Lys (Boc)-OH was fixed in 4-methyl-trityl resin, afterward deprotected by Hat reagent, exposing amino group, then the next protected amino acids were added for condensation. In this work, use of coupling reagent (NMM: DMF = 1:5 v / v) can enhance the yield (yield of peptide received per step $\geq$ 84%). Adding ether to precipitate the crude peptide can avoid using hydrogen fluoride and other toxic agents, reducing pollution, and improve the yield. Using C18 (or C8) column for the separation and purification can avoid applying TFA, reducing waste (Chiara *et al.*, 2007), and the total yield is 25%-35%. The purity of the octapeptide obtained is high. The process of separation and purification has no impact on the biologically active products. The relative molecular mass of GHGKHKNK octapeptide which is determined by flight mass spectrometer is not very different from the theoretical value. It also displayed a high and specific activity against tumor metastasis (Xiao *et al.*, 2012). Therefore, the preparation process of GHGKHKNK octapeptide proposed in this study is stable and has short production cycle, low production costs, less waste, high yield, stable quality, and large-scale production capacity.

ACKNOWLEDGMENTS

This work was funded by project 31201061 supported by the National Natural Science Foundation of China, project 20110729, 20130522051JH supported by Jilin Province Sci-tech Department (China) and project 2013625030 supported by Jilin City Sci-tech Bureau (China).

REFERENCES

Ariamala G., Hui Y. & John W. (2000) Parallel Solid-Phase Synthesis of Vitronectin Receptor(v3) Inhibitors. *Bioorganic & Medicinal Chemistry Letters*, 10(15),1715–1718.

Merrifield R.B. (1986) Foreign pharmaceutical synthetic medicine, biochemical drugs, formulations. *Solid phase synthesis*, 7(5), 295–300.

Mian L., George B., & David L. (2005) Parallel solid-phase synthesis of mucin-like glycopeptides. *Carbohydrate Research*, 340, 2111–2122.

Kawasaki M., et al. (2003) Effect of His-Gly-Lys motif derived from domain 5 of high molecular weight kininogen on suppression of cancer metastasis both in vitro and in vivo. *J Biol Chem*, 278, 49301–49307.

Oyston P.C., et al.(2009) Novel peptide therapeutics for treatment of infections. *J Med Microbiol*, 58(Pt 8), 977–987.

Pantarotto D., et al.(2002) Solid-Phase Synthesis of Fullerene-peptides. *American Chemical Society*, 42(5),12543–12549.

Xiao H., et al. (2012) GHGKHKNK octapeptide (P-5m) inhibits metastasis of HCCLM3 cell lines via regulation of MMP-2 expression in in vitro and in vivo studies. *Molecules*, 17(2),1357–1372.

Chiara F., et al. (2007) Synthesis and biological activity of stable branched neurotensin peptides for tumor targeting. *Mol Cancer Ther*, 6(9), 2441–2448.

Medicine Sciences and Bioengineering – Wang (Ed.)
© 2015 Taylor & Francis Group, London, ISBN: 978-1-138-02684-1

The anti-inflammatory activity of a natural occurring coumarin: Murracarpin

Wei-mei Shi, Hai-qing Liu, Lin-fu Li & Long-huo Wu[*]
College of Pharmacy, Gannan Medical University, Jiangxi, China

ABSTRACT: Murracarpin, a natural occurring couamrin, exhibits anti-inflammatory activity. By using Discovery Studio software, the 3D model of 5-LOX was successfully homology built. Molecular docking researches found that murracarpin positioned in the active site of COX-2 and interacted with Val-523 in a strong hydrogen bond, interacted with 5-LOX in two hydrogen bonds. In carrageenin pleurisy model, murracarpin could effectively inhibit the elevation of IL-1β, TNF-α, and PGE2. These biological efforts might underline the anti-inflammatory mechanism of murracarpin, which could be a good lead compound for further research.

1 INTRODUCTION

The two enzymes Cyclooxygenases (COXs) and Lipoxygenase (LOXs) are both included in the metabolism of Arachidonic Acid (AA). COXs are the rate-limiting enzymes that convert AA to Prostaglandins (PGs). Of three COX isozymes (Bazan, 2002), COX-2 has become the focus of growing attention, because selective COX-2 inhibitory drugs target its high inducibility by inflammation. However, it has been pointed out that inhibiting COX pathway could shunt the metabolism of AA toward the 5-LOX pathway, increasing the formation of Leukotrienes (LTs), and leading to inflammation (Asako, 1992). Therefore, it is expected that dual inhibitors against both COX-2 and 5-LOX should present an enhanced anti-inflammatory potency without risks of serious side effects (Scholz, 2008). Coumarins, have been revealed to posses multiple biological and pharmacological properties, including anti-inflammatory and anti-oxidant activities (Wu, 2009). Murracarpin, 8-(1′-methyloxy-2′-hydroxy-3′-methylbut-1′-enyl)-7-methyloxy-2H-1-chromen-2-one, had been reported to have moderated activities in anti-leukemia and anti-proliferation (Norihito, 2004).

To explore the mechanisms of the anti-inflammatory activity of murracarpin, we used the software Discovery Studio (DS) 2.1 to dock COX-2 and 5-LOX with murracarpin, and duplicated carrageenin pleurisy model to evaluate the contents of proinflammatory cytokines such as IL-1β, TNF-α, and PGE2. We found that murracarpin exhibited anti- inflammatory activity by inhibiting COX-2, 5-LOX, IL-1β, TNF-α, and PGE2.

2 EXPERIMENTAL SECTIONS

2.1 *General*

KunMing strains of male rats weighing 200 ± 20 g were obtained from the animal house of Nanchan University. All experimental procedures were approved by the Institutional Animal Ethical Committee of Gannan Medical University. Murracarpin was dissolved in 1% tween-80 to give a final concentration of 50, 25, and 12.5 mg/kg for intraperitoneal injection for each rat. The ELISA kits of IL-1β, TNF-α, and PGE2 were purchased from U.S. R&D System.

---

[*]Correspondence and reprint request to Dr. L.H. Wu: longhw@126.com

2.2 Molecular modeling

The 3D model of 5-LOX was constructed by employing Discovery Studio (DS) software, version 2.1. Alignments the sequence of human 5-LOX with the structures of 15-LOX, 3-LOX, and 1-LOX were carried out. Homology model of 5-LOX was built according to the template 15-LOX. Molecular modeling studies were carried out using DS 2.1. Docking simulations were performed inside the murine COX-2 (PDB entry 6COX) and the human 5-LOX enzymes. The binding mode with the best fit as well as the function score was selected.

2.3 Carrageenin Pleurisy model

Pleurisy was induced in male rats by intrapheural injection of 0.2 ml of 2% λ-carrageenin under 3% pentobarbitone anesthesia (Harada, 1996). Murracarpin and hexadecadrol were intraperitoneal injection 30 min before the injection of carrageenin. 6 h later, the rats were exsanguinated under anesthesia at given times. The pleural fluid was harvested, and its volume was measured. The pleural fluid was then centrifuged at 3000 g for 10 min at 4°C. The resulting supernatant was collected and applied to the ELISA determinations of IL-1β, TNF-α, and PGE2.

2.4 Data analysis

Results were expressed as mean ± S.D. Statistical analyses were performed with one-way ANOVA followed by Student's t-test.

3 RESULTS AND DISCUSSION

3.1.1 Docking in COX-2 and 5-LOX models

5-LOX has been developed as a major target for the discovery of anti-inflammatory agents. Although various 5-LOX inhibitors have been synthesized or discovered to date, the mechanism by which they interact with 5-LOX is poorly understood due to the deficiency of structural information about 5-LOX. It has been reported that 120 amino acids in N-terminal were not essential for catalytic activity in LOXs (Zheng, 2006). For structural integrity, we herein kept these 120 residues and used 15-LOX as the template for creating a 3D model of human 5-LOX.

Built by homology module, the 3D model of human 5-LOX was obtained after energy minimization (Figure 1). The Profile-3D compatibility scores for the initial and final 3D model were 235.17 and 258.03, respectively. Further checked by Procheck software and Prostat (online) (Zheng, 2006), the final 5-LOX model (after equilibrium and reminimizatioin) showed that more 90.7% residue φ-ψ angels were in the 'core' regions of Ramachandran plot, the Z-score was -10.36, and the overall G-factor was -0.03, indicating again that the final human 3D model of 5-LOX was acceptable.

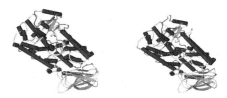

Figure 1.   Comparisons of secondary structure of 15-LOX model (left) with that of the 5-LOX structure (right). α-Helices were represented as cylinders, β-sheets as flat ribbons, and coils as strands. Each secondary structural element in 15-LOX is denoted the same color as the corresponding part of 5-LOX.

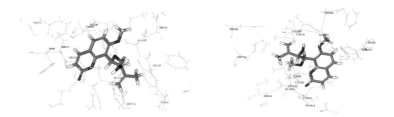

Figure 2. Docking of murracarpin into the COX-2 (upper) and the 5-LOX (lower) active sites. Different regions of the active site as well as key residues were explicitly shown.

The structural shape of murracarpin was very similar to 'T'. When docked in the COX-2 active site (Figure 2), the coumarin nucleus occupied the upper part of the channel. The hydrophilic groups like carbonyl group and hydroxyl group in the side chain were directed to side pocket. Although no groups were fully inserted into the side pocket, the hydroxyl group interacted with Val-523 in a strong hydrogen bond (d = 2.01205 Å). On the opposite side, the methoxyl group came near to Ser-530.

In contrast to COX enzymes, structural knowledge about the 5-LOX active site is much more limited. The active site is a deep cleft, bent in shape, which includes the catalytic non-heme iron and a positively charged residue (Lys-409) at its entrance. It appears to be preponderantly hydrophobic in nature with some polar residues. The binding mode proposed for murracarpin was shown in Figure 2. The side chain at C-8 position inserted into the hydrophobic channel, the hydroxyl group interacted with the oxygen atom in Ala-606 in hydrogen bond (d = 2.31468 Å). The coumarin nucleus blocked up at the entrance, the carbonyl group interacted with the nitrogen atom in Leu-414 in a strong hydrogen bond (d = 1.86907 Å), and with Lys-409 in a weak hydrogen bonding interaction (d = 2.77914 Å).

3.1.2 *Effects on cytokines levels in pleurisy exudates*

Rat pleurisy is the most widely accepted model suitable for collection and analysis of cells and exudates from the inflammatory site (Harada, 2001). Elevated levels of inflammatory mediators have been detected within pleural infusions, such as neutrophils, eosnophills or lymphocytes, including lipid mediators, cytokines and proteins. Intrapleural injection of carrageenin could significantly cause leukocyte infiltration, plasma exudation and increase in the level of proinflammtory cytokines (Jana, 2008). COX products were involved in the plasma exudation during the first 5 h, and the high level of PGE2 was kept until 48 h, which provide major contribution in causing the plasma exudation to initiate the accumulation of the pleural exudates in the first 5 h. In this paper, animals were killed at 6 h after carrageenin injection. Intrapleural injection of carrageenin injection caused the accumulation of a volume of pleural exudates that reached 2.98 ± 0.25 ml in the control group. Murracarpin dose dependently suppressed the accumulation of pleural exudates significantly. At the dose of 50 mg/kg, murracarpin showed the highest activity, the volume of pleural exudates decreased to 0.79 ± 0.12 ml, much less than that in hexadecadrol group 1.65 ± 0.07 (P < 0.05) ml (Figure 3).

It was reported that TNF-α and IL-1β, two important proinflammatory cytokines, were detectable in the pleural exudates 1 h after carrageenin injection, and their level peaked 2 and 5 h, respectively (Jana, 2008). At 6 h after carrageenin injection, murracarpin (50 mg/kg) could significantly down-regulate the level of IL-1β (100.7 ± 4.92 pg/ml, P < 0.05) in pleural exudates, stronger than that in hexadecadrol group 121.01 ± 7.08 pg/ml. Similarly, murracarpin dose dependently decreased the contents of TNF-α to 50.01 ± 4.89 pg/ml (P <0.05), 73.18 ± 4.51 pg/ml (P < 0.05), and 84.94 ± 8.42 pg/ml (P < 0.05) at the dose of 50, 25, and 12.5 mg/kg, respectively. In contrast, the content of TNF-α in control group was 100.07 ± 6.64 pg/ml (Figure 4).

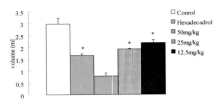

Figure 3.   The volume of carrageenin-induced pleural exudates at 6 h after injection. Murracarpin was administrated at the doses of 50, 25, and 12.5 mg/kg. Hexadecadrol (0.5 mg/kg) was as reference.

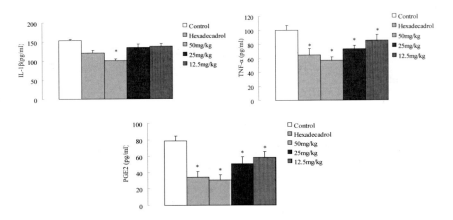

Figure 4.   The contents of IL-1β, TNF-α, and PGE2 in pleural exudates at 6 h after injection, Murracarpin was administrated at the doses of 50, 25, and 12.5 mg/kg.

PGE2, the major metabolite of COX-2, can be up-regulated by TNF-α and IL-1β. Harada (1996) reported that the maximum level of PGE2 in pleural exudates was at 5 h after carrageenin injection, and the level of COX-2 kept high level between at 3 h and 7 h. PGE2 indirectly become a pointer for the expression of COX-2. In the pleural exudates model, murracarpin dose dependently decreased the synthesis and release of PGE2, and reached statistical significance. Administration of 50 mg/kg murracarpin, the content of PGE2 in the pleural exudates was 30.34 ± 6.87 pg/ml ($P < 0.05$) (Figure 4), which was much lower than that in the control groups. These might suggest that murracarpin could effectively inhibit the activity of COX-2.

4   CONCLUSIONS

In the present study, we had examined the molecular docking of murracarpin with COX-2 and 5-LOX, and the effect on the inflammatory mediators. Our results showed that the 3D model of 5-LOX was successfully homology built; murracarpin showed strong interacting with COX-2 and 5-LOX in hydrogen bonds, and anti-inflammatory activity by decreasing the contents of IL-1β, TNF-α, and PGE2.

ACKNOWLEDEMENTS

This study was financially supported by the National Science Foundation of China (81360277), the National Science Foundation of Jiangxi Province (20142BAB215047 and 20142BAB215069), and Scientific Research Fund of Jiangxi Provincial Education Department (GJJ13669) award to Wu L.H.

REFERENCES

Asako,H., Kubes, P., Wallace, J., et al. Granger. (1992) Indomethacin- induced leukocyte adhesion in mesenteric venules: role of lipoxytenase products. Am J Physiol, 262(5 Pt 1), G903–908.

Bazan, N.G., Flower R.J.. (2002) Lipid signals in pain control. Nature, 420, 135–138.

Harada, K., Kawamura, M., Murai, N., et al. (2001) FR167653, a cytokine synthesis inhibitor, exhibits anti-inflammatory effects early in rat carrageenin-induced pleurisy but no effect later. J Pharmacol Exp Ther, 229, 519–527.

Harada, Y., Hatanaka, K., Kawamura, M., et al. (1996) Role of prostaglandin H synthase-2 in prostaglandin E2 formation in rat carrageenin-induced pleurisy. Prostaglandins, 15, 19–33.

Jana, B., Kozlowska, A., Andronowska, A., et al. (2008) The effect of tumor necrosis factor-α (TNF-α), interleukin (IL)-1β and IL-6 on chorioamnion secretion of prostaglandins (PG)F2α and E2 in pigs. Reproductive Biology, 8, 57–68.

Norihito, C., Kazuko, T., Yuriko, T., et al. (2004) Antiproliferative constituents in plants 14. Coumarins and acridone alkaloids from Boenninghausenia japonica Nakai. Biol Pharm Bull, 27(8), 1312–1316.

Scholz, M., Ulbrich, H.K., Dannhardt, G.. (2008) Investigations concerning the COX/5-LOX inhibiting and hydroxyl radical scavenging potencies of novel 4,5-diaryl isoselenazoles. Eur J Med Chem, 43, 1152–1159.

Wu, L., Wang, X., Xu, W., et al. (2009) The structure and pharmacological functions of coumarins and their derivatives. Curr Med Chem, 16, 4236–4260.

Zheng, M., Zhang, Z., Zhu, W., et al. (2006) Essential structural profile of a dual functional inhibitor against cyclooxygenase-2 (COX-2) and 5-lipoxygenase (5-LOX): Molecular docking and 3D-QSAR analyses on DHDMBF analogues. Bioorg Med Chem, 14, 3428–3437.

Medicine Sciences and Bioengineering – Wang (Ed.)
© 2015 Taylor & Francis Group, London, ISBN: 978-1-138-02684-1

Complete structural assignment of a new natural product from the roots of Raphanus Sativus L.

Feng Wang, Huan Chen, Yi-bo Wang & Shu-mei Wang*
College of Traditional Chinese Materia Medica, Guangdong Pharmaceutical University, Guangzhou, China

ABSTRACT: One new natural product was isolated from the roots of *Raphanus sativus* L. by successive chromatographic procedures, such as open silica gel, Sephadex LH-20 and open RP-18 column chromatograph. The structure of the isolated compound was elucidated as Cis-(1-methylazetidin-2-yl)methanol on the basis of spectral data analysis. The new natural product would be potential candidates for early anti-migraine drug study.

1 INTRODUCTION

Migraine is a severe and persistent headache which can cause nausea and light sensitivity, and one in five people in the world are suffering from this disease. Some migraineurs also experience an "aura" around objects which warns them an attack is on the ways (Natoli, Manack and Dean, 2010). *Raphanus sativus* L. is a plant from Cruciferae family, which is not only a delicious food, but also a medicine used as antitumor, antimicrobial and antiviral agents (Hanlon and Barnes 2011). Furthermore, according to the ancient Chinese medical books, the juice of *Raphanus sativus* L. can treat migraine through intranasal administration. However, little research were conducted on the effective ingredients and the pharmacological mechanism of *Raphanus sativus* L. Besides, the existing anti-migraine drugs, such as sumatriptan and aspirin, were expensive or just analgesic, which couldn't heal the disease but eased the pain temporarily (Moon and Kim, 2012). *Raphanus sativus* L. might be a good candidate for anti-migraine drug study.

2 EXPERIMENTAL

2.1 General experimental procedures

ESI-MS and HR-ESI-MS data were obtained using a Q-Tof Micro mass spectrometer (Waters, USA). NMR spectra were recorded on Avance DRX-500 MHz spectrometer (Bruker, Germany) with TMS as the internal standard. Analytical HPLC was performed on Waters e2695/2998 Series HPLC system equipped with a C_{18} column (4.6×250 mm, 5 μm, SunFire™, Waters, USA). HPLC-grade solvents were purchased from Merck (Germany). Silica gel (100-200 and 200-300 mesh, Qingdao Haiyang Chemical Co., Ltd., Qingdao, China) and Sephadex LH-20 gel (GE Healthcare, USA) were both used for column chromatography. TLC analysis was run on GF254 precoated silica gel plates (Merck, Germany), and spots were visualized at 110°C after spraying 10% H_2SO_4-EtOH. All solvents used for extraction and isolation were at least of analytical grade.

---

*Prof. Shumei Wang, department of Traditional Chinese Medicine, Guangdong Pharmaceutical University, is the corresponding author of this research. (Tel:020-39352559; E-mail:shmwang@sina.com)

2.2 Plant material

The *Raphanus sativus* L. (Yantai, Shandong, China) was purchased from Guangzhou Carrefour (Franch) in July 2013 and botanically identified by Prof. Honghua Cui from Guangdong Pharmaceutical University, Guangzhou, China. A voucher specimen (LF20130811) is kept at College of Traditional Chinese Materia Medica, Guangdong Pharmaceutical University, China.

2.3 Extraction and isolation

The juice (70 kg), from the roots of fresh *Raphanus sativus* L. (100 kg), was concentrated under reduced pressure to give dry extracts (2424 g) at 60°C. This crude extracts were then suspended in H_2O (2 L) and partitioned successively with n-hexane (3 batch ×2 L), CH_2Cl_2 (3×2 L), EtOAc (3×2 L), and n-BuOH (3×6 L). The n-BuOH fraction (98.0 g), which exhibited strong anti-migraine activity, was chromatographed over a silica gel column (9 × 40 cm; 200-300 mesh) and eluted with gradient mixtures of CH_2Cl_2-MeOH (100:1, 100:2, 100:3, 100:5, 100:7, 100:15, 100:20, 100:30, 100:50, 100:100, 0:100, H_2O, each 11 L) to yield 19 pooled fractions (D-1, D-2,...,D-19). D-8 (1.817 g) was chromatographed over a silica gel column to give nine fractions (from D-8-1 to D-8-9). Fraction D-8-8 was chromatographed over a Sephadex LH-20 column (10 × 150 mm) using MeOH as the eluting solvent to give five subfractions (form D-8-8-1 to D-8-8-5). D-8-8-2 was further purified by Pre-HPLC using 30% MeOH in water with the detector of 254 nm to yield compound **1** (6 mg).

3 RESULTS AND DISCUSSION

One new natural products was isolated from the n-BuOH extracts of *Raphanus sativus* L. The structure of the compound was determined by MS, 1D-NMR and 2D-NMR data analysis.

Compound **1** was obtained as colorless needle crystals; its molecular formula was determined as $C_5H_{11}NO$ from the HR-ESI-MS data (*m/z* 102.1288, calcd for $C_5H_{12}NO$, 102.0919). The structural formula of **1** was shown in Figure 1. In the ^1H NMR spectrum, the signals of ten H which linked to C were given and *d* 2.71 (3H, s, H-6) was assigned to methyl group. In the ^{13}C NMR spectrum, five C signals were given. Therefore, it was forecasted that there is one methyl, three methylenes of which one was linked by hydroxy for higher chemical shift and one methine in the molecule. The ^1H and ^{13}C NMR data were assigned by the HSQC and HMBC spectra (Table 1). A four-membered ring, which was formed by two methylenes, one methine and N, was found to exist in the molecule on the basis of the fact that there is one degree of unsaturation but lack unsaturated bond. The conclusion was supported by the correlation between δ 3.81 (1H, m, H-2) with C-3 (δ 27.3), C-4 (δ 43.8) and C-5 (δ 59.2) in the HMBC spectrum. Furthermore, the correlations between *d* 2.71 (3H, s, H-6) and C-2 (δ 40.0), C-4 (δ 43.8) revealed that methyl group was lined to N. So, CH_2OH (δ 59.2, C-5) was unambiguously located at C-2.

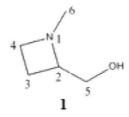

1

Figure 1.   Structure of compound **1**.

Table 1.   Spectral data of compounds **1** and **2** (CD$_3$OD).

position	Compound **1**	
	δ_H	δ_C
1	–	–
2	3.81 (1H, m)	40.0
3	2.46 (1H, m, α) 2.01 (1H, m, β)	27.3
4	3.42 (1H, m, α) 3.57 (1H, m, β)	43.8
5	3.02 (1H, dd, J = 13.5, 5.0 Hz) 3.17 (1H, dd, J = 13.5, 9.5 Hz)	59.2
6	2.71 (3H, s)	38.8

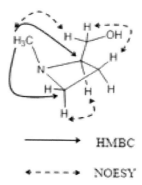

⟶ HMBC

◆ - - - - ◆ NOESY

Figure 2.   Selected HMBC and NOESY correlations of compound 1.

The relative configuration of **1** was established from NOESY experiments (Figure 2). Two substituent groups, a methyl and a hydroxymethyl, both located at one side of the four-membered ring according to the NOESY cross-peaks between CH$_3$ and d 3.02H-5a and between CH$_3$ and H-5b and significant absence of the correlation between H-2a and CH$_3$. The configuration of remaining four H assigned to two methylenes was indicated by the correlations in NOESY spectrum between H-2a and H-4a and between H-5b and H-3b. Thus, the structure of compound **1** was determined to be Cis-(1-methylazetidin-2-yl)methanol.

4   CONCLUSIONS

The preliminary procedure for extraction and isolation of components from *Raphanus sativus* L. was established. One new natural product from *Raphanus sativus* L. was identified as Cis-(1-methylazetidin-2-yl)methanol, and its full spectral data was given for the first time. The compound would be helpful for further research about their potential anti-migraine, anti-tumor activity and other pharmacological activities.

ACKNOWLEDGMENTS

This work was financially supported by the Funds National Natural Science Foundation of China (No. 81202884) and Guangdong Province College students' innovative entrepreneurial training project (1057312035).

REFERENCES

Akerman, S., Holland, P.R. & Hoffmann, J. (2013) Pearls and Pitfalls in Experimental in Vivo Models of Migraine: Dural Trigeminovascular Nociception. *Cephalalgia*, 33(8), 577–592.

Hanlon P.R. & Barnes D.M. (2011) Phytochemical Composition and Biological Activity of 8 Varieties of Radish (*Raphanus sativus* L.). *J. Food Sci.*, 76(1), 185–187.

Moon P.D. & Kim H.M. (2012) Anti-inflammatory Effect of Phenethyl Isothiocyanate, an Active Ingredient of *Raphanus sativus* L. *Food Chemistry*, 131(4), 1332–1333.

Natoli, J.L., Manack, A. & Dean, B. (2010) Global Prevalence of Chronic Migraine: A Systematic Review. *Cephalalgia*, 30(5), 599–609.

Medicine Sciences and Bioengineering – Wang (Ed.)

Pharmacokinetic analysis of five rhubarb aglycones in rat plasma after oral administration and the influence of borneol on their pharmacokinetics

Feng Wang, Qin-xiao Guan, Li Lu, Lu Zhao, Xian-shuai Guo, Sheng-wang Liang &
Shu-Mei Wang*
Department of Traditional Chinese Medicine, Guangdong Pharmaceutical University, Guangzhou, China

ABSTRACT: It was proved that the optimum ratio of five rhubarbs aglycones showed potent effect on ischemic cerebral apoplexy, but their pharmacokinetics are ambiguous in rats. A simple and sensitive high-performance liquid chromatographic method was developed for the simultaneous determination and comparative pharmacokinetic analysis of aloe-emodin, rhein, emodin, chrysophanol, and physcion in rat plasma after oral administration with or without borneol. The results demonstrated that the assay had remarkable reproducibility with acceptable accuracy and precision and borneol may slow down the absorption of the five rhubarb aglycones and accelerate their elimination in rats.

1   INTRODUCTION

Rhubarb is one of the common Traditional Chinese Medicine (TCM) and its main active components are known as rhubarb aglycones, such as aloe-emodin, rhein, emodin, chrysophanol, and physcion. The pharmacological research on rhubarb have revealed its diverse pharmacological properties, including liver protecting and cholagogic (Xing *et al*, 2011), reducing blood lipid (Wang *et al*, 2008), and protection of cerebral ischemia (Li *et al*, 2003).

Our group conduced the Support Vector Machine regression to investigate the interactions among the different ratio of five rhubarb aglycones and pharmacological actions by analyzing neural symptoms, infarction area, contents of brain water, ATP, lactic acid, and the number of normal neurons. As a result, the optimum ratio of five rhubarbs aglycones was determined as 1.32:2.00:1.00:2.76:1.79 by weight, which showed potent effect on ischemic cerebral.

Pharmacokinetic studies of the active constituents in TCM are essential to clinical application. Meanwhile, the simultaneous determination of the content of five aglycones from rhubarb in plasma and tissue and pharmacokinetic study of these compounds were rarely reported.

Many reports have confirmed that borneol play a significant role in improving the transdermal absorption of drugs (Xu *et al*, 2001), accelerating the opening of blood–brain barriers, and the distribution of drugs in brain tissue (Xiao *et al*, 2007). The effects of borneol on pharmacokinetic of rhubarb aglycones in rats in vivo were not reported so far To reveal pharmacokinetic characteristics of the optimum proportion of rhubarb aglycones in rats in vivo, the method of high-performance liquid chromatography with diodearray detection (HPLC-DAD) was developed for the pharmacokinetic studies of five rhubarb aglycones in rat after oral administration with or without borneol.

*corresponding author, Tel:020-39352559; E-mail:shmwang@sina.com, Prof. Shumei Wang, department of Traditional Chinese Medicine, Guangdong Pharmaceutical University, is the corresponding author of this research.

2 MATERIALS AND METHODS

2.1 *Materials*

Rhubarb aglycones were bought from the Institute for Phytochemistry, Huaihai City, Jiangsu Province. Reference standards of aloe-emodin, rhein, emodin, chrysophanol, physcion, and 1, 8-dihydroxyanthraquinone (Internal standard, IS) were purchased from the National Institute for the Control of Pharmaceutical and Biological Products (Beijing, China). The purity of was above 98.0%. Borneol was obtained from Huangpu Chemical Reagent Co. Ltd. (Guangzhou, China). SD rats, including 12 males (300 ± 20 g) and 12 females (250 ± 20 g), were provided by Guangdong Provincial Experimental Animal Center. All animal experiments were approved by the institutional ethics committee prior to the study. All the animals were clinically healthy and hematologically and biochemically normal throughout the experimental period. Before using, animals were housed in experimental environment provided with standard feed and water. Animals were fasted for 24 h before and after the oral administration.

2.2 *Experimental method*

2.2.1 *Apparatus and chromatographic conditions*

Analyses were performed by HPLC system (Waters2695 Separations Module, Waters2996 Photodiode Array Detector) with diode array detector. Detection wavelengths were 254 nm. A Venusil XBP C_{18} (250 mm × 4.6 mm, 5 μm) was used with a flow rate of 1.0 ml/min. The injection volume was 20 μl, and the column temperature was at 25°C. The mobile phase was composed of aqueous phosphoric acid (0.1%, *V/V*) and methanol (28:72, *V/V*).

2.2.2 *Standard solutions preparations*

Standard solutions of the five compounds were dissolved with methanol, respectively, to get a concentration of 0.04260 mg/ml (aloe-emodin), 0.07213 mg/ml (rhein), 0.06616 mg/ml (emodin), 0.05927 mg/ml (chrysophanol), and 0.03163 mg/ml (physcion). 1,8-Dihydroxyan-thraquinone was used as the internal standard and its stock solution was prepared with methanol to 0.05002 mg/ml. Mixed standard working solutions were prepared daily by mixing and diluting the stock solutions with methanol. The solutions were filtered through a 0.45 μm membrane prior to injection.

2.2.3 *Pharmacokinetic studies of rhubarb aglycones in rats*

Twenty-four healthy SD rats were randomly divided into four groups, with each including 3 males and 3 females. Three groups were planned to be orally administrated high, middle, and low dose of the optimum ratio rhubarb aglycones suspended in 5 ml of 0.5% CMC-Na solution respectively and the other would be orally administrated middle dose of the mixture of the optimum ratio rhubarb aglycone and borneol (0.6 g/kg) suspended in 5 ml of 0.5% CMC-Na solution. About 0.5 ml of blood samples via the orbital cavity were collected into a heparinized tubes at 0.083, 0.167, 0.25, 0.33, 0.5, 0.75, 1, 1.5, 2, 4, 8, 12, and 24 h before and after oral administration of the optimum ratio rhubarb aglycone. During sampling, rats were anesthetized with ether. Blood samples were centrifuged immediately for 10 min (3500 revolutions/min, 4°C) to separate the supernatant of plasma, which were stored at −20°C until analysis.

The internal standard solution (0.5 μg/ml) and 600 μl of acetonitrile were added into 200-μL plasma sample. After vortex-mixing and centrifuging, the separated supernatant was mixed with triple volume of aqueous phosphoric acid (0.1%, *V/V*) and then was disposed through solid phase extraction C_{18} column, which was eluted with 2ml mixture composed of methanol and acetonitrile (1:1). The eluent were evaporated to dryness at 37 °C under a gentle stream of N_2 and the residue was reconstituted in 100 μl of methanol to produce a solution, which was centrifuged at 15000 revolutions/min and 4°C for 10 min to separate the supernatants of plasma sample.

2.2.4 *Statistical analysis*

The pharmacokinetic parameters were calculated using the DAS2.1.1 software (Mathematical Pharmacology Professional Committee of China).

3 RESULTS

3.1 *Bioanalytical method*

The calibration curves in rat plasma were constructed by plotting the peak area ratio (y) of corresponding standard substances to IS versus the spiked concentrations (x) of the analytes. All the calibration curves showed good linearity (r $\geq$ 0.9982). The limit of detection under the chromatographic conditions were determined by injecting a series of standard solutions until the signal-to-noise (S/N) ratio for each compound was 3 for LLOD (the lower limit of detection). The linear regression equation of analytes is shown in Table 1. LLOQ (the lower limit of quantification) and LLOD for analytes are revealed in Table 1 too. No significant interference was detected at the retention times of the analytes in the blank plasma chromatograms (Figure 1), indicating that the method was specific for the determination of targeted compounds.

Table 1. The results of standard curves, linear range, LLOD, and LLOQ of rhubarb aglycone in rat plasma.

Compound	Regression equation	γ	Linear range	LOD	LOQ
			μg/ml		
Aloe-emodin	y = 1.6001x + 0.0038	0.9991	0.0170 − 1.704	0.00852	0.0170
Rhein	y = 1.8196x − 0.013	0.9989	0.0721 − 7.213	0.00902	0.0721
Emodin	y = 1.2793x + 0.08	0.9993	0.0159 − 1.588	0.00795	0.0159
Chrysophanol	y = 2.0235x + 0.018	0.9982	0.0143 − 1.4225	0.00715	0.0143
Physcion	y = 0.9737x + 0.0033	0.9986	0.0127 − 1.2652	0.00635	0.0127

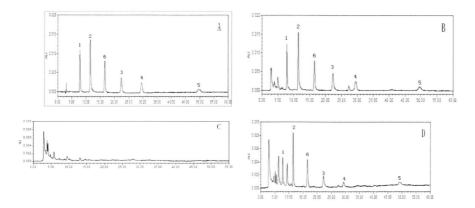

Figure 1. HPLC of rhubarb aglycones in rat plasma: (A) mixed references; (B) mixed references in blank plasma; (C) blank plasma; (D) plasma sample after intragastric administration.

The intra- and interday precision were determined by calibration samples during a single day and on five consecutive days, respectively (see Table 2). The mean values and the relative standard deviation (RSD) for quality control (QC) samples at three concentration levels were calculated over three validation runs. Overall intra- and interday variations were less than 8.51%. Stability of each compound with three different concentration levels was tested under such procedures as storing analytes at room temperature for 24 h, at 4°C for 2 days, and at −20°C for 7 days, respectively. RSDs of stability were not more than 9.66% for all analytes. The nominal plasma concentrations of QC samples were 0.8520, 0.1702, 0.0341 μg/ml for aloe-emodin, 3.6065, 0.7213, 0.1443 μg/ml for rhein, 0.7940, 0.1985, 0.0318 μg/ml for emodin, 0.7113, 0.1423, 0.0285 μg/ml for chrysophanol, and 0.6326, 0.1265, 0.0253 μg/ml for physcion. The results indicated that the present method had a satisfactory precision.

The plasma samples at different levels recorded above, each including five replicates, were prepared for the determination of extraction recovery. Mean recoveries of five compounds were 82.32%–91.75% at low concentration level, 84.82%–90.09% at middle concentration level, and 83.22%–93.03% at high concentration level. Elaborate experimental data of extraction recovery were listed in Table 3.

Table 2.   The precision of five rhubarb aglycones at three concentration levels in rat plasma ($n = 5$).

Compound	Intraday(μg/ml)		Interday(μg/ml)	
	Found conc.	RSD (%)	Found conc.	RSD (%)
Aloe-emodin	0.0291	5.01	0.0284	6.82
	0.1513	3.32	0.1309	5.68
	0.7612	2.95	0.6754	4.83
Rhein	0.1401	4.11	0.1369	6.03
	0.6337	3.16	0.6821	4.37
	3.2755	3.58	3.2901	4.62
Emodin	0.0284	5.24	0.0297	5.12
	0.1701	4.19	0.1643	6.56
	0.7441	4.51	0.6382	6.68
Chrysophanol	0.0228	4.32	0.0231	8.51
	0.1255	5.67	0.1129	7.03
	0.6137	5.53	0.6020	7.31
Physcion	0.0199	5.14	0.0188	6.47
	0.1138	3.22	0.1172	5.76
	0.5809	4.59	0.5937	5.63

Table 3.　The extraction recovery of five rhubarb aglycones at three concentration levels in rat plasma.

Compound	Spiked conc. (μg/ml)	Found conc. (μg/ml)	Mean extract recovery (%)	RSD%
Aloe-emodin	0.0287	0.0341	84.16	4.86
	0.1457	0.1702	85.61	4.76
	0.7090	0.8520	83.22	3.18
Rhein	0.1324	0.1443	91.75	5.07
	0.6498	0.7213	90.09	3.92
	3.3552	3.6065	93.03	4.84
Emodin	0.0275	0.0318	86.48	4.21
	0.1756	0.1985	88.46	5.43
	0.7109	0.7940	89.53	3.72
Chrysophanol	0.0235	0.0285	82.32	6.38
	0.1216	0.1423	85.43	5.97
	0.5972	0.7113	83.97	5.66
Physcion	0.0217	0.0253	85.77	5.82
	0.1073	0.1265	84.82	6.05
	0.5579	0.6326	88.19	4.77

3.2　*Pharmacokinetic studies*

The LC-DAD method developed was used to investigate the pharmacokinetics after oral administration of rhubarb aglycones with or without borneol to rats. The kinetic curve of plasma concentrations of five rhubarb aglycones with or without borneol in oral administration to rat was shown in Figure 2. The concentrations of aloe-emodin, rhein, and emodin in plasma and their elimination from plasma followed the two-compartment model when low, middle, and high dose were administrated to rats. Changes in plasma levels of chrysophanol could be fitted to the one-compartment open model at middle- and high-dose administration and the two-compartment model at low-dose administration. The pharmacokinetic parameters of physcion conformed to the one-compartment open model at high-dose administration and the two-compartment model at low- and middle-dose administration. When the optimum ratio of rhubarb aglycones with middle-dose concentration was administrated to rats with borneol, the concentrations of all five rhubarb aglycones abided by

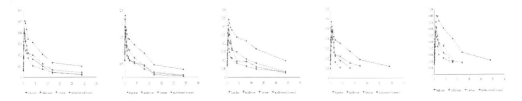

Figure 2.　Plasma concentration–time curves for A (aloe-emodin), B (rhein), C (emodin), D (chrysophanol), and E (physcion) in rat plasma after oral administration with or without borneol.

the two-compartment model except for chrysophanol whose pharmacokinetics parameters were calculated by one-compartment open model. The pharmacokinetic parameters for all compounds are calculated and listed in Tables 4 and 5.

The pharmacokinetic parameter values of Ka, T_{max}, and C_{max} showed that these rhubarb aglycones were rapidly absorbed in the intestines and stomach, but the pharmacokinetic differences

Table 4.   The main pharmacokinetic parameters of five rhubarb aglycones at three concentration levels.

Parameters	Aloe-emodin	Rhein	Emodin	Chrysophanol	Physcion
	0.5047	2.2971	0.3411	0.05726	0.04512
C_{max} (µg/ml)	0.4296	1.8725	0.2852	0.04841	0.03658
	0.4127	1.7536	0.2602	0.04711	0.03317
	0.75	0.33	0.75	0.5	1.00
T_{max} (h)	0.50	0.25	0.50	0.5	0.75
	0.50	0.25	0.33	0.5	0.75
	2.043	6.983	2.345	9.709	2.481
Ka (1/h)	3.253	6.294	3.138	7.573	2.073
	3.375	5.75	4.169	2.236	3.837
	14.301	5.615	8.628	232.894	154.748
CL/F (L/h/kg)	16.553	8.01	13.731	320.099	259.21
	15.097	6.826	13.621	623.596	265.445
	83.789	30.15	99.627	2748.049	1937.913
V1/F (L/kg)	53.711	21.478	81.263	1864.201	1209.100
	59.777	14.565	49.727	647.987	1398.275
	4.498	17.080	4.312	0.563	0.532
AUC0-t (mg/L*h)	2.606	9.039	2.279	0.244	0.203
	1.709	6.995	1.491	0.088	0.114
	4.823	20.000	6.510	0.783	0.713
AUC0-∞ (mg/L*h)	3.156	9.176	2.706	0.436	0.244
	1.765	7.505	1.857	0.113	0.225
	8.533	7.811	9.468	8.828	8.768
MRT0-t (h)	7.458	5.941	8.062	4.757	4.529
	6.833	5.887	8.619	1.495	3.28
	10.192	13.41	21.977	18.315	16.848
MRT0-∞ (h)	12.632	6.297	12.707	14.682	6.963
	7.604	7.741	13.915	2.569	11.605

Table 5. The main pharmacokinetic parameters of five rhubarb aglycones at middle-dose level in rat plasma after oral administration with borneol.

Parameters	Aloe-emodin	Rhein	Emodin	Chrysophanol	Physcion
C_{max} (µg/ml)	0.4296	1.8725	0.2852	0.04841	0.03658
	0.4021	1.7465	0.2808	0.04725	0.03612
T_{max} (h)	0.50	0.20	0.50	0.5	0.75
	0.50	0.50	0.75	1.00	1.00
Ka (1/h)	3.253	6.294	3.138	7.573	2.073
	3.300	3.477	1.888	3.344	3.621
CL/F (L/h/kg)	16.553	8.01	13.731	320.099	259.21
	22.303	9.429	17.068	510.977	304.147
V1/F (L/kg)	53.711	21.478	81.263	1864.201	1209.100
	58.403	21.715	78.374	2014.787	2002.01
AUC0-t	2.606	9.039	2.279	0.244	0.203
	2.166	6.930	1.898	0.167	0.149
AUC0-∞	3.156	9.176	2.706	0.436	0.244
	2.197	7.228	2.069	0.249	0.219
MRT0-t (h)	7.458	5.941	8.062	4.757	4.529
	6.182	5.518	7.633	2.997	3.113
MRT0-∞ (h)	12.632	6.297	12.707	14.682	6.963
	6.515	6.199	9.786	7.22	6.967

between five rhubarb aglycones were observed due to their disparate absorption strength, structure, transport carrier species, and quantity. Meanwhile, CL/F and MRT_{0-t} indicated that five rhubarb aglycones were tardily eliminated in rats. The rhubarb aglycones, especially chrysophanol and physcion were widely distributed in rats because of their lipophillc characteristic, which facilitate those compounds to penetrate the cell membrane.

4 DISCUSSION

The pharmacokinetic characteristics of the optimum ratio of five rhubarb aglycones are not consistent with those reported in literatures (Zhang *et al*, 2010; Tan *et al*, 1998; Zhang *et al*, 2005; Shi *et al*, 2010; Song *et al*, 2009) and the differences possibly arose from animal species, drug dose, proportion of rhubarb aglycones, and interaction between rhubarb aglycones, such as synergy or competitive effect, which will be further investigated.

After administration of rhubarb aglycones at middle dose with borneol, several pharmacokinetic parameters change, including T_{max}, V1/F, CL/F, and MRT_{0-t}. Borneol extended the reach peak time of rhein, emodin, chrysophanol; reduced the absorption rate of rhein, emodin, chrysophanol, physcion in rats; and reduced the reach peak concentration. These changes observed the concern that borneol could competitively occupy absorption site, which consequently influence the diffusion and hinder the absorption rate of rhubarb aglycones. Moreover, borneol increased the apparent distribution volume of aloe-emodin, rhein, emodin, physcion; broaden the distribution; and accelerated the elimination of five rhubarb aglycones in rat. It is the reason that borneol induced the activity of P450 (Hu *et al*, 2005).

5 CONCLUSIONS

In our study, administration of the optimum ratio of rhubarb aglycones with borneol can prevent the side effect from long-term administration of rhubarb aglycones. The method presented here circumvents the need for MS instrumentation and provides reproducible and specific analysis for the pharmacokinetic study of five active components from rhubarb.

ACKNOWLEDGMENTS

This work was supported by National Natural Science Foundation of China (No. 81073024, 81274060, and 81202884).

REFERENCES

Hu, L.M., Jiang, M., Wang, S.X., Gao, X.M. & Zhang, B.L .(2005). Impact of Borneolum Syntheticum on Contents of YP450 in Rat Liver and Expression of CYP3A1 mRNA. *Tianjin Journal of Traditional Chinese Medicine*, 22,284–286.

Li, J.S., Hou, X. J., Zheng, X.K., Li, X.L. & Wang, Z.W. (2003). Protective Effect of Rhubarb and Its Extraction on Cerebral Ischemia in Rats. *Liaoning Journal of traditional Chinese Medicine*, 30,338–340.

Shi, Y., Wang, B.J., Lin, X.K., Huang, S.X. & Lin, K.Q. (2010). Determination of rat serum emodin level by microemulsion liquid chromatography with direct sample loading. *Journal of Southern Medical University*, 30, 2759–2761.

Song, Z.F., Peng, J. & Ma, C .(2009). LC-MS/MS determination of plasma and brain concentration of emodin in rats. *Chinese Journal of Pharmaceutical Analysis*, 29,926–930.

Tan, L., Yuan, Y.S. & Yang. J.W. (1998). Determination of rhein in human plasma by HPLC and the study of its pharmacokinetics. *Bulletin of Jinling Hospital*, 11,112–115.

Xiao, Y.Y., Ping, Q.N. & Chen, Z.P.(2007). The enhancing effect of synthetical borneol on the absorption of tetramethylpyrazine phosphate in mouse. *International Journal of Pharmaceutics*, 337, 74–79.

Xing, X.Y.,Zhao, Y.L., Kong, W.J.,Wang, J.B.&Jia,L.(2011). Investigation of the "dose–time–response" relationships of rhubarb on carbon tetrachloride-induced liver injury in rats. *Journal of Ethnopharmacology*, 135,575–581.

Xu, B.L., Wang, H. & Xu, W.M.(2001). Enhancing Effect of Synthetic Borneol on Skin Permeation of Ligustrazine Hydrochloride. *Chinese Traditional Patent Medicine*, 23,864–867.

Wang, Y.M., Tian, L.H. & Zhang, J.(2008). Effects of Rhubarb polysaccharide on blood glucose, blood lipids, hepatic lipase activity in rats with diabetic atherosclerosis. *China Journal of Modern Medicine*, 10,6–9.

Zhang, J.W., Wang, G..J., Sun, J.G.., Xie, H.T. & Hao, H.P. (2005). Determination of Rhein in Plasma by HPLC-Fluorescence Detection and its Parmacokinetics in Rats. *Chinese Journal of Natural Medicines*, 3,238–241.

Zhang, J.W., Wei, Y.H., Wu, Q.Y., Li, B.X., Duan, H.G.. & WU, X.A.(2010). Simultaneous determination of aloe-emodin,emodin and chrysophanol in rat plasma by HPLC-CPE. *Chinese Journal of Hospital Pharmacy*, 30,911–915.

Bioinformatics and Biomedical Engineering

Medicine Sciences and Bioengineering – Wang (Ed.)
© 2015 Taylor & Francis Group, London, ISBN: 978-1-138-02684-1

Study actuality of immune optimization algorithm

Yu Miao, Hua-min Yang, Wei-li Shi*, Li-yuan Zhang & Yan-ni Cao
School of Computer Science and Technology, Changchun University of Science and Technology, Changchun, China

ABSTRACT: This article introduces an optimization algorithm based on immune principle, explains its basic theory and process, and discusses immune algorithm's advantage. It introduces several better algorithms based on immune algorithm and presents application in optimization problems. Finally, we propose immune algorithm's further development.

1 INTRODUCTION

The immune system is one of the most intricate bodily systems. It is a very important to make sure a healthy living. The immune system is very complex protects the body from a large variety of bacteria, viruses, and other pathogens.

2 SEVERAL IMPROVEMENT OPTIMIZATION ALGORITHMS

Vaccination is very important for immunization. Immunity obtained by vaccination destroys many serious diseases worldwide, for example, smallpox, measles, and infantile paralysis. With sufficient knowledge about an epidemic virus, people develop vaccines to prevent and cure the epidemic, using the concept of vaccine to improve the immune algorithm performance.

In evolution and selective procedure, the "vaccine inoculation" and the "immune selective" has been used to guide research procedure and obtain the better optimization performance. Figure 1 shows the algorithm flow chart.

The extraction vaccine in reason is the key in immune operate number. Generally speaking, there are two methods to decide the selective vaccine. One is based on the character information of the problems and the other is based on the analyses of the problems. They can reduce original problem's size and increase some local constraints for predigesting problems. Actually, after calculated the ancestor knowledge sufficiency, the algorithm can make it more pertinence to reduce calculate time.

Wang Lei *et al.* (2000) have carried out the simulation experiment using this method to the TSP (Traveling Salesman Problem) question, which can be compared with general genetic algorithms. This kind of immune optimization algorithm can solve the degenerated phenomenon well, which appears in the existing algorithm, and also enable the convergence rate to have remarkable enhancement. Result demonstration: the vaccine choice has tremendous influence on the algorithm performance, but it cannot provide the algorithm the astringency; this algorithm has good search ability and auto-adapted ability.

The following paragraphs explain the feasible solution diversity. The data structure of the genes can be depicted as shown in Figure 2. According to Figure 2, there are N antibodies with M genes in the antibody pool. N is presented as the number of antibodies (candidates for unit commitment) in a generation, and M is the number of units.

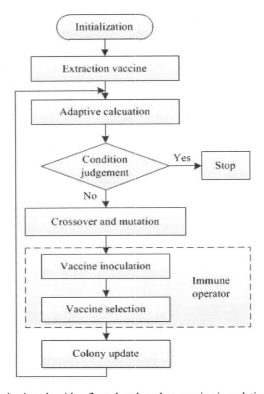

Figure 1.   Immune optimization algorithm flow chart based on vaccine inoculation.

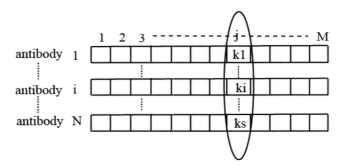

Figure 2.   Model of antibody.

Assume that antibody pool is composed of N antibodies having M genes. From the information entropy approach, we can get

$$H_j(N) = \sum_{i=1}^{S} -P_{ij} \lg P_{ij} \qquad (1)$$

$H_j(N)$ is the number j information entropy in number N antibodies. P_{ij} is the probability of the k_i allele coming from the jth gene.

The mean of the information entropy $H(N)$ is defined as

$$H(N) = \frac{1}{M} \sum_{j=1}^{M} H_j(N) \tag{2}$$

where M is the size of the gene in antibody. The entropy can illustrate the diversity of the antibody population.

The expression observes the diversity between two antibodies as follows:

$$a_{vw} = \frac{1}{1 + H(2)} \tag{3}$$

where a_{vw} is the affinity between two antibodies v and w, and $H(2)$ is the information entropy of antibodies v and w. The larger the a_{vw}'s value, the more the matching between antibodies v and w. Calculate the concentration c_v of antibody v.

$$c_v = \frac{1}{N} \sum_{w=1}^{N} ac_{vw} \tag{4}$$

where

$$ac_{vw} = \begin{cases} 1 & a_{vw} \geq T_{ac} \\ 0 & otherwise \end{cases}$$

The expected breeding ratio e_v of antibody v guides to promote or suppress antigens. a_{v0} expresses affinity between antibody v and antigen.

$$e_v = \frac{a_{v0}}{c_v} \tag{5}$$

The greater the unit adaptation, higher the expected breeding ratio. The greater the unit's concentration, lower the expected breeding ratio. The advantage of utilizing information entropy is keeping units that have higher adaptation, at the same time, making unit's diversity, and improving the speed of convergence.

1. In order to adopt information entropy evaluate similarly of the colony solution, the information entropy is more impersonality than Hamming distance.
2. Based on the concentration, selection mechanism encourages higher suitable feasible solution, and suppresses higher concentration solution; makes sure algorithm convergence and solution colony diversity. The algorithm is suitable to resolve optimization function problem that has many peak values.
3. Introduce the threshold value function. Utilizing immune recognize diversity, namely BALDWIN domino effect (encourages the antigen reproduce that has higher matching) and improving the algorithm performance.

Article (Su Caihong et al., 2002) utilized information entropy immune algorithm which solves the Rosenbrock function overall situation maximum value computation question. Then it drew the

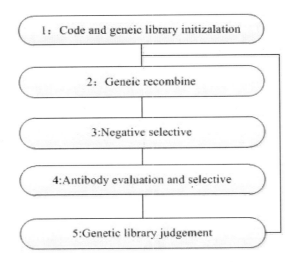

Figure 3. IAIR base flow chart.

conclusion: This algorithm enhanced the overall situation and the partial search ability, improved the flaw of immature convergence, and enhanced the convergence rate.

IAIR base flow can be depicted as shown in Figure 3. IAIR base process is similar to genetic algorithm and it can deal with the solution data directly, via coding express as gene string structure data. Normally utilizing binary-code structure, we regard elements of the problem as gene fragment, and take all feasible values initializing the gene library. Therefore, all combination results germ library equal to all solution space. The solution-finding process of IAIR need no other exterior information. The function uses the value to evaluating antibodies or solution according as evaluating result to process the immune operation.

Genetic rearrangement, Negative selective (NS), and Gene library adjust are 3 main immune operations of IAIR.

1. Genetic rearrangement: Each gene fragment randomly select corresponding allele from gene library, composing a legal antibody (solution of the problem). The objective of genetic rearrangement is to improve the whole search capability.
2. Negative selective (NS): Utilizing genetic rearrangement to produce new antibody, the antibody maybe a better solution, or a worse solution. NS can exclude the worse solution via self-selection and improve the search speed and algorithm time performance.
3. Gene library adjust: Utilizing mature antibody to modify concentration of corresponding gene in gene library, increase concentration of the better antibody gene, and decrease concentration of the worse one. And improve probability to produce the better antibody in next gene rearrangement.

3 CONCLUSION AND PROSPECT FORECAST

The immunity evolution algorithm improved the basic immunity algorithm to have the strong overall importance-thick search, lacked high-accuracy search ability in the partial region. It carries on overall large adjacent-field search, evaluates value high area, and then carries on the local accuracy search in this area. From thick to accuracy, the two adjacent-field search had achieved its overall search optimize solution and local-seek accuracy solution. Immune genetic algorithm has inherited the immune algorithm, and genetic algorithm merit can be more effective in finding the overall situation optimal solution. Wu Xiaojin and Zhu Zhongyin (2005) designed an improvement immune genetic algorithm, introduced the pattern memory library, caused a more effective renewal of memory cell, and has solved the problem which the general immunity genetic algorithms is short of memory function.

3.1 *Development and prospect forecast*

According to immune algorithm research experience, external violation examination and internal study mechanism become two big difficulties (Cai Zixing and Gong Tao, 2004). At present, the external violation examination algorithm is extremely simple, has the very big disparity with organism function, cannot satisfy the need of the actual optimized question application. Present immune algorithm general establishment in precise mathematical model or in formula foundation. The mathematical model, no doubt, is simple and easy to realize, but the function is not strong, with often distorting results, low intelligence , and not advantageous for improvement.

REFERENCES

Fu Haidong, Wang Feng. "Intrusion detection system model based on mathematic statistic and immunlogical principle". Computer Engineering and Design. Vol. 29, No. 12, pp.3037–3039, 2008.

G.-X. TAN, Z.-Y. MAO. "Study on Pareto Front of Muliti-Objective Optimization using Immune Algorithm". Proceedings of the Fourth International Conference on Machine Learning and Cybernetics pp. 2923–2928, 2005.

Jiao Licheng, Du Haifeng. "Development and Prospect of the Artificial Immune System". Acta Electronica Sinica. Vol. 32, NO. 10, pp. 1540–1548, 2003.

J.-S. Chun, H.J and S.-Y. Hahn. "A Study on Comparison of Optimization Performances between Immune Algorithm and other euristie Algorithms", IEEE TRANSACTIONS ON MAGNETICS vol. 34, pp. 2972–2975, 1998.

Mo Hongwei, Jin Hongzhang. "Immune algorithm and application". Aeronautical Computer Technique. vol. 32, No.4, pp. 49–51, 2002.

Medicine Sciences and Bioengineering – Wang (Ed.)
© *2015 Taylor & Francis Group, London, ISBN: 978-1-138-02684-1*

Zinc oxide nanorod biosensor for detection of Alpha Feto Protein in blood serum

Anishkumar Manoharan & Simon S. Ang
High Density Electronics Center, University of Arkansas, Arkansas, USA

ABSTRACT: A zinc oxide nanorod biosensor for the detection of Alpha Feta Protein (AFP) has been fabricated and tested. A low-cost solution growth technique was used to grow the zinc oxide nanorods which serve as the transducer. To enhance signal detection, a Wheatstone bridge microelectrode configuration is applied. A real-time detection limit of AFP target cells of 1 ng/ml has been demonstrated using an electrochemical detection method.

1   INTRODUCTION

The need for clinical diagnostics and accurate detection of cancer target cells are much in demand. Early detection of cancer enhances the chance of a patient being cured of the cancer. Biosensors which have the ability to detect specific biological analytes and to determine drug effectiveness at various target levels accurately are much needed. Alpha-fetoprotein (AFP), a glycoprotein, is produced by a variety of tumors including hepatocellular carcinoma, hepatoblastoma, and non-seminomatous germ cell tumors of the ovary and testis. Most studies report elevated AFP concentrations in approximately 70% of patients with hepatocellular carcinoma and in 50% to 70% of patients with nonseminomatous testicular tumors (Sturgeon, 2008). However, concentrations of AFP above the reference range (<6ng/ml) also have been found in serum of patients with benign liver disease (e.g., viral hepatitis, cirrhosis), gastrointestinal tract tumors and, along with carcinoembryonic antigen in ataxia telangiectasia. Reference values are for non-pregnant women only; fetal production of AFP elevates values in pregnant women. This assay is intended only as an adjunct in the diagnosis and monitoring of alpha-fetoprotein (AFP)-producing tumors and is recommended to be confirmed by other tests or procedures (Mayo Clinic, 2014).

A solid phase direct sandwich enzyme-linked immunosorbent assay (ELISA) has been used in measuring blood AFP concentrations. ELISA is an antibody assay involving sample preparation, several incubations, and washing steps, and is laboratory-intensive and difficult for real-time detection. As such, alternate detection method is needed that should exhibit a high sensitivity, a low detection limit, rapid analysis time, and portability and ease of use important for labor-free and on-site monitoring of these cancer biomarkers. One dimensional (1-D) nanostructures, such as nanowires, nanotubes, and nanorods have received great interests due to its unique properties, such as their high surface areas, and comparatively improved performance in wide range of applications. Zinc oxide (ZnO) can be fabricated into 1-D nanostructures using various methods and growth of different structures such as nanoparticles and nanorods (Kumar, 2006) were reported for biological applications. The selection of the transducer material and the design of the microelectrodes play a very important role in bio-detection (Wang, 2011). Zinc oxide nanorods are used as the transducer materials due to their biocompatibility properties and high electron transfer rate (Cui 2010, Sau 2010, Shankar 2009 & Wang, 2010). The high electron transfer rate helps in the faster reactivity during the immobilization of biomaterials. Quantum dots on zinc oxide nanorods substrate has been reported (Kwon 2013) to increase the immobilization sites, and thereby, improve the sensitivity of the sensor. A FFT admittance voltammetry principle for the target cell detection using ZnO nanoparticles was reported (Norouzi, 2011). Florescent based nanorod biosensors have also been reported (Hu 2011, Lu 2008).

In this paper, we report a low cost zinc oxide nanorod based biosensor that is capable of detecting AFP target cells up to 1 ng/ml using the Wheatstone bridge principle and electrochemical-impedance spectroscopy (EIS) technique. The zinc oxide nanorods were grown using a solution process technique. Zinc oxide seed layer was first grown on a silicon wafer with a silicon dioxide (SiO$_2$) layer. Wheatstone bridge based interdigitated electrodes were fabricated on top of this zinc oxide seed layer. Zinc oxide nanorods were then grown in between these electrodes. AFP specific antibodies were then immobilized onto these nanorods using covalent bonds. The detection limit of AFP antigens of 1 ng/ml, in real time, was achieved using the EIS method.

2 EXPERIMENT

2.1 Synthesis of zinc oxide nanorods

A biosensor consists of two parts, namely the transducer part and the detection part. The detection part consists of the biological components, AFP antibodies, in this case, captures the target cells present in the solution medium passing over it. The transducer part, zinc oxide nanorods in our case, converts biological signals into electrical signals. A bottom-up approach was used to fabricate our biosensor. As an initial step, acetone cleaned SiO$_2$ wafer was spin coated with 5 layers of zinc oxide seed solution consisting of 0.1M zinc acetate and 0.1M ethanolamine in ethanol. The as-formed seed layer was then annealed at 350°C for 1 hour in a vacuum oven. A four quadrant pattern was formed over the seed layer using a photolithography process followed by etching the seed layer in a solution bath consisting of 0.5:500ml of DI H$_2$O:HCl. Wheatstone bridge interdigitated microelectrodes were then formed using a gold lift off process. Growth of zinc oxide nanorods on top of the seed layer and between the microelectrodes was accomplished using a solution mixture of 0.025M zinc nitrate and 0.025M hexamethylenetetramine with 80ml DI water inside a conventional oven at 90°C for 4 hours.

2.2 Immobilization of AFP Antibodies and Antigens

After the construction of transducer part (zinc oxide nanorods) of the biosensor, AFP antibodies (the detector part) were immobilized onto the transducer using covalent bonds. This is accomplished by adding a 0.1M/0.4M ethyl (dimethylaminopropyl) carbodiimide/ N-Hydroxysuccinimide (EDC/NHS) onto layers of synthesized nanorods where the EDC layer gets attached to the ZnO surface with the help of hydroxyl groups and the NHS ester increases the coupling efficiency and strengthens the bond. After the solution dried, AFP antibodies (30µg/ml) were immobilized onto the nanorods via the covalent bonds of EDC/NHS. The antibodies along with the zinc oxide nanorods complete the fabrication of biosensor. The fabricated zinc oxide nanorod biosensors were then tested for capturing of AFP target cells (1ng/ml) by passing the solution over the device. The target cells gets captured on antibodies based on a lock and key process, meaning AFP antibodies can capture only AFP target cells and not any other target cell types.

3 RESULTS

3.1 Zinc oxide nanorods synthesis

Figure 1(a) shows the SEM of four quadrant seed layers with the ZnO nanorods in between the microelectrodes. The grown zinc oxide nanorods are hexagonal in shape and are densely packed resulting in a high surface area. Figure 1(b) shows an x-ray diffraction (XRD) plot of these ZnO nanords with peaks at (002), indicating that the material is zinc oxide in hexagonal shape. These

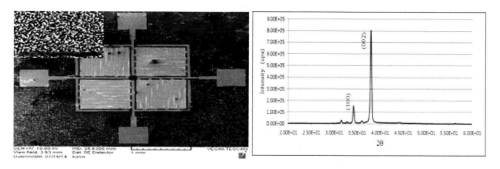

Figure 1. (a) SEM of four quadrant zinc oxide seed layer with Cr/Au microelectrodes and ZnO nanorods growth, (b) XRD plot of the zinc oxide nanorods

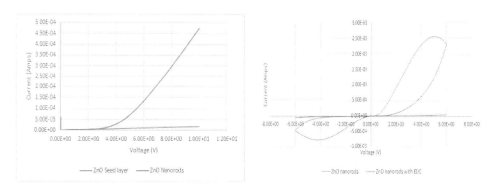

Figure 2. (a) Current-voltage curve at different stages of biosensor fabrication, (b) Cyclic voltammetry curves showing effect of EDC binding onto the ZnO nanorods

data match with the standard data of ZnO (ICDD #00-036-1451), confirming that these nanorods are crystalline in nature.

Figure 2(a) shows the current-voltage characteristics that confirm the growth of the ZnO nanorods onto the seed layer. Since ZnO is an n-type material, as the nanorods grow onto the seed layer, the number of electrons increase leading to an increase in current as seen in Figure 2(a). The next step in the fabrication of biosensor is the immobilization of AFP antibodies onto ZnO nanorods using covalent bonds. Figure 2(b) shows the increase in current of the cyclic voltammetry curves as ZnO nanorods with EDC/NHS crosslinking from that without the covalent bonds. This increase in current is due to the negative charges present on these cross linkers.

3.2 AFP Antibody and Antigen Immobilization

Figures 3(a) and 3(b) show the real-time current-voltage plots during the immobilization of p-type AFP antibodies (30μg/ml) and target cells (1 ng/ml). When a p-type and an n-type material are present on the same surface, an increase in conductivity can be observed in response to time (Zheng 2011). AFP antibodies possess a positive charge and they interact with the n-type ZnO material. As such, its conductivity increases causing an increase in current as shown in Figure 3(a). The peak occurred immediately as antibodies were added and an increase in current of a few hundreds of microamps (μA) was observed.

Figure 3(b) shows the real-time detection of target cells (1ng/ml) binding over the antibodies. An increase of a few microamps (μA) of current was measured within a few seconds after the target

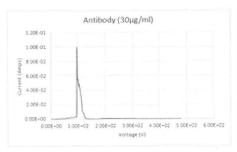
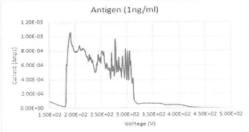

Figure 3.   Real time detection of AFP a) Antibody (30μg/ml) and b) Target cells (1 ng/ml) immobilization.

cells passed through, indicating that the binding of target cells over the antibodies took place. As mentioned above, the normal level of AFP in a human body is <6 ng/ml and if it increases even by 1ng/ml, an early stage of cancer development is indicated. Our device has demonstrated the sensitivity of being able to detect these target cells at a very low concentration accurately in real time.

4   CONCLUSION

An AFP cancer specific biosensor that enables the early detection of this cancer marker in real time was fabricated. Zinc oxide nanorods were grown using a low cost solution process method. Interdigitated microelectrodes in the form of a Wheatstone bridge configuration were shown to enhance the detection of this cancer marker. The detection limit was found to be 1 ng/ml of AFP target cells within a few seconds. As such, a real-time and low detection limit biosensor for AFP was demonstrated.

REFERENCES

C.M. Sturgeon, M.J. Duffy, & U.H. Stenman, et al. (2008) National Academy of Clinical Biochemistry laboratory medicine practice guidelines for use of tumor markers in testicular, prostate, colorectal, breast, and ovarian cancers. Clinical Chemistry, 54 (12), 1–79.

D.N. Kumar & J. Hahm (2006) Nanoscale ZnO-enhanced fluorescence detection of protein interactions. Advanced Materials, 18, 2685–2690.

D.N. Kumar & J.I. Hahm (2006) Highly sensitive biomolecular fluorescence detection using nanoscale ZnO platforms. Langmuir, 22, 4890–4895.

G. Zheng & C. M. Lieber (2011) Nanowire biosensors for label free, real time, ultrasensitive protein detection. Methods Mol. Biol., 790, 223–227.

Mayo Clinic (2014) [online] Available from: http://www.mayomedicallaboratories.com/test-catalog/Clinical+and+Interpretive/8162.

P. Norouzi, V.K. Gupta, F. Faridbod, M.P. Hamedani, B. Larijani & M.R. Ganjali (2011) Carcinoembryonic antigen admittance biosensor based on Au and ZnO nanoparticles using FFT admittance voltammetry. Anal. Chem., 83, 1564–1570.

Q. Wang, D.B. Rihtnesberg, A. Bergstrom, S. Almqyist, A.Z.Z. Zhang, W. Kaplan & J.Y. Anderson (2011) Compacted nanoscale sensors by merging ZnO nanorods with interdigitated electrodes. Proceedings of SPIE, 8031, 80312J–1–80312J–8.

S. Kwon, J.K. Park & I. Park (2013) Quantum dot labelled zinc oxide nanowires. Transducers 2779–2782.

S.S. Shankar, L. Rizzello, R. Cingolani, R. Rinaldi & P.P. Pompa. (2009) Micro/nanoscale patterning of nanostructured metal substrates for plasmonic applications. ACS Nano, 4, 893–900.

T.K. Sau, A.L. Rogach, F. Jäckel, T.A. Klar & J. Feldmann (2010) Properties and Applications of Colloidal Nonspherical Noble Metal Nanoparticles. Adv. Mater, 22, 1805–1825.

W. Hu, Y. Liu, H. Yang & C. M. Li (2011) ZnO nanorods enhanced fluorescence for sensitive microarray detection of cancers in serum without additional reporter amplification. Biosensors and Bioelectronics, 26, 3683–3687.

X. Cui, K. Tawa, K. Kintaka & J. Nishii (2010) Enhanced Fluorescence Microscopic Imaging by Plasmonic Nanostructures: From a 1D Grating to a 2D Nanohole Array. Adv. Funct. Mater., 20, 945–950.

X. Lu, H. Bai, P. He, Y. Cha, G. Yang, L & Tan, Y. Yang (2008) A reagentless amperometric immunosensor for α-1-fetoprotein based on gold nanowires and ZNO nanorods modified electrode. Analytica Chimica Acta, 615, 158–164.

Y. Wang, B. Liu, A. Mikhailovsky & G. C. Bazan (2010) Conjugated Polyelectrolyte–Metal Nanoparticle Platforms for Optically Amplified DNA Detection. Adv. Mater. 22, 656–659.

Medicine Sciences and Bioengineering – Wang (Ed.)
© 2015 Taylor & Francis Group, London, ISBN: 978-1-138-02684-1

Region-Of-Interest tomography with noisy projection data

Renzhen Ye

College of Sciences, Huazhong Agricultural University, Wuhan, Hubei, China

Yi Tang*

School of Mathematics and Computer Science, Yunnan Minzu University, Kunming, Yunnan, China

ABSTRACT: In Region-Of-Interest(ROI) tomography, image reconstruction is an ill-conditioned inverse problem due to the presence of additive noise and incomplete projection data. To improve reconstructed image quality, this paper is aimed at reconstructing a small portion of an object from noisy observations of its projections sampled in and near the ROI. The proposed method can divided into two steps to reconstruct ROI of an object from a set of its noisy projection lines that passed through ROI. First, we introduce filter matrices to filter noisy projection data in multiresolution local tomography. Second, we apply total variation(TV) methods to make reconstructed image deblurring. Experimental results show that the proposed method outperforms state-of-the-art method.

1 INTRODUCTION

In practical application the primary disadvantage of X-ray CT is ionizing radiation, which may induce cancer and cause genetic damage. A major method for reduction of the radiation dose is so-called local CT, which is to reconstruct ROI in a patient from, or primarily from, locally collected projection data. low-dose X-ray computed tomography (CT) imaging is clinically desired and has been deteriorate under investigation in the last decade (Sahiner, B., Yagle, ,A. E. 1995). However the low-dose CT images are susceptible to noise. Recently, many noise-reduction strategies have been proposed to address this problem (Osher, S. J., Rudin, L. I. 1990). In ROI tomography, A slice of an object is represented by a two-dimensional image f. An estimation of f must be computed with a tomographic reconstruction procedure from projection data which are sampled in or near ROI, denoted G, and defined as $G = Af + W$ $A = \{A_{ij}\}$, where weight matrix A is composed of each of weight A_{ij} and A_{ij} is the weight factor that represents the contribution of the *jth* cell to the *ith* ray integral. Here we assume that W is Gaussian noise. However image reconstructed is an ill-conditioned inverse problem, due to the presence of additive noise and incomplete projection data. In general ROI tomography without noisy projection data, a great deal of attention has been given to the wavelet approach in local CT. The application of wavelet theory to local tomography was introduced in Olson, T., DeStefano, J. 1994. Likewise there are many studies which are designed to reconstruct images from noisy projections in CT-(Lee, Lucier, B. (2001)). One of the major strategies models the data noise property by a cost function in image space and then minimizes the cost function for image reconstruction by iterative numerical algorithms (Elbakri, I. A., Fessler, J. A. 2003). An alternative strategy models the noise property by a cost function in sinogram space, seeks an optimal solution for the Radon transform, and then inverts the Radon transform for image reconstruction by filtered backprojection (FBP) algorithm (Li, T. *et. al.* 2004). However there are few studies on ROI tomography with noisy projection data.

---

*The corresponding author is Yi Tang

This paper is aimed at reconstructing a small portion of an object (an ROI) from noisy projection data. We combined two ideas to reconstruct ROI of an object from a set of its noisy projection lines that passed through ROI. Firstly we introduce filter matrices to filter noisy projection data in multiresolution local tomography. Secondly we apply total variation(TV) methods to make reconstructed image clear.

2 FILTER MATRICES INTRODUCED AND MULTIRESOLUTION ROI TOMOGRAPHY

Because there exist the noise in projection data which are sampled in ROI or near ROI, we introduced filter matrices to reduce the noise. Filter matrices are given together with their both filtering and regularization effects. We define the noisy projection data which are sampled in ROI or near ROI as G. And the linear approximation problem can be represented as $Af = G'$, $G = G' + W$, where weight matrix $A \in R^{m \times n}$ has rank $r \leq n$, G' is non-noisy projection data, W is mean-zero Gaussian noise, and f is density function vector responding to ROI which are passed through by projection lines. We assume that $m \geq n$ for simplicity. We try to let noisy projection data G to approximate to G' in order to reconstruct function f. Hence, the problem we use is the Tikhonov problem

$$\min_f \|Af - G\|^2 + \mu^2 \|f\|^2 \tag{1}$$

where $\|\cdot\|$ is the 2-norm. The regular solutions to the Tikhonov problem(1) may be written as $f_{reg} = A^{\#}G$, where

$$A^{\#} = \left(A^T A + \mu^2 I\right)^{-1} A^T \tag{2}$$

is the Tikhonov regularized inverse and $\mu > 0$ is a regularization parameter. We introduced filter matrices which are defined as

$$P_R = AA^{\#} \tag{3}$$

And we can get

$$Af_{reg} = I_r P_R G = G^n \tag{4}$$

It is clear from equation (2) and equation(3) that the weigh matrix plays an important role in reconstructing filter matrices P_R. Each weight can be represented accurately by introducing a Bessel-Kaiser function in order to obtain a perfect reconstruction. Because the Bessel-Kaiser function can be tuned in both the spatial and the frequency domain and has a finite spatial extent and a closed form solution for the ray integral (Beilei, W., Barner, K. 2003). The intensities of the pixels can be solved according to a set of algebraic equations and the measured projections. $p_i = \sum_{j=1}^{N} f_j \cdot A_{ij}$ $1 \leq i \leq M$ where weight A_{ij} represents the influence that the jth pixel f_j has on the ith projection line p_i. Weight matrix A is composed of each of weight A_{ij}. Weight factor A_{ij} can be expressed in the spatial domain as follows (Beilei, W., Barner, K. 2003)

$$A_{ij} = \alpha \sqrt{2\pi/\beta} \cdot \left(1-(r/\alpha)^2\right)^{m+1/4} I_{m+1/2}\left(\beta\sqrt{1-(r/\alpha)^2}\right)\Big/I_m(\beta) \tag{5}$$

Here, r is the shortest distance from a pixel to an projection line, α determines the extent of the function, β controls the trade-off between the width of the main lobe and the amplitude of the side lobes of the Fourier transform of the window (Beilei, W., Barner, K. 2003), m is the dimension of the object, and $I_m(\cdot)$ is the modified Bessel function of the first kind and order. Following Lewitt, R. M. 1990, the function f can be recovered from the filtered projection data G'' from equation(4) by using the inverse Radon transform defined as

$$f(\vec{x}) = \int_0^\pi \int_{-\infty}^{+\infty} \hat{G}''(\omega)|\omega| e^{i2\pi\omega(\vec{x}\cdot\vec{\theta})} d\omega d\theta \tag{6}$$

where $\hat{G}''$ are Fourier transforms of the filtered noisy projection data G''. Insertion of an approximate band-limiting window $w(\omega)$ into the equation(5) yields the filtered back-projection formula(Rashid-Farrokhi, F., Liu, K., Berenstein, C. A., & Walnut, D. 1997). $f_w(\vec{x}) = \int_0^\pi \int_{-\infty}^{+\infty} (\hat{G}'')(\omega)(w(\omega)|\omega|)e^{i2\pi\omega(\vec{x}\cdot\vec{\theta})} d\omega d\theta = \int_0^\pi G'' * F^{-1}(w(\omega)|\omega|)d\theta$ where $w(\omega)$ is a smoothing window, $*$ denote convolution. and F^{-1} is inverse Fourier transforms. the ramp filter $|\omega|$ in equation(6) is replaced by a general angle dependent filter $h_\theta(s)$ to get the formula of reconstructed ROI $f_r(x,y) = \int_0^\pi (h*G'')(\vec{x})d\theta$.

3   THE TV MINIMIZATION ALGORITHM FOR IMAGE DEBLURRING

The importance of minimizing total variation for image processing purposes was first noticed by Osher, S. J., Rudin, L. I. 1990. The argument is that images, seen as functions of two variables, are at most piecewise smooth and important data like edges are discontinuities. Thus image restoration techniques using regularization by smoothing will destroy on one hand noise and on the other important features(e.g. edges, textures). By working in the space of functions of bounded total variation we allow discontinuities in the result of the minimization and thus preserve sharp boundaries. Let f be reconstructed image defined on an open subset Ω of R^2 (Ω is usually a rectangle). The TV minimization algorithm seeks the solution of the following optimization problem:

$f = \arg\min\left(\int_\Omega |\nabla f|^p \, dx + \lambda \int_\Omega |f-f_0|^2\right),\quad f(0) = f_0$ Where λ is a Lagrange multiplier. The reconstructed image becomes blurring in ROI tomography due to noise. We apply the TV minimization algorithm to make the reconstructed image deblurring.

4   IMPLEMENTATION AND SIMULATION RESULTS

To verify the efficiency of the method introduced above, we reconstructed the image from projection data which are sampled in or near ROI. Without loss of generality, we assume the ROI is at the center of the image and reconstruct a local region 35×35 pixels in radius in a 256×256 image. In order to avoid the artifacts, we assumed that noisy projection lines which pass through the interior 35 pixels and a margin of 26 pixels close to ROI can be acquired. On first step, we filter noisy projection data by using filter matrices from equation(4). And we reconstruct image from the filtered noisy projection data on second step. Figure 1(a) shows the original 256×256 pixels mid-plane image of the phantom. Figure 2 shows the results reconstructed from noisy projection data by using the method in (Ye, R., Lu, X., & Liu, H. 2013). Figure 2(a)(b)(c)(d) show the 35×35 pixels mid-plane image by the method in (Ye, R., Lu, X., & Liu, H. 2013) when the power of the output noise in projection data are 40 dBW, 30 dBW, 20 dBW, 10 dBW respectively.

From Figure 2., we can find that above four reconstructed image are blurring due to noise. Figure 3(a)(b)(c)(d) show the 35×35 pixels mid-plane image by our method when the power of the output noise in projection data are 40 dBW, 30 dBW, 20 dBW, 10 dBW respectively. It can be seen that Figure 3(a)(b)(c)(d) has a high contrast and more clear than Fig.2(a)(b)(c)(d).

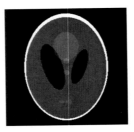

Figure 1.   The original image of a 256×256 shepp-logan phantom.

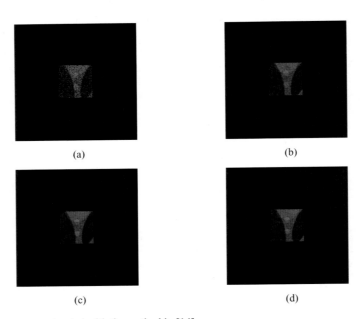

(a)

(b)

(c)

(d)

Figure 2.   Image reconstructed with the method in [14].

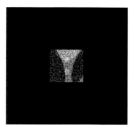

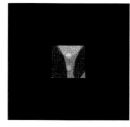

(a) deblurring image from Figure 2(a),   (b) deblurring image from Figure 2(b),

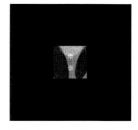

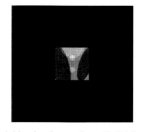

(c) deblurring image from Figure 2(c)   (d) deblurring image from Fig2 (d)

Figure 3.   TV Image reconstructed with our method.

ACKNOWLEDGEMENTS

This paper is partly supported by the National Natural Science Foundation of China (Grant Nos. 61300142 and 61105051).

REFERENCES

Beilei, W., Barner, K. (2003) Fast, accurate and memory-saving ART based tomosynthesis. *IEEE 29th Annual, Proceedings of Bioengineering Conference, Newark, NJ, 2003*.

Elbakri, I. A., Fessler, J. A. (2003) Efficient and accurate likelihood for iterative image reconstruction in X-ray computed tomography. *Proc.SPIE Med. Imag.*, 5032,1839–1850.

Lee, Lucier, B. (2001) Wavelet methods for inverting the radon transform with noisy data. *IEEE Trans. Image. Processing*, 10, 79–94.

Lewitt, R. M. (1990) Multidimensional digital image representations using generalized Kaiser-Bessel window functions. *J. Opt. Soc. Amer. A*, 7(10), 1834–1846.

Li, T., Li, X., Wang, J., Wen, J., Lu, H., Hsieh, J. & Liang, Z. (2004) Nonlinear sinogram smoothing for low-dose X-ray CT. *IEEE Trans. Nucl. Sci.,* 51(5), 2505–2513.

Olson, T., DeStefano, J. (1994) Wavelet localization of the Radon transform. *IEEE Trans. Signal Processing*, 4, 2055–2067.

Osher, S. J., Rudin, L. I. (1990) Feature-oriented image enhancement using shock filters. *SIAM J. Numer. Anal.*, 27, 919–940.

Rashid-Farrokhi, F., Liu, K., Berenstein, C. A., & Walnut, D.(1997) Wavelet-based multiresolution local tomography. *IEEE Transactions on Image Processing*, 6, 1412–1430.

Sahiner, B., Yagle, ,A. E. (1995) Region-of-interest tomography using exponential radial sampling. *IEEE Trans.Image Processing*, 4(8), 1120–1127.

Ye, R., Lu, X., & Liu, H. (2013) Local Tomography Based on Gray System Model, *Neurocomputing*, 101(4), 10–17, 2013.

Medicine Sciences and Bioengineering – Wang (Ed.)
© *2015 Taylor & Francis Group, London, ISBN: 978-1-138-02684-1*

Gene biclustering based on Independent Component Analysis and Non-negative Matrix Factorization

Li-qiang Zhao, Shu-juan Wan, Zhi-guang Zhang, Huan Jiang, Xiao-rui Jia & Yan-hong Zhou
School of Mathematics and Information Science & Technology, HeiBei Normal University of Science & Technology, Qinhuandao, Hebei Province, China

ABSTRACT: This article presents a biclustering method to deal with gene expression data based on Independent Component Analysis (ICA) and Non-negative Matrix Factorization (NMF). ICA is used to select genes to reduce the dimensionality of dataset and eliminate the influence from noisy or irrelevant genes, and NMF to deal with the chosen genes to achieve biclustering. The testing result on the gene expression datasets of Iris and Yeast indicates the efficiency of this method.

1   INTRODUCTION

Usually, gene expression matrix is analyzed in two directions. One is the direction of gene to analyze the gene expression mode by comparing the rows of gene expression in the matrix. Other is in the direction of sample to analyze the expression mode of the samples by comparing the columns of gene expression in the matrix. Biclustering, i..e., a piece of clustering, was first used in gene expression data analysis by Cheng and Church (2000). Biclustering is a special clustering method that was carried out both in rows and columns. Compared with the traditional clustering, biclustering has the following features:

- Locality. The genes in biclustering have high similarity in the part conditions, rather than in the whole conditions.
- Multiplicity. A gene can exist in multiple biclustering classes (cross clustering is allowed, i.e., it can de overlap between biclustering classes). And it cannot be in any biclustering classes.

Non-negative matrix factorization (NMF) is a group of algorithms in multivariate analysis where a matrix V is factorized into two matrices W and H, with the property that all three matrices have no negative elements. From biological sense, each column of matrix W corresponds to a biological process, each item of matrix V can be a weighted sum of gene expression patterns in various biological processes, and weight vector is the corresponding column H.

Biclustering is to cluster genes and samples at the same time, and to find a gene subset so that the genes in the subset can communicate or coordinate with each other only under the certain experimental conditions, but they are unrelated under other conditions (Leo and Björn, 2012). So biclustering is essentially consistent with NMF.

2   USE OF INDEPENDENT COMPONENT ANALYSIS (ICA) TO SELECT GENES

2.1   *The ICA model of gene expression data*

Biological signals from multisensor detection are a number of unknown source signals aliasing, and gene expression noises exist in the operation process of gene expression experiments. Compared with the traditional filter method, ICA does little damage to details of other signals while eliminating noise. Here is a brief introduction for the mathematical model of ICA.

Matrix X of $p \times n$ ($p >> n$) represents the dataset of gene expression. The element x_j of X is the expression level of the ith gene in the jth experiment ($1 \pounds i \pounds p$, $1 \pounds j \leq n$).

The ICA model of X is shown as follows:

$$X_{p \times n} = S_{p \times n} A_{p \times n} \qquad (1)$$

Here S is an active matrix of $p \times n$, and A is a mixed matrix of $n \times n$. The S_q is called statistical independent component of S (ICs). We can multiply both sides of formula (1) by the inverse of mixed matrix A. Namely

$$S = XA^{-1} = XW \qquad (2)$$

Then using ICA algorithm to find a matrix W and making the columns of S as independent as possible. Then a set of new base vectors (rows of A) is selected for gene expression profile to cells classification.

2.2 *The genes selection method based on ICA*

It is easy to get the local optimal solution for ICA factorization (Junying Zhang, 2008). To overcome this defect, this article first processes the gene expression data with standardization and bleaching, and then determines the number of independent components via principal component analysis. Finally it uses ICA to select m genes. The steps are as follows:

1. Calculate the covariance matrix cov(X) of $X_{p \times n}$.
2. Calculate nonzero eigenvalues $\{\lambda_i\}$ of cov(X) and arrange them in descending order.
3. Determine the number z of ICs via the cumulative percentage >0.85.
4. In ICA factorization $X = SA$, S is the matrix formed by independent components.
5. Calculate the maximum number of the gene ($l = 1, \cdots, p$) projection in each principal direction. Let $g_l = \max_{j \in \{1,2,\ldots,m\}} |s_{1j}|$.
6. Arrange $\{g_l\}$ of the p genes in descending order and take the first m genes. And record the rank of each gene.
7. Operate ICA 100 times under different initial conditions. According to steps (5) and (6) select m genes. And then calculate the frequency of each gene chosen. Finally, take the m genes that appear most times.

3 BICLUSTERING BASED ON NMF

3.1 *The relation between biclustering and NMF*

From a mathematical view, the gene expression is a large non-negative matrix. Biclustering is to cluster genes and samples at the same time, and to find a gene subset so that the genes in the subset can communicate or coordinate with each other only under certain experimental conditions, but they are unrelated under other conditions (Yifeng Li, and Jim Jing 2013).

NMF method can be used to deal with this potential cross-clustering, and have an advantage such as dimensionality reduction and the lower complexity of the calculation at the same time. The aim of NMF is to decompose it approximately to a product of two nonnegative matrices $W_{m \times k}$ and $H_{k \times n}$.

$$V \approx WH \qquad (3)$$

Here k is an integer known or unknown, $k << \min(n, m)$ and it represents the number of classes in $V_{m \times n}$. The selection of k is a hard nut to crack. There is an effective method to search gradually a more reasonable value of k based on consensus clustering. First, operate NMF algorithm 30 times with each k within the specified interval, and get a connection matrix C_k of $n \times n$. For each element c_{ij} of C_k, $c_{ij} = 1$ when sample i and j belong to one class and $c_{ij} = 0$ when they do not. Then average C_k and get the consistent matrix $\overline{C}$. Calculate the correlation coefficient

$\rho_k(\overline{C}) = \dfrac{1}{n} \sum_{i=1}^{n} \sum_{j=1}^{n} 4(\overline{c_k}(i, j) - \dfrac{1}{2})^2$. Select k of maximum correlation coefficient by comparing the

correlation coefficients of different values of k.

The process of NMF can be expressed as the optimization problem (Liviu Badea, 2008). The common objective function is

$$\min_{W, H} f(W, H) \equiv \frac{1}{2} \sum_{i=1}^{n} \sum_{j=1}^{m} (V_{ij} - (WH)_{ij})^2 \tag{4}$$

The minimum of the objective function is 0 if and only if $V = WH$.

3.2   *The implementation of biclustering based on NMF*

Biclustering processes on the two non-negative decomposition matrices $W_{m \times k}$ and $H_{k \times n}$ produced by the NMF for $V_{m \times n}$. Gene clustering processes in the row direction of $W_{m \times k}$, sample clustering in the column direction of $H_{k \times n}$. In this way, we can achieve the biclustering for $V_{m \times n}$. The methods used in clustering are hierarchical clustering (HC), k-means, and self-organizing maps (SOM). Considering the running time and accuracy, k-means is better than the other two. Therefore, we use k-means for clustering.

3.3   *Experimental method*

In conclusion, biclustering of the gene expression data matrix $X_{p \times n}$ is outlined below.

1. Use ICA with $X_{p \times n}$ for gene selection. Choose m genes to form $V_{m \times n}$ to avoid fall into local optimal solution.
2. Process non-negative decomposition on $V_{m \times n} \approx W_{m \times k} H_{k \times n}$.
3. Process clustering on $W_{m \times k}$ in the direction of row, namely gene clustering. And process clustering on $H_{k \times n}$ in the direction of column, namely sample clustering. In this way, we can achieve the biclustering of $V_{m \times n}$.

The flow chart of this method is shown as Figure 1: The flow chart of experimental methods.

4   EXPERIMENT

The testing dataset is the gene expression data of Yeast. The dataset can be found in http://arep. med.harvard.edu/biclustering/. The purpose that we use the same dataset as Cheng and Church is to compare the biclustering results. This dataset contains 2884 genes and 17 samples. The data is between 0 and 600, and the missing data is replaced by −1.

First, bleaching and standardization of Yeast's gene expression data. Then the number z of ICs is determined by PCA. We can know the best number for z is 16 from Figure 2: Distribution of the eigenvalues of the covariance matrix in PCA.

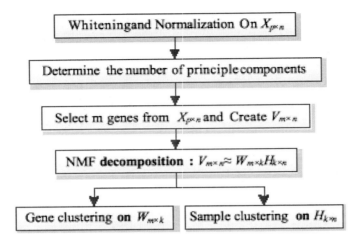

Figure 1. The flow chart of experimental methods.

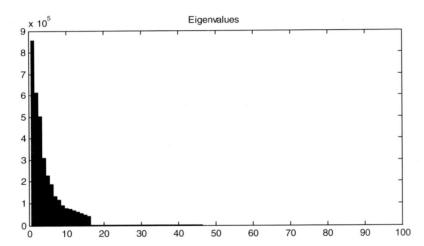

Figure 2. Distribution of the eigenvalues of the covariance matrix in PCA.

Next, process the Yeast data in FastICA and select 16 principal elements and 300 genes. Let the class number k = [2, 3, ..., 9], respectively, to calculate the corresponding coefficients. The result is as shown in Table 1: The corresponding coefficient corresponds to k.

Because the corresponding coefficients are lager when k are 3 and 8, non-negative decomposition should separately proceed for $k = 3$ and $k = 8$.

Process nonnegative decomposition on the 300 gene data filtered. Process k-means clustering on W in the direction of row, namely gene clustering. And process k-means clustering on H in the direction of column, namely sample clustering. The clustering result of 3 genes is shown in Figure 3: The gene clustering result of $k = 3$. The clustering result of 8 genes is shown in Figure 4:

Table 1. The corresponding coefficient corresponds to k.

k	2	3	4	5	6	7	8	9
Corresponding coefficient	0.6512	0.8697	0.6945	0.7601	0.8307	0.8459	0.8539	0.8013

K-Means Clustering of Profiles

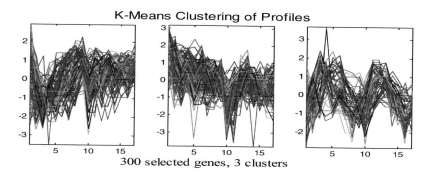

300 selected genes, 3 clusters

Figure 3.   The gene clustering result of k = 3.

K-Means Clustering of Profiles

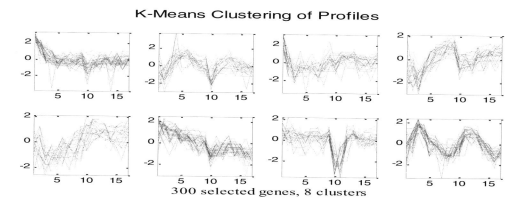

300 selected genes, 8 clusters

Figure 4.   The gene clustering result of k = 8.

K-Means Clustering of Profiles

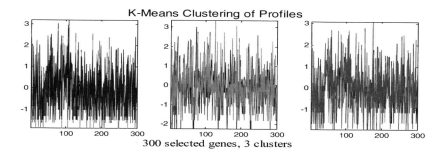

300 selected genes, 3 clusters

Figure 5.   The samples clustering result of k = 3.

The gene clustering result of k = 8. The clustering result of 3 samples is shown in Figure 5: The samples clustering result of k = 3. The clustering result of 8 samples is shown in Figure 6: The samples clustering result of k = 8. From the clustering results, we can find the spectral curves have a good consistency.

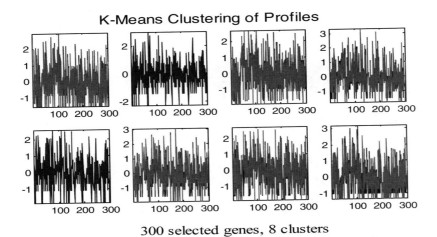

K-Means Clustering of Profiles

300 selected genes, 8 clusters

Figure 6.   The samples clustering result of k = 8.

5   CONCLUSION

This article mainly aims at the complexity of gene regulation and the noise in gene expression experimental operating. Combination of two techniques, FastICA and NMF, is used for preprocessing the gene expression data, to eliminate the influences of noise or unrelated genes on clustering, and to achieve to reduce the dimension of data and the complexity of calculation, and then use biclustering in the data. In application to two testing datasets of Iris and Yeast, we show that FastICA+NMF are able to recover biologically significant phenotypes and identify the potential cross clustering.

ACKNOWLEDGMENTS

This work was supported by Doctor Fund of HeiBei Normal University of Science & Technology (No. 2011YB-006), and Project of Hebei Science and Technology Agency (No. 13212003).

REFERENCES

Y.Cheng and G. (2000) Church. Biclustering of expression data. *The 8th International Conference on Intelligent Systems in Molecular Biology*, pp. 93–103.

Leo Taslaman and Björn Nilsson. (2012) A Framework for Regularized Non-Negative Matrix Factorization, with Application to the Analysis of Gene Expression Data. *PLoS One*. [Online]: 2012, 7(11): e46331. Available from: http://www.ncbi.nlm.nih.gov/pmc/articles/PMC3487913/[Accessed Nov 2, 2012].

Junying Zhang, Le Wei, etc. (2008) Pattern Expression Nonnegative Matrix Factorization: Algorithm and Applications to Blind Source Separation. *Computational intelligence and neuroscience*. [Online]: 2008 (2008). doi: 10.1155/2008/168769. Available from: http://www.ncbi.nlm.nih.gov/ [Accessed 12th June 2008].

Yifeng Li and Alioune Ngom. (2013) The non-negative matrix factorization toolbox for biological data mining. *Source Code Biol Med*. [Online]: 2013, 8: 10. Available from: http://www.ncbi.nlm.nih.gov/pmc/articles/PMC3487913/[Accessed Apr 16, 2013].

Jim Jing-Yan Wang, Xiaolei Wang, & Xin Gao. (2013) Non-negative matrix factorization by maximizing correntropy for cancer clustering. *BMC Bioinformatics*. [Online]: 2013, 14: 107. doi:10.1186/1471–2105-14–107. Available from: *http://www.biomedcentral.com/1471-2105/14/107* [Accessed 24th March 2013].

Liviu Badea, Doina Tilivea. (2008) Nonnegative Decompositions with Resampling for Improving Gene Expression Data Biclustering Stability. In: *Proceedings of the European Conference on Artificial Intelligence ECAI 2008, 21-25 August 2008*, Patras, Greece. pp. 152–156.

Medicine Sciences and Bioengineering – Wang (Ed.)
© *2015 Taylor & Francis Group, London, ISBN: 978-1-138-02684-1*

A recognition method based on curvature feature for identifying dental anatomical reference points from 3D digital models

Ao Lv & Bing-Wei He
School of Mechanical Engineering and Automation, Fuzhou University, Fuzhou, China

Jun Yao & Dan Tong
The Affiliated Stomatological Hospital of Fujian Medical University, Fuzhou, China

ABSTRACT: Traditionally, dental anatomical reference points are chosen from a 3D digital model by the dental doctor with a mouse so that the whole process has low accuracy and repeatability. In this paper, we present a digital recognition method based on the curvature feature to automatically identify the dental anatomical reference points. First, the plaster casts are scanned to acquire the 3D digital dental models. Second, the point curvature features of the 3D dental models are obtained. Then, we use the values of Gaussian curvature kK and mean curvature kH together to identify the dental anatomical reference points. According to the result of curvature analysis, points with smaller absolute magnitude of Gaussian curvature and larger mean curvature are identified as reference points. In this way, the dental parameters are measured. To evaluate the reliability and validity of this method, a comparison between curvature analysis and manual method is presented using the intraclass correlation coefficient (ICC) and the Bland–Altman statistical test. Results show that the measurement method based on the curvature feature performs well in identifying the dental anatomical reference points.

1 INTRODUCTION

Orthodontic treatment outcome and treatment change have traditionally been recorded with study plaster casts, which offer the gold standard for orthodontic diagnosis (Bell *et al*, 2003). Patients' orthodontic data such as arch widths, arch lengths, and arch perimeters are typically obtained from measurements of dental casts by a digital caliper manually (Quimby *et al*, 2004). Technological advances have led to vast improvements in diagnostics tools, the most recent of which is the advent of digital technology; the introduction of digital models offers the orthodontist an alternative to the plaster study models routinely used (Stevens *et al*, 2006). Several other methods of measurement have been proposed over the years with the introduction of digital models, which indicates that digital models have remained as an acceptable substitute for plaster casts. The digital measurement method allows the investigator to click the mouse pointer either within or on the outside surface of teeth. For ease and accuracy of measurements, the 3D digital models were magnified and rotated on screen to aid the identification of landmarks manually. Although the method is simple and easy, it has low precision and reliability (Santoro *et al*, 2003). Therefore, it is important to develop a method to address this problem, which includes the ability to recognize the dental anatomical reference points reliably.

In this paper, we aim at describing a method to identify 3D dental anatomical reference points by calculating the Gaussian and mean curvatures and evaluating the reliability and validity of this method compared with the traditional manual method.

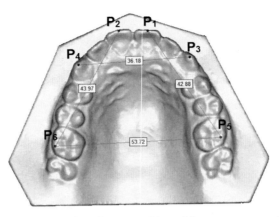

Figure 1. The six anatomical landmarks points (P_1 to P_6) used for measurement of dental parameters: the midincisal points of incisors, canine's cusp tips, and distobuccal cusp tips of the first molars.

2 DESCRIPTION OF THE TRADITIONAL MANUAL METHOD FOR CHOOSING DENTAL REFERENCE POINTS FROM THE 3D MODEL AND ITS DRAWBACKS

Nowadays, the dental anatomical reference points are chosen manually based on the digital models. For this method, first the plaster casts are scanned from different views to acquire the 3D digital models. Triangular mesh models are constructed according to the cloud point data. Based on the 3D digital dental model, each view of the model can be enlarged using the magnifying tool until it is accurately seen on the computer screen. According to the doctor's experience, the cursor is positioned over the landmark in the proper position and the point (e.g., P_1) is chosen by clicking the mouse under this magnifying view. Other landmarks points (P_2, P_3, P_4, P_5, and P_6) are chosen in the same way, as shown in Figure 1.

As long as dental anatomical reference points are carefully selected on the computer screen, it would be reasonable to believe that the digital measurements are more valid than those made by calipers on plaster casts (Stevens *et al*, 2006). The measurement precision largely depends on the accuracy of the selected reference points. And these points are influenced by the operator's skill and learning curve. In order to improve the selecting accuracy and stability of the reference points, we present a digital recognition method based on the curvature feature to identify these feature points automatically.

3 DESCRIPTION OF THE TRADITIONAL MANUAL METHOD FOR CHOOSING THE DENTAL REFERENCE POINTS FROM THE 3D MODEL AND ITS DRAWBACKS

Curvature has only recently been exploited to its full potential, due mainly to the advent of computer technology. Calculating the maximum and minimum principals and Gaussian and mean curvatures provides the basis for a complete characterization of the geometry of folded surfaces and allows some application in 3D images. Curvature attribute is a recently introduced method for geologic structure interpretation and reservoir analysis by measuring stratum bending.

3.1 *Obtaining the curvatures of 3D points on the dental model*

Two partial differential equations define the so-called First and Second Fundamental Forms of differential geometry and uniquely determine how to describe the shape of a parameterized surface in 3D space. The Gaussian curvature k_K and the mean curvature k_H are calculated by the differential geometry (Roberts, 2001):

$$k_K = \frac{LN - M^2}{(EG - F^2)} \qquad k_H = \frac{EN - 2FM + GL}{2(EG - F^2)} \tag{1}$$

The principal curvatures k_{min} and k_{max} are calculated by the Gaussian curvature k_K and the mean curvature k_H:

$$k_{min} = k_H - \sqrt{k_H^2 - k_K} \qquad k_{max} = k_H - \sqrt{k_H^2 - k_K} \tag{2}$$

3.2 *Recognizing the dental anatomical reference points based on the curvature feature*

Gaussian curvature $k_K = k_{min} \times k_{max}$ is one of the two important quantities that are useful for geometric surface description. If only one principal curvature is zero, the surface locally is cylindrically shaped. If both principal curvatures are zero, the surface is a plane. If $k_K > 0$, the two principal curvatures have the same sign and the surface at this point will have a local extremum, making it either a dome or a basin. If $k_K < 0$, then the signs of the two principal curvatures are opposite and the surface locally forms a saddle (Figure 2).

Surfaces with equal Gaussian curvature can be distinguished based on a second important quantity, named mean curvature $k_H = (k_{min} + k_{max})/2$. The orientation of a point also can be determined using the mean curvature. Take the Gaussian curvature $k_K > 0$ for example; the mean curvature can distinguish between a dome ($k_H > 0$) and a bowl ($k_H < 0$). Similarly, when the Gaussian curvature $k_K = 0$ the cylindrical surface can be flat ($k_H = 0$), shaped like a cylindrical anticline ($k_H > 0$), or shaped like a cylindrical syncline ($k_H < 0$) (Figure 2).

Based on the curvature features, ideally the dental anatomical reference points we choose have a local extreme. That is to say, the area shape of the feature point is closed like a dome ($k_K > 0$). In most cases, the point that $k_K > 0$ nearby does not exist because of the triangle mesh structure. In this study, we took into account the values of Gaussian curvature k_K and mean curvature k_H together as a whole to aid in the identification of the dental anatomical reference points. A certain feature point with a smaller absolute magnitude of Gaussian curvature ensured that one of the principal curvatures should be relatively smaller, showing that the area shape was flat at a particular path. On the other hand, the larger mean curvature ensured that the two principal curvatures should be relatively larger, meaning that the area shape at the principal curvature directions was steep. In this situation, the plane nearly reached the dome. And this procedure was repeated until all the dental anatomical reference points were identified automatically.

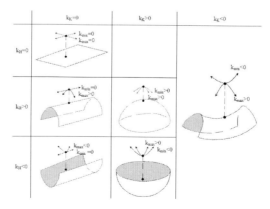

Figure 2. Geologic curvature classification. The local shape of a folded surface can be described by the Gaussian curvature and mean curvature of the point on the surface.

4   ANALYSES OF BOTH METHODS AND RESULTS

For easy measurements, four dental parameters (P_1P_5, P_2P_6, P_3P_4, and P_5P_6) were constructed to evaluate reliability and repeatability between traditional manual method and our proposed method. The traditional method was repeated three times and averaged manually. In our method, the parameter distance could be easily acquired according to the coordinate value of identified points. The reliability of each method was estimated using the ICC and the Bland-Altman test. The ICC was used to determine how well the two methods were correlated. The Bland–Altman analysis was undertaken to determine the agreement between methods.

The Bland–Altman plot (Figure 3) is used to compare the magnitude of error between the manual method and our proposed method. In an evaluation between two sets of measurements made by different methods, the mean of the pair of measurements taken on each specimen is plotted against the actual two measurement values. Such plots make it possible to quickly see if there is any systematic difference between observers or whether the size of error changes over the measurement ranges (Simon *et al*, 2006). The reliability and repeatability with which a measurement can be made is expressed as the mean difference between methods, together with its 95% confidence interval around the mean difference. All the tests were performed separately for the four parameters P_1P_5, P_2P_6, P_3P_4, and P_5P_6.

Table 1.   ICC for manual method (T1) and curvature analysis method (T2).

Parameter (mm)	T1 Mean	SD	T2	T1 × T2 ($n = 20$) R
P_3P_4	35.9110	1.9507	35.9685	0.9873
P_5P_6	55.5535	2.2006	55.5020	0.9885
P_1P_5	41.9685	2.1023	41.9035	0.9836
P_2P_6	41.9230	2.0035	41.8860	0.9824

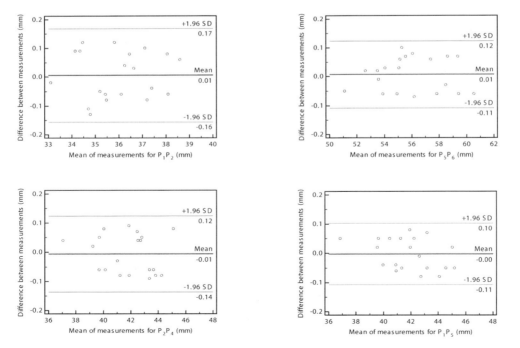

Figure 3.   Bland–Altman plot for manual method and curvature analysis method.

394

The results of and comparisons between the manual method and the curvature analysis method in choosing the dental anatomical landmarks points were obtained and are presented in Table 1 and Figure 3, showing that the curvature analysis method had the highest reliability. In our proposed method, ICC analysis revealed strong linear correlation to the manual measurements, with r values ranging from 0.9824 to 0.9885. For the Bland-Altman statistical test, the limits of agreement were $(-0.16, 0.17)$, $(-0.11, 0.12)$, $(-0.14, 012)$, and $(-0.11, 0.10)$ for the four dental parameters. All points were clustered around the mean difference of zero, within two standard deviations of the difference, indicating good reliability for this method.

5 CONCLUSIONS

We have presented a novel digital identification method to recognize dental anatomical reference points based on the curvature feature and evaluated the reliability and validity of two methods. The digital measurement method identifies the dental anatomical reference points from similar structural areas and facilitates the selection of the points. The reliability and repeatability for manual and curvature analysis methods are estimated by the ICC and the Bland-Altman statistical test. Excellent agreement was found between the measurements with conventional and digital recognition methods. And the curvature analysis method can be an alternative to the manual method. Future studies are necessary to verify the reliability for other dental parameters.

ACKNOWLEDGMENTS

This study is supported by the Education Department of Fujian Province (grant number: JA11010), Science and Technology Department of Fujian Province (grant number: 2012Y4007), and Overseas Studies Scholarship of Fujian Province.

REFERENCES

Bell, A., Ayoub, A.F. & Siebert. P. (2003) Assessment of the accuracy of a three-dimensional imaging system for archiving dental study models. *J Orthod*, 30(3), 219–223.

Quimby, M.L., Vig, K.W., Rashid, R.G. & Firestone A.R. (2004) The accuracy and reliability of measurements made on computer-based digital models. *Angle Orthod*, 74, 298–303.

Roberts, A. (2001) Curvature attributes and their application to 3D interpreted horizons. *First Break*, 19, 85–100.

Santoro, M., Galkin, S., Teredesai, M., Nicolay, O. & Cangialosi T. (2003) Comparison of measurements made on digital and plaster models. *Am J Orthod Dentofacial Orthop*, 124, 101–105.

Simon, H., Charles, F., Helen, F. (2005) Alternative dental measurements: proposals and relationships with other measurements. *Am J Phys Anthropol,* 126, 413–426.

Stevens, D.R., Flores-Mir, C., Nebbe, B., Raboud, D.W., Heo, G. & Major P.W. (2006) Validity, reliability, and reproducibility of plaster vs. digital study models: comparison of peer assessment rating and Bolton analysis and their constituent measurements. *Am J Orthod Dentofacial Orthop*, 129, 794–803.

Medicine Sciences and Bioengineering – Wang (Ed.)
© *2015 Taylor & Francis Group, London, ISBN: 978-1-138-02684-1*

Bioinformatics analyses for the Mycobacterium *tuberculosis* secreted proteins prediction

Liang Wang[a] & Zhe Jin[*]
Shenzhen University School of Medicine, Shenzhen, Guangdong, China
Shenzhen Key Laboratory of translational Medicine of Tumor, the Shenzhen University School of Medicine, Shenzhen, Guangdong, China

Ze Sun
China Telcom Co. Ltd. Shenzhen Branch, Shenzhen, Guangdong, China

ABSTRACT: The aim of this article is to establish a bioinformatics strategy for Mycobacterium *tuberculosis* (H37Rv) secreted protein prediction. The whole protome of H37Rv was scanned by SignalP and TMHMM. A protein date analysis system based on Visual FoxPro was established to process the data output from SignalP and TMHMM and to identify the secreted proteins. The sequences of the secreted proteins were aligned by BLASTp. 179 secreted proteins were identified, where 12 of them were found to be unique inH37Rv. Bioinformatics approaches can be used as an assistant tool in secreted protein research.

1 INTRODUCTION

Proteins secreted by Mycobacterium *tuberculosis* (Mtb) are the unique proteins which can induce protective immunity to M. *tuberculosis* (Horwitz, Harth, Dillon, *et al.* 2005). Two different experimental approaches have been used for the research of proteins secreted by M. *tuberculosis*. One is the analysis of the protein composition of M. *tuberculosis* culture filtrates by using two-dimensional polyacrylamide gel electrophoresis, then to identify the secreted proteins by N-terminal sequencing or by immunological methods (Weldingh, Rosenkrands, Jacobsen, *et al.* 1998. Malen, Berven, Fladmark, *et al.* 2007; Liu, Han, Sun, *et al.* 2011). The other is a genetic approach involving the screening of libraries of fusions of M. *tuberculosis* genes to reporter genes encoding enzymes that become active upon translocation across the cell membrane (Braunstein, Griffin, Kriakov, *et al.* 2000). As a result of the combined efforts of several laboratories, more than 30 secreted proteins of M. *tuberculosis* have been characterized, however, there are still much more secreted proteins have not yet been identified.

Many proteins of *M. tuberculosis* are secreted via the classical sec-dependent (type II) pathway. A signal peptide with N-domain, H-domain and C-domain is the main character in the N-terminal of these proteins. The N-domain located at N-terminal of signal peptide contains one to three positively charged amino acid residues. The H-domain is composed of predominantly hydrophobic residues and alanine and lacks strongly polar of charged residues. The C-domain is usually less hydrophobic and contains the signals that are recognized by signal peptidases (Kostakioti and Stathopoulos. 2006). The conserved features of signal peptides make them amenable to be identified by sequence analysis.

---

*Correspondence: Zhe Jin, Shenzhen University School of Medicine. Phone: 0755-86671902; email address: zhejin1995@yahoo.com,[a] & *These authors contributed equally to this work.

Both secreted proteins and transmembrane proteins have signal peptides. However, secreted proteins have not hydrophobic trans-membrane helix. In general export pathway (GEP), signal peptide was cut by signal peptidases at C-domain after secreted protein was transferred outside of the membrane. Transembrane proteins have not only signalled peptide but also hydrophobic trans-membrane helix which anchors them in the cytoplasmic membrane (Jittikoon, East, Lee. 2007). Thus, in this article, we set out to identify proteins of *M. tuberculosis* secreted via the GEP by using bioinformatics methods.

2   METHODS

2.1   *Signal petides and trans-membrane helix analysis*

Complete proteome sequences of H37Rv were analyzed for secretory signal peptides and trans-membrane helixes with two computer programs, SignalP and TMHMM.

2.2   *Establish database*

Based on the data features, we established a software system named "Analyze system for protein data" to deal with the analyzed result of SignalP and TMHMM (Figure 1).

2.3   *Identify secreted proteins and trans-membrane proteins*

Identify secreted proteins and trans-membrane proteins automatically by using the database mentioned above (Figure 2).

2.4   *BLASTp analysis, acquire secreted proteins unique to H37Rv*

Each secreted protein identified by this strategy was compared with all proteins which amino acid sequences are known already by using the BLASTp in NCBI.

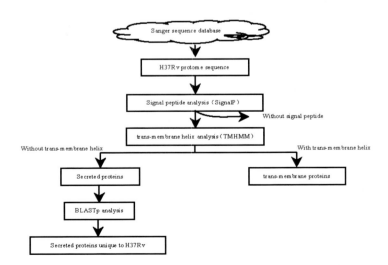

Figure 1.   Flow chart of prediction strategy.

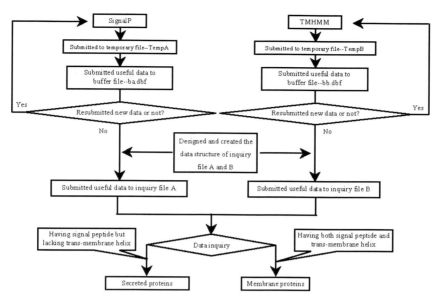

Figure 2.   Flow chart of program design.

3   RESULTS

The typical features of signal peptides (including N-domain, H-domain and C-domain) and trans-membrane helixes analyzed by SignalP and TMHMM were identified automatically by "Analyse system for protein data". We found 179 secreted proteins and 150 trans-membrane proteins. 12 of them were found to be unique to $H_{37}Rv$ based on the results of sequence comparison studies (Table 1).

4   DISCUSSION

SignalP and TMHMM, used in this research, are very efficient in signal peptide and trans-membrane helix prediction (Menne, Hermjakob, and Apweiler, 2000; Moller,. Croning, and Apweiler, 2001). SignalP can identify signal peptide by analyzing the main character in the N-terminal of secreted proteins (N-domain, H-domain and C-domain) (Emanuelsson, Brunak, and. von Heijne, *et al.* 2007). TMHMM can identify both the features of hydrophobic trans-membrane helix and the feature of signal peptide (Kall, Krogh, and Sonnhammer, 2004). The two programs assigned scores to potential signal peptides and trans-membrane helixes for all of the $H_{37}Rv$ proteins. 329 proteins were found to have the typical feature of the signal peptide. Of the proteins in this group, 150 were putative membrane proteins, for they contained hydrophobic trans-membrane helix. The remaining 179 proteins were classified as secreted proteins. These proteins contained one signal peptide, no additional membrane-spanning segments.

Generally, if two proteins have similar sequences, especially the similarity is between functional domains, it is indicated that two proteins may have the same function. Therefore, the crucial problem in bioinformatics is to analyze unknown proteins by sequence alignment. In this article, we found 179 proteins with features of secreted proteins, 12 of them were found to be unique to $H_{37}Rv$ based on the results of sequence comparison studies—BLASTp. It is conceivable that these 12 proteins may be valuable for *M. tuberculosis* clinical diagnoses. Because they are secreted proteins, they may also be protective antigens and be used as targets in *Mycobacterium tuberculosis* vaccine research.

Table1.　H$_{37}$Rv unique secreted proteins.

Gene name	SignalP score	Cleavagesite	Number of trans-membrane helix	SignalP-predicted signal peptide sequence
Rv0179c	0.990	44–45	0	MWIRAERVAVLTPTASLRRLTACYAALAVCAALACTTGQPAARA^AD
Rv0203	1.000	27–28	0	MKTGTATTRRRLLAVLIALALPGAAVA^LL
Rv0398c	1.000	28–29	0	MGVIARVVGVAACGLSLAVLAAAPTAGA^EP
Rv1174c	1.000	28–29	0	MRLSLTALSAGVGAVAMSLTVGAGVASA^DP
Rv1799	1.000	34–35	0	MSVKSKNGRLAARVLVALAALFAMIALTGSACLA^EG
Rv1974	1.000	28–29	0	VQRQSLMPQQTLAAGVFVGALLCGVVTA^AV
Rv2297	0.842	19–20	0	MAMEMAMMGLLGTVVGASA^MG
Rv2330c	1.000	30–31	0	VRRQRSAVPILALLALLALLALIVGLGASG^CA
Rv2341	0.645	37–38	0	MPVGGRQHVFEKLASILGLVAAPLMLLGLSACGRSAG^KT
Rv2452c	0.998	29–30	0	VAFRDILVLFSMKTLTLTLAMAAASSTALT^TV
Rv3491	0.997	20–21	0	VNIRCGLAAGAVICSAVALG^IA
Rv3675	0.876	20–21	0	MFTLLVSWLLVACVPGLLML^AT

This prediction strategy is based on general export pathway (GEP), though GEP is the main protein secretion pathway, there are some other pathways for secretion. Some proteins, which can be transported outside of the membrane without signal peptides (van Bloois, Nagamori, Koningstein *et al.* 2005), cannot be identified by this system. In addition, some trans-membrane proteins have ⊠ sheet, not ⊠ helix, as their hydrophobic trans-membrane domains (Tamm, Arora, and Kleinschmidt. 2001). So these trans-membrane proteins could be miss identified as secreted proteins by this strategy. Despite with some insufficient aspects, as a primary bioinformatics prediction strategy, this method is valuable for further research.

ACKNOWLEDGEMENTS

This study was supported by the Science and Technology Bureau of Shenzhen City grant JC201006010727A, JCYJ20120613165853326, GJHS20120621154321244, National Nature Science Foundation of China 81171921, 81172282, the Shenzhen Peacock Plan KQCX20130621101141669, the Planned Science and Technology Project of Shenzhen GJHS20120621142654087, the Key Laboratory Project of Shenzhen ZDSY20130329101130496, Natural Science Foundation of SZU 201108 and T201202.

REFERENCES

E. van Bloois, S. Nagamori, G. Koningstein, et al. (2005) The Sec-independent function of Escherichia coli YidC is evolutionary-conserved and essential. *J Biol Chem*, 280(13):12996–13003.

H. Malen, F.S. Berven, K.E. Fladmark, et al. (2007) Comprehensive analysis of exported proteins from Mycobacterium tuberculosis H37Rv. *Proteomics*, 7(10):1702–1718.

J. Jittikoon, J.M. East, A.G. Lee. (2007) A fluorescence method to define transmembrane alpha-helices in membrane proteins: studies with bacterial diacylglycerol kinase. *Biochemistry*, 46(38):10950–10959.

K. Weldingh, I. Rosenkrands, S. Jacobsen, et al. (1998) Two-dimensional electrophoresis for analysis of Mycobacterium tuberculosis culture filtrate and purification and characterization of six novel proteins. *Infect Immun*, 66(8):3492–3500.

K.M. Menne, H. Hermjakob, R. Apweiler. (2000) A comparison of signal sequence prediction methods using a test set of signal peptides. *Bioinformatics*, 16(8):741–742.

L. Kall, A. Krogh, E.L. Sonnhammer. (2004) A combined transmembrane topology and signal peptide prediction method. *J Mol Biol*, 338(5):1027–1036.

L.K. Tamm, A. Arora, J.H. Kleinschmidt. (2001) Structure and assembly of beta-barrel membrane proteins. *J Biol Chem*, 276(35):32399–32402.

M. Braunstein, T.I. Griffin, J.I. Kriakov, et al. (2000) Identification of genes encoding exported Mycobacterium tuberculosis proteins using a Tn552'phoA in vitro transposition system. *J Bacteriol*, 182(10):2732–2740.

M. Kostakioti, C. Stathopoulos. (2006) Role of the alpha-helical linker of the C-terminal translocator in the biogenesis of the serine protease subfamily of autotransporters. *Infect Immun*, 74(9):4961–4969.

M.A. Horwitz, G. Harth, B.J. Dillon, et al. (2005) Enhancing the protective efficacy of Mycobacterium bovis BCG vaccination against tuberculosis by boosting with the Mycobacterium tuberculosis major secretory protein. *Infect Immun*,73(8):4676–4683.

O. Emanuelsson, S. Brunak, G. von Heijne, et al. (2007) Locating proteins in the cell using TargetP, SignalP and related tools. *Nat Protoc*, 2(4):953–971.

S. Liu, W. Han, C. Sun, et al. (2011) Subtractive screening with the Mycobacterium tuberculosis surface protein phage display library.*Tuberculosis (Edinb)*, 91(6):579–86

S. Moller, M.D. Croning, R. Apweiler. (2001) Evaluation of methods for the prediction of membrane spanning regions. *Bioinformatics*, 17(7):646–653.

Medicine Sciences and Bioengineering – Wang (Ed.)
© *2015 Taylor & Francis Group, London, ISBN: 978-1-138-0-02684-1*

Analyzing method of exercise intensity based on wavelet frequency band energy quotient

Xie-feng Cheng & He Yang
College of Electronics, University of Posts and Telecommunications, Nanjing, China
Jiangsu Province Engineering Lab of RF Integration & Micropackage, Nanjing, China

Wei Jiang
College of Electronics, University of Posts and Telecommunications, Nanjing, China

ABSTRACT: Human PCG and ECG signals change significantly before and after taking exercise. This paper presents a new method called wavelet frequency band energy quotient as a physiology evaluation parameter of human exercise intensity. Firstly, the paper analyzes the characteristics of PCG and ECG signals, then puts forward a frequency band energy quotient algorithm based on wavelet packet decomposition, and verifies its validity and applicability by making three groups of simulation experiments. Finally, combined theory with practice, a new kind of human exercise intensity detector is designed. This paper not only has made a qualitative analysis of PCG and ECG signals, but also made detailed quantitative analysis. Experimental results demonstrate that the human exercise intensity detector has good classification and recognition effects, with simple and reliable hardware design as well as good adjustability on detecting standard, the detector can evaluate the human exercise intensity correctly and properly.

1 INTRODUCTION

In recent years, the events of sudden death, sometimes occur in China among those people who take their exercises, especially with the largest proportion of students. According to the statistics, the annual rate of sudden death among people who take their exercises is 1/250 000 (Zhang, 2011). It is necessary to test and evaluate exercise intensity and physiological parameters of students to prevent these accidents, especially to those students who have poor health. PCG and ECG as two of the most important human physiological signals contain a large number of physiological and pathological information about the human heart and blood vessels (Cheng, 2012). Both of them can well reflect cardiac contractility and cardiac reserve situation, and has a non-invasive, high sensitivity and specificity, can be repeated using objective and quantitative characteristics (Guo, 2006). Detecting and analyzing PCG and ECG signals is an indispensable way to understand the health of the human heart (Yuan, 1981). These properties of the two physiological signals can be applied to a variety of sports occasions and realize the real-time monitoring of the physical fitness evaluation and exercise training on the human body.

2 METHODS AND INSTRUMENTS

2.1 *Characteristics of PCG and ECG*

As one of the most important human physiological signals, PCG consists of the first PCG (S1) and second PCG (S2), third PCG (S3), and the fourth PCG (S4). The first and second PCG signals are strong enough and can be detected through the stethoscope auscultation. While the third and fourth PCG signals are weak and cannot be detected by hearing. Once the heart function become abnormal, 'the additional sound' or 'noise' will be added in PCG (Cheng, 2010). According to the analysis, normal PCG frequency is mainly less than 250HZ, but the frequency of noise and the additional sound are higher. Thus, it is possible to judge the health of heart based on the PCG signal frequency distribution. ECG is the basis of clinical heart disease intelligent diagnosis revealing cardiac electrical activity in the human body. The ECG is a non-linear and non-stationary weak signal, the frequency range of 0.05–100HZ, 90% of ECG spectral energy is concentrated in less than 35 HZ. The normal ECG includes P wave, QRS wave group, T wave, U wave and J point of integration (Zhou, 2005). To study the frequency distribution of the individual components of the ECG wave can determine the characteristic of this signal from qualitative and quantitative analysis.

2.2 Methods and instruments

Wavelet packet transforms two-scale equation:

$$w_{2n}(t) = \sqrt{2} \sum_{k \in Z} h_{0k} w_n(2t - k) \tag{1}$$

$$w_{2n+1}(t) = \sqrt{2} \sum_{k \in Z} h_{1k} w_n(2t - k) \tag{2}$$

Where: when n=0, Scaling function is $w_0(t) = \phi(t)$, Wavelet function is $w_1(t) = \psi(t)$. Defined function sequences $\{w_n(t)\}$ (n $\square$ Z) wavelet packet $w_0(t) = \phi(t)$ identified on the ground. Wavelet packet formula reconstruction:

$$d_l^{j,n} = \sum_k \left[h_{0(2l-k)} d_k^{j+1,2n} + h_{1(2l-k)} d_k^{j+1,2n+1} \right] = \sum_k g_{0(l-2k)} d_k^{j+1,2n} + \sum_k g_{1(l-2k)} d_k^{j+1,2n+1} \tag{3}$$

Where: h and g are the scale function $\phi(t)$ and wavelet function $\psi(t)$ corresponds to the low-pass and high-pass filter. Signal after wavelet packet decomposition corresponds to the wavelet packet node, the distribution of the frequency band is not continuous, there is interlacing. According to study, this is determined by Mallat algorithm.

Mallat algorithm is defined as follows: Let $a_j(k), d_j(k)$ as a discrete approximation coefficient in multi-resolution analysis, $h_0(k), h_1(k)$ are two filters which meet the two-scale difference equation, then $a_j(k)$ and $d_j(k)$ have the following recurrence relations:

$$a_{j+1}(k) = \sum_{n=-\infty}^{\infty} a_j(n) h_0(n - 2k) = a_j(k) * \overline{h}_0(2k) \tag{4}$$

$$d_{j+1}(k) = \sum_{n=-\infty}^{\infty} a_j(n) h_1(n - 2k) = a_j(k) * \overline{h}_1(2k) \tag{5}$$

Where: $\overline{h}(k) = h(-k)$. In fact, due to the characteristics of Mallat algorithm, there are band staggered phenomena of multi-layer wavelet packet decomposition in each layer, after decomposition we need to find the right band order. There are more or less noise in both PCG and ECG signals. The noise is existed in normal individuals (benign noise, such as children and youth, sports, pregnancy), also can be found in patients with heart disease (Guo, 2006). The study indicates that the benign murmur frequency is similar with normal PCG frequency, both belong to

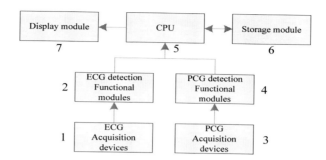

Figure 1.   Structure diagram of instrument.

the low-frequency, while patients murmur generally distributed in the high-frequency domain. Therefore, after the wavelet packet decomposition, the heart condition can be inferred by analyzing the normalized ratio of the size of the energy band of the total energy of the low frequency component. This is the basis of detecting the intensity of human exercise by wavelet packet decomposition band energy quotient method. Defined the wavelet packet decomposition band energy quotient:

$$R = \frac{E(i)}{E} \infty 100\% \qquad (6)$$

where: $E(i) = \left|g_i(k)\right|^2$ Expressed as a band normalized energy: $E = \sum_{k=1}^{n} \left|g_n(k)\right|^2$ Expressed as a layer of band energy sum, $n = 0,1,2,...,2^m - 1$ n is the band number.

Figure 1 is the structure diagram for this instrument. Part 1 represents plane, palm type electrode. Part 2 on behalf of the ECG signal detection module. Part 3 is double auscultation head PCG sensor. Part 4 on behalf of the PCG signal detection module. Part 5 is the central control unit. Part 6 represents a data storage unit. And Part 7 on behalf of the liquid crystal displays module. According to the structure diagram, Part 1 was formed by two metal circular electrodes which fixed at intervals in the same plane and connected to the Part 2 represent ECG signal detection module. The acquired ECG signal was delivered to the Part 5 to be processed, and the results can be stored either in Part 6 or can be displayed in liquid crystal display module. There is another device to collect PCG signal: The Part 3, double auscultation head PCG sensor, can be used to obtain PCG signal, and then connected to PCG signal detection function module Part 4, The acquired PCG signal was delivered to the Part 5 to be processed, and the results can be stored either in the part 6 or can be displayed in liquid crystal display module. Before exercise, users will put their hands closely to the center of the palm of two metal circular electrodes (Part 1) to detect the ECG signals. The acquired ECG signal was delivery to the part 5 to be processed, and the results can be stored either in Part 6 or can be displayed in Part 7. And they can take another test after their warm-up exercises using the same method, in this way an evaluation or suggestion about human exercise intensity will be given. For example, before the PE exam, students were asked to participate in this test, and then teachers can judge the students if fit to take part in physical examination.

2.3   Experiment

Verify the reasonableness of using PCG wavelet packet quotient method to detect the exercise intensity of human. A group data of 80 human PCG signals was selected as an experimental object. Half of them were normal PCG data and the other were collected from disease patients.

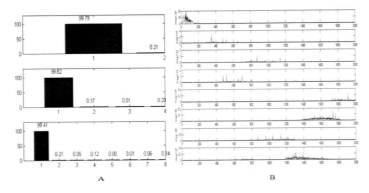

Figure 2.   Wavelet packet energy- band interleaved of PCG.

Experimental data were processed by the wavelet packet decomposition method with db6 wavelet and frequency band energy of wavelet packet was calculated using wave energy instruction and db6 wavelet. The layers of wavelet packet decomposition depend on the accuracy of time-frequency analysis of experiment signal. The less the decomposition layer number is, the faster analysis speed is, but the frequency resolution is low, it is the same if vice versa. The Nyquist frequency is 2000 HZ due to the experimental data of PCG signal sampling rate for 4000 HZ. As known the normal PCG signal frequency mainly concentrates in 250 HZ, so three layers were decided to decompose the PCG signal. The following is the decomposition band distribution of the third layer: 0–250HZ, 250–500 HZ, 500 HZ–750 HZ, 750–1000 HZ, 1000–1250 HZ, 1250–1500 HZ, 1500–1750 HZ, and 1750–2000 HZ. The band distribution indicates that the first band of the third decomposition just in the range of normal PCG frequency. Therefore, the normalized energy of the first band of the third decomposition was selected to define the PCG wavelet packet decomposition band energy quotient. Namely:

$$R_1 = \frac{E(1)}{E} \infty 100\% \tag{7}$$

In order to prevent band interleaved, which brings inaccuracy in band energy quotient calculation, it is necessary to reconstruct experimental PCG data in wavelet packet decomposition, and the reconstruction signal in each band can reflect each band frequency distribution order under

Table 1.   Audio frequency band energy business statistics of PCG

The third layer decomposition		Abnormal data	Normal data	
Mean		92.58	99.84	
Maximum		99.51	100	
Minimum		65.24	99.04	
Standard deviation		9.47	0.19	
First detected		X/65.24≥1	Qualified	
		X/65.24<1	Unqualified	
Second detection		X/99.04≥1	Qualified	
		X/99.04<1	Unqualified	
Overall	Data number	Correct number	Error number	Accuracy
	80	78	2	97.5%

406

Fourier transformation. From the diagram 1 B, we can see the band sequence after band inter-leaved (1, 2, 4, 3, 7, 8, 6, 5). It is clear that the order of the first band (minimum band in the third band) did not confuse, so the result can be used in the next step.

3 CONCLUSION

PCG and ECG as two kinds of human important physiological signal, include much pathological information of human body. In recent years, the PCG and ECG research change from qualitative analysis to the quantitative analysis phase due to the improvement of signal technology. The appli-cation of computer technology for detection can well reflect the heart health, playing a critical role in today's clinical medicine. Therefore, the analysis advantage of PCG and ECG signals combined with exercise intensity detecting not only embodies the value of the current medical research but also meets the demand of people's health. In this paper, band energy quotient as a quantitative analysis of the PCG signals and a kind of characteristic parameters was proposed by using wavelet packet decomposition. And a computer simulation experiment proves this method in the detec-tion of the intensity of human whether has better ability, the main program has high efficiency in temporal and it is easy to adjust the threshold. Then, a simple and reliable project of hardware equipment is proposed based on the above theory research.

ACKNOWLEDGMENT

This work is supported by the National Natural Science Foundation of China (Grant No.61271334) "Research and application on the heart sound feature extraction for identification".

REFERENCES

Cheng Xiefeng, Ma Y, Liu C, et al. Research on PCG identification technology [J].2012, (42):237–251.
Cheng X F, Ma Y, etc. Three-step identity recognition technology using PCG based on information fusion [J]. *Chinese Journal of Scientific Instrument (in Chinese), 2010.* 8(31):1712–1720.
Guo X M, Yan Y,et al. Used for heart change trend of the evaluation based on probabilistic neural network recognition algorithm of PCG [J]. *Journal of Biomedical Engineering*,2006(05).112–118.
Yuan S Y. Electrocardiogram diagnosis knowledge [M]. *Tianjin: Tianjin Science and Technology Press*, 1981,52–52.
Zhou J, Yang Y M, He W. PCG signal analysis and feature extraction methods [J]. *Chinese Journal of Biomedical Engineering*,2005,24(6):682–689.
Zhang J L, Jiang H, Kan D S, et al. The PCG signals based on wavelet analysis and feature extraction [J]. *Computer and Information Technology*,2011,19(1). 756–762.

Medicine Sciences and Bioengineering – Wang (Ed.)
© *2015 Taylor & Francis Group, London, ISBN: 978-1-138-02684-1*

Neuroprotective effects against ischemia injury derived from Smad7-modulated ActA/Smads pathway activation

Yan-kun Shao
Department of Neurology, China-Japan Union Hospital, Jilin University, Changchun, China

Zhong-hang Xu, Yi-ming Wang & Yong-tao Wang
Norman Bethune Health Science Center Of Jilin University, Changchun, China

Jiao-qi Wang
Department of Neurology, China-Japan Union Hospital, Jilin University, Changchun, China

Chun-li Mei
Beihua University, Jilin City, Jilin, China

Jing Mang* & Jin-ting He*
Department of Neurology, China-Japan Union Hospital, Jilin University, Changchun, China

ABSTRACT: To assess the role of Smad7, which mediate the activation of ActA/Smads pathway against ischemia neural injury. The model of PC12 cells with Oxygen Glucose Deprivation(OGD) was built to simulate the process of ischemia neural injury in vitro, Smad7 gene was silenced by using RNA-interfering technology, apoptosis of PC12 cells from ischemia injury was analyzed with DAPI, the expression of p300 and procaspase-3 gene was observed by real-time PCR. Smad7-siRNA can inhibit the expression of Smad7 and reduce the apoptotic rate of PC12 cells caused by ischemia injury, whereas Smad7-siRNA can promote the expression of procaspase-3 protein and downstream gene of signal protein transcription activating factor: p300. Target-silencing Smad7 gene can enhance the signal transduction pathway of ActA/Smads and reduce the sensitivity of PC12 cell to OGD injury.

1   INTRODUCTION

Ischemic cerebrovascular disease is one of the most common causes of death and long-term disability in the world. The ischemic neural injury is often accompanied with series of signal transduction pathways changes and produce relevant biological functions (Meschia *et al.*, 2011). As a member of the superfamily of transforming growth factor-beta (TGF-β), Activin A (ActA) triggers a cascade reaction downstream by activating the transmembrane receptor-mediated cell signal transduction pathway of Smads and thus protect nerve cells from hypoxic-ischemic injury (Schmierer *et al.*, 2007; He *et al.*, 2011). ActA has been found to perform neuroprotective effects against ischemia injury resulting from brain stroke. Signal transduction of ActA was mainly depended on Smads: Smad2 and Smad3 are the direct substrates of activin receptor of type I, which can be phosphorylated to form a complex substance with Smad4 to regulate gene expression after transferred into the nucleus (Wang *et al.*, 2013). Smad7, as the I-Smad, can competitively bind the phosphorylated ActRI and suppress ActA/Smads pathway (KATO *et al.*, 2001). However, as one of the inhibitory Smads, whether Smad7 is related to the regulation of ActA/Smads pathway in the process of ischemic neural injury has not been reported. In this study, we

---

*Author to whom correspondence should be addressed: Jing Mang, mangjing@jlu.edu.cn, Tel: +8615844031118 and Jin-Ting He, hejinting333@sina.com.

explore the function of Smad7 in brain ischemic injury in vitro, which may provide considerable insight into mechanism of ischemic cerebrovascular disease related to cell signaling pathway.

2 MATERIALS AND METHODS

2.1 Cell culture and Oxygen–Glucose Deprivation (OGD)

PC12 cells were purchased from Cancer Cell Bank of Chinese Academy of Medical Sciences, which were routinely cultured in high glucose DMEM (Dulbecco's modified Eagle's medium) containing 5% horse serum and 10% fetal bovine serum. It is then incubated with 50 ng/mL nerve growth factor (NGF) for 7 days, and then cultured in the absence of sugar and 1.0 mmol/L NaS2O4 in hypoxic tank (37°C, 5% CO2 and 95% N2) for 0, 3, 6, 12, 16, and 24 h, setting control group OGD 3h, 6h, 12h, 16h, 24 h group separately.

2.2 Si-RNA transfection determination and grouping

The designation of siRNA was based on the sequence of Rat Smad7 (NM030858.1) refer to Dharmacon siDESIGN Center. The target sequence of siRNA is 5′-AACGAUCUGCGC UCGUCCGGCGU-3′, sense 5′-AACGAUCUGCGCUCGUCCGGCGUDTDT-3′, antisense 3′-DTDTUUGCUAGACGCGAGCAGGCCGCA-5′. FITC-labeled positive siRNA was used to transfect PC12 cells to determine siRNA transfection efficiency and optimal transfection concentration. According to the instruction, transfection was conducted when adherent PC12 cells reach 80% in 24-well plates. According to the experimental requirements, this research includes siRNA transfection group, negative transfection group, and control group.

2.3 Real-time RT-PCR

Total RNA from PC12 cells was extracted using Trizol Kit. C-DNA was synthesized by reverse transcription and the premier was designed according the gene bank. The sequences of primers for smad7 and p300 were as follows: smad7, sense: 5′-AACCCCATCACCTTAGTCG-3′; antisense: 5′-TGCTCCGCACTTTCTGTACC-3′; p300: sense: 5′-GGGCTCAACCGACAA GAC-3′; antisense: 5′-GGAGGCAGAGGCAATCAA-3′. The conditions for amplification were 45 s at 94 °C, 45 s at 56°C, and 1 min at 72°C for 29 cycles. An RNA control tube containing all RT reagents except the reverse transcriptase was included as a negative control to monitor genomic DNA contamination. The detection of smad7 was conducted 16 h after OGD.

2.4 Western blot analysis

The cells were collected and counted in group: OGD 0 h, OGD 16 h, siSmad7-OGD 16 h separately, and then the precooling cell lysis buffer was added (Mei et al., 2011). The mixture was laid on ice for 30 min until the cells split completely, decentered in 12000 rpm and 4°C for 10 min, and tested the concentration by method of BCA(2-Quinolinecarboxylic acid). Another cell lysis buffer, including equal volume of protein, was mixed with electrophoretic buffer solution and boiled at 100°C for 5 min; then the mixture was centrifuged, separated by electrophoresis in 12% SDS-PAGE. The membrane was blocked with 5% skim milk. The primary antibodies were diluted with 5% skim milk for one night. The PVDF(polyvinylidene fluoride) membrane was washed with TBST(Tris-Buffered Saline and Tween 20) three times (each time for 10 min), second antibody was added, incubated at room temperature for 1 h. PVDF membrane was washed with TBST for three times, (each time for 10 min), then was exposed by the ECL color reagent.

2.5 Detection of apoptosis

PC12 cells were fixed by formaldehyde at room temperature for 10 min, washed twice with PBS, added 300 μL DAPI solution, protecting from light at room temperature for 10 min, then added 500 μL PBS, and observed by fluorescence microscope to detect cell activation.

2.6 Statistical analysis

SPSS software was used for statistical analysis. Values are presented as means ± SD. An ANOVA was used. P-values less than 0.05 were considered to be significant.

3 RESULTS

3.1 Transfection efficiency of siRNA

Fluorescence microscope observation showed that whole green fluorescence can be found in each siRNA group and scRNA group 24 h after transfection. The occurrence rate was higher than 73%.

3.2 Detection of apoptosis

Control group (OGD 0-h group): fluorescence in the nucleus showed blue, oval, and uniform density of nuclear chromatin; OGD 16-h groups: visible nuclear shrinkage, chromatin condensation, nuclear fragmentation, morphological changes; siSmad7-OGD 16-h group: significant reduction of apoptotic bodies compared with ischemia group. (Figure 1)

3.3 Detection of ActA and P300 transcriptional co-stimulating factor

The mRNA expression in OGD 16-h group is the highest and siSmad7-OGD 16-h group is the lowest. (Figure 2-a) ActA and p300 mRNA expression of siSmad7-OGD 16-h group was the highest, OGD 0-h group was the

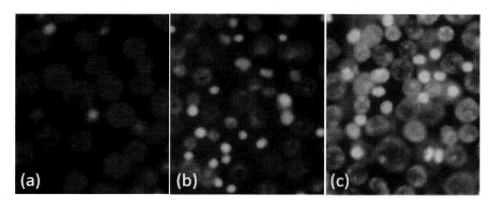

Figure 1. Apoptosis was analyzed by DAPI (×400). (a) Control group, (b) siSmad7 group, and (c)OGD 16-h group.

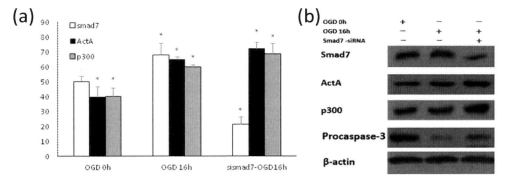

Figure 2. (a) mRNA expression of different groups. (b) Protein expression of different groups.

lowest (P < 0.05). As for the protein expression of ActA and p300, siSmad7-OGD 16 h was the highest and OGD 0 h was the lowest (P < 0.05). Compared to OGD16-h group, the expression of Procaspase-3 is higher in group sismad7-OGD16 h. Smad7-siRNA upregulated Procaspase-3 protein on the nerve cell protective effect of ischemic injury. (Figure 2-b).

4   DISCUSSION

According to the role of Smad proteins in TGF-β signal pathway, it can be classified into 3 categories: receptor-activated Smads (R-smad), common mediator Smads (Co-Smad), and inhibitory Smads (I-smad), Smad7 is a kind of I-Smad, which play negative regulatory function in TGF-β signaling (KATO et al., 2001). Smad7 can regulate TGF-β/Smad signal pathway and maintain its balance. Contrary to Smad2 and Smad3, Smad7 is capable of binding activated Activin receptor and prevents Smad2 and Smad3 in combining with TGF-β receptor and the following phosphorylation (Shi et al., 2004).

It has been indicated that target-silencing Smad7 can downregulate the transcription and expression of Smad7. Our results showed that the expression of ActA and p300 was increased after OGD 16 h and higher after silencing Smad7. p300 is an important co-transcription factor downstream, which can bind to more than 100 types of transcription-associated protein (Antonio et al., 1999). p300 protein is widely distributed in the neuron system and plays an important role in gene expression in hypoxia (Ogawa et al., 2001). The expression of p300 and the function of relative protein combination can influence the selective expression of hypoxia-related genes (Chevillard-Briet et al., 2002). In the initial stage of neuronal apoptosis, p300 can be degraded by Caspase. The binding rate to p53 and NF-KB can influence the survival of neuron under DNA injury. Increase in p300 protein can significantly improve the survival rate of neurons (Yamashita et al., 2004). This research indicated an elevation of p300 16 h after OGD, which is similar to the result of the former report (Tang, 2005). A higher level of p300 after smad7 silencing indicated an improvement of cell survival when sismad7 and smad7 play a negative effect in the regulation of p300 protein content. Besides, in the process of neuron protection, the function of p300 must be involved. When combined with p300, p300-binding protein can be connected to a same gene-promoter region with specific DNA elements and regulate the expression of same gene. Whether the combination function of p300 is influenced by smad7 and its mechanism still needs further exploration.

Therefore, this result confirms ActA/Smads signaling pathway is activated after focal cerebral ischemia. Besides, the activation of ActA/Smads can be elevated by the target-silencing Smad7 by siRNA. Our former work indicated that the expression of ActA increased in the OGD 16-h group, which is in accordance to this result (Mang et al., 2013). The elevation of ActA and p300 after siRNA can prove the negative regulatory function of Smad7 in another facet and provide a clue for further exploring the ActA/Smads signaling pathway on ischemic brain injury in the mode of action and signal transduction mechanisms.

There are both neuronal apoptosis and necrosis after stroke. By detecting apoptotic bodies, the level of apoptosis can be better understood (JAZAG et al., 2005). As for a kind of signaling protein, the biological function of Smad7 is through the ActA/Smads signal transduction pathway. The extracellular to intracellular signal transduction is a series of physiological changes occurring within the cell producing a certain function. Apoptosis cascade is regulated by a series of reaction of Caspase, and Caspase-3 is a key protein in this process. After target-silencing Smad7 by siRNA in ischemic cell, the morphological pathological condition is significantly improved and the number of apoptotic bodies reduced. Caspase-3 is a key enzyme of downstream apoptosis. Its activation means inevitable cell apoptosis. Caspase-3 is biologically synthesized as pro formation that is inactivated. We found that the expression of Procaspase-3 decreased 16 h after OGD and increased after siRNA silencing, which means the amount of activated caspase-3 is elevated after OGD and reduced after Smad7-siRNA. Smad7-siRNA attenuated apoptosis and Caspase cascade program, and decreased ischemic neuronal apoptosis rate significantly. Therefore, Smad7-siRNA plays a protective function in ischemic neuronal injury.

5 CONCLUSION

Target-silencing Smad7 gene can enhance the activation of ActA/Smads signal transduction, which play a protective role against ischemic neuronal injury.

ACKNOWLEDGMENT

Supported by the Innovation Project by College students (2014) of Jilin University in China.

REFERENCES

Antonio, G., & Maria, L.A. (1999) P300 and CBP: Partners for Life and Death. *J. Cell. Physiol.*, 181, 218–223.

Chevillard-Briet, M., Trouche, D. & Vandel, L. (2002) Control of CBP co-activating activity by arginine methylation. *EMBO J*, 21(20), 5457–5466.

He, J.T., Mang, J. & Mei, C.L.(2011) Neuroprotective Effects of Exogenous Activin A on Oxygen-Glucose Deprivation in PC12 Cells. *Molecules*, 17(1), 315–27.

JAZAG, A., & KANAI, F.(2005) Single small-interfering RNA expression vector for silencing multiple TGF-β pathway components. *Nucleic Acids Research*, 33(15),131–140.

KATO, S., UEDA, S. & TAMAKI K.(2001) Ctopic expression of Smad7 inhhibit strans-forming growth factor responses in vascular smooth muscle cells. *Life Sci*, 69(22), 2641–2652.

Mang, J., He, J.T. & Wang, J.Q.(2013) ActA and ActRIIA expression in Smads signaling pathway in ischemia brain injury. *J Apoplexy and Nervous Diseases*. 2013, 30(1):15–18.

Mei, C.L., He, J.T. & Mang, J.(2011) Nerve growth factor (NGF) combined with oxygen glucose deprivation (OGD) induces neural ischemia tolerance in PC12 cells. *AJBR*, (5)10, 315–320.

Meschia, J.F., Nalls,M. &Matarin M.(2011) Siblings with ischemic stroke study: Results of a genomewide scan for stroke loci. *Stroke*, 42, 2726–2732.

Ogawa, H., Nishi, M., & Kawata, M.(2001) Localization of nuclear co-activators P300 and steroid receptor co-activator 1 in the rat hippocampus. *Brain Res*, 890(2), 197–202.

Schmierer, B. & Hill, C.S. (2007) TGF beta-SMAD signal transduction: molecular specificity and functional flexibility. *Nat Rev Mol Cell Biol*, 8(12), 970.

Shi, W., Sun, C., & He, B. (2004) GADD34-PP1c recruited by Smad7 dephosphorylates TGFbeta type I receptor. *J Cell Biol*, 164(2), 291–300.

Tang, X.L. (2005) Effect of p300 and p300-binding properties on the neuron injury during hypoxia. [Dissertation]*Chongqing: Third Military Medical University.*

Yamashita, S. (2004) Ontogenic expression of estrogen receptor coactivators in the reproductive tract of female mice neonatally exposed to diethylstilbestrol. *RePro Toxi*, 18(2), 275–284.

Wang, J.Q., He, J.T. & Mang, J.(2013) Effects of SARA on oxygen-glucose deprivation in PC12 cell line. *Neurochem Res*,38(5),961–71.

Medicine Sciences and Bioengineering – Wang (Ed.)
© 2015 Taylor & Francis Group, London, ISBN: 978-1-138-02684-1

Structure of clustering based on inquiry of TCM data storage management system in wireless sensor network

Jian-qing Liang & Jian-cheng He*
School of Basic Medicine, Shanghai University of TCM, Shanghai, China

ABSTRACT: Objective: To find the structure of clustering based on inquiry of TCM data storage management system in wireless sensor network. Methods: The article about data centric and cluster–based routing, design an Inquiry of TCM data storage management system, which suits cluster-routing of wireless sensor network. Results: From the perspective of data storage and data inquiry, this article surveys the system, and verifies the improvement on energy consumption, and inquires speed of the system by clinical experiment. Conclusion: it provides a good way on Inquiry of TCM data storage and management.

1 INTRODUCTION

Wireless sensor network is a wireless network composed of sensor, stationary or moving, in a self-organizing and multi hop manner, to collaborate perception, acquisition, processing, and transmission of network covering the geographical area–perceived objects, and finally puts the information sent to the network owner. Wireless sensor network is the current concern in the international community, involving a high degree of cross-multidisciplinary, highly integrated knowledge of the hot research field (Jalil Jabari Lotf, 2010). Inquiry of TCM has long been engaged in research of this task group, which plans to use the wireless sensor network technology, and the realization of intelligent TCM interrogation.

2 THE CLUSTER-BASED ROUTING PROTOCOLS

Wireless sensor network must use the cluster-based routing protocols. The data management system of traditional Chinese medicine diagnosis is based on clustering. In the cluster-based routing protocols, network is divided into clusters. Network node cluster is the associated sets, each cluster consists of a cluster head and a plurality of intracluster members, the cluster head low-level network is a network of cluster members, where the higher-level cluster heads communicate with the base station. This algorithm divides the whole network into connected regions, as shown in Figure 1. Wireless sensor network responsible for the cluster of interrogation information collecting and processing data fusion and inter cluster forwarding.

3 CLUSTERING ROUTING ALGORITHM

The definition of Technology Information Process (TIP) to predict the node temperature, increased biological cluster-based wireless sensor networks, and take GA (Genetic algorithm, a randomized algorithm simulation sequences characteristics) cluster head to judge network optimal order

---

*Corresponding author: HE Jian-cheng, Email: hejc8163@163.com.

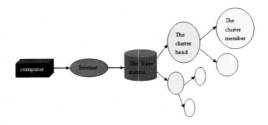

Figure 1.   Clustering routing protocol system structure.

(Qinghui Tang, 2005). The wireless sensor network node energy consumption model is assumed in this article (Soro S, 2005), such as type (1)–(3) as shown:
Data transmission:

$$E_{TX}(k,d) = \begin{cases} E_{elec}K + \varepsilon_{fs}KD^2, d \le d0, \\ E_{elec}K + \varepsilon_{fs}KD^2, d \le d0. \end{cases} \tag{1}$$

Data reception:

$$ERX(k) = E_{elec}K, \tag{2}$$

Data fusion:

$$EGX(k) = E_{gather}K, \tag{3}$$

4   TRADITIONAL CHINESE MEDICINE DIAGNOSIS DATA COLLECTION

4.1   *Literature sources*

Chinese biomedical literature database (CBMdisk), Chongqing VIP (VIP), and Chinese HowNet (CNKI), included Wan Fang database with data of all the literatures of interrogation. "*Plain Questions*," "*Classic of Acupuncture*," "*A-B Classic of Acupuncture and Moxibustion*" and other books provide information; self-symptom questionnaire was used to collect the symptoms.

4.2   *Inclusion and exclusion criteria*

1. Has a complete and accurate information about "inquiry of TCM symptoms/signs," description document, and its treatment, medicine, cure (whether complete or not), all included in the data collection
2. Duplicate content in published articles or documents repeated in references (such as medical cases and inquiry Monograph), only one is used, the rest is excluded.

4.3   *Methods of data processing and input*

On the basis of standardized syndrome and symptoms, computer search and manual search are combined based on a comprehensive collection and the correct understanding of the literature

416

data, to establish database interrogation differentiation. EpiData 2.1 software was used for data entry—double-independent input, and to check, modify, select 10% manual checking—to ensure accurate data input.

5   INTERROGATION OF DATA STORAGE AND QUERY

Before establishing the inquiry of TCM database, the consistent treatment of the first to standardize the selected symptoms, the symptoms were qualitative ("disease" [hypochondriac pain, diarrhea] and "syndrome" [liver stagnation and spleen deficiency syndrome] as examples). Each property name is represented by a database field, and the specific permit various symptoms of standard code name had included in accordance with the unified character. Meanwhile, in the specific application, symptom code symbols can be converted to the corresponding TCM symptoms and syndrome-type name card. In the database, symptoms are of dendritic distribution. And then through the Internet, the doctor and the patient can exchange the disease symptoms, see Figure 2.

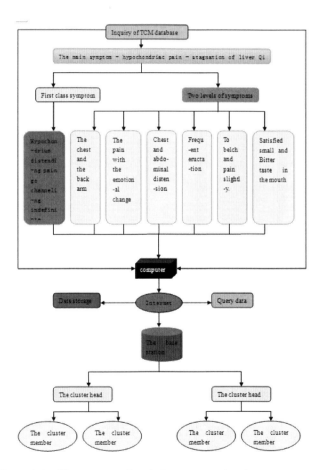

Figure 2.   TCM diagnosis intelligent system for wireless sensor networks.

6   CLINICAL APPLICATION OF CLUSTERING IN WIRELESS SENSOR NETWORK INTELLIGENT SYSTEM BASED ON TCM INTERROGATION

This work is based on the clustering of wireless sensor network to support the system applied to clinical and medical resource sharing. For example, consider the case of Li Ming, male, 64 years old. Primary symptom (4 points): hypochondriac pain; one-level symptoms (2 points): swelling, pain, walk up indefinite (solid, hot); the disease location is hypochondriac (inside). The secondary symptoms (1 point): feeling pain with changes in emotion, which increase or decrease, small and bitter taste in the mouth. Preliminary diagnosis (7 points): hypochondriac pain (Qi Stagnation). Accompanied symptom (3 points): Diarrhea. One-level symptoms (2 points): Bowel and abdominal distension, abdominal pain (virtual, cold). Disease location is belly (inside). Secondary symptoms (0.5 point): flatus. Preliminary diagnosis of 2 (5.5 points): diarrhea (liver stagnation and spleen deficiency syndrome, as shown in Figure 3).

7   THE PROSPECT OF THE DEVELOPMENT OF TCM DIAGNOSIS INTELLIGENT SYSTEM FOR WIRELESS SENSOR NETWORKS

Medical symptoms and syndrome of TCM in ancient Chinese form the dominant position, the name of the concept, is "to logical thinking method name" (REN Xiu-ling, 2011), that is not conducive to international exchange and dissemination of TCM. With the advance in time, the traditional Chinese medicine is also to "advance with the times," which absorb modern outstanding civilization achievements, continuous innovation, and continuous development. Therefore, research on TCM symptom is the foundation to achieve accurate differentiation, making the

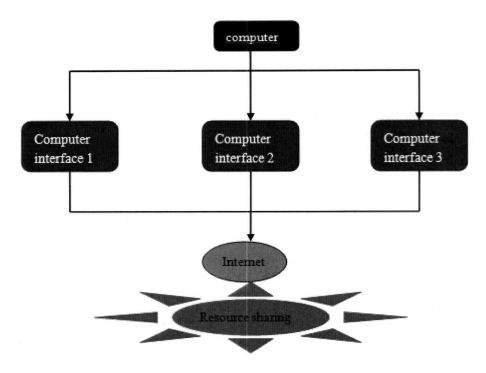

Figure 3.   Interrogation-intelligent clinical operating system.

diagnostic criteria for the disease domain (HUANG Bi-qun, 2011). In this guidance, the clinical symptoms and the TCM interrogation of computer programming included in the establishment of database, which is a successful construction of inquiry of TCM diagnosis database, at the same time to cluster based routing, design a kind of wireless sensor networks suitable for traditional clustering routing that asked diagnosis data storage management system. First, the data storage and query of two aspects of the data storage management system are described, and then verified by clinical application, the energy consumption and the query speed of data storage management system with good effect are considered, which provide reference and ideas for the development of digital TCM interrogation, worthy of further clinical application.

ACKNOWLEDGEMENTS

This paper is one of the achievements such as the Twelve and Five support program of National (No.2012BAI25B05), Special Expo of Shanghai Municipality (No.06dz05815), The third phase of the key subject of Shanghai TCM diagnostics project (No.S30302).

REFERENCES

HUANG Bi-qun. The standardization of TCM symptoms with Necessity.Chinese Journal of traditional Chinese medicine and pharmacy, 2011,26(3):429–432.

Jalil Jabari Lotf. Seyed Hossein Hosseini Nazhad Ghazani. Overview on routing protocols in wireless sensor networks //The 2nd Int Conf on Computer Engineering and Technology (ICCET), Vol 3. Piscataway, NJ:IEEE, 2010:610–614.

Qinghui Tang, Tummala N, Gupta S K S. Communication scheduling to minimize thermal effects of implanted biosensor networks in homogeneous tissue [D], Schwiebert L, biomedical Engineering [J]. IEEE Transactions,2005,52(7):1285–1294.

REN Xiu-ling.Form of the theory concept of TCM by yixingzhengming.Chinese Journal of traditional Chinese medicine and pharmacy, 2011,26(4):644–646.

Soro S, Heinzelman W B. Prolonging the lifetime of wireless sensor networks via unequal clustering[A]. Proc. of the 19th IEEE Int'l on Parallel and Distributed Processing Symposium[C]. San Francisco: IEEE Computer Society Press, 2005:236–240.

Medicine Sciences and Bioengineering – Wang (Ed.)
© 2015 Taylor & Francis Group, London, ISBN: 978-1-138-02684-1

A simple enzyme glucose biosensor based on Ag doped Fe_3O_4 nanoparticles

Yue-yun Li, Jian Han, Ping Wang, Kai Li & Yun-hui Dong
School of Chemical Engineering, Shandong University of Technology, Zibo, China

ABSTRACT: A simple amperometric enzyme biosensor for the determination of glucose was constructed. Glucose Oxidase (GOX) was covalently bonded with Ag doped Fe_3O_4 nanoparticles (GOX-Ag@Fe_3O_4) via Glutaraldehyde (GA) and Chitosan (CS) was used to immobilize the modified electrode. The performance of GOX-Ag@Fe_3O_4 assembled electrode was studied by Electrochemical Impedance Spectroscopy (EIS) and Cyclic Voltammetry (CV). The detection limit of the biosensor was 0.02 mM (S/N = 3). A good linear relationship between the current signals and the concentrations of glucose was achieved from 0.06 to 23 mM. In addition, the sensor has some important advantages such as simple preparation, fast response and good stability. Therefore, this proposed strategy could be applied to detect glucose in human serum sample.

1 INTRODUCTION

Diabetes is a worldwide public health problem (Magner, 1998). Its diagnosis and management require tight monitoring of blood glucose levels and the normal level of blood glucose is 4.4–6.6 mM (Dai *et al.*, 2009). In recent years, different methods have been used for glucose analysis, such as fiber optic sensor (Brondani *et al.*, 2009), chemiluminescence (Yang *et al.*, 2010), and electrochemical method (Yan & Chuan, 2009). Among these methods, electrochemical biosensors have unique advantages for the detection of glucose due to its simplicity, fast response time, high sensitivity, and excellent selectivity (Yang & Zhu, 2006). GOX is widely employed as an analytical reagent with its relatively low cost and good stability, which makes the glucose/GOX system a very convenient model for enzyme-based biosensors. More recently, iron oxide nanoparticles (Fe_3O_4NPs) have been paid more attentions owing to their interesting inherent magnetic property which can be utilized to immobilize biomolecules on substrate surfaces and thus construct magnetically controllable bioelectrochemical systems (Gao *et al.*, 2007). AgNPs have an activity for high intensity electron transfer (Chen *et al.*, 2007) and they can facilitate the electron transfer from the redox center of a protein in the electrode surface (Huang & Miao, 2008). CS has been widely used for the immobilization of various enzymes in recent years (Wan & Yuan, 2010). CS has lots of advantages, such as excellent membrane-forming ability, good biocompatibility, and susceptibility to chemical modification arising from the presence of reactive amino and hydroxyl functional groups (Yan & Chuan, 2009).

In this paper, we synthesize Fe_3O_4NPs and AgNPs are doped on Fe_3O_4NPs (Ag@Fe_3O_4) by in situ reduction. GOX is covalently bonded with Ag@Fe_3O_4 via crosslinking agent, glutaraldehyde (GA) which provides the reactive aldehyde groups. The mixture is used to modify the GCE and CS is immobilized on the modified electrode via robust covalent bonds. And the fabricated biosensor was applied successfully to the detection of glucose.

2 EXPERIMENTAL SECTION

2.1 *Chemicals*

GOX and CS were purchased from Sigma Aldrich (USA). $AgNO_3$ and sodium citrate were purchased from Shanghai reagent (Shanghai, China). All other chemicals were of analytical reagent grade. Phosphate buffered saline (PBS, 0.1 M) was used as an electrolyte for all the electrochemistry measurements. Ultrapure water was used in the process of the experiments. CS was dissolved in 1% acetic acid to give a final mass fraction of 0.5%.

2.2 *Apparatus*

TEM images were obtained from an H-800 microscope (Hitachi, Japan). The UV-Vis absorbance spectra were examined with a Lambda 25 UV-Vis Spectrophotometer (PerkinElmer, American). All the electrochemical measurements were performed on CHI760D electrochemical workstation (Chenhua Shanghai Co., Ltd., China) and used conventional three-electrode system. The conventional three-electrode system included GCE as working electrode, a saturated calomel as reference electrode (SCE), and a platinum wire as auxiliary electrode.

2.3 *Preparation of Mesoporous Fe$_3$O$_4$NPs*

Mesoporous Fe_3O_4NPs were synthesized following the method reported previously (Guo, & Wang, 2009). In brief, 1 g of $FeCl_3 \times 6H_2O$ was dissolved in 20 mL of ethanediol to form a transparent solution. Next, 3 g of sodium acetate and 10 mL of ethylenediamine were added to the solution. After stirring for 30 min, the mixture was transferred into an autoclave and heated for 8 h at 200°C. When cooled down to room temperature, the amino-group functionalized Fe_3O_4NPs was collected on the vessel wall with a permanent magnet and then washed three times with ultrapure water and vacuum dried at 50°C overnight.

2.4 *Preparation of GOX-Ag@Fe$_3$O$_4$*

$Ag@Fe_3O_4$ was synthesized by situ reduction. Briefly, 30 mg of Fe_3O_4NPs and 30 mg of $AgNO_3$ were dissolved in 30 mL of ultrapure water and stirred for 24 h. Then, the precipitate was collected on the vessel wall and 0.2 M HCl was used to adjust the pH less than 2. After stirring for 30 min, 1 mL of 50 mM sodium citrate was added into the mixture. Finally, the resulting material was vacuum dried at 50°C overnight.

In this work, the amino-group functionalized $Ag@Fe_3O_4$ (1 mg) was dispersed in 0.6 mL of PBS (pH 7.4) and 0.2 mL of 2.5 wt% GA solution was added into this $Ag@Fe_3O_4$. After stirring for 1 h and magnetic separation, 2.5 mg of GOX was added into the solution and the mixture was allowed to react at room temperature and kept stirring for 24 h. The resulting GOX-$Ag@Fe_3O_4$ was collected by magnetic separation and dispersed in PBS (pH 7.4) and stored at 4°C when not in use.

2.5 *Fabrication of the biosensor*

A GCE (4 mm) was polished to a mirror-like finish with 1.0, 0.3 and 0.05 μm alumina powder and then thoroughly cleaned before use. Then 6 μL of the prepared GOX-$Ag@Fe_3O_4$ was dropped onto the electrode surface and dried at 4°C. Following that, 10 μL of 2.5 wt% GA was dropped onto the modified electrode and dried at 4°C. After the electrode was washed with ultrapure water, 0.5% CS was dropped onto the modified electrode. When not in use, the electrode was stored at 4°C in a refrigerator.

3 RESULTS AND DISCUSSION

3.1 Characterization of Fe₃O₄NPs and Ag@Fe₃O₄

Figure 1A showed the TEM of the prepared Fe_3O_4NPs. It can be seen that Fe_3O_4NPs owned an average size of about 50 nm and had mesoporous structures. The TEM of Ag@Fe_3O_4 (Figure 1B) further indicated the successful synthesis of Ag@Fe_3O_4. The formation of Ag@Fe_3O_4 was also characterized by UV-Vis absorption spectra (Figure 1C). It was evident that the absorbance intensity of the Fe_3O_4NPs was relatively stable with increasing light wavelength in the range of 300–800 nm (curve a). When AgNPs were reduced on the surface of Fe_3O_4NPs, a new absorption peak centered at 390 nm was clearly observed (curve b). Curve c showed the UV-Vis absorbance spectra of AgNPs and its characteristic absorption peak was approximately at 390 nm. Compared with curve c, curve b indicated that the formation of Ag@Fe_3O_4.

3.2 Optimization of experimental conditions

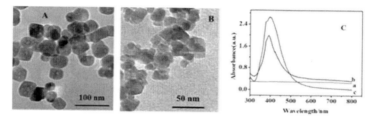

Figure 1. TEM images of the Fe_3O_4NPs (A) and Ag@Fe_3O_4 (B); (C) the UV-Vis spectra of Fe_3O_4NPs (a), Ag@Fe_3O_4 (b), and AgNPs (c).

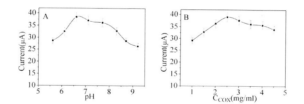

Figure 2. Effect of pH (A) and the concentration of GOX (B) on the response of the biosensor to 5 mM glucose Error bar = RSD (n = 3).

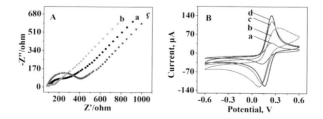

Figure 3. (A) EIS of 2.5 mM Fe(CN)63−/4− and 0.1 M KCl at (a) bare GCE; (b) GCE/Ag@Fe_3O_4; (c) GCE/GOX-Ag@Fe_3O_4. (B) CV of different modified electrodes in 10 mM Fe(CN)63−/4−: (a) bareGCE; (b) GCE/Fe_3O_4; (c) GCE/GOX-Ag@Fe_3O_4; (d)GCE/Ag@Fe_3O_4.

The activity of the enzyme GOX was heavily affected by the pH of substrate solution. Therefore, the pH effect on the biosensor performance was also investigated by measuring the current response to 5 mM glucose. As clearly seen in Figure 2A, the optimal amperometric response was achieved at pH 6.5. The reason was that the highly acidic or alkaline surroundings would damage the activity of immobilized protein (Guo et al, 2006). The amperometric response of the measuring system was related to the concentration of GOX (Figure 2B). As shown in Figure 2B, the optimal concentration of GOX was chosen as 2.5 mg/mL.

3.3 Evaluation of the electrochemical performance of the glucose biosensor

The electrochemical performance of Ag@Fe_3O_4 modified GCE was characterized using EIS. The corresponding results were shown in Figure 3A. The bare GCE exhibited a small semicircle domain (curve a), When Ag@Fe_3O_4 was modified onto GCE, the GCE presented the smaller semicircle domain (curve b) which indicated that faster electron transfer resistance of $[Fe(CN)_6]^{3-/4-}$ on GCE/Ag@Fe_3O_4. However, the presence of GOX-Ag@Fe_3O_4 via GA, remarkably increased the electron transfer resistance (curve c), indicating the larger obstruction effect of GOX on the flow of electrons. These experimental results not only proved that the surface of GCE has been successfully modified with Ag@Fe_3O_4 but also demonstrated that the GOX was successfully linked onto the Ag@Fe_3O_4.

To further investigate the feasibility of the electrochemical assay, the CV has been performed. As shown in Figure 3B, for the bare GCE, the well-defined oxidation and reduction peaks caused by the Fe^{3+}/Fe^{2+} redox couples were noticed in forward and reverse scan (curve a). After the electrode was modified by Fe_3O_4NPs, an obvious increase in reduction and oxidation peak is observed (curve b). The peak current was further increased after the electrode was modified by Ag@Fe_3O_4 (curve d) compared to GCE/Fe_3O_4 (curve b), indicating that AgNPs can promote the conductivity of Fe_3O_4NPs. After the electrode was modified by GOX-Ag@Fe_3O_4, the peak current was decreased (curve c). The reason was that GOX acted as an inert block layer to hinder the electron transfer.

3.4 Response of the biosensor to glucose

Under the optimal conditions, a linear relationship between the current and glucose concentration was obtained from 0.06 to 23 mM ($R^2 = 0.9947$) The detection limit was estimated to be 0.02 mM at a signal/noise ratio of 3. The results demonstrated that the proposed method could be used to detect glucose concentration quantitatively.

3.5 Reproducibility and selectivity of the biosensor to glucose

To evaluate the reproducibility of the biosensor, five electrodes were prepared for the detection of 5 mM glucose. The relative standard deviation (RSD) of the measurements for the five electrodes was 4.6%, suggesting the precision and reproducibility of the proposed biosensor was quite good. To examine the specificity of the fabricated biosensor, interferences study was performed using ascorbic acid, uric acid, Na-ascorbate and urea. The 5 mM of glucose solution containing 100 mM of interfering substances was measured and the RSD of the measurements was under 5.0%. The results indicated that the selectivity of the biosensor was acceptable.

4 CONCLUSION

We constructed a biosensor based on GOX-Ag@Fe_3O_4/CS composites for the detection of glucose. AgNPs can promote the conductivity of Fe_3O_4NPs and enhance the detection sensitivity. The proposed biosensor showed high sensitivity and long-term stability. The simple proposed method may lead to an attractive approach for the other analyte determination.

REFERENCES

Brondani, D., Scheeren, C.W., Dupont, J., & Vieira, I. C. (2009) Biosensor based on platinum nanoparticles dispersed in ionic liquid and laccase for determination of adrenaline. *Sensors and Actuators B: Chemical*, 140(1), 252–259.

Chen, Z.P., Peng, Z.F., Luo, Y., Qu, B., Jiang, J.H., Zhang, X.B., Shen, G.L. & Yu, R.Q. (2007) Successively amplified electrochemical immunoassay based on biocatalytic deposition of silver nanoparticles and silver enhancement. *Biosensors and Bioelectronics* 23(4), 485–491.

Dai, Z.H., Shao, G.J. & Hong, J.M.(2009) Immobilization and direct electrochemistry of glucose oxidase on a tetragonal pyramid-shaped porous ZnO nanostructure for a glucose biosensor. *Biosensors and Bioelectronics,* 24(5), 1286–1291.

Gao, L.Z.,Zhuang, J., Nie, L., Zhang, J.B., Zhang, Y., Gu, N., Wang, T.H., Feng, J., Yang, D.L., Perrett, S., &Yan, X.Y. (2007) Intrinsic peroxidase-like activity of ferromagnetic nanoparticles. *Nature nanotechnology*, 2, 577–583.

Guo, S.J., Li, D., Zhang, L.X., Li, J. & Wang, E.K. (2009), Monodisperse mesoporous superparamagnetic single-crystal magnetite nanoparticles for drug delivery. *Biomaterials*, 30(10), 1881–1889.

Guo, W., Lu, H.Y. & Hu, N.F. (2006) Comparative bioelectrochemical study of two types of myoglobin layer-by-layer films with alumina: Vapor-surface sol–gel deposited Al_2O_3 films versus Al_2O_3 nanoparticle films. *Electrochimica Acta* 52(1), 123–132.

Magner, E. (1998), Trends in electrochemical biosensors. *Analyst*, 123, 1967–1970.

Nan, C.F., Zhang, Y., Zhang, G.M., Dong, C., Shuang, S.M. & Choi, M.M.F. (2009) Activation of nylon net and its application to a biosensor for determination of glucose in human serum. *Enzyme and Microbial Technology,* 44(5), 249–253.

Wan, D.,Yuan, S.J., Li, G.L., Neoh, K.G., & Kang, E.T. (2010) Glucose Biosensor from Covalent Immobilization of Chitosan-Coupled Carbon Nanotubes on Polyaniline-Modified Gold *Electrode.Applied Materials & Interfaces* 2(11), 3083–3091.

Yang, C.Y., Zhang, Z.J., Shi, Z.L., Xue, P., Chang, P.P., & Yan,R.P. (2010) Application of a novel co-enzyme reactor in chemiluminescence flow-through biosensor for determination of lactose. *Talanta,* 82(1), 319–324.

Yang, H.P. & Zhu, Y.F. (2006) Size dependence of SiO_2 particles enhanced glucose biosensor. *Talanta*, 68(3), 569–574.

Medicine Sciences and Bioengineering – Wang (Ed.)
© 2015 Taylor & Francis Group, London, ISBN: 978-1-138-02684-1

Design and implementation of a cursor control system based on steady-state visual evoked potential

Xia Zou, Qing-guo Wei* & Zong-wu Lu
Department of Electronic Engineering, Nanchang University, Nanchang, China

ABSTRACT: This article presents a two-dimensional (2D) cursor control system, which is an important and challenging issue in EEG-based Brain–Computer Interfaces (BCIs). The system was designed and implemented based on Steady-State Visual Evoked Potential (SSVEP). This system consists of three parts: an EEG acquisition platform, a PC real-time processing system, and a Graphical User Interface (GUI). In the cursor control system, the SSVEP is transformed into a control command to control cursor movement or select a target of interest on the GUI. Nine subjects attended an online experiment to perform 2D cursor control tasks. The average accuracy rates of single task and dual-task are 90% and 87.5%, respectively, which indicates that the cursor control system has high recognition performance and can satisfy the demand of disabled people for the operation of computers.

1 INTRODUCTION

A Brain–Computer Interface (BCI) is a communication and control pathway to directly translate brain activities into control commands (Wolpaw et al, 2002). In recent years, BCI has attracted increasing attention from multiple disciplines, such as neural engineering, artificial intelligence, and pattern recognition (Mellinger et al, 2007, Pfurtscheller et al, 2000, Weikophf et al, 2004). An important issue in BCI research is cursor control, where the goal is to map brain signals to the movements of a cursor on a computer screen. Its potential applications include computer mouse control, web browser, and e-mail. In the BCI field, the research of 1D cursor control was paid much attention to, which was implemented by motor imagery–based BCIs.

Compared with 1D cursor control, 2D cursor control has more advantages, for example, greatly enhancing the ability of human-computer interaction and bringing a much wider range of applications. But so far, most of the existing 2D cursor control BCI systems are invasive (Hochberg et al, 2006), or require expensive devices for brain signal acquisition, such as magnetoencephalography (MEG) (Gervena & Jensenb, 2009) and near-infrared spectroscopy (NIRS) (Nicdas-Alonso & Gomez-Gil, 2012). The first work on EEG-based 2-D cursor control attracted a lot of attention. The authors showed that users could be guided to regulate two particular EEG rhythms to obtain two independent control signals (Wolpaw & McFarland, 2004). However, this approach requires users to have a lot of training.ga

In this article, a 2D cursor control system is proposed that adopts a discrete control paradigm using SSVEP. It can be defined as periodically evoked potential induced by rapidly repetitive visual stimulation, typically at frequencies greater than 6 Hz. When a person is gazing at such stimulation, an SSVEP component generates in the occipital area of his/her brain. It normally comprises the fundamental frequency of the visual stimulus as well as its harmonics (Shen et al, 2009). The SSVEP-based BCI has many advantages over other BCIs, including shorter training time required to enable a user to operate the BCI, larger number of selectable targets, and higher information transfer rate (ITR). These advantages make it a promising option in practical applications.

---

* Corresponding author, email: wqg07@163.com

2 MATERIALS AND METHODS

2.1 *System components*

The cursor control system contains three parts: an EEG acquisition platform consisting of an EEG amplifier and an electrode cap, a PC real-time processing system and a graphical user interface (GUI). Figure 1 shows the schematic diagram of the cursor control system. The GUI is designed to provide a few visual stimulus sources, and a workspace for cursor control. When the user is looking at a particular stimulus, the EEG signal is recorded by the scalp electrodes, amplified and digitized by the EEG amplifier, and then transferred to the PC real-time processing system based on TCP/IP protocol, where the EEG signal is processed to determine which stimulating target is pointed at. Finally, the command associated with the stimulus target is sent to the GUI to control cursor movement in specific directions.

2.2 *PC real-time processing system*

The PC real-time processing system, developed based on Visual C++ 6.0 development environment, is a core component of the cursor control system and a significant link to connect the EEG amplifier and the GUI. Its main functionalities include EEG signal preprocessing, SSVEP frequency detection, and command recognition. The block diagram of the PC real-time processing system is shown in Figure 2, which consists of a ring buffer and a signal-processing module. EEG data as the input is stored in the ring buffer, and a fixed-length data segment is intercepted for signal processing, whose result is converted into control commands for cursor movement.

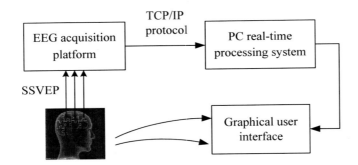

Figure 1.   Schematic diagram of the cursor control system.

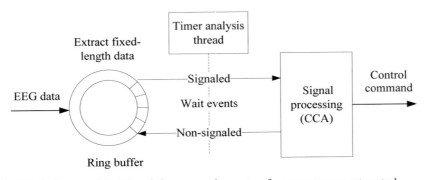

Figure 2.   Block diagram of the PC real-time processing system for cursor movement control.

To avoid data overflow, a ring buffer is adopted to store the EEG data continuously. It is mainly responsible for receiving EEG data derived from the EEG amplifier. EEG data is stored in the ring buffer in the order of time so that the previous data can be used for signal processing. In the signal-processing module, the EEG data is taken out of the ring buffer and processed at a certain time interval, which is set to 2 seconds in the system. The processing results are converted into control commands as the output. A mechanism of asynchronous processing is introduced for data extraction to reduce the possibility of obstruction to some extent and for improving the real-time ability of signal processing.

In our system, canonical correlation analysis (CCA) is employed for signal processing. CCA method focuses on the relationship between the stimulus signals and EEG signals derived from multiple channels in a local area. CCA method is explained in detail by Wei et al, 2014. Besides, there is a timer analysis thread triggered by the "START" button in the signal-processing module. The "START" button triggers to turn the real-time analysis thread on, while the "STOP" button turns that off. After being turned on, the thread waits until an event signal triggers signal-processing operation. Once the fixed-length data segment is successfully extracted, the event is set to be signaled. The processing results are then converted into control commands and transferred to the GUI to control the operations of the cursor in the GUI.

2.3   Graphical User Interface

The GUI for 2D cursor control was developed based on Visual C++ 6.0 platform. Figure 3(a) shows the design drawing of the GUI and Figure 3(b) shows a screenshot of the GUI. Five flashing buttons are located at the horizontal and vertical edges of the screen, which represent the five different operations of cursor movement control: move upward (↑), move downward (↓), move left (←), move right (→), and select (•). The rectangular central area of the GUI denotes the workspace of cursor movement control with a dimension of 820 pixels × 560 pixels. The ball and the square inside the rectangle represent a cursor and a target, respectively. In each cursor-control trial, the cursor and the target appear randomly inside the workspace. The ratio of the size of the cursor, the size of the target, and the size of workspace is fixed to be 1:3.57:1190.

In the cursor-control system, five visual stimuli are provided by the computer LCD screen that corresponds to five aforementioned operations of cursor control. Compared with cathode ray tube (CRT) or independent LED displays, LCD is more stable, lightweight, and beneficial to make more miniature and portable BCI devices. The principle of LCD stimulators is to divide the monitor's refresh rate of 60 Hz by an integer multiple. To avoid the harmonic relation between stimulating frequencies, the five frequencies, 6.67 Hz, 8.57 Hz, 10 Hz, 12 Hz, and 15 Hz, were selected as the stimulus frequencies. In the Windows environment, it is difficult

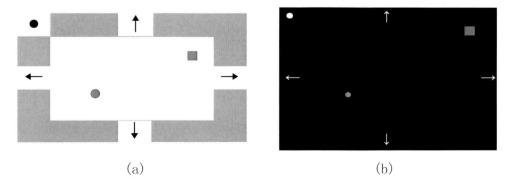

(a)   (b)

Figure 3.   GUI for 2-D cursor control: (a) the design drawing of GUI; (b) a screenshot of the GUI.

to generate a frequency-stable stimulation only with software timing mode. Therefore, DirectX software development kit (SDK) was adopted to implement the stimulation interface, importing the static link libraries like ddraw, dinput, dxguid, and calling some functions to draw the flashing square on the screen.

In a cursor-control system, two tasks are required to complete: the first task is to move the cursor to the target location on the screen and the second task is to select the target. In each trial, subjects should move the cursor to the target position first, and then make a decision of selecting or rejecting a target. In this GUI, we use SSVEP signal to control both the vertical and the horizontal movements of the cursor. For example, if the user wants to move the cursor up, then he needs to focus on the "move upward" button. Once the system detects his/her SSVEP corresponding to this button, the cursor is moved upward.

When the cursor arrives at target position, it should exert a choice to select or reject the target according to the color of the square. If the square is white, the user needs to focus on the "select" button to select the target. When the system detects his/her SSVEP signal corresponding to this button, the cursor will overlap the target, and the square will become green at the same time. On the other hand, if the square is gray, the user should ignore all the flashing buttons to reject the target, and then the square becomes red.

3 CURSOR CONTROL EXPERIMENTS

Nine volunteers with normal or corrected-to-normal vision participated in the experiment for testing the system, whose ages ranged from 20 to 28 years. All subjects were seated comfortably in an armchair in a dim and quiet environment without any distractions. At the beginning of the experiment, the subjects had 10 minutes to be familiar with the system, adapted themselves to the flicking stimulation. In our system, two computers are adopted, one of which serves as a visual stimulator, and the other is responsible for data acquisition and processing. Figure 4 shows the screenshot of a subject doing the cursor-control experiment.

In each trial, the target randomly appeared at one of the four corners, while the starting position of the cursor was fixed at the center of the GUI. Every subject was required to carry out 40 trials and complete two tasks consecutively for each trial. The first task was to move the cursor to the target location on the screen (called 2D cursor movement control). Note that one trial would be failing, if the user could not move the cursor to the target location in 2 minutes; the second task was to select the target (called the target selection). If the user could not hit or reject the target in 4 seconds, that trial would be a failure.

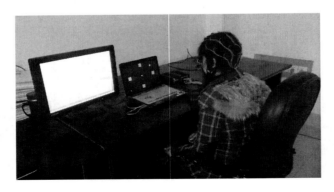

Figure 4.   A screenshot of a subject doing the cursor-control experiment.

4 RESULT ANALYSIS AND DISCUSSION

Table 1 shows the average online experimental results of the nine subjects over 40 trials. In the table, single task denotes that these subjects successfully completed the 2D cursor movement control only, while dual task means that these subjects successfully completed two consecutive tasks—2D cursor movement control and target selection. The average accuracy rates of single task and dual-task are 90% and 87.5%, respectively, and the average time of dual-task is 52.18 seconds. The experimental results indicate that the proposed cursor control system has high recognition performance and fast cursor movement control speed.

To make a further analysis, the experimental data of the nine subjects were recorded for offline analysis. According to the online experimental results, we compared the SSVEP responses to visual stimuli between the best subject CT and the worst subject WZH. Figure 5 shows the power spectrum of the experimental data derived from subjects CT and WZH. The stimulus frequency is 12 Hz. From the figure, we can observe an obvious spectral peak at frequency 12 Hz for subject CT, whereas there are more noise interferences in the vicinity of the spectral peak for subject WZH. This means that it is harder for subject WZH to recognize the stimulus frequency than for subject CT. Therefore, from the offline analysis, we can conclude that subject CT has higher recognition accuracy rate for SSVEP frequency than subject WZH. Therefore, the offline analysis verifies the online experiment results well.

Meanwhile, the offline analysis also illustrates the differences between the subjects. The response of each subject to stimulus frequencies is different. The strength of the SSVEP signal induced by the subject WZH is weaker than that induced by subject CT. This leads to different recognition accuracy rate for different subjects. In addition to the factors of users themselves, the recognition accuracy rate is determined by the design of visual stimulator and the algorithm for SSVEP frequency detection. Improving stimulation effect of the LCD stimulator could improve the SNR of SSVEP. Moreover, advanced signal preprocessing method could lead to higher accuracy rate.

In our system, the cursor moves only in a few fixed directions, for example, walk straight upward and downward in the vertical direction, and the speed of the cursor is a constant. Under these conditions, the movement of the cursor is unsmooth and discrete. Real-world applications often require 2D movement of a cursor between two arbitrary positions. Therefore, two brain signals, SSVEP, and motor imagery could be combined for 2D control. The user controls the vertical movement by an SSVEP paradigm and at the same time, the user also uses a motor imagery-based paradigm to control the horizontal movement.

Table 1. Average online experimental results of the nine subjects over 40 trials and their mean.

Subject	Average time for each trail (seconds)	Accuracy rates of dual task (%)	Accuracy rates of single task (%)
CT	41.55	95	95
WJ	45.3	92.5	92.5
YZR	42.65	90	92.5
ZAD	51.6	90	90
HY	47.4	87.5	90
LXK	55.45	85	90
XK	57.1	85	87.5
ZX	62.5	82.5	87.5
WZH	66.1	80	85
Average	52.18	87.5	90

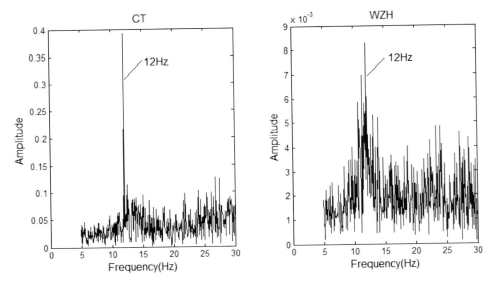

Figure 5.   Power spectrum derived from subjects CT and WZH.

5   CONCLUSION

We have designed and implemented a cursor-control system based on an SSVEP BCI. Nine subjects attended an online experiment to perform 2D cursor movement control tasks. The average accuracy rates of single task and dual task are 90% and 87.5%, respectively, and the average time of dual task is 52.18 seconds. The experimental results suggested that the SSVEP-based cursor-control system is feasible for disabled people. The proposed cursor-control system can satisfy the demand of disabled people for the operation of computers. After improving the algorithm for signal processing and using an additional motor imagery-based EEG signal, the 2D cursor movement control system would become more practical for real-world use.

ACKNOWLEDGMENTS

This project was funded by National Natural Science Foundation of China (# 61365013) and Science and Technology Support Program of Jiangxi Provence, China (# 20132BBE50050).

REFERENCES

Gervena M. V. and Jensenb O. (2009) Attention modulations of posterior alpha as a control signal for two-dimensional brain-computer interfaces, *J. Neurosci. Methods*, 179, 78–84.

Hochberg L. R., Serruya M. D., Friehs G. M., et al. (2006) Neuronal ensemble control of prosthetic devices by a human with tetraplegia, *Nature*, 442(13), 164–171.

Mellinger J., Schalk G., Braun C., Preissl H., et al. (2007) An MEG-based brain-computer interface (BCI), *NeuroImage*, 36, 581–593.

Nicolas-Alonso L F. and Gomez-Gil J. (2012) Brain computer interfaces, a review, *Sensors*, 12(2), 1211–1279.

Pfurtscheller G., Neuper C., Guger C., et al. (2000) Current trends in Graz brain-computer interface research, *IEEE Trans. Rehabil. Eng.*, 8(2), 216–218.

Shen H., Zhao L., Bian Y., Xiao L. T. (2009) Research on SSVEP-Based controlling system of multi-DoF manipulator, *Lecture Notes in Computer Science* , 5553, 171–177.

Wei Q., Zou X., Lu Z. W., Wang Z. (2014) Design and implementation of a mental telephone system based on steady-state visual evoked potential, *Journal of Computational Information Systems*, 10(2), 547–554.

Weiskopf N., Scharnowski F., Veit R., et al. (2004), Self-regulation of local brain activity using real-time functional magnetic resonance imaging (fMRI), *J. Physiol Paris*, 98, 357–373.

Wolpaw J. R., Birbaumer N., McFarland D. J., et al. (2002) Brain-computer interface for communication and control, *Clin. Neurophysiol.* 113 (6), 767–791.

Wolpaw J. R. and McFarland D. J. (2004) Control of a two-dimensional movement signal by a noninvasive brain-computer interface in humans, Proc. Natl. Acad. Sci. USA, 2004, 101(51), 17849–17854.

Medicine Sciences and Bioengineering – Wang (Ed.)
© *2015 Taylor & Francis Group, London, ISBN: 978-1-138-02684-1*

Design of a tonometer pressing force measuring device

Jian-hang Zhao
School of Electronic Information & Engineering, Anhui University, China

Yi-jie Wang, Jin Zhang & Jian-guo Ma
Huainan Normal University, Huainan, Anhui, China

ABSTRACT: A design method of the diagonal type cantilever structure of applanation tonometer pressing force measuring device is presented. The entire structure of diagonal cantilever beam-measuring device, pressure measurement module and A/D conversion module are introduced. The pressure measurement module mainly includes diagonal type fasteners, resistance bridge pressure sensor, and optical pressure head. Stress on the diagonal type cantilever beam pressure measuring device is analyzed and calculated, and the actual calibration and performance test of the whole device is carried out. The experimental results show that the entire diagonal type cantilever beam pressure measuring device, compared with the same type abroad, the performance is more stable, the measurement precision had obtained the very big promotion.

1   INTRODUCTION

The eyes in order to accomplish the normal visual function, Intraocular Pressure (IOP) must be maintained at a certain level. The normal IOP is in 8–21 mmHg (1 mmHg = 0.133 kPa). It belongs to a kind of sickness if the IOP is too high or too low. Measurement of IOP is beneficial to clinical analysis and diagnosis of glaucoma, cataracts and other diseases in the Department of Ophthalmology. Therefore, the study of IOP detection and accurate measurement of IOP value is very important in the clinical treatment of diseases in the Department of Ophthalmology (Zhang Xueyong *et al.*, 2011).

The traditional instrument for measuring IOP is mainly divided into indentation tonometer and applanation tonometer, as the need for a certain depth of corneal indentation in using indentation tonometer. This method may cause some damage to the cornea. In view of this, the ophthalmology profession actively advocated the use of applanation tonometry (Katuri, 2008). In 1954, American Goldmann designed the Goldmann Applanation Tonometer (GAT; Goldmann, 1957). GAT considered the pressure meter with highest precision so far, and the results of measurement are looked as "the gold standard" in the Department of Ophthalmology circles. In 1965, the British Perkins invented and produced the Perkins tonometer, it is actually GAT portable handheld product (Perkins, 1965).

At present, most hospitals generally use applanation tonometer, calculation of IOP is achieved by measuring the applanation area and pressing force (Kaufmann *et al.*, 2003). Measuring the accuracy of the pressing force in tonometry measuring device early is not high enough, or complex structure, in view of the development, research situation at home and abroad over. We referred a Paul S.Yang patented (Paul S.Yang, US6413214B1) and designed pressing force measuring device diagonal type cantilever beam structure. Different from the traditional measurement method, the device has the advantages of simple structure, suitable for miniaturization, to facilitate later intelligence, research and design of portable tonometer.

2 THE OVERALL STRUCTURE

Pressing force measuring device diagonal cantilever structure is presented in this paper, using resistance strain gauge manometry and cantilever beam structure. The overall structure is shown in Figure 1, including the diagonal type cantilever beam load structure, 24 bit A/D conversion circuit, MCU part and the PC machine. Diagonal type cantilever beam pressure structure in the process of flattening the cornea, optical pressure head bearing force balance the rebound and flatten the cornea, piezometric head with eye contacting will be pressing force through the hard way links without loss to a resistance bridge pressure sensor diagonal cantilever structure, the hanging side deformation of resistance bridge pressure sensor is large, changing into voltage signal through a bridge circuit internal pressure sensor, the voltage signal received through the A/D conversion after the original digital signal, the digital signal sampled by MCU and processed to get the actual pressure force, pressure will be outputted to the PC by MCU analysed for the observer.

3 THE OVERALL DESIGN

3.1 Mechanical design of diagonal type cantilever beam structure

Diagonal cantilever structure which is shown in Figure 2, structure design uses the symmetrical, optical pressure heads through a switching tube with the screw thread and the connecting plate, resistance bridge pressure sensor is fixed by screws in the upper connecting plate, the other end is connected by screw at the bottom of the shell. The pressure head and the connecting plate drum, the center point O are in a straight line. This structure is mainly realized flatten the cornea, pressure transfer and piezoelectric signal conversion functions.

3.2 Stress analysis of diagonal cantilever structure

We use the Solid-Works software focusing on resistance bridge pressure sensor diagonal cantilever stresses in the structure to analyze Finite Element Analysis (FEA). Due to the actual measured pressure force basically maintained at levels below 10g (Katuri, 2008), we selected 0.5g, 1g, 2g,

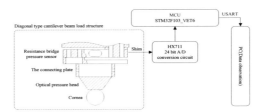

Figure 1. Applanation tonometer pressing force diagram of measuring device.

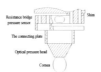

Figure 2. Diagonal type cantilever beam structure section.

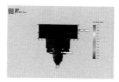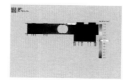

Figure 3. The stress distribution of the corresponding of 0.5g pressure.

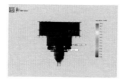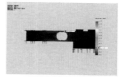

Figure 4. The stress distribution of the corresponding of 1g pressure.

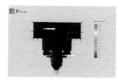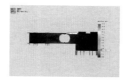

Figure 5. The stress distribution of the corresponding of 2g pressure.

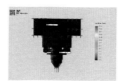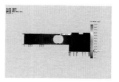

Figure 6. The stress distribution of the corresponding of 5g pressure.

5g of pressure on the overall structure and the resistance bridge pressure sensors to respectively analyse in stress. The results are shown in Figure 3–6.

The analysis results show that the pressing force is transmitted to the resistance bridge pressure sensor through a hard link, the transmission loss in the affordable range.

3.3 *Pressure sensor and A/D conversion module*

The pressure sensor is an important measurement part of the structure. Advantages of resistance bridge pressure sensor are precision and high sensitivity, long service life and less stringent requirements on the environment. Considering the actual situation following IOP instrument for high precision and the complex environment variables, our design uses the resistance bridge pressure sensor. Resistance bridge as shown in Figure 7, the DC power supply, voltage is E, the ΔU_{BC} of Resistance bridge is (1).

Four arms of resistance bridge are respectively connected to a working strain gauge, involved in the mechanical deformation and the same temperature field, temperature affects offset each other, the voltage output of high sensitivity. When the gauges and materials of the four strains are the same, deduced the following formula (2), the output voltage of the bridge is only related to the input voltage.

$$\Delta U_{BC} = (\frac{R_2}{R_1 + R_2} - \frac{R_3}{R_3 + R_4})E \qquad (1)$$

$$= \frac{R_2 R_3 - R_1 R_4}{(R_1 + R_2)(R_3 + R_4)}E$$

$$\Delta U_{BC} = \frac{EK}{4}(\varepsilon_1 - \varepsilon_2 + \varepsilon_3 - \varepsilon_4) \qquad (2)$$

$$= EK\varepsilon_1$$

The HX711 is a high precision 24 bit A/D converter chip. Channel A programmable gain Gu to 128dB or 64dB. According to the schematic shown in Figure 8 of the A/D conversion circuit, to the maximum number of excitation voltage, A/D converter chip full range of maximum outputted voltage and output by A/D conversion values were calculated, According to the calculation procedure to determine the conversion algorithm of data in a program. The output reference voltage V_{BG} 1.25V, $R_1 = 20\ K$, $R_2 = 8.2\ K$, V_{AVDD} is about 4.3V.

Sensitivity δ of 20g resistance bridge pressure sensor is 1.0 ± 0.15 mV/V. The formula (3) to get the V_{AVDD} into the formula (4), then calculate the full-scale outputted maximum voltage value V_{Max} is 4.3 mV. After 128 times, the gain amplification and A/D conversion, V_{Max} output 24bit digital maximum formula for (5).

$$V_{AVDD} = \frac{V_{BG}(R_1 + R_2)}{R_2} \qquad (3)$$

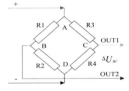

Figure 7.   Resistance bridge principle diagram.

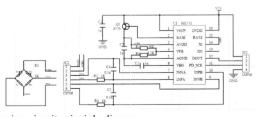

Figure 8.   The A/D conversion circuit principle diagram.

$$V_{Max} = V_{AVDD} \times \delta \tag{4}$$

$$D_{out} = \frac{V_{Max} \times Gu \times 2^{24}}{V_{AVDD}} \tag{5}$$

The above calculated of $V_{AVDD} = 4.3\,V$, $V_{Max} = 4.3\,mV$, $Gu = 128$ dB are put into the formula (5), then get the value of D_{out} is about 2147484.

4 DEVICE CALIBRATION AND ANALYSIS

The circuit is the actual connection test which found that the maximum number of A/D converts the output value $D_{out} = 2147484$. Finally, a numerical change almost has no effect on the test results, and used the first six numerical. Download the best program package to MCU, and the program flow is shown in Figure 9. Record the data view results in the PC serial debugging tools.

Calibration of test data is required to derive directly from the PC, and carries on the analysis, calculation and processing. Finally, we get the calibration results as shown in Table 1.

According to the system calibration, the results show that 1mg corresponds to the value 0.0777, testing program flow is shown in Figure 9, boot A/D conversion, MCU reads the initial load value (because the resistance bridge pressure sensor has its own weight, so the need for no-load value recording), and storage. Calculation of a scaling relationship of 1 mg corresponds to 0.0777. The actual measurement results are given in Table 2.

Due to flatten force in the actual instruments IOP to measure less than 10^{-2} N (Katuri K C, 2008). So we chose 0.5g, 1g, 1.5g, 2g, 3g, 5g as the actual measurement of the sample. The actual measurement results show (Table 2) that software correction control can be pressing force measurement error precision which is about 2.030%.

5 CONCLUSION

IOP measurement is very important for glaucoma, cataracts and other diseases in the Department of Ophthalmology Clinical Analysis and Diagnosis. This paper proposes the design method of the diagonal type cantilever beam structure applanation tonometer pressing force measuring device.

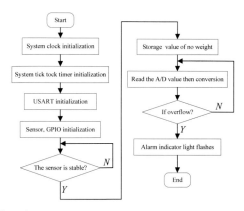

Figure 9. The program flow chart.

Table 1. Calibration test results.

Test group	Test results(A/D converts the digital value)						Number/1mg
	Empty	0.5g	1g	2g	3g	5g	
First	114900	114940	114977	115055	115132	115288	
Second	114899	114940	114977	115054	115133	115287	
Third	114900	114939	114979	115054	115132	115289	
Fourth	114900	114938	114976	115055	115134	115287	
Fifth	114900	114940	114976	115054	115135	115289	
Sixth	114900	114938	114976	115053	115133	115286	
The test results processing							
Measurement of mean	114899.8	114939.2	114977.2	115054.2	115133.2	115287.7	
And the load difference	0	39.333	77.333	154.333	233.333	387.333	
Number/1mg		0.0786	0.0773	0.0772	0.0778	0.0776	**0.0777**

Table 2. The actual test results.

Test group	Test results(A/D converts the digital value)							The error precision(%)
	Empty	0.5g	1g	1.5g	2g	3g	5g	
First	38	509	1016	1526	2062	3056	5075	
Second	12	512	1016	1527	2059	3062	5082	
Third	25	516	1016	1522	2054	3065	5083	
Fourth	25	508	1029	1525	2046	3058	5076	
Fifth	12	507	1029	1524	2052	3056	5086	
Sixth	25	506	1029	1525	2056	3061	5082	
The test results processing								
Measurement of mean	22.83	508.67	1022.5	1524.83	2054.83	3059.67	5080.67	
And the load difference	22.83	9.67	22.50	24.83	54.83	59.67	80.67	
The error precision (%)	——	1.93	2.25	1.66	2.74	1.99	1.61	**2.030**

Its structure is simple, easy to use. This paper analyzes the rationality of the measurement device, introduces the design scheme of A/D conversion module, and calibrates the device on this basis, measures practically. The measurement results show that we can control the error precision of pressing force at around 2.030%. The measurement precision of pressing force is improved.

REFERENCES

Goldmann H, Schmidt T. Ueber Applanationstonometrie [J].Ophthalmologica, 1957, 134:221–242.
Jia Guo Ma et al., A miniaturized applanation tonometer, IEEE Transactions on BiomedicalEngineering, Vol.46, pp. 947–9 51, 1999.

Jianguo Ma, Jin Zhang, "An Improved Maklakoff's Method for Measuring the Intraocular Pressure- Volume Relationship," Proc. Applied Mechanics and Materials, 2012, 103:518–524.

Katuri K C, Asrani S, Ramasubramanian M K. Intraocular Pressure Monitoring Sensors [J]. IEEE Sens J, 2008, 8(1):12–19.

Kaufmann, C., Bachmann, L. M., Thiel, M. A. Intraocular pressure measurements using dynamic contour tonometry after laser in situ keratomileusis. Invest. Ophthalmol. Vis. Sci., 44(2003), 3790.

Nakamura, M., et al, A.Agreement of rebound tonometer in measuring intraocular pressure with three types of applanation tonometers. Am. J. Ophthalmol., 142(2006), 332.

Paul S.Yang, "Applanation Tonometer"[p]. American Patent: US6413214B1.

Perkins E S. Hand-held applanation tonometer [J].Br J Opthalmol,1965, 49: 591–593.

Recep, O. F, et al, Relation between corneal thickness and intraocular pressure measurement bynoncontact and applanation tonometry. J. Cataract. Refract. Surg., 27(2001), 1787.

Zhang Xueyong, Ma Jianguo, Lu Rongsheng. State of arts of intraocular pressure measurement technology [J].Journal of hefei University of Technology,2011, (7):976–981.

Medicine Sciences and Bioengineering – Wang (Ed.)
© 2015 Taylor & Francis Group, London, ISBN: 978-1-138-02684-1

From "unusual sequences" to human diseases

Fei-juan Huang & Zheng-zhi Wu*
First Affiliated Hospital of Shenzhen University, Shenzhen, China
Shenzhen Institute of Gerontology, Shenzhen, China

ABSTRACT: Special regions in protein sequences with biased compositions of amino acids beyond restricted criteria are simply defined as "unusual sequences." The presence of these unusual sequences has shown not rare and of great importance in human diseases. The present work reviewed the distribution, abundance, structure, and functional features of these unusual sequences with an emphasis on polyQ, polyA, Leu-rich, and tryptophan–aspartic acid (WD) repeats and their association with human diseases as well as other relevant medical significance.

1   INTRODUCTION

The occurrences of these 20 common amino acids in a large scale of proteomes are generally expected to be randomly similar, estimated from 1 to 10% (Doolittle, 1989). However, many previous studies have observed that the compositional biases in protein sequences are very frequently present in proteomes. The statistics analysis of the composition of proteins in the SwissProt database reported that surprisingly, up to 1/4 proteins in the database contain at least one such compositionally biased fragment (Wootton, 1994a). Due to the great abundance and diversity of these compositional biases, they are arbitrarily termed as several nicknames according to their compositional features. Particularly, some of them highly rich in only one certain residue type, such as the most common glutamic acid, asparagines, aspartic acid, alanine, proline, and serine are particular defined as "single-residue rich sequences" (SRRs), single amino acid repeats (SAARs), or just as "homopolymers" (Katti *et al.*, 2000). The sequences that are rich in several different amino acids are generally termed as "simple sequence(s)/repeats," "low-complexity sequences," or "unusual sequences" (Wootton, 1994b). All the sequences with remarkable compositional biases in one or several residues are simply collectively marked as "unusual sequences" herein.

However, it is still hard to give a thorough description of all the frequencies of residue repeats in an organism; some general common features are shared and exhibited in different taxonomical groups in a large scale. As demonstrated in Figure 1, the predominant residue types are primarily those of uncharged polar amino acids glutamine (Gln), serine (Ser), asparagine (Asn); the small residues glycine (Gly) and alanine (Ala); the acidic amino acid aspartic acid (Asp); or the nonpolar amino acid proline (Pro) (Faux et al., 2005). Nevertheless, the individual frequency and prevalence of one certain type of unusual sequences also could differ dramatically even between species.

2   UNUSUAL SEQUENCES AND HUMAN DISEASES

To date, many severely diseases have been found to be associated with these unusual sequences. Only the expansion of a single residue has been reported to be responsible for more than twenty heritable diseases, with the majority of them being neurological diseases. These neurological

---

*To whom correspondence should be addressed: Tel: (86)755-25533018; Fax: (86)755-25622938; email: szwzz001@163.com

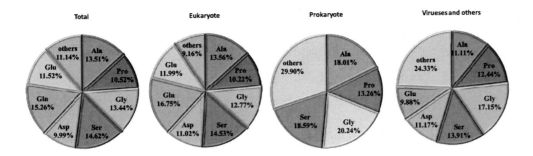

Figure 1. The percentage of remarkable SRRS in the proteomes of tree taxa groups those were available in the nonredundant protein database from NCBI of 2005 (Faux, 2012). Note: Those with percentage less than 8% are not present with their values.

diseases exhibit partial loss of memory, verbal span, motor function and executive function, acknowledges ability, alteration in complex visuoperceptual and visuoconstructive abilities, disorientation, and psychiatric symptoms.

2.1 PolyQ diseases

The polyQ proteins lead to a few diseases. To date, up to 9 progressive neurodegenerative diseases that induced by the unusual sequences of polyglutamine (polyQ) is identified. The members in this disease group include Kennedy's disease (KD), Huntington disease (HD), spinocerbellar ataxia (SCA) 1, 2, 3, 6, 7, and 17, and dentatorubral-pallidoluysian atrophy (DRPLA). Among them, Kennedy's disease, also known as spinal and bulbar muscular atrophy (SBMA), which is a progressive neurodegenerative disease characterized by muscle and limbs weakness and atrophy, is the first identified polyQ disease (Zajac & Fui, 2012, Orr, 2012). The enrichment of glutamines in HTT protein induces the aggregation of this protein and causes the production of fibrous in the brain, resulting in progressive neuronal cell death, dementia, and even psychiatric symptoms. The long polyQ fragments in Ataxin (ATXN)-1, 2, and 3 proteins cause the spinocerebellar ataxia 1 and 2 and ataxin 3 (Machado–Joseph disease, MJD), respectively, which characterized by ataxia and progressive motor deterioration (Kang and Hong, 2009).

2.2 PolyA diseases

PolyA stretches in a few of proteins are also the pathogenesis for several diseases. These diseases include the oculopharyngeal muscular dystrophy and cleidocranial dysplasia. The patients of the former disease suffer from painful swallowing and progressive paralysis of the eyelids and the patients of cleidocranial dysplasia are characterized by shortness of the hands and feet and minor craniofacial features (Faux, 2012). The expansion of polyA regulated by transcription factor gene *FOXL2* was identified to influence the development of craniofacial and ovarian (Cocquet *et al.*, 2003).

2.3 Leu-rich proteins

A typical family of the four-member leucine-rich repeat transmembrane (LRRTM) proteins, predominately expressed in the human vertebrate nervous system playing roles in cell surface signaling and cell adhesion as transmembrane receptor, single transporter, and DNA repairing proteins, is implicated to be involved in behavioral variability and psychiatric disease (Francks, 2011, Lauren *et al.*, 2003). Typically, each one LRRTM protein contains 10 extracellular Leucine-rich repeats (LRRs) with a length of around 20–30 residues rich in leucines, which build up an arched surface with β-strands in it and α-helices out of it. The unique surface has been identified as the interface of the interaction between LRRTMs and their partners (Loimaranta *et al.*, 2009). It should be noted that sometimes the α-helix inside of the arc could be replaced by $3_{(10)}$-helix, and pII helix, while β-strand could be β-$3_{(10)}$ or β-pII units; furthermore, the radii of the LRR arc with* β–α units are smaller than those with β-$3_{(10)}$ or β-pII units (Enkhbayar et al., 2004).

2.4 *WD-repeat proteins*

WD-repeat proteins are defined by the presence of several regions of approximately 40 residues ending with tryptophan–aspartic acid (WD). As demonstrated by the crystal structure of a G-protein beta gamma dimer at 2.1Å resolution (Sondek *et al.*, 1996), all the WD-repeat proteins showed to form a circularized antiparallel β-sheet framework within the "WD fragments" (as shown in Figure 2). The importance of these proteins is recognized as they are associated with several human genetic diseases (Li and Roberts, 2001). They played critical roles in a few of essential biological processes including cell division, transmembrane signaling, transcription regulation, and cell apoptosis (Neer *et al.*, 1994).

3 SUMMARY

These unusual sequences with low complexity, high richness in one or several certain residues, such as glutamine, asparagines, glutamic acid, and alanine, posed to be relatively rare but of great biological and medical significance. These observed unusual sequences were analyzed in relation to their impact on human diseases as well as their special structural framework (as shown in Table 2). Moreover, the results have organized in the form of different types of disease, which would be of

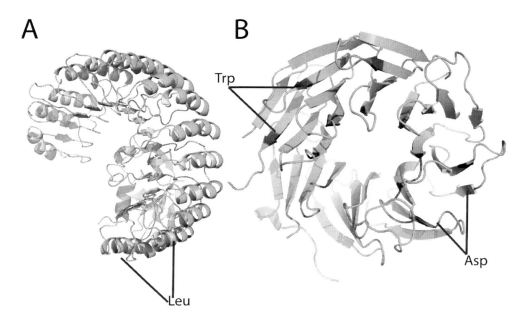

Figure 2. The structural models for LRRTM and WD repeats. (A) The structure of porcine ribonuclease inhibitor, one of LRRTMs, (PDB code: 1DFJ, Leu highlighted in yellow color), showed an arched surface with β-strands inside and α-helices outside. (B) The structure of TBL1XR1 WD40 repeats (PDB code:4LG9) with emphasis of the WD fragments marked as blue (Trp) and pink color (Asp) exhibited a circularized anti-β sheets.

Table 1. Diseases caused by the presence of "unusual sequences." The length details of the unusual sequences were obtained from reference Faux (2012).

Protein	Disease	Repeats	Length	Structural features
Huntingtin (HTT)	Huntington's disease	PolyQ	30–130	Aggregates
Androgen receptor (AR)	Kennedy's disease	PolyQ	40–50	Aggregates
Atrophin-1	Dentatorubral-pallidoluysian atrophy (DRPLA)	PolyQ	50–90	Aggregates
Ataxin (ATXN)-1	Spinocerebellar Ataxia-1	PolyQ	40–80	Aggregates
Ataxin (ATXN)-2	Spinocerebellar Ataxia-2	PolyQ	36–52	Aggregates
Ataxin (ATXN)-3	Ataxin-3 (MJD)	PolyQ	55–84	Aggregates
Voltage-dependent calcium channel α-1A subunit	Spinocerebellar Ataxia-6	PolyQ	21–25	Aggregates
Ataxin (ATXN)-7	Spinocerebellar Ataxia-7	PolyQ	38–240	Aggregates
TATA box-binding protein	Spinocerebellar Ataxia-17	PolyQ	38–240	Aggregates
PolyA-binding protein-2	Oculopharyngeal muscular dystrophy	PolyA	8–13	Aggregates
Runt-related transcription factor 2	Cleidocranial dysplasia	PolyA	27	Aggregates
Homeobox D13	Syndactyly, type II	PolyA	20–30	Aggregates
LRRTMs	Behavioral variability and psychiatric disease	Leu-rich motifs	20–30	Arch surface with β-strands inside and α-helices outside
G proteins	Genetic diseases	WD	~40	Circularized antiparallel β-sheet

Note: Q – Gluatmine, Ala-Alanine, Leu-Leucine, WD-tryptophan and aspartic acid

great interest to the research community and useful for the further discovery of disease's biomarker. At current stage, these unusual sequences have demonstrated to be the hallmark for the corresponding disease. Development of the medicine agent that target to these unusual sequences could be a promising direction for the diagnosis and therapy of these severely diseases.

ACKNOWLEDGMENTS

We thank Prof. Hongzhe Sun from the University of Hong Kong, Dr. Wei Xia from the Harvard University, and Dr. Claudia Blindauer from Warrick University for helpful discussions. This work was supported by National Science Foundation Grant (30973779 and 30772757).

REFERENCES

COCQUET, J., DE BAERE, E., CABURET, S. & VEITIA, R. A. (2003) Compositional biases and polyalanine runs in humans. *Genetics,* 165, 1613–7.

DOOLITTLE, R. F. (1989) Redundancies in protein sequences. *Prediction of protein structure and the principles of protein conformation.* Springer.

ENKHBAYAR, P., KAMIYA, M., OSAKI, M., MATSUMOTO, T. & MATSUSHIMA, N. (2004) Structural principles of leucine-rich repeat (LRR) proteins. *Proteins,* 54, 394–403.

FAUX, N. (2012) Single amino acid and trinucleotide repeats: function and evolution. *Adv Exp Med Biol,* 769, 26–40.

FAUX, N. G., BOTTOMLEY, S. P., LESK, A. M., IRVING, J. A., MORRISON, J. R., DE LA BANDA, M. G. & WHISSTOCK, J. C. (2005) Functional insights from the distribution and role of homopeptide repeat-containing proteins. *Genome Res,* 15, 537–51.

FRANCKS, C. (2011) Leucine-rich repeat genes and the fine-tuning of synapses. *Biol Psychiatry,* 69, 820–1.

KANG, S. & HONG, S. (2009) Molecular pathogenesis of spinocerebellar ataxia type 1 disease. *Mol Cells,* 27, 621–7.

KATTI, M. V., SAMI-SUBBU, R., RANJEKAR, P. K. & GUPTA, V. S. (2000) Amino acid repeat patterns in protein sequences: Their diversity and structural-functional implications. *Protein Science,* 9, 1203–1209.

LAUREN, J., AIRAKSINEN, M. S., SAARMA, M. & TIMMUSK, T. (2003) A novel gene family encoding leucine-rich repeat transmembrane proteins differentially expressed in the nervous system. *Genomics,* 81, 411–21.

LI, D. & ROBERTS, R. (2001) WD-repeat proteins: structure characteristics, biological function, and their involvement in human diseases. *Cell Mol Life Sci,* 58, 2085–97.

LOIMARANTA, V., HYTONEN, J., PULLIAINEN, A. T., SHARMA, A., TENOVUO, J., STROMBERG, N. & FINNE, J. (2009) Leucine-rich repeats of bacterial surface proteins serve as common pattern recognition motifs of human scavenger receptor.

NEER, E. J., SCHMIDT, C. J., NAMBUDRIPAD, R. & SMITH, T. F. (1994) The ancient regulatory-protein family of WD-repeat proteins. *Nature,* 371, 297–300.

ORR, H. T. (2012) Polyglutamine neurodegeneration: expanded glutamines enhance native functions. *Curr Opin Genet Dev,* 22, 251–5.

SONDEK, J., BOHM, A., LAMBRIGHT, D. G., HAMM, H. E. & SIGLER, P. B. (1996) Crystal structure of a G-protein beta gamma dimer at 2.1A resolution. *Nature,* 379, 369–74.

WOOTTON, J. C. (1994a) Sequences with 'unusual' amino acid compositions. *Curr Opin Struct Biol,* 4, 413–421.

WOOTTON, J. C. (1994b) Sequences with 'unusual'amino acid compositions. *Curr Opin Struct Biol,* 4, 413–421.

ZAJAC, J. D. & FUI, M. N. (2012) Kennedy's disease: clinical significance of tandem repeats in the androgen receptor. *Adv Exp Med Biol,* 769, 153–68.

Medicine Sciences and Bioengineering – Wang (Ed.)
© *2015 Taylor & Francis Group, London, ISBN: 978-1-138-02684-1*

Modeling of virtual spine based on multi-body dynamics

Fei Pan, Zhan Gao, Chen Ding, Jun-ze Wang & Jie-Hua Wang
School of Computer Science and Technology, Nantong University, Nantong, Jiangsu, China

ABSTRACT: To accomplish simulation of virtual spinal orthopedic surgery, a spine model has been developed as a rigid-flexible multi-body system based on the theory of multi-body dynamics and recursive spine systematic construction. The rigid-flexible multi-body system integrated centrum and intervertebral disc has been constructed and visualized by the Simbody platform. The main purpose of this paper is to actually model functional spinal unit average stiffness simulation and the lumbar spine's basic movements, including flexion, extension, bending, and rotation.

1 INTRODUCTION

With the rapid development of computer technology, virtual surgery has been developed and is widely used in medical research. Virtual surgery is useful for the training of medical students (Ahmed *et al.*, 2011) (Tanoue *et al.*, 2008). Compared with other parts of the human body, the deformations and movements of the spine are complex. Because of the difficulty of spinal surgery, it is necessary to simulate, analyze, and evaluate orthopedic strategies and procedures for such surgery (Balakrishnan *et al.*, 2011). Use of appropriate analytical methods and efficient kinematic simulation algorithms is the key element of achieving kinematic simulation of the virtual spine (Kim *et al.*, 2010). In this article, a rigid-flexible coupled multi-body dynamic model is proposed to simulate the kinematic behavior of the spine (Jia-zhen *et al.*, 2008). Based on the spine's anatomy and biomechanical characteristics and according to the theory of rigid-flexible multi-body dynamics, vertebrae are treated as rigid bodies, whereas intervertebral discs are treated as flexible bodies.

2 MODELING SPINE BASED ON RIGID-FLEXIBLE MULTI-BODY DYNAMICS

The human spine can be divided into the cervical zone (C1–C7), the thoracic zone (T1–T12), the lumbar zone (L1–L5), the sacral zone (S1–S5), and the coccyx. It is composed of vertebra, intervertebral discs, and ligaments. The inside of the intervertebral discs is a semi-liquid nucleus pulposus, and the outside is composed of fibrous rings. Ligaments are elastic and connect vertebrae or fibrous tissue. The spine can be considered as a system with a tree structure constituting of rigid bodies coupled with flexible bodies. Here, the lumbar spine is taken as an example to illustrate how to construct a multi-body model of the spine.

Using a laser scanning technique, a triangular mesh model of the spine was obtained, as shown in Figure 1. To reduce computational cost, this model was simplified using an assemblage of primitive geometrical elements such as cylinders and beams.

Simbody is an open-source dynamic physics simulation engine developed by the SimTK research team (Michael *et al.*, 2011). Simbody includes contact modeling, matrix computation, numerical calculation, redundant constraint processing, optimization and solving, visualization, and real-time interactive functions. Simbody was used here to implement multi-body dynamic modeling. Within the Simbody framework, an inertial reference base O was created. The root object (SAC) was fully constrained in six degrees of freedom (rotation in the X, Y, and Z directions

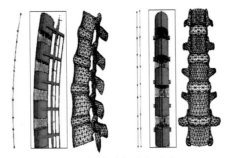

Figure 1.   Simplified Model and triangular mesh Model of the Spine.

and translation in the X, Y, and Z directions). The hinges of the vertebrae were of the spherical hinge type. The vertebrae were constrained in three degrees of freedom (translation in the X, Y, and Z directions) in their local coordinate systems. Constraint equations were then established to limit relative movement between adjacent bodies.

The adjacency relation between L4 and L5 is taken as an example. The hinge joints on L5 and L4 are P and Q, and R and S are concretion joints on L5 and L4. Hinge joints are always coincident with concretion joints. The constraint equation is

$$\underline{\Phi}^{(d3)}(h) = \underline{0} \cdot$$ (1)

$d_i(i = \text{L5,L4})$ are two vectors fixed to L5 and L4. $l_i^m(i = \text{L5,L4}; m = P,Q,R,S)$ are radius vectors of C_i $(i = \text{L5,L4})$. C_i is the base point of m's body-fixed base, and

$$d_{\text{L5}} = \text{RP} = l_{\text{L5}}^P - l_{\text{L5}}^R$$ (2)

$$d_{\text{L4}} = \text{SQ} = l_{\text{L4}}^Q - l_{\text{L4}}^S.$$ (3)

The body-joint vector h is

$$h = \text{QP} = r_{\text{L5}} + l_{\text{L5}}^P - r_{\text{L4}} - l_{\text{L4}}^Q.$$ (4)

Substituting equation (4) into (1), the constraint equation is determined as

$$\underline{\Phi}^{(d3)}(h) = r_{\text{L5}} + l_{\text{L5}}^P - r_{\text{L4}} - l_{\text{L4}}^Q = 0.$$ (5)

By differentiating this equation, the corresponding velocity and acceleration constraint equations can be obtained. By determining vectors d_{L5} and d_{L4}, the spatial position of the lumbar spine can be obtained, and the constraint equation according to h based on the establishment of adjacency can be established between the vertebrae.

In the lumbar segments, B_i is followed by B_j $(j = 1,\cdots,5)$. By use of a lumped-mass finite-element method, B_j is divided into units l. As the node of k $(k = 1,\cdots,l)$, the mass m_j^k is concentrated in node k and is not deformed when in the position of radius vector $p_{l j0}^k$. The node translation vector is u_j^k. By establishing the absolute reference base $\underline{e}$ in O and establishing a floating coordinate system $\underline{e}^j$ in the center of mass C_j, B_j is not deformed. The absolute radius vectors of C_j and k are r_j and r_j^k respectively.

For element k, the modal coordinates to describe the unit deformation are

$$u_j^k = \underline{\Phi}_j^k \underline{a}_j \tag{6}$$

where $\underline{\Phi}_j^k$ and $\underline{a}_j$ are node k's modal vector and the modal coordinate of B_j respectively. The relationship between the relative radius vector of node k and the extent of deformation is

$$\rho_j^k = \rho_{j0}^k + u_j^k \tag{7}$$

The relationship between the absolute radius vector and the relative radius vector of node k is

$$r_j^k = r_j + \rho_j^k. \tag{8}$$

By performing primary and secondary differentiation on this equation, the velocity and acceleration constraint equations can be obtained.

In a flexible multi-body system, the system energy is an important indicator of the correctness of the simulation process. The flexible-system energy includes kinetic and potential energy, with potential energy including gravitational potential energy and elastic potential energy. For B_j, the expressions for these energies are:

$$T_j = \sum_{k=1}^{l} \frac{1}{2} m_j^k \dot{\underline{r}}_j^{kT} \dot{\underline{r}}_j^k, \tag{9}$$

$$V_j^{\mathrm{g}} = -\sum_{k=1}^{l} m_j^k \underline{g}^T \underline{r}_j^k, \tag{10}$$

$$V_j^{\mathrm{u}} = \frac{1}{2} \underline{a}^T \underline{K}_a^j \underline{a}, \tag{11}$$

where T_j is the kinetic energy of B_j, V_j^{g} is the gravitational potential energy of B_j, V_j^{u} is the elastic potential energy of B_j, $\underline{g}$ is the coordinate matrix of gravity in the inertial base, and $\underline{K}_a^j$ is the modal stiffness matrix of B_j.

In the modeling process, vertebrae are treated as rigid bodies, whereas intervertebral discs and ligaments are treated as flexible bodies. A mass-spring model is used to represent an intervertebral disc. The rigid-flexible coupling of vertebrae and intervertebral discs can be modeled by springs and dampers. The application points μ and v of the spring and damper are on L5 and L4 respectively, and $\overrightarrow{v\mu}$ is d:

$$d = r_{\mathrm{L5}}^{\mu} - r_{\mathrm{L4}}^{v} = (r_{\mathrm{L5}} + l_{\mathrm{L5}}^{\mu}) - (r_{\mathrm{L4}} + l_{\mathrm{L4}}^{v}). \tag{12}$$

The stiffness and damping coefficients of the spring and damper are k and c, and the original length of the spring is $|d_0|$. The active force of L4 to L5 is F^{L5}, and the damping force of L4 to L5 is opposite to F^{L5}. Therefore,

$$F_{L5}^{\mu} = -[k(1 - \frac{|d_0|}{|d|}) + c\frac{d \cdot v_r}{|d|^2}]d + \frac{F^{L5}}{|d|}d. \tag{13}$$

According to Newton's first law, the resultant force of L5 to L4 is

$$F_{L4}^{v} = -F_{L5}^{\mu}, \tag{14}$$

and $v_r = \dfrac{d}{dt}r_{L5}^{\mu} - \dfrac{d}{dt}r_{L4}^{v}$ is the velocity of μ relative to v.

Let vertebra $i(i = L5, L4, L3, L2, L1)$ exert an external force acting on point m and denoted by F_i^m. The torque of the vertebral-body centroid is $M_i^m = l_i^m \times F_i'$.

Based on the dynamic model defined above, Simbody was used to build a spine multi-body dynamic model and to perform visualization. Figure 2(a) shows the lumbar spine's flexion and extension in the sagittal plane, Figure 2(b) shows the lumbar spine's lateral bending in the coronal plane, and Figure 2(c) shows the lumbar spine's rotation in the horizontal plane.

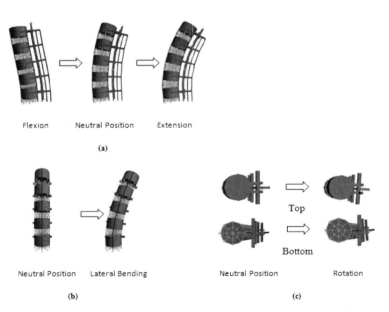

Figure 2. Multi-Body Dynamic Simulation of Spine : (a) Flexion / Extension; (b) Lateral Bending; (c) Rotation.

3 DISCUSSION AND CONCLUSIONS

This paper has presented a modeling method for the virtual spine based on rigid-flexible multi-body dynamics. Dynamic system equations for a spine with a tree structure were developed based on the theory of multi-body dynamics. Constraint equations and adjacency relations were established using springs and dampers. Thus, a spine model based on rigid-flexible multi-body dynamics was constructed. Future experiments will validate the accuracy of this method. Such finding will be used to improve simulation models in a physically consistent way, for training and planning application.

REFERENCES

Ahmed Y., Scott I. U., Greenberg P. B. (2011) A survey of the role of virtual surgery simulators in ophthalmic graduate medical education. *Graefes Archive for Clinical and Experimental Ophthalmology*, 249(8): 1263–1265.

Balakrishnan K. Y., Rathinam K. A., Su-Tung T, et al. (2011) Virtual Method to Compare Treatment Options to Assist Maxillofacial Surgery Planning and Decision Making Process for Implant and Screw Placement. Visual Informatics: Sustaining Research and Innovations, 7066:361–367.

Jia-zhen H, Yong-zhu L (2008) Modeling Methods of Rigid-Flexible Coupling Dynamics. *Journal of Shanghai Jiaotong University*, 42(11):1923–1926.

Kim T. H., Zhan G, Ian G., et al. (2010) Haptically Integrated Simulation of A Finite Element Model of Thoracolumbar Spine Combining Offline Biomechanical Response Analysis of Intervertebral Discs. *Computer-Aided Design*, 42(12):1151–1166.

Michael A. S., Ajay S., Scott L. D. (2011) Simbody: Multibody Dynamics for Biomedical Research. *Procedia IUTAM*, 2:241–261.

Tanoue K., Ieiri S., Konishi K., et al. (2008) Effectiveness of Endoscopic Surgery Training for Medical Students Using A Virtual Reality Simulator Versus A Box Tainer: *A Randomized Controlled Trial. Surgical Endoscopy*, 22(4):985–990.

Medicine Sciences and Bioengineering – Wang (Ed.)
© 2015 Taylor & Francis Group, London, ISBN: 978-1-138-02684-1

Image registration based on weighted residual complexity using local entropy

Juan Zhang, Ming-hui Zhang, Wei-Yang & Zhen-tai Lu*
School of Biomedical Engineering, Southern Medical University, Guangzhou,China

ABSTRACT: In this paper, we propose a novel intensity-based similarity measure to match medical images with intensity distortions. A specifically designed weighting function was incorporated into the residual term in residual complexity to weight the residual image between reference image and warped floating image adaptively. The weighting function is modeled by a function of the local entropy difference after mapping images to local entropy space respectively. The experimental results show that our proposed approach has achieved more accurate and robust performance than mutual information and residual complexity.

1 INTRODUCTION

The basic principle of medical image registration is to search a transformation that maximizes a criterion. There are some intensity-based similarity measures, sum of squared differences, sum of absolute differences (Hill DL et al., 2001), and mutual information (William M. Wells et al., 1996). They assumed that the intensity relationship between pixels is independent and stationary. However, none of them can process images with intensity distortion because of its violation on the assumption. The intensity distortion is mainly caused by intensity bias field in MRI or contrast agent. It is a challenge task.

To deal with this problem, the bulk of methods have been proposed over these years. Local measure–based method utilizes sum of local measures (Soatto ZYaS, 2009), which is sensitive to noise and outliers. Probabilistic models are utilized to model higher order pixel interdependence. It heavily relies on the definition of local intensity interactions (Wyatt PP & Noble JA, 2003). Intensity distortion correction–based method corrects intensity distortions simultaneously with image registration. It requires defining intensity correction function accurately. Andriy Myronenko (Andriy Myronenko & Xubo Song, 2010) et al. proposed residual complexity measure to solve the intensity correction field. However, it is sensitive to parameter, noise and outliers. Inspired by the robust estimation (Li SZ: Markov, 2001), Weighted Residual Complexity using Local Entropy (WRCLE), an extension to residual complexity, was presented in this paper. It uses a designed weighting function to constraint the residual term in residual complexity. After mapping the reference image and floating image to local entropy space respectively, the weighting function is constructed by a function of local entropy difference. It weights residual image automatically to ensure the accuracy and robustness of the registration.

2 METHOD

2.1 *Residual complexity*

A model to express the intensity relationship between reference image I and floating image J :

$$I = J(\tau) + S + \eta \tag{1}$$

*Corresponding author: Zhentai-Lu, Email: xylzj123@126.com.

where S is an intensity correction field, η denotes zero mean Gaussian noise. τ is the spatial transformation. We can estimate S and τ by maximizing the posteriori probability:

$$P(\tau, S \mid I, J) \propto P(I, J \mid \tau, S) P(\tau) P(S) \tag{2}$$

$P(S)$ can be formulated as $P(S) \propto e^{-\beta \|PS\|^2}$. Maximization of (2) is equivalent to minimize (3)

$$E(\mathbf{S}, \tau) = \|\mathbf{I} - \mathbf{J}(\tau) - \mathbf{S}\|^2 + \beta \|\mathbf{PS}\|^2 \tag{3}$$

$\mathbf{I}$, $\mathbf{J}$, and $\mathbf{S}$ are in column-vector form of I, J, and S, respectively. Compute the correct field $\mathbf{S}$ and substitute it back to (3), $\mathbf{P}^T\mathbf{P} = \mathbf{Q}\Lambda\mathbf{Q}^T$, $\Lambda = \mathrm{d}[\lambda_1, ..., \lambda_N]$, $\lambda_i \square 0$, Then:

$$E(\tau) = \mathbf{r}^T \mathbf{Q} \mathrm{d}(\beta\lambda_i / (1 + \beta\lambda_i)) \mathbf{Q}^T \mathbf{r} = \mathbf{r}^T \mathbf{QLQ}^T \mathbf{r} = \mathbf{r}^T \mathbf{Ar} \tag{4}$$

$\mathbf{A} = \mathbf{QLQ}^T$, $\mathbf{L} = \mathrm{d}(l_1, ..., l_N) = \mathrm{d}(\beta\lambda_i / 1 + \beta\lambda_i)$, $1 \square l_i \square 0$. $\mathbf{r} = \mathbf{I} - \mathbf{J}(\tau)$ is residual vector (residual image). $\mathrm{d}()$ is the diagonal matrix, If choose a proper $\mathbf{L}$, then $\mathbf{A}$ is known:

$$E(\mathbf{L}, \tau) = (\mathbf{Q}^T\mathbf{r})^T \mathbf{L}(\mathbf{Q}^T\mathbf{r}) + \alpha R(\mathbf{L}); 1 \square l_i \square 0 \tag{5}$$

L is a regularization term, $R(\mathbf{L}) = -\Re_i p_i \log(p_i / l_i) + l_i - p_i$. $\mathbf{Q} = [\mathbf{q}_1, ... \mathbf{q}_N]$, $\mathbf{q}_i$ are eigenvectors in Q. α is a parameter. Set the derivative of l_i to zero and substitute result into (5). Then:

$$E(\tau) = \sum_{n=1}^{N} \Re \log((\mathbf{q}_n^T\mathbf{r})^2 / \alpha + 1); \quad \mathbf{r} = \mathbf{I} - \mathbf{J}(\tau) \tag{6}$$

2.2 Weighted residual complexity using local entropy

Local entropy expresses the local complexity or unpredictability of a local region in an image. It is not sensitive to noise due to the contribution of all pixels in local region. Given a location x, local entropy is

$$H_l(\boldsymbol{x}) = -\sum_{i=1}^{k} \Re p_{N_x}(i) \log p_{N_x}(i) \tag{7}$$

$P_{N_x}(i)$ is the probability of the pixel value i in local region N_x. Figures 1(a)–(b) show local entropy image of post- and precontrast enhanced CT image. The residual value between post- and precontrast enhanced CT image is big in misregistration region in Figure 1(c). Generally, the pixels with large residual value can be viewed as outliers or noise points. It makes statistics results serious challenges. So, we need to design a weighting function to deduce the influence of outliers.

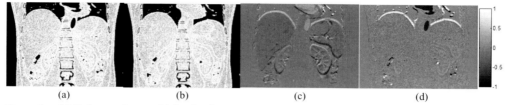

(a)   (b)   (c)   (d)

Figure 1.   (a) Reference image, (b) floating image, (c) residual image, and (d) local entropy difference.

Inspired by M estimation, outliers and noise points are constraint by small penalties and others by big penalties. We find out that the misregistration region with large residual value corresponds to the region with large value in local entropy difference in Figure 1(d). Here, local entropy is used to construct the weighting function. It assigns low value to the pixel with big gray value in residual image, and vice versa. The weight (Mahapatra D & Sun Y., 2008) $\omega(i)$ for the *ith* pixel in the residual image is:

$$\omega(i) = (\frac{\exp(H_l^I(i) - H_l^{J(\tau)}(i))}{1 + \exp(H_l^I(i) - H_l^{J(\tau)}(i))})^{-1} \tag{8}$$

H_l^I is the normalized local entropy of reference image I, $H_l^{J(\tau)}$ is the normalized local entropy of the warped floating image $J(\tau)$. Then, we substituted the weighting function to residual complexity in (6). Thus, the new similarity measure WRCLE is:

$$E(\tau) = \Re_{n=1}^{N} \log((\mathbf{q}_n^T(\mathbf{r}\omega))^2 / \alpha + 1); \tag{9}$$

Here, $\omega(i)$ is the element of weight matrix ω. The expression for the gradient of WRCLE is

$$\Box E = -\mathbf{q}^{-1} \notin \frac{2\mathbf{q}(\mathbf{r}\omega)/\alpha}{\copyright(\mathbf{q}(\mathbf{r}\omega))^2 / \alpha + 1} \div \mathbf{J}(\tau) \frac{\Box \tau}{\Box \theta}; \ \mathbf{r} = \mathbf{I} - \mathbf{J}(\tau) \tag{10}$$

$\mathbf{q}$ and $\mathbf{q}^{-1}$ are forward and inverse discrete cosine transform basis, respectively. $\Box \mathbf{J}$ is the intensity image gradient. θ represents the transform parameters.

3   EXPERIMENTS AND RESULTS

The registration is implemented using a hierarchical FFD (Kapur JN. *et al.*, 1985) transformation model based on cubic B-spline. A gradient descent method was used to iteratively optimize transformation parameters.

3.1   *The registration of nonuniformity image with Gaussian noise*

A cross slice (256 ∞ 256 pixels) of T1-weighted MRI volume on BrainWeb phantom (Collins DL *et al.*, 1998) is used. We generated synthetic example by both geometric distortions with thin-plate spline transformation and intensity distortions. Moreover, Gaussian noise was taken in Figure 2.

457

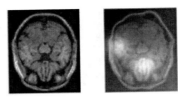

Figure 2. Left: reference image with $\mu_N = 0$, $\sigma_N = 0.01$; Right: floating image with $\mu_N = 0$, $\sigma_N = 0.001$.

The warped floating image and deformed mesh are wrong when using MI in Figure 3(a). There is misregistration region in pons and folding effect in deformed mesh when RC is used in Figure 3(b). However, the satisfied result is achieved when using WRCLE, also there is no folding effect in the deformed mesh in Figure 3(c). MI is sensitive to noise and intensity distortion. The poor robustness of RC results in undesirable registration results. WRCLE weights residual image by a function of local entropy difference to achieve the satisfactory results.

3.2 Artificial deformation examples

We used the DCE–MRI of breast from the same patient at different times with sizes 384×384 (pixels). The image at one time is defined as reference images in Figure 4(a). The floating image was obtained by artificially deforming the image at another time, as is shown in Figure 4(b). Figures 4(c)–(e) show the residual gray maps between reference image and final warped floating image when using MI, RC, and WRCLE. Here, we observe that there are many dark or bright pixels in residual map when using MI. Although the number of pixels with dark or bright value decreased when using RC, it still registered not well. However, there are little dark or bright pixels in the residual map when WRCLE is used. Intuitively, WRCLE performed well and outperformed the similarity measure RC.

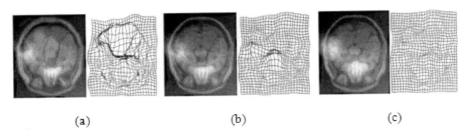

(a)   (b)   (c)

Figure 3. The warped floating image and deformed mesh after registration (a) MI, (b) RC, and (c) WRCLE.

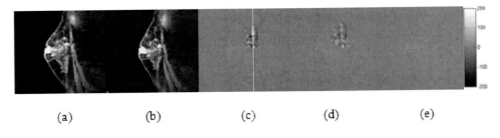

(a)   (b)   (c)   (d)   (e)

Figure 4. (a) Reference image, (b) floating image, and (c)–(e) residual gray maps after registration using MI, RC, and WRCLE.

458

3.3 *Patient examples in 3D*

A set of pre- and postcontrast enhanced CT data were acquired using a Philips Brilliance 64-Slice CT scanner from the same patient shown in Figure 5. The size is 512 ∞ 512 ∞ 397, the voxel size is 0.68 ∞ 0.68 ∞ 0.50 mm. In this experiment, the proposed WRCLE was compared to RC.

The residual color map before and after registration in three views are demonstrated in Figure 6. The first row shows the cross view in the 60th slice. The 100th slice in sagittal view is displayed on the second row. The last row demonstrates the 70th slice in coronal view. Intuitively, the result before registration shows a relative motion due to patient movement in Figure 6(a), which could be reduced after registration. WRCLE achieve better results than RC, since less motion is found in Figure 6(c). Overall, WRCLE is a more efficient similarity measure than RC.

4 SUMMARY

In this paper, we proposed WRCLE for nonrigid medical image registration. Residual complexity is modified by taking local entropy, which can be achieved by mapping reference image and floating image to local entropy space respectively. Then, the residual term in residual complexity is weighted by a function of local entropy difference. The new similarity measure weight residual image adaptively, which ensures the accuracy and robustness of the registration.

In the current work, we only consider the registration of monomodality images with intensity distortion. Hence, future work will extend the proposed registration algorithm to multimodality images.

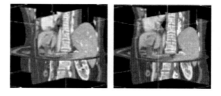

Figure 5.   Left: postcontrast enhanced CT data as fixed volume. Right: precontrast data as floating volume.

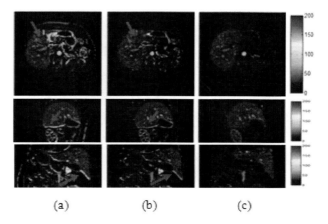

(a)   (b)   (c)

Figure 6.   The blank space between rows separates view: cross view, coronal view, and sagittal view. (a) Before registration, (b) registration using RC, and (c) registration using WRCLE.

ACKNOWLEDGMENTS

This work is supported by the Special Funded Projects of Pearl River in Guangzhou City of Nova of Science and Technology No. 2012J2200041, the Major State Basic Research Development Program of China (973 Program, No. 2010CB732500), and National Natural Science Foundation of China (No. 81101109).

REFERENCES

Hill DL, Batchelor PG, Holden M, Hawkes DJ. (2001) Medical image registration. *Physics in Medicine and Biology*. 46(3), R1–R45.

William M. Wells, Paul Viola, Hideki Atsumi, Shin Nakajima, Ron Kikinis. (1996) Multi-modal volume registration by maximization of mutual information. *Medical Image Analysis*. 1(1), 35–51.

Soatto ZYaS. (2009)Nonrigid registration combining global and local statistics. In: *IEEE Conference on Computer Vision and Pattern Recognition*. Miami, Florida, USA. pp. 2200–2207.

Wyatt PP, Noble JA. (2003) MAP-MRF joint segmentation and registration. *Medical Image Analysis*. 7(4), 539–552.

Andriy Myronenko, Xubo Song. (2010) Intensity-Based Image Registration by Minimizing Residual Complexity. *IEEE Transaction on Medical Imaging*. 29(1), 1882–1891.

Li SZ: Markov. (2001) *Random Field Modeling in Image Analysis*. second edition: 149–151.

Mahapatra D, Sun Y. (2008) Nonrigid registration of dynamic renal MR images using a saliency based MRF model. *Medical Image Computing and Computer assisted Intervention*. 11(1), 771–779.

Kapur JN., Sahoo PK, Wong AKC. (1985) A new method for gray-level picture thresholding using the entropy of the histogram. *Computer Vision, Graphics, and Image Processing*. 29(3), 273–285.

Collins DL, Zijdenbos AP, Kollokian V, Sled JG, Kabani NJ, Holmes CJ, Evans AC. (1998) Design and construction of a realistic digital brain phantom. *IEEE Transaction on Medical Imaging*. 17 (3), 463–468.

Medicine Sciences and Bioengineering – Wang (Ed.)
© 2015 Taylor & Francis Group, London, ISBN: 978-1-138-02684-1

Preparation of modified TiO$_2$ nanorods and research of light photocatalytic activity

Miao-jing Li
Mudanjiang Medical University, Mudanjiang, China
Harbin Medical University, Harbin, China

Xin-yu Cui, Yong-kui Yin, Sheng-zhong Rong & Xiu-dong Jin
Mudanjiang Medical University, Mudanjiang, China

Qun-hong Wu* & Yan-hua Hao
Harbin Medical University, Harbin, China

ABSTRACT: To improve visible-light photocatalytic activity of nano TiO$_2$, N,W-codoped TiO$_2$ nanorods were prepared by hydrothermal method. The prepared samples were characterized by SEM, XRD, and TEM. The results showed that the N,W-codoped TiO$_2$ nanorods exhibited a higher photocatalytic activity under visible-light irradiation compared with undoped TiO$_2$, because the codoping of N and W ions extended the visible-light absorption.

1 INTRODUCTION

TiO$_2$ nanoparticles have charge separation and transport properties of highly efficient, TiO$_2$ nano-particles' (VII.L. Gonzalez-G,I.Gonzalez-V, M.Lira-Cantu, A. Barrancoa, A.R. Gonzalez-E, 2011. IX.T. Tachikawa, M.Fujitsuka, T.Majima, 2007. III.I.Gonzalez-Valls, M. LiraCantu, 2010.) application in the photocatalytic degradation of pollutants in the field. However, owing to the large band gap (3.2 eV), their activity is largely restricted to the ultraviolet region, which only contributes about 4% of the entire solar spectrum (VIII.M.M. Rashad, A.E. Shalan, 2012. J.Zhang, Y. Wu, M. Xing, S. Leghari, and S. Sajjad, 2010. V.J. Xu, Y. Ao, M. Chen, and D. Fu, 2010).

One way to counter this limitation and shift absorbance into the visible region is to alter the band gap of TiO$_2$ through selective doping (VI.K. Fan, W. Zhang, T. Peng, J. Chen, F. Yang, 2011). A common approach in shifting the absorption edge of TiO$_2$ to the visible region is to modify its electronic structure by substituting the oxygen in the lattice with anionic dopants (I.A. Hauch, A. Georg, 2011). Among these dopants, use of nitrogen has been found to be the most effective strategy, and it can narrow the band gap of TiO$_2$ to 2.6 eV, which consequently gives rise to visible light–driven photo catalytic activity (II.B.H. Lee, M.Y. Song, S.Y. Jang, S.M. Jo, S.Y. Kwak, D.Y. Kim, 2009). However, nitrogen doping inevitably induces oxygen vacancies as electron-hole recombination centers, which has a negative influence on catalytic activity.

In this study, N,W-codoped TiO$_2$ nanorods were synthesized by a simple one-step hydrothermal method. Then, the obtained catalyst could increase the absorption of visible light and further improve the visible-light photodecomposition of dye.

2 EXPERIMENTAL

2.1 *Preparation of N,W codoped TiO2 nanorods*

A total of 2.20 g titanium tetrachloride and 1.74 g ammonium tungstate are added in 50 mL distilled water at room temperature with stirring until dissolved. It is then transferred to a hydrothermal

---

*Corresponding author. E-mail addresses: limiaojing@aliyun.com (Qunhong Wu).

reaction kettle at 180°C for 14 h and cooled down naturally. Then washed several times with distilled water, and dried at 50°C for 6 h. Finally, the sample calcined at 400°C for 2 h in air. Use the same method for the preparation of undoped TiO_2 samples.

2.2 *Characterization*

The phase of the as-prepared products was determined by a Rigaku D/Max 2400 X-ray diffractometer (XRD) equipped with graphite-monochromatized Cu Kα radiation. The morphology of the prepared samples was observed using scanning electron microscopy (SEM, Quanta 200 FEG) and transmission electron microscopy (TEM, Tecnai-F30).

3 RESULTS AND DISCUSSION

3.1 *Structure and morphology characterization*

3.1.1 *XRD spectra*
As shown in Figure 1, all diffraction peaks belong to the anatase phase TiO_2. These indicate that there is virtually no phase change in TiO_2 during the doping process. The intensity of the anatase (101) peak at 25.38° decreased and its peak width became broader after the N,W-codoping. According to the TiO_2 (101) diffraction peak position, the calculated crystal size of TiO_2 and N,W-doped TiO_2 were 19.8 nm and 11.6 nm by the Scherrer equation, size decreased.

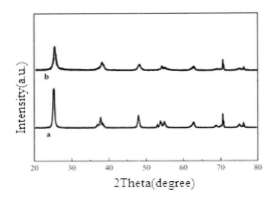

Figure 1.   XRD patterns of TiO_2 samples a and N,W codoped TiO_2 nanorods b.

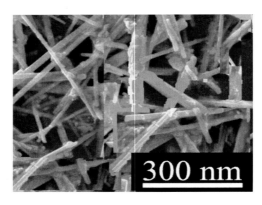

Figure 2.   SEM image of N,W-codoped TiO_2 nanorods.

3.1.2 *SEM and TEM diagram*

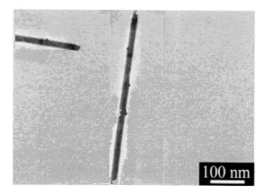

Figure 3. TEM image of N,W codoped TiO2 nanorods.

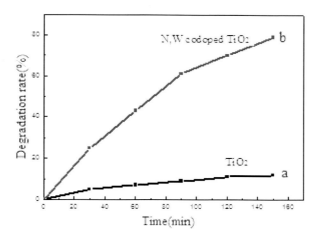

Figure 4. Comparison curves of efficiency on the photocatalytic degradation of RhB under visible-light irradiation. (a): TiO_2 sample, (b) N,W-codoped TiO_2 nanorods.

As shown in Figure 2, there are a large range of nanorods, and their structure is relatively uniform. The nanorods have a length of about 0.4 μm and width of about 20 nm (Figure 3).

3.2 *Visible-light photocatalytic activity test*

The photocatalytic degradation performance of N,W-codoped TiO_2 nanorod tungsten was tested on rhodamine B (RhB), under visible-light irradiation. As can be seen from Figure 4, after 150 min irradiation, degradation rate of TiO_2 on RhB is 7%, N,W-codoped TiO2 nanorods degradation of RhB rate is 79%.

4 CONCLUSION

(1) N- and W-codoped TiO2 nanorods were successfully prepared by the hydrothermal method.
(2) Detailed study of the surface morphology, phase composition, and structural properties of these samples reveals successful doping of N and W ions into the TiO_2 nanocrystals.
(3) The photocatalytic activities of the as-prepared samples were investigated under visible-light irradiation. It was found that codoping could significantly improve the visible-light photocatalytic activity of TiO2.

ACKNOWLEDGEMENTS

This work was financially supported by the 2014 Young Teachers Project of Heilongjiang Province (No. 1254G062); The Postdoctoral Science Foundation of Heilongjiang Province (No. LBH-Z13161); Science Foundation of Mudanjiang Medical University (No. ZS201325); Science Foundation of Mudanjiang (No. Z2014s027)

REFERENCES

A. Hauch, A. Georg, Diffusion in the electrolyte and chargetransfer reaction at the platinum electrode in dye-sensitized solar cells[J]. Electrochim. Acta, 2011, 46:3457–3465.

B.H. Lee, M.Y. Song, S.Y. Jang, S.M. Jo, S.Y. Kwak, D.Y. Kim, Charge transport characterization of high efficiency dye sensitized solar cells based on electrospun TiO2 nanorod photoelectrodes[J]. J. Phys. Chem. C, 2009, 113: 21453 21461.

I. Gonzalez-Valls, M. Lira-Cantu, Dye sensitized solar cells based on vertically-aligned ZnO nanorods: effect of UV light on power conversion efficiency and lifetime[J]. Energy Environ. Sci. 2010, 256:789–795.

J. Zhang, Y. Wu, M. Xing, S. Leghari, and S. Sajjad, "Development of Modified N Doped TiO2 Photocatalyst with Metals, Nonmetals and Metal Oxides[J]. Energy Environ. Sci., 2010,3(6):715–722.

J. Xu, Y. Ao, M. Chen, and D. Fu, "Photoelectrochemical Property and Photocatalytic Activity of N-Doped TiO2[J] Nanotube Arrays, Appl. Surf. Sci., 2010,256 (13): 4397–4403.

K. Fan, W. Zhang, T. Peng, J. Chen, F. Yang, Application of TiO2 fusiform nanorods for dye-sensitized solar cells with significantly improved efficiency[J]. J. Phys. Chem. C, 2011, 154:1721–1729.

L. Gonzalez-G, I. Gonzalez-V, M. Lira-Cantu, A. Barrancoa, A.R. Gonzalez-E, Aligned TiO2 nanocolumnar layers prepared by PVD-GLAD for transparent dye sensitized solar cells[J]. Energy Environ. Sci. 2011,4: 3426–3432.

M.M. Rashad, A.E. Shalan, Synthesis and optical properties of titania–PVA nanocomposites[J]. Int. J. Nanopart, 2012, 192:159–166.

T. Tachikawa, M. Fujitsuka, T. Majima, Influences of adsorption on TiO2 photocatalytic one-electron oxidation of aromatic sulfides studied by time-resolved diffuse reflectance spectroscopy[J]. J. Phys. Chem, 2007, 111:5259–5265.

Medicine Sciences and Bioengineering – Wang (Ed.)
© 2015 Taylor & Francis Group, London, ISBN: 978-1-138-02684-1

Gradient projection method on Electrical Impedance Tomography

Dan-yang Jiang, Hui Xu, Zhou Zhou & Nan Li
School of Electronic Science and Engineering, National University of Defense and Technology, ChangSha, China

ABSTRACT: In comparison with conventional medical imaging techniques, such as X-rays, Computerized Tomography and Molecular Imaging, Electrical Impedance Tomography (EIT) is a novel imaging modalities which approximates the spatial conductivity changes inside a body from voltage measurements through a set of electrodes on its surface. Whereas, the ill-posed nature of the EIT inverse problem requires the use of regularization methods that incorporate priori information. However, most of the proposed approaches have excluded the conductivity bounds of in vivo tissues. To solve this problem, a novel Gradient Projection method is proposed and applied to the image reconstruction of EIT. Compared to traditional Gauss-Newton method, this method has better robustness, which improves resolution of EIT images.

1 INTRODUCTION

Electronic Impedance Tomography (EIT) is an attractive method for monitoring patients' abnormal biological tissues or organs, it can provide a non-invasive continuous image of internal conductivity changes, indicating the distribution of various tissues or different functional states of one tissue. The conductivity changes within a body could be obtained by measuring the voltages at electrodes on the body surface caused when a number of different currents are passed through the body (Adler A. *et al.*, 2009). The image reconstruction problem in EIT is a nonlinear inverse problem which minimize the sum of squares error (Vauhkonen M. *et al.*, 1998)

$$\|V_{meas} - F(s)\|^2 \tag{1}$$

where $\|\cdot\|$ is the standard 2-norm, V_{meas} is the boundary voltage measurements and F represents the forward operator of unknown conductivity distribution s.

As (1) is ill-posed, it is necessary to incorporate further information about the desired solution to stabilize the problem and single out a useful solution (Hansen P.C., 1994). One of the most common and well-known approach is to use regularization techniques, a regularized version of (1) can be generalized in the form of

$$\min_s \left\{ f(s) = \|V_{meas} - F(s)\|^2 + \alpha^2 \|L(s - s_{ref})\|^2 \right\} \tag{2}$$

where L is called regularization matrix, α is a regularization parameter and s_{ref} denotes reference conductivity.

Conventional Newton-type methods search for a global minimizer of $f(s)$, with no restriction at all on the value of s (Vauhkonen M. *et al.*, 1998; Cheney M. *et al.*, 1990). An apparent drawback of these methods is they failed to consider the fact that the conductivity of in vivo tissues have certain values or explicit constraints (Table 1) which can be obtained from tissue samples.

Table 1:　Resistivity of different tissues at 10 kHz

Tissue	Resistivity $\rho(\Omega m)$
Blood	1.50
Neural tissue	5.80
Gray matter	2.84
White matter	6.82
Lungs(out-in)	7.27–23.63
Skeletal muscles (longitudinal)	1.25
Skeletal muscles (transverse)	18.00
Fat	27.20
Bone	166.00

Therefore, we employed the Gradient Projection (GP) method in EIT image reconstruction problem and combined it with GN to acquire more precise reconstructed images.

2　METHOD

2.1　Gauss-Newton method

The Gauss-Newton (GN) method has been widely applied to the EIT inverse problems (Cheney M. *et al.*, 1990). For difference imaging, (2) can be reformulated as

$$\min_{s}\left\{ f(s) = \|\Delta V - J\Delta s\|^2 + \alpha^2 \|L\Delta s\|^2 \right\} \tag{3}$$

where J is the Jacobian matrix of forward operator F, ΔV and Δs are differences of voltage measurements and conductivity, respectively.

The linearized, one-step inverse solution of problem (3) is

$$(J^T J + \alpha^2 L)\Delta s = J^T \Delta V \tag{4}$$

where $J^T J + \alpha^2 L$ is the Hessian matrix of GN form excluding the second-order derivative of the residual error. Nevertheless, the approximated Hessian will never be able to calculated directly in large-scale inverse problems, and the solution Δs^* can only be approached by a sequence $\left\{\Delta s_k\right\}$.

2.2　Gradient projection method

GP method looks for a Cauchy point Δs^c along the search path projected onto the constraints. Unlike GN, we added a single inequality constraint to problem (3). Accordingly, we restricted our attention to the following bound-constrained problem (Nocedal J. & Wright S.J., 2006):

$$\min_{s}\left\{ f(s) = \|\Delta V - J\Delta s\|^2 + \alpha^2 \|L\Delta s\|^2 \right\}$$
$$\text{subject to } l \leq \Delta x \leq u \tag{5}$$

where l and u are vectors of lower and upper bounds on the components of Δs.

In our inverse problem model, GP was done in two stages. First we sought the first local minimizer of $f(s)$ in the feasible region along the steepest descent direction. During this process, a piecewise linear path is created by the projection of the gradient. We then regarded x^c as an initial point and located a global solution of problem (3) by the use of nonlinear Gauss-Newton iteration method.

3 RESULTS AND DISCUSSION

We implemented simulations of the two reconstruction methods mentioned above. The finite element model (FEM) of a cylindrical tank is generated with 22795 elements. Voltage measurements are simulated by a ring of 16 circular electrodes with adjacent pair drive, adjacent pair measurement protocol. To simulate an inhomogeneous model, we placed two ball perturbations in (–0.25, 0.5, 0.5) and (0.25, –0.5, 0.5) respectively (Figure 1), these two balls are different in conductivity but same in diameter (0.15 cm). In addition, we added white Gaussian noise of signal-to-ratio (SNR) 40 dB in measurements.

Given the large size of the FEM, we adopted the Generalized Minimal Residual (GMRES) method in the calculation of Δs (Saad Y. & Schultz M.H., 1986). On the other hand, as the quality of reconstructed image is sensitive to the choice of regularization parameter, the L-Curve method is introduced to seek a fair balance between regularization error and perturbation error (Hansen P.C. & O'Leary D.P., 1993).

Figure 2 and Figure 3 illustrate the reconstructed images of GN as well as GP. Several effects can be seen from these images. Despite the resolution around two targets is relatively high and the two perturbations are visible, GN reconstruction produces distinct smearing artefacts in the homogenous background. Moreover, the blurring image of GN indicating that this approach is

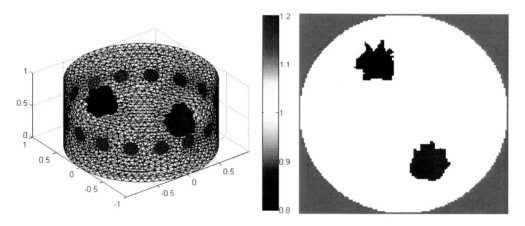

Figure 1: Simulation model and horizontal slice at z = 0.5.

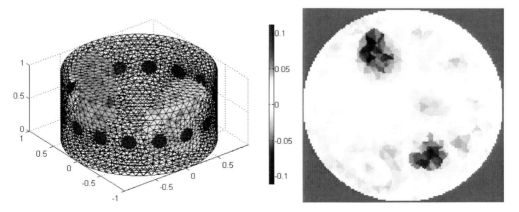

Figure 2: Reconstructed images using GN.

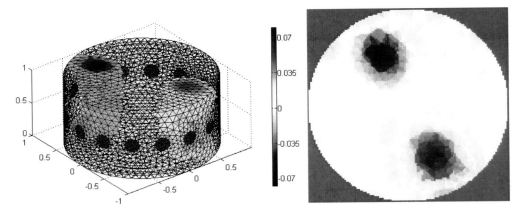

Figure 3:   Reconstructed images using GP.

easy to be interfered by additive noise, which limits its application in clinical practice. Compared with GN, GP provides a better reconstruction image with more constant resolution and less arte-facts. However, the size of reconstructed perturbations in GP is larger than GN, which implies GP enlarges the perturbation to its neighbor fields.

4   CONCLUSION

This paper applied GP method in EIT inverse problem. GP method requires priori information of the tissues' conductivity which can be estimated empirically or obtained by clinical research. The simulation results of GP demonstrated superior image quality results than the GN method, which provide an new method for EIT image reconstruction.

REFERENCES

Adler, A., et al. (2009) GREIT: a unified approach to 2D linear EIT reconstruction of lung images. Physiological measurement, 30(6), S35–S55.
Cheney, M., et al. (1990) NOSER: An algorithm for solving the inverse conductivity problem. In-ternational Journal of Imaging Systems and Technology, 2(2), 66–75.
Hansen, P.C. (1994) Regularization tools: A Matlab package for analysis and solution of discrete ill-posed problems. Numerical algorithms, 6(1), 1–35.
Hansen, P.C. & O'Leary, D.P. (1993) The use of the L-curve in the regularization of discrete ill-posed problems. SIAM Journal on Scientific Computing, 14(6), 1487–1503.
Nocedal, J. & Wright, S.J. (2006) Numerical optimization: Springer series in operations research and financial engineering. New York, Springer-Verlag Publishing.
Saad, Y. & Schultz, M.H. (1986) GMRES: A generalized minimal residual algorithm for solving nonsymmetric linear systems. SIAM Journal on scientific and statistical computing, 7(3), 856–869.
Vauhkonen, M., et al. (1998) Tikhonov regularization and prior information in electrical impedance tomography. IEEE Transactions on Medical Imaging, 17(2), 285–293.

Medicine Sciences and Bioengineering – Wang (Ed.)
© *2015 Taylor & Francis Group, London, ISBN: 978-1-138-02684-1*

Multidimensional multigranularity data mining for health-care service management

Johannes K. Chiang[1] & Chia-Chi Chu[2]
Department of Management Information Systems, Cloud Computing and Operation Innovation Center, National Chengchi University, Taipei, Taiwan

ABSTRACT: Data Mining is getting increasingly important for discovering association patterns for health service innovation and Customer Relationship Management (CRM). Yet, there are deficits of existing data mining techniques. First of all, most of them perform a plain mining based on a predefined schemata through the data warehouse; however, a re-scan must be done whenever new attributes appear. Second, an association rule may be true on a certain granularity but fail on a smaller one and vice versa. Last but not least, they are usually designed to find either frequent or infrequent rules. In this article, we are going to invent more efficient and accurate approach with novel data structure and multidimensional mining algorithm to explore association patterns on different granularities and to find out portfolios of health-care service management.

1 INTRODUCTION

Nowadays, Health-care institutions are eager to target patients with new portfolios of service variances so that they can improve their performance and offer better quality of services. For example, offering lessons of disease prevention for people to inform them that change habits to prevent chronic illness and physical checkup periodically can improve their health quality.

Researchers identified simple yet useful insights using association rules on services (G. Shmueli, N.R. Patel & P.C. Bruce, 2007). Significant examples are finding new therapies and drugs for cancer cure as well as new portfolios of rationale services. However, the conventional mining approaches lie in the assumption that the rules derived should be effective throughout a database as a whole. Different association rules can be found in different segments of the database. As a result, meaningful rules that are partially true may be ignored.

After a survey of a category of significant health services, we propose a data mining algorithm alone with a forest data structure to solve aforementioned weaknesses at the same time. At first, we construct a forest structure of concept taxonomies that can be used for representing the knowledge space. On top of it, the data mining is developed as a compound process to find the large-itemsets, to generate, to update, and to output association rules that can represent service portfolio. After a set of benchmarks derived to measure the performance of data mining algorithms, we present the performance with respect to efficiency, scalability, information loss, etc. The results show that the proposed approach is better than existing methods with regard to the level of efficiency and effectiveness.

[1] jkchiang@nccu.edu.tw
[2] jkchiang@nccu.edu.tw

2 BASELINE OF THE RESEARCH

2.1 *Data mining for healthcare services*

Data mining technology can help hospitals learn more about patients' illness status, and improve quality of service (QoS). Regarding data mining technology, they are now exploring five constructs for better service such as patient segmentations with respect to different types of service, different insurance reimbursement for various types of patients, chronic illness, self-pay treatment, and physical checkup services.

2.2 *Multidimensional data mining*

Finding association rules involving various attributes efficiently is an important subject for data mining. Association Rule Clustering System (ARCS) was proposed in, where association rule clustering is proposed for a two-dimensional space. But, it takes massive redundant scans to find all rules. The method proposed in the work by P.S.Tsai & C.M.Chen (2004), which mines all large itemsets at first and then use a directed graph to assign attributes according to the user-given priorities of each attribute. Since the method is meant to discover the large itemsets over a database as the whole, it may loss some rules that hold only in specific segments of the database. In this article, we also proposed multidimensional mining algorithms to solve above-mentioned problem.

2.3 *Apriori algorithm*

The Apriori algorithm is a level-wise iterative search algorithm for mining frequent itemsets with respect to association rules. The key drawback of the Apriori algorithm is that it requires k passes of database scans when the cardinality of the longest frequent itemsets is k. In addition, the algorithm is computation intensive in generating the candidate itemsets and computing the support values, especially for applications with very low support threshold and/or vast amount of items. In this algorithm, if the number of the first itemsets element is k, the database will be scanned k times. So, it is not efficient enough. The key point for improving the algorithm is to reduce the number of itemsets.

3 METHODOLOGY

3.1 *Representation schema and data structure*

For the sake of comprehension and compatibility, we use the forest structure consisting of Concept-Taxonomies to represent the overall searching space, i.e., the set of all the propositions of the concepts. On top of this structure, the sets of association patterns can be formed by selecting concepts from individual taxonomies. The notions can be clarified with examples as follows:

3.1.1 *Taxonomy*
A category consists of domain concepts in a latticed hierarchical structure, while each member per se can be in turn taxonomy, an example for customer's characteristics can be age, sex, marital status, and urbanization (e.g., sex can be male/female and marital status can be married/unmarried).

3.1.2 *Forest of concept taxonomies*
A hyper-graph for representing the universe of discourse or the closed world of interests is built with taxonomies under consideration. An example of forest of taxonomies consists of two subtaxonomy: age and sex.

3.1.3 *Association rule*

An association rule typically refers to a portfolio's pattern, which consists of elements taken from various concept taxonomies such as [(Location=branch1), (Sex=female)].

3.1.4 *Element patterns and generalized patterns*

An element pattern is composed of dimension atoms. If at least one of them is a dimension compound which combine several dimension atoms, we call this pattern a generalized pattern. For example, [web, Female] is an element pattern, [branch1, Any] is a generalized pattern, and both them are multidimension patterns. More notations to be used in the following text are shown in Table 1.

3.2 *The multidimensional multigranularity data mining algorithm*

The input of the mining process involves 5 entities, namely (1) a multidimensional transaction database (MD), (2) a set of concept taxonomies for each dimension (CTs), (3) a minimal support, and a minimal confidence, and (4) a match ratio m for the relaxed match.

The most significant feature of the algorithm is its capability to discover both frequent and infrequent associations rules R_{Ei} (based on different levels of granularities) in the element segment T[Ei] for each element pattern Ei. After it, R_{Ei} is used to update R_{Gj}, i.e., the set of association patterns for every generalized pattern Gj which includes Ei. The heuristic regarding each element pattern is to find the large itemsets per se and acknowledge its super generalized patterns with the result. The task of each generalized pattern is to decide which rules hold within it, according to the acknowledgments from the element patterns. The mining procedure needs only to work on each element segment to determine which rules hold in the compound segments. Thus, it is not necessary to scan all of the potential segments for finding the rules.

```
 1)  Input:
 2)      Multidimensional Transaction Database MD
 3)      Concept taxonomies for each dimension: CTx(X= 1-n)
 4)      User given threshold: minsup. minconf. match ratio m
 5)  Procedure:
 6)      Phase0:
 7)          to generate all Ei and Gj by CTx (x = 1 to n):
 8)          build the pattern table:
 9)      Phase1:
10)          For all Ei ⊂ G
11)              to discover all association rules r in T[Ei] as R_Ei
12)      Phase2:
13)          for all Ei
14)              for all Gj that Ei ⊂ Gj
15)                  to update R_Gj using R_Ei:
16)      Phase3:
17)          for all Gj
18)              For all r (which satisfy m) in R_Gj
19)                  output (Gj, r):
20)  Output:
21)      all multidimensional association rules(p, r)
```

Figure 1.   Outline of the proposed algorithm.

3.3 Pattern generation and the pattern table

Being a preprocessing mechanism, the algorithm generates at first all elementary and generalized patterns with the given forest, where a pattern table for recording the belonging relationship between the elementary and generalized patterns is built.

3.4 Update process

To be more optimization algorithm, we proposed full match and relaxed match method for update process. For a full match, the update is done by intersection of the set R_{Gj} and the set R_{Ei}, where Ei belongs to Gj, let $R_{Gj} = R_{Ei}$ if R_{Gj} is updated for the first time. After all the intersections, the association pattern r left in R_{Gj} holds in all element segments covered by T[Gj].

For the relaxed match, a counter for each rule in R_{Gj} is set. While using R_{Ei} for updating R_{Gj}, the counters of both R_{Gj} and R_{Ei} are incremented by one and the rules, those appear in R_{Ei} but not in R_{Gj}, will be added to R_{Gj} while setting the counter to one. After all the update process, the association rule r in R_{Gj} whose counts exceed m|T[Gj]| holds in at least m *100% of the element segments $T[E_i]$ that are covered by T[Gj], and thus (Gj, r) is a multidimensional association rule for the relaxed match in MD.

3.5 Design of metrics for measuring data mining

To design metrics for measuring the mining performance, a one-step look-ahead strategy based on Shannon's Entropy Function is adopted and the capacity of ICT systems can be described in the following form (J.K.Chiang, 2007 & W. Stallings, 2004):

$$C = B \cdot [\log 2(1 + S / N)] \cdot \tag{1}$$

Drawing on this equation, the function for the performance of data mining can be formulated as follows: C=|D| [log2 (1+information lost ratio)], where |D| is the number of transactions in whole transaction database (J.K.Chiang, 2007).

Thereafter, the definitions of information loss are

$$\text{discrete ratio} = \frac{|\{r \mid r \text{ holds in } T[Gj] < Gj, r > \text{doesn't hold in MD}\}|}{|\{r \mid r \text{ holds in } T[Gj]\}|} \tag{2}$$

$$\text{lost ratio} = \frac{|\{< Gj,r > | < Gj,r > \text{holds in MD r doesn't hold in T[Gj]}\}|}{|\{< Gj,r > | < Gj,r > \text{holds in MD}\}|} \tag{3}$$

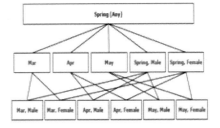

	(Mar)	(Apr)	(May)	(Spring, Male)	(Spring, Female)	(Spring)
(Mar, Male)	1	0	0	1	0	1
(Mar, Female)	1	0	0	0	1	1
(Apr, Male)	0	1	0	1	0	1
(Apr, Female)	0	1	0	0	1	1
(May, Male)	0	0	1	1	0	1
(May, Female)	0	0	1	0	1	1

Figure 2. & 3. Belonging relationships between patterns and pattern table shows an example of the belonging relationship between 12 patterns in a lattice structure. The relationships are recorded in the form of bit map as shown in Figure 3, a "1" indicates that the element pattern belongs to the corresponding generalized pattern and "0" indicates the case vice versa.

4 EXPERIMENT AND EVALUATION

4.1 *Experiment scenario on a case of hospital*

Data from different departments of the medical center and the website are gathered for the experiment. We take five attributes in the database of patients' records that may influence the health-care behaviors, viz., address, sex, occupation, age, and marriage, as the dimensions for the test. Adding with the therapy/service catalog and the cost records, there are 7 dimensions, *i.e.,* 7 concept-taxonomies for each dimension. There are 110 multidimensional patterns with respect to these taxonomies, where 40 of them are element patterns and the remaining 70 are generalized patterns. The proposed mining tool should find all large itemsets for the 70 generalized patterns.

4.2 *Results of experiment*

The default value of MinSup is 0.5%, match ratio $m = 1$, and the number of element patterns is 40. All of this kind of algorithms is sensitive to the minimum support; the smaller the minimum support, the longer the execution time.

The results of the measure on discrete ratio are shown in Figures 4 and 5. The results show that the algorithm can prune rules which only hold in element segments belonging to the domain effectively. The results of the measurement of lost ratio are shown in Figure 6. According to the result, the algorithm can discover rules which only hold in parts of the database.

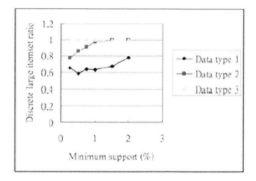

Figure 4.   Effects of MinSup on discrete large itemsets ratio.

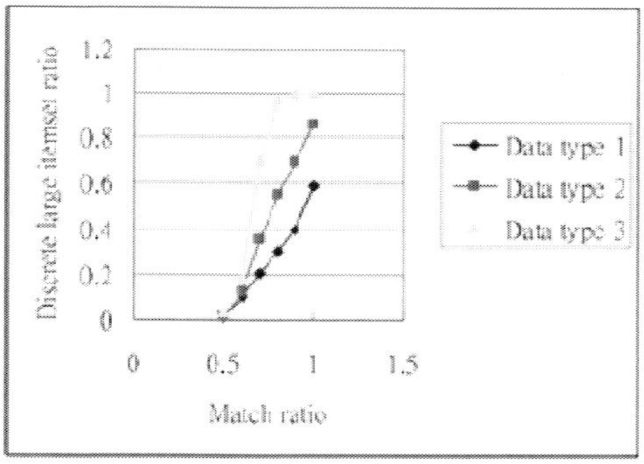

Figure 5.   Effects of match ratio on discrete large itemsets ratio.

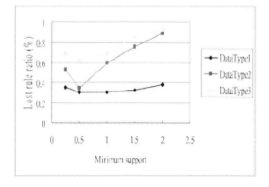

Figure 6.   Effects of match ratio on lost itemsets. (Right).

5 SUMMARY

This article presents at first the categories of innovative health-care services as well as the way to find new service patterns. Then, we propose a data mining approach for managing such new health-care services, including a novel data structure and an effective algorithm for multidimensional mining association rules on various granularities. It is proved to be very useful for discovering new service patterns. The advantages of this approach over existing approaches is that (1) it is more effective with finding rules hold in different granularity levels, (2) it is capable of finding frequent patterns and infrequent patterns while users can choose the full match and the relaxed match, (3) it has low information loss rate, and (4) it is capable of incremental mining of association rules to avoid unnecessary re-scan.

Consequently, it is a very effective and useful way to find out patterns of multigranularities in whole data warehouse. It also can help health-care service management to find out service portfolios. In our case, discovered when women over the age of 50 need blood transfusion, blood with higher ratio of blood platelet is needed.

REFERENCES

B. Lent, A. Swami and J. Widom (1997). *"Clustering Association Rules,"* in Proceedings of the 13th International Conference on Data Engineering.

J. Han and M. Kamber (2006). *Data Mining - Concepts and Techniques*, 2nd ed., Morgan Kaufman.

J. K. Chiang (2007). *"Developing an Approach for Multidimensional Data Mining on various Granularities ~ on Example of Financial Portfolio Discovery,"* in ISIS 2007 Proceedings of the 8th Symposium on Advanced Intelligent Systems, Sokcho City, Korea.

J. K. Chiang and J. C. Wu (2005). *"Mining Multi-Dimension Rules in Multiple Database Segmentation-on Examples of Cross Selling,"* in Proceedings of the 16th International Conference on Information Management, Taipei, Taiwan.

R. Agrawal and J. C. Shafer (1996). *"Parallel Mining of Association Rules,"* IEEE Transactions on Knowledge and Data Engineering, vol. 8, no. 6, pp. 962–969.

R. Agrawal and R. Srikant (1994). *"Fast Algorithms for Mining Association Rules in Large Databases,"* in Proceedings of the 20th International Conference on Very Large Data Bases.

R. Agrawal, T. Imielinski and A. N. Swami (1993). *"Mining Association Rules between Sets of Items in Large Databases,"* in Proceedings of the 1993 ACM SIGMOD International Conference on Management of Data.

T. M. Cover and J. A. Thomas (2006). *Elements of Information Theory*, 2nd ed., Wiley.

Medicine Sciences and Bioengineering – Wang (Ed.)
© *2015 Taylor & Francis Group, London, ISBN: 978-1-138-02684-1*

Packed fiber solid-phase extraction of monoamine neurotransmitters in human plasma using composite nanofibers composed of polyvinyl pyrrolidone and polystyrene as sorbent prior to HPLC-fluorescence detection

Xiao-Xiao Wu & Kang-Wei Shen
Key Laboratory of Child Development and Learning Science, Southeast University, Nanjing, China

Jian-Jun Deng
Suzhou Dongqi Biological Technology Co. LTD, Suzhou, China

Yu Wang, Lei Ma & Xue-Jun Kang*
Key Laboratory of Child Development and Learning Science, Southeast University, Nanjing, China

ABSTRACT: A simple and high-efficiency method was developed for the Packed Fiber Solid-Phase Extraction (PFSPE) of monoamine neurotransmitters in human plasma using composite nanofibers composing of polyvinyl pyrrolidone and polystyrene as sorbent. The plasma samples without protein precipitation and derivatization were loaded on the PFSPE column and the analytes were eluted from the solid-phase with sulfuric acid-methanol mixture (1:9, V/V) before separation and fluorescent detection by HPLC. The extraction recovery of the composite nanofibers was between 60.3% ~ 72.5%.

1   INTRODUCTION

Monoamine neurotransmitters (MANTs) mainly consist of Catecholamines (CAs) Norepinephrine (NE), Epinephrine (E), Dopamine (DA), and Indoleamine Serotonin (5-HT). They are involved in many brain processes, such as fear memory, learning and pain, or neuropathologies, such as schizophrenia, epilepsy, depression and Parkinson's disease (Parrot, 2011). Currently, MANTs are often used as valid clinical biomarkers for the diagnosis of related diseases, and they have been widely studied in different biological samples, for instance, blood, plasma, urine or dialysate (Kovac, 2014). Therefore, it is essential to develop methods that can effectively quantify very low concentrations of MANTs in biological samples.

The determination of MANTs requires a sample pretreatment to remove potentially interfering compounds, enrich the analytes and enhance the detection sensitivity. Solid phase extraction (SPE) is widely used for the purification of MANTs not only because of its easy operation but also due to the wide range of sorbent material (Augusto, 2011). The traditional adsorbent usually performs with activated alumina, cation exchange adsorbents, or phenylboronic acid (Grossi et al., 1991), and the operation seems a little time-consuming and labor intensive. During the operation, some loss of MANTs maybe inevitable due to their instability to light, pH, oxygen and heat, therefore it is recommended to use short-time and gentle extraction methods.

In recent years, it has been demonstrated that the electrospinning nanofibers may be good candidates for the adsorbents used in the SPE, offering a reduced volume of both the solid phase and desorption solvent and a simple operation compared to the conventional particle-packed SPE cartridge (Kang, 2007). In this study, using composite nanofibers composing of polyvinyl pyrrolidone

---

*Corresponding author: Xue-Jun Kang, Key Laboratory of Child Development and Learning Science, Nanjing, 210096, China. Tel: + 86 25 83795664, E-mail: xjkang64 @ 163.com.

and polystyrene (PVP-PS) as adsorbent, we developed a new method for the determination of four MANTs in human plasma by HPLC with fluorescence detection.

2 EXPERIMENTAL SECTION

2.1 *Instrumentation and reagents*

The HPLC system used consisted of a LC-20AD pump, RF-10AXL fluorescence detector and a SIL-20AC autosampler (Shimadzu, Japan). A high-voltage power supply (model DWP 403-1AC, Tianjin, China) was used for the electrospinning, A Hitachi S-3000N scanning electron microscope (SEM, Tokyo, Japan) was used to examine the nanofibers. An Orion model SA 720 PH meter (Orion Research, USA), and a High Speed Tabletop Centrifuge (Ruijiang, Wuxi, China) were used during the experiments.

Standards of monoamine neurotransmitters were purchased from Sigma-Aldrich (St. Louis, MO, USA). HPLC-grade methanol was obtained from Shandong Yuwang Chemical. PVP and PS were purchased from Shanghai Chemical Agents Institute. All other reagents were of analytical grade. The 1 mg mL^{-1}standard solutions of MANTs were prepared by dissolving appropriate amounts of these chemicals in water and stored in the dark refrigerator at 4°C.

2.2 *Fabrication of nanofibers*

The PVP-PS composite nanofibers were fabricated as the typical procedures. The electrospinni-ng solution was prepared by dissolving appropriate amounts of PVP and PS in proportion as 1:2 in the mixture of N, N-Dimethylformamide and tetrahydrofuran (1:1, V/V). The fibers were spun in the following condition: an anodic voltage of 18 kV, the feeding rate of 1.0 ml h^{-1} for precursor solution, appropriate temperature and humidity. The random nanofibers were collected by a piece of aluminum.

2.3 *Chromatographic conditions*

The column used was VP-ODS Shimadzu C$_{18}$ (5 μm, 150 mm × 4.6 mm) and the column temperature was set for 30°C. The mobile phase was a mixture of 5% methanol and 95% 0.1 mol L^{-1} acetate sodium (V/V) containing 0.2 mmol L^{-1} EDTA and was adjusted to pH 5.50 with glacial acetic acid. Fluorescence excitation and emission wavelength were set at 285 nm and 320 nm. The flow rate was 1.0 mL min^{-1} .The injection volume was 20 μL.

2.4 *Sample preparation*

The plasma samples were kept at -80°C in the refrigerator after collection, thawed at low temperature and centrifuged (12000 r min^{-1}) for 5min before analysis. The packed-fiber solid phase extraction (PFSPE) cartridge was prepared by packing 10 mg nanofibers tightly into the tip of SPE column as shown in Figure 1. The nanofibers column was activated by 100 μL methanol and 200 μL water before extraction. 1mL plasma sample after centrifugation was loaded on and pushed through the PFSPE column at a low flow rate by the pressure of air forced by a gastight plastic syringe. The target analytes adsorbed on the fibers were eluted with 100 μL sulfuric acid-methanol mixture (1:9, V/V) and 20 μL eluate was injected into the HPLC via an autosampler.

3 RESULTS AND DISCUSSION FIGURES

3.1 *Characterization of nanofibers*

The SEM image of PVP-PS composite nanofibers is illustrated in Figure 2. The nanofiber is network structure, and the diameter is 400 ~ 600nm.

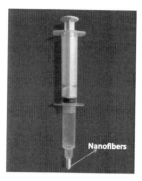

Figure 1.   PFSPE column.

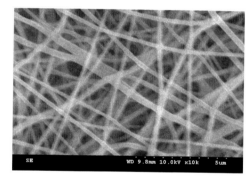

Figure 2.   The SEM image of PVP-PS composite nanofibers.

3.2   *Optimization of extraction conditions*

In our study, we found that PVP-PS nanofiber could effectively adsorb four MANTs in human plasma directly without adjusting PH or changing ion concentration. Elution solvent is also an important factor affecting extraction efficiency. During the experiment, methanol, glacial acetic acid, 10% perchloric acid and sulfuric acid-methanol mixture (1:9, V/V) were used as elution solvent, and their desorption efficiency is showed in Figure 3. The results indicated the analytes could be eluted from the surface of the nanofiber by strong acidic solution and sulfuric acid-methanol mixture (1:9, V/V) had proved to be the best choice.

3.3   *The absolute extraction recovery of the composite nanofibers*

To further verify the viability of the method, we evaluated the absolute extraction recovery by the spiked solution under optimized conditions, and the recovery was determined to be 72.5% for DA, 67.0% for E, 68.1% for NE and 60.3% for 5-HT.

3.4   *The chromatograms of the analytes and the validation of the method*

The chromatograms are displayed in Figure 4. We can see that the target analytes in the plasma sample extracted by the PFSPE column were clearly visible and the signal were enhanced. Furthermore, most of the interfering substances in the plasma sample were removed, which reflected a good characteristic of selective extraction for MANTs.

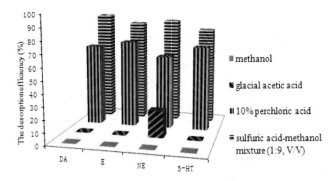

Figure 3. The desorption efficiency of different elution solvents.

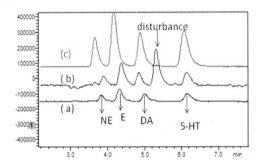

Figure 4. Chromatograms: (a) standard solution (b) spiked plasma sample (c) eluate of spiked solution.

We also evaluated the quality parameters of this new method. The limits of detection (signal to-noise ratio=3) were 1.2 ~ 3.5ng mL^{-1}. Good linearity of the analytes was achieved in the range 3 ~ 300 ng mL^{-1} with correlation coefficients of 0.9983 ~ 0.9992. The intra-day precision ($n=6$) and the inter-day precision ($n=6$) were less than 4.2% and 8.6%.

3.5 The possible extraction mechanism

We successfully used the PFSPE column packed with PVP-PS composite nanofibers to extract the MANTs in human plasma in this research, while our previous studies have demonstrated PS nanofibers could hardly adsorbe them. Therefore, we speculate that the PVP-PS composite nanofibers containing many carboxides adsorb MANTs predominantly through very strong hydrogen bond, with multiple attachment sites. The schematic diagram is described in Figure 5.

4 CONCLUSION

A convenient and selective method using PVP-PS composite nanofibers as adsorbent was presented for extracting four MANTs in plasma samples. The possible adsorption mechanism was proposed in the paper based on the molecular structure. This new method coupled with HPLC-fluorescence detection can achieve the determination for actual plasma samples without protein precipitation and derivatization.

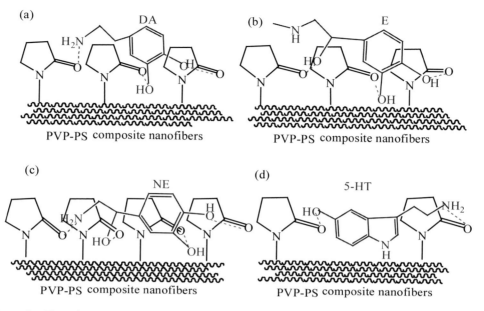

Figure 5. The schematic diagram of interactions between MANTs and PVP-PS composite nanofibers. The red dotted lines represent hydrogen bonds.

ACKNOWLEDGEMENTS

This work was supported by the National Basic Research Program (973 Program No. 2012CB933302), the National Natural Science Foundation of China (No. 81172720, and No. 21307086) and Colleges and Universities in Jiangsu Province plans to graduate research and innovation projects (CXLX12_0121).

REFERENCES

Augusto, F., Carasek, E., Silva, R. G. C., Rivellino, S. R., Batista, A. D. & Martendal, E. (2011) New sorbents for extraction and microextraction techniques. *Journal of Chromatography A*. [Online] 1217(16), 2533–2542. Available from: http://dx.doi.org/10.1016/j.chroma.2009.12.033 [Accessed 17th May 2014].

Christensen, T. T., Frystyk, J. & Poulsen, P. L. (2011) Comparison of plasma metanephrines measured by a commercial immunoassay and urinary catecholamines in the diagnosis of pheochromocytoma Scand. *J. Clin. Lab. Invest.* [Online] 71(8), 695–700. Available from: doi: 10.3109/00365513.2011.6 22410 [Accessed 17th May 2014].

Grossi, G., Bargossi, A. M., Lucarelli, C., Paradisi, R., Sprovieri, C. & Sprovieri, G. (1991) Improvements in automated analysis of catecholamine and related metabolites in biological samples by column-switching-high-performance liquid chromatography. *Journal of Chromatography*. [Online] 541, 273–284. Available from: doi: 10.1016/S0021-9673(01)95999-0 [Accessed 17th May 2014].

Kang, X., Pan, C., Xu, Q., Yao, Y., Wang, Y., Qi, D. & Gu, Z. (2007) The investigation of electrospun polymer nanofibers as a solid-phase extraction sorbent for the determination of trazodone in human plasma. *Analytica Chimica Acta*. [Online] 587(1), 75–81. Available from: http://dx.doi.org/10.1016/ j.aca.2007.01.021 [Accessed 17th May 2014].

Kovac, A., Somikova, Z., Zilka, N. & Novak, M. (2014) Liquid chromatography-tandem mass spectrometry method for determination of panel of neurotransmitters in cerebrospinal fluid from the rat model for tauopathy. *Talanta*. [Online] 119, 284–90. Available from: doi: 10.1016/j. talanta. 2013. 10.027 [Accessed 12th May 2014].

Parrot, S., Neuzeret, P. C. & Denoroy, L. (2011) A rapid and sensitive method for the analysis of brain monoamine neurotransmitters using ultra-fast liquid chromatography coupled to electrochemical detection. *Journal of Chromatography B*. [Online] 879(32), 3871–3878. Available from: http://dx. doi.org/10.1016/j.jchromb.2011.10.038 [Accessed 12th May 2014].

Sabbioni, C., Saracino, M. A., Mandrioli, R., Pinzauti, S., Furlanetto, S., Gerra, G. & Raggi, M. (2004) Simultaneous liquid chromatographic analysis of catecholamines and 4-hydroxy-3–methoxyphenylethylene glycol in human plasma comparison of amperometric and coulometric detection. *Journal of Chromatography A*. [Online] 1032(1-2), 65–71. Available from: doi: 10.1016/j.chroma.2004.01. 008 [Accessed 17th May 2014].

Medicine Sciences and Bioengineering – Wang (Ed.)
© *2015 Taylor & Francis Group, London, ISBN: 978-1-138-02684-1*

Exploring the treatment laws of Sinomenium Acutum through text mining

Na Ge

Shenzhen Affiliated Hospital, Guangzhou University of Traditional Chinese Medicine, Shenzhen, China

Guang Zheng

School of Information Science Engineering, Lanzhou University, Lanzhou, China

Ai-rong Qi, Dong Yang, Shu-dong Yang, Wen-jing Wang & Shun-min Li*

Shenzhen Affiliated Hospital, Guangzhou University of Traditional Chinese Medicine, Shenzhen, China

ABSTRACT: The study summarized the treatment laws of *Sinomenium Acutum* (SA) (Menispermaceae) using text mining techniques. First, we proposed text mining by collecting related literatures about SA from Chinese Biomedical Literature (CBM) Database, and then the ACCESS database was constructed. Second, structured query language was used to do data processing as well as data stratification. Algorithm was adopted to analyze the basic laws of symptom, Traditional Chinese Medicine (TCM) pattern, TCM herb compatibility, and drug combination. Our study indicates that text mining could be used to analyze the treatment laws of SA and provide a good reference for clinical application and intensive research.

1 INTRODUCTION

Sinomenium Acutum Rehder et Wilson (Menispermaceae, SA), first recorded in *Ben-Cao-Gang-Mu* (*Compendium of Materia Medica*), is widely used to treat various rheumatic diseases, allergy, dropsy, and acesodyne in China. SA, also called Qing Vine and Xun Feng Vine, refers to the vines and leaves of Menispermaceae plants as well as wind cane plants. SA should be harvested in winter. It is bitter, pungent, and neutral, and it distributes to the liver and spleen meridian. SA has the function of dispelling wind-damp, unblocking channels and promoting urination. This article summarized the treatment laws of SA with text-mining techniques (Zheng, G.,2001). The diseases, symptoms, and TCM syndromes that are treated with SA and herb compatibility as well as drug combination were all explored in our study. As the results came from the mass literature data on medical database, they might be good references for both clinical practice and medical research.

2 MATERIALS AND METHODS

2.1 *Data collection and pretreatment*

All the literatures collected in this study are mined from Sinomed (CBM, http://sinomed.cintcm .ac.cn/index.jsp). We used "Qingfengteng (SA)" as the keyword to search under the theme search, and then received a total of 400 documents (Search Date: May 4, 2014). In addition, we selected "Details" and "Show All" in the "Display Format" to show the serial number, title, abstract, keywords, and other information of each article. All the data were saved in TXT file coded with ANSI. The semistructured data were transferred into structured database file (Microsoft access) with the

---

*Corresponding Author: Shunmin Li, Equal contributions to this work: Na Ge, Guang Zheng.

proprietary tool. Within the data, keywords (core or not) were retrieved together with the article ID for further calculation. Provided that the contribution of each article was the same, repeated keywords of each article were counted only once. Data-cleaning work was preceded according to the previously described method.

2.2 *Data analysis and Data visualization*

The data stratification algorithms based on the frequency of sensitive keywords was used to calculate and explore the basic laws of SA. Based on the principle of co-occurrence, we built and calculated the concurrent keyword pairs. The network of concurrent keyword-pairs was drawn using Cytoscape 3.1 software. The basic treatment laws of SA were visually obtained.

3 RESULTS

3.1 *Symptom, TCM syndrome, and diseases treated with SA*

Diseases treated with SA were sorted by frequency in descending order as shown in Fig.1. Rheumatoid arthritis (RA) was the first. The second, Bi Zheng, is a TCM concept referred to as joint diseases. RA, spondylitis, ankylosing spondylitis, gouty arthritis, and osteoarthritis all belong to the categories of rheumatoid disease and Bi Zheng. SA was also used to treat arrhythmia, nephritis, chronic glomerulonephritis, hypertension, diabetes mellitus, and hepatitis. The network based on the concurrent disease pairs in Fig.2 showed that RA, Rheumatoid disease, and TCM Bi Zheng were the main diseases treated with SA. TCM syndromes treated with SA were shown in Fig.3. Wind-cold-dampness Bi Zheng and wind-dampness-heat Bi Zheng were the main syndromes. Network of TCM pathological factors in Fig.4 indicated that dampness-heat, wind-dampness, cold-dampness, sputum, stasis, and deficiency were the main pathological factors. We also calculated the frequency of symptoms treated with SA (Fig. 5). Ache, swelling, and stiffness were the main symptoms. Network of symptom (Fig. 6) also shows a consistent result.

3.2 *Herb compatibility and medicine combination*

Herbs with frequency more than 6 were listed in Table. 1. We found that these herbs were always bitter, pungent, and distributed to liver, kidney, gallbladder, and spleen meridian. Network of herbs in Fig.7 showed consistent result. Drugs combined with SA in Fig.7 could be classified as dispelling wind-damp, dredging collaterals, activating blood stasis, warming meridian, tonifying Qi

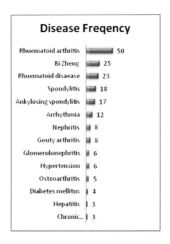

Figure 1.   Diseases treated with SA.

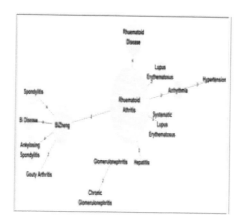

Figure 2.   Disease Network.

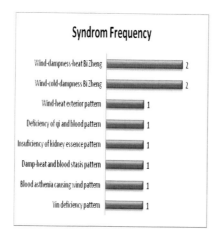

Figure 3.   TCM Syndrome.

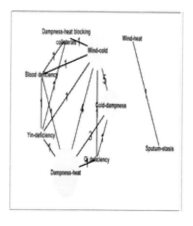

Figure 4.   Pathological factors Network.

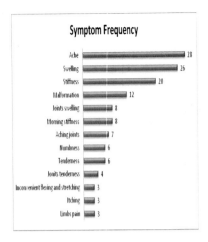

Figure 5. Symptom frequency.

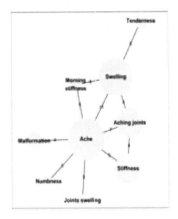

Figure 6. Symptom Network.

and blood, and nourishing liver and kidney. As SA belongs to Fang Ji family, after checking out the original data, we found Fang Ji (second line in Table 1.) was a noise.

Frequencies of Chinese patent medicine in our study were shown in Fig. 8. Zheng Qing Feng Tong Ning, the patent medicine of SA, was the first. Functions of the patent medicine in Fig. 8 could be classified as nourishing kidney, dredging collaterals, and dispelling cold. We also explored the laws of Western medicine. Sinomenine, the main component of SA, was the first in Fig. 9. The following drugs were immunomodulators, analgesics, and blood pressure modulators. Network was shown in Fig. 10. Zheng Qing Feng Tong Ning, the sinomenine patent medicine, was always used with Tripterygium Glycosides and Huo Luo Pill. Fig. 10 shows the correlation between sinomenine and morphine as well as sodium hydrogen phosphate (SHP). We checked out the original data and found that sinomenine could inhibit the withdrawal response of morphine dependence. SHP was the agent used to test the content of sinomenine with HPLC. Therefore, morphine and SHP in Fig.10 were noises.

Table 1. Herbs and frequencies in diseases treated with SA

Herb	Chinese	Note	Frequency	Property and Flavor	Meridian	Function
Sinomenium Acutum	青风藤	Qing Feng Teng	400	Bitter, pungent, neutral	Liver, spleen	Dispelling wind damp and dredging collaterals
Radix Stephaniae Tetrandrae	防己	Fang Ji	29	Bitter, pungent, cold	Bladder, kidney, spleen	Dispelling wind damp and dredging collaterals
Angelica Sinensis	当归	Dang Gui	26	Sweet, pungent, warm	Liver, heart, spleen	Nurishing and activating blood
Tripterygium Wilfordii	雷公藤	Lei Gong Teng	21	Bitter, pungent, cool	Liver, kidney	Dispelling wind damp and dredging collaterals
Radix Paeoniae Alba	白芍	Bai Shao	20	Bitter, sour, cool	Liver, spleen	Nurishing Yin and blood
Gentiana Macrophylla	秦艽	Qin Jiao	17	Bitter, pungent, cool	Stomach, liver, gallbladder	Dispelling wind damp and dredging collaterals
Glycyrrhiza	甘草	Gan Cao	17	Sweet, neutral	Heart, lung, spleen, sotmach	Nurishing Qi
Radix Angelicae Pubescentis	独活	Du Huo	17	Pungent, bitter, warm	Liver, kidney, gallbladder	Dispelling wind damp and dredging collaterals
Astragalus Membranaceus	黄芪	Huang Qi	16	Sweet, warm	Spleen, lung	Nurishing Qi
Ramulus Cinnamomi	桂枝	Gui Zhi	16	Pungent, sweet, warm	Heart, lung, gallbladder	Warming meridians
Asarum Sieboldii	细辛	Xi Xin	12	Pungent, warm	Lung, kidney	Dispelling wind,removing cold and warming kidney
Radix Clematidis	威灵仙	WeiLing Xian	12	Pungent, sault, warm	Gallbladder	Dispelling wind damp and dredging collaterals
Caulis Spatholobi	鸡血藤	Ji Xue Teng	12	Bitter, sweet, warm	Liver	Activating blood stasis and dredging collaterals
Ligusticum Wallichii	川芎	Chuang Xiong	11	Pungent, warm	Liver, gallbladder, pericardium	Activating blood stasis and dispelling wind
Chinese Starjasmine Stem	络石藤	Luo Shi Teng	11	Bitter, cool	Heart, liver	Dispelling wind damp and dredging collaterals
Rhizoma seu Radix Notopterygii	羌活	Qiang Huo	10	Pungent, bitter, warm	Gallbladder, kidney	Relieving exterior syndrome and dispelling wind damp
Golden Cypress	黄柏	Huang Bai	10	Bitter, cold	Kidney, gallbladder, large intestine	Clearing heat and eliminating damp
Radix Paeoniae Rubra	赤芍	Chi Shao	10	Bitter, cool	Liver	Clearing heat and activating blood stasis
Eucommia Ulmoides	杜仲	Du Zhong	9	Sweet, warm	Liver, kidney	Nourishing liver and kidney and strengthening bone
Kadsura Pepper Stem	海风藤	Hai Feng Teng	9	Pungent, bitter, warm	Liver	Dispelling wind damp and dredging collaterals
Radix Achyranthis Bidentatae	牛膝	Niu Xi	8	Bitter, sour.neutral	Liver, kidney	Activating blood stasis and nourishing liver and kidney
Honeysuckle	金银花	Jin Yin Hua	7	Sweet, cold	Lung, stomach, large intestine	Clearing heat and detoxifying
Earthworm	地龙	Di Long	7	Sault, cold	Liver, spleen, gallbladder	Cleaing heat, dispelling wind,dredging collaterals and
Salvia Miltiorrhiza	丹参	Dan Shen	7	Bitter, cool	Heart, pericardium, liver	Activating blood stasis
Rhizoma Cibotii	狗脊	Gou Ji	6	Bitter, sweet, warm	Liver, kidney	Nourishing liver and kidneyn,strengthening bone and dispelling wind damp

4 DISCUSSION

Text mining is a branch of data mining (Jeffrey W. Seifert, 2004). Our study showed the powerful function of text mining in exploring treatment law of SA. Our SA results would give an objective and comprehensive reference for SA clinical application and intensive research.

4.1 *The treatment law of SA could be well interpreted by ancient TCM theory*

The study indicated that SA could treat diseases with symptoms like ache, swelling, stiffness, and malformation. The pathological factors were wind, cold, damp, heat, sputum, stasis, and deficiency. The results could be explained with our ancient TCM theories. In *Ben Cao Hui Yan*, SA

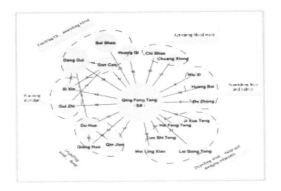

Figure 7. Network of herbs.

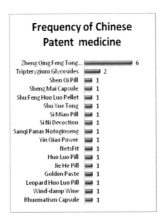

Figure 8. Patent medicine.

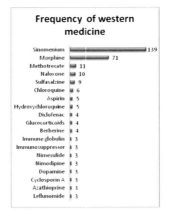

Figure 9. Western medicine.

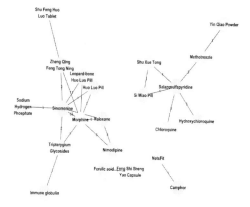

Figure 10.   Medicine network.

was recorded with the function of dispelling wind-cold-dampness, activating blood, dredging collaterals, and nourishing bone marrow. It is effective in the treatment of wind disease such as Li Jie and Bi Zheng. The compatibility results showed SA always matched herbs with the function of dispelling wind-damp, nourishing and activating blood, dredging collaterals, warming meridians, and tonifying kidney. *Angelica sinensis*, *Tripterygium wilfordii*, and *Radix paeoniae alba* were the main herbs. With TCM theory, Bi Zheng should be treated with additional methods such as regulating Qi and blood, and nourishing liver and kidney. In the TCM book *Yi Zong Bi Du*, there was a record *treating blood before treating wind; when blood circulates smoothly, the wind naturally disappears*. So our result of compatibility has an ancient theoretical foundation. Well, a modern research about sinomenine and paeoniflorin indicates that sinomenine could significantly improve the bioavailability of paeoniflorin in rats (Liu, Z. Q., 2005). This also gives the herb compatibility (SA and *Radix paeoniae alba*) a scientific explanation.

4.2   *Diseases treated with SA have modern research foundation*

Our study showed that SA could treat a lot of modern diseases such as rheumatoid diseases, nephritis, arrhythmia, hypertension, diabetes mellitus, and hepatitis. The results could also find modern research foundation. The mechanism that SA could treat rheumatoid arthritis might be relevant to the antinociceptive, anti-inflammmation, antiangiogenic, and apoptosis suppression function of sinomenine (Mu, H., 2013; Ju, X. D., 2010). SA could inhibit renal interstitial fibrosis, modulate expression of renal nephrin and podocin, and protect podocytes (Zhao, Z., 2013). Study also (Nishida, S., 2007) showed that sinomenine could maintain the cardiovascular functions due to modulation of cardiac ionic channels and blood vessels.

5   CONCLUSION

The study systematically summarized the treatment laws of SA with text-mining techniques. Our results could not only be interpreted with ancient TCM theories but also with modern researches. Text-mining technology could comprehensively analyze the treatment laws of SA and the results could provide objective reference for clinical application and intensive research.

REFERENCES

Jeffrey W Seifert. (2004). Data mining: An overview. CRS Report for Congress, Order Code RL31798.

Ju, X. D., Deng, M., Ao, Y. F., Yu, C. L., Wang, J. Q., & Yu, J. K., et al. (2010). Protective effect of sinomenine on cartilage degradation and chondrocytes apoptosis. Yakugaku Zasshi, 130(8), 1053–1060.

Liu, Z. Q., Zhou, H., Liu, L., Jiang, Z. H., Wong, Y. F., & Xie, Y., et al. (2005). Influence of co-administrated sinomenine on pharmacokinetic fate of paeoniflorin in unrestrained conscious rats. J Ethnopharmacol, 99(1), 61–67.

Mu, H., Yao, R. B., Zhao, L. J., Shen, S. Y., Zhao, Z. M., & Cai, H. (2013). Sinomenine decreases MyD88 expression and improves inflammation-induced joint damage progression and symptoms in rat adjuvant-induced arthritis. Inflammation, 36(5), 1136–1144.

Nishida, S., & Satoh, H. (2007). Cardiovascular pharmacology of sinomenine: the mechanical and electropharmacological actions. Drug Target Insights, 2, 97–104.

Zhao, Z., Guan, R., Song, S., Zhang, M., Liu, F., & Guo, M., et al. (2013). Sinomenine protects mice against ischemia reperfusion induced renal injury by attenuating inflammatory response and tubular cell apoptosis. Int J Clin Exp Pathol, 6(9), 1702–1712.

Zheng, G., Jiang, M., He, X., Zhao, J., Guo, H., & Chen, G., et al. (2011). Discrete derivative: a data slicing algorithm for exploration of sharing biological networks between rheumatoid arthritis and coronary heart disease. BioData Min, 4, 18.

Medicine Sciences and Bioengineering – Wang (Ed.)
© *2015 Taylor & Francis Group, London, ISBN: 978-1-138-02684-1*

Biomechanical research on treatment of fracture of femoral shaft

Xiao-yong Wang
Sichuan Provincial Hospital of orthopedics, Chengdu, China

Ji-he Zhou
Faculty of Sports Medicine, Chengdu Sport University, Chengdu, China

ABSTRACT: Early fixed restoration technique in the treatment of femoral fractures is an inconvenience in practice. Most patients have fear in early bone injury; coupled with the reduction of pain, severe muscle activity, sometimes with muscle spasms, often leads to lack of good cooperation between patients and doctors. After reduction of the fracture and the shift, or even multishift, this aggravated the psychological burden of the patient, which delayed fracture healing. In recent years, some biomechanics research had been conducted on the treatment of closed femoral shaft fracture patients, with heavy rapid traction reduction and splint fixation for the treatment, and obtained better results. The basic theory and methods of treatment of 13 patients were reported as follows:

1   GENERAL DATA

A total of 13 patients were treated in recent years—10 males and 3 females of age 13–75 years, mean age 29.9 years; the fracture site in 1 case was in the upper 1/3 of the bone, 11 cases had the fracture in the middle 1/3, and 1 case had it in the lower 1/3. Fracture types: transverse fractures in 6 cases, oblique fracture in 4, and comminuted fractures in 3 cases. Except for 1 case of old fracture in a hospital after injury, the rest were admitted within five days after injury.

2   THE TREATMENT RESULTS

Thirteen patients were treated with the above method, according to the national unified standard to judge the curative effect: 7 cases are excellent, 4 cases are good, 1 case fair, and 1 case with poor effect. Excellent effect accounted for 84.6% of the total cases; the average clinical healing time was 60 days.

3   METHODS OF TREATMENT

3.1   *The traction and traction frame, position adjustment*

Considering to use heavy traction, with steel skeletal traction in all patients, its position in the femoral condyle, we can obtain the same effect with Blanc's frame or Thoma stand in principle; it is important to be clear traction limb every point and direction of the force reduction, according to the fracture photographs, regulate the limb traction frame position, with heavy traction, the dislocation of the fracture dislocation overlap restoration, usually have four kinds of cases, the femur of 1/3 as an example, such as fracture of the distal proximal forward backward, and overlapping, adjustable traction frame to make the hip flexion angle reduced, in distal behind plus pad, the use of body gravity, and interaction along the femoral axis traction, plays the composite effect (as is shown in Figure 1). If the fracture of the distal proximal forward, backward dislocation, regulating the traction frame, the hip flexion angle increased, placing 2 kg weight at the distal limb, help to reset (as is shown in Fig. 2).

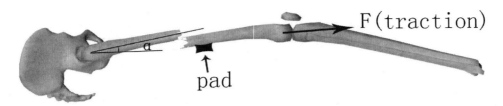

Figure 1.   Traction with pad (smaller α).

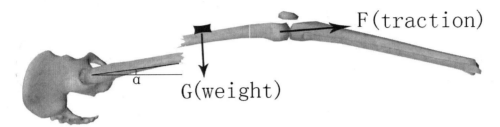

Figure 2.   Traction with weight (bigger α).

If the fracture of the distal and proximal malposition in two sides, also let a padded thigh adduction or abduction, then can achieve the same reduction effect. In short, to make the heavy pound and padded or pressure force to reset. Some oblique fracture and has big fractures in the broken position of a rotating need some auxiliary means apex before reset to the traction direction.

3.2   *Traction weight and time*

Lay the wire, adjust the traction frame, starting with a weight of 2 kg and traction for 2–3 hours, to allow the patient to gradually adapt to the pain caused by traction; then use the patient's healthy limb thigh circumference (unit: cm) multiplied by the coefficient 0.18 to get the number (unit: kilogram) as price basis, generally 8–10 kg. Heavy traction time is not long, generally 2–3 days. If the X-ray found that the traction effect is not good on the second day, we can increase or decrease the weight by 1–2 kg. The traction weight and time principle is (1) young patients have a good muscle tension, and the traction weight is slightly heavier, the elderly and children have lighter. (2) If the patient has long-time fracture, then traction weight is heavier and traction time longer. For example, for an old fracture traction weight is 12 kg, traction for 3 days. (3) Heavy traction for a proximal distal fracture. (4) Slightly larger traction weight for a serious longitudinal fracture dislocation.

After the fracture of paper pressure pad is fixed with a small splint mixture, transverse fractures reduce the average weight, oblique fracture and comminuted fracture day minus 0.5–1 kg to drawing a week or so, and then take 3-4 kg amount to maintain traction, the drawing time is about 5 to 7 weeks, and then can get rid of traction.

3.3   *The fixed method*

After 2 to 3 days' traction, we had external fixation with a small splint. According to the anatomic characteristics of femur, internal, lateral splint flat pad of cotton paper pad pressure. For transverse fractures, fracture pressure pad placed on the front, thickened outer splint, to prevent bending. Splint paper pad plus cotton pad was used if femur bending is slightly raised. In addition, based on the photos, we may place 2–3 point pressure pads. In the not-too-affecting blood circulation situation, splint external cloth is tied tight as possible, especially in the first week of traction. During this period, patients should strengthen the ankle and the stock for myo exercises, make use of muscle longitudinal tension and pressure pad splint binding effect to make the traction fracture reduction. We should promptly make the patients take ossicular conduction sound and X-ray examination. If the reduction is good, we can adjust the tightness of cloth.

3.4 *The technique of auxiliary application*

General transverse and oblique fracture do not require auxiliary application to reset; in this group of 13 patients, 10 cases were of natural restoration, 3 cases with extrusion. Take off the splint, increase 2 kg, according to the displacement direction, applying some techniques, reducing weight after reset, the comminuted fracture splint, daily rounds with the palm of the hand squeeze across the splint, and the fracture after reduction, separation, or manipulation, than in the past the traditional manual reduction effort, also does not need to match the assistant, so the hospital staffs save effort, and for the patients it's more psychologically acceptable.

3.5 *The functional exercise*

The treatment from small splint on both sides, the body can do ankle back stretch and thigh muscle exercise. We can get rid of traction after 5−7 weeks, gradually to practice hip/knee joint activities in bed, according to the condition of fracture healing, then the patients can practice standing, crutch, and single-throw walking.

4 DISCUSSION

The design and application of this treatment is based on the biological mechanics principle and methodology of modern medicine.

Biomechanics has proved that muscle stress−strain relations do not obey Hooke's law. A load−deformation curve is shown in Figure 3. After the muscle stiffness, linear relationship between BC segment load and elongation, modulus of elasticity of muscle is approximately Tan α, nonlinear relationship between the load and elongation in the CD segment. Muscle instantaneous stiffness gradually dropped to zero. Until the muscle rupture. Usually AB segment is a normal physiological stage, this stage is the normal physiological state of muscle loads under the BC section, has been extended to D point load strength reserve that can be. We use the traction, the starting weight is 2 kg, equivalent to AB load, which is a kind of psychological adaptation for the patient, because the muscles in the extraordinary physiological condition, load and elongation is not linear relationship, so to add the pounds traction, we should make sure the muscle is not damaged under

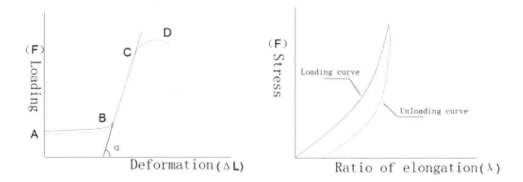

Figure 3. Load−deformation curve.   Figure 4. Relationship curve when upload and download.

the design load, therefore, based on past experience, with reference to the relevant literature, we designed the healthy limb circumference by 0.18 coefficient as a reference of the weight traction, and the application has achieved good results.

Muscle unloading stress–strain curve and the stress–strain curves are different (as is shown Figure 4), under the same load, unload curve elongation ratio "λ" (ratio of the length of the original length under loading condition) is bigger than the "λ" value of the loading process, and the longer the time between loading and unloading, the bigger the difference of "λ", that is to say, the muscle elastic component deformation recovery started relatively quickly, but the real deformation recovery is more slow. The subsequent deformation muscle, is the inherent characteristic of viscoelastic , thus, pulling wrapped muscles fracture overlapping part, not only need not injury cases with heavy traction, also need to pay attention to that the heavy trac tion time will not too long, otherwise the fracture muscles loose deformation, after bone healing in a corner or bone nonunion. Therefore, for different ages, sexes, and body condition of subjects, the traction weight is slightly different, and for heavy pound, generally only 2−3 days. Also, skin traction and skeletal traction produces shear strain of the thigh muscle. But the skin traction is different from the than skeletal traction .Moreover, with heavy skin traction, the skin is also easy to damage. So, the heavy pound is suitable for bone traction.

Dietrik et al. made a very significant stress test in 1948, and the results showed that after short-term bone stress, bone matrix appearing in the alkaline, dissolved in the matrix with alkaline phosphates precipitate. Therefore, inorganic salt in the bone increased, the compressive performance will be increased; on the contrary, if the stress is reduced, the bone matrix is acidic, it will dissolve part of inorganic salt in the bone, and the salt excreted. If the stress level in a long time to maintain the new level, not only the inorganic salt content change in the bone, and also will the change of bone shape and cross section size, continued function under relatively high stress, a part of bone cells into osteoblasts. To reduce the stress in the bone on the role of bone cells, which become the osteoclasts. The bony stress caused by recycling mechanism, Fukada first found it is due to collagen fibers produces piezoelectric, according to this theory, the femoral reconstruction in small splint reduces the traction load , hip, thigh, knee joint is not fixed, which is conducive to the early function exercise, enhance its physiological stress, contribute to the callus remodeling. Thus shorten the healing time.

Biomechanics study on vascular indicates that, vessel wall with creep, relaxation and hysteresis viscoelastic properties. Since then, the vessel wall is anisotropic, and has no compression properties. Under certain stress it will relax faster, and then slow down in a logarithmic form. Vein and artery are similar in constitutive relation. The capillary wall is very thin; some people think that it is only a layer of endothelial cells. Its role is to separate the blood and the surrounding tissue, so the capillary is not under pressure, blood pressure basically bear by the surrounding tissue. From this point, capillary can be a channel as in the organization. When the femur fracture, nearby tissue tension decreases, blood vessel rupture and bleeding of blocked blood circulation. We made an experiment and choose just admitted severe swelling of the femoral shaft fracture patients' limb lay the needle, and test the blood of injured limb in no load condition and compared it with healthy limb in load traction. The test results show that, with 2-kg load traction, blood flow of the injured limb increased 14% than bond limbs; with 4 kg of traction loads increase 46%; and 6 kg load, blood flow increased 83% than that of the healthy limb; continue to increase load of 2 kg to 12 kg, blood flow decreased by 22%. This may be due to excessive traction, muscle reflex contraction, or a block in blood vessel. I think this experiment indicated that suitable heavy traction can relieve the spasm muscle damage and increases muscle and blood vessels, blood flow also increases. Experts think, repair key fracture is the formation of new blood vessels and adequate blood supply. Obviously, heavy traction on limb swelling plays a very positive role, such as reducing pain, and improving the nutritional supply of limb.

Using the principle of biomechanics to the treatment of femoral fractures, we should organically combine the three basic principles of fracture treatment—reduction, fixation, and functional exercise. This can reduce psychological burden of patients in the treatment process. What prompted us to explore the core idea of the method is: we can't just look at the femoral fracture treatment itself, but the patients' physical and mental comprehensive consideration, the treatment of the patient in a relatively natural environment, play the patient's subjective dynamic role, set up faith in conquering disease, and traditional tedious manual reduction and plaster fixation, easy to cause the patient's fear mood.

About the drug treatment, the medicine directly to callus growth mechanism was not seen in the literature, in addition to some antibiotics and blood stasis pain medications, we rarely use medicines.

The treatment is not limited to the equipment conditions, and it also can be carried out in local hospitals, the key of this method is to master good traction weight and time; pressure pad splint resettlement; traction angle adjustment, and to check the reset condition in a timely manner. This method cannot importune blockbuster traction for a long time, in accordance with the principle of "blockbuster, short-term", if the reset result is bad; we can consider using gimmick reset or operation.

Above is our preliminary summary of the treatment of closed femoral fractures; further study of open fractures and other long tube in the future is required in the clinical setting.

RERERENCES

Jingming Wu, The exploration of the causes of failure of internal fixation for femoral shaft fracture with bio-mechanical principles, *China Journal of reparative and reconstructive surgery*, 1994-05-15.
Pengjian Wang, Analysis of the causes of failure of femoral shaft fracture of internal fixation, *Chinese Orthopedic Journal* [J], 2003-07-30.

Medicine Sciences and Bioengineering – Wang (Ed.)
© *2015 Taylor & Francis Group, London, ISBN: 978-1-138-02684-1*

Locating robot capsule looped by magnet ring

Wan-an Yang* & Yan Li
School of Computer and Information Engineering, Yibin University, Sichuan, China

Chao Hu
School of Information Science and Engineering, Ningbo Institute of Technology, Zhejiang, China

Feng-qing Qin
School of Computer and Information Engineering, Yibin University, Sichuan, China

ABSTRACT: Accurate position of Wireless Capsule Endoscope (WCE) is essential for function improving of current passive moving WCE. This article proposes that a magnet ring with about a length of 18 mm and thickness of 1 mm is looped around the capsule. The magnetic sensors around the human body measure the magnetic fields. With these data and quaternion describing rotation, the model about the capsule position and orientation is established. The optimization algorithm Levenberg-Marquardt (LM) is used to search for the solution of the model. Experiment states that the algorithm has good precision, high speed, strong initial guess error tolerance, and anti-noise ability.

1   INTRODUCTION

WCE is famous for its painless check for the entire gastrointestinal track (D. E. Fleischer, 2010; Gavriel Iddan *et al*, 2000; A. Moglia *et al*, 2009). However, the lack of accurate localization function makes it less beneficial. To make it more widely used and operated conveniently, many scholars studied the localization system for WCE and provided some localization schemas (Than T.D. *et al*, 2012; C. Hu *et al*, 2010).

To monitor the magnetic marker, Weitschiles *et al.* devised a localization system by using a 37-channel Superconducting Quantum Interference Device sensor system (W. Weitschies *et al*, 1994). Using 16 Hall sensors, Schlageter *et al.* also developed a system to detect position and orientation of a small magnet (V. Schlageter *et al*, 2002). Inspired by other localization systems, C. Hu *et al.* devised a complex magnetic localization system, which consisted of four magnetic sensor planes that forms 0.5 m × 0.5 m × 0.5 m cubic space (C. Hu *et al*, 2010). The position accuracy can reach up to 1.8 mm and orientation accuracy can get to 1.6°. The proposed system has a common view that the cylindrical magnet or magnetic marker is inserted into the capsule. The magnetic source is regarded as dipole, and the localization model is established. However, the space of capsule is limited, which makes it rather challenging, and the expansion of capsule will make it hard to swallow. So we present a new approach that the capsule is looped by a permanent magnet ring. The localization model should be re-established and corresponding algorithm should be found.

2   LOCALIZATION MODEL OF MAGNET RING

2.1   *Magnetic fields of permanent magnet ring*

As shown in Figure 1, the inner and outer radii and height of magnet ring is r_{in}, r_{out}, and h, respectively. The top and bottom plane is charged with a surface magnetic pole density $+\sigma^*$ and $-\sigma^*$; The magnetic field $\bar{H}'_u(r', z')$ created by the top plane at any observation point P(r', z') is given

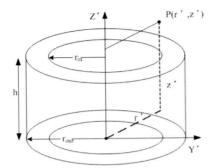
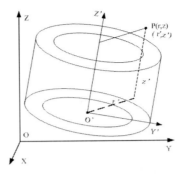

Figure 1.   Geometry of the ring systems.   Figure 2.   World and objective coordinate.

by Eq.(1) (R. Ravaud *et al.* 2008), and the magnetic field $\vec{H}'_l(r',z')$ created by bottom plane of the magnet ring at the same point is given by Eq.(2).

$$\vec{H}'_u(r',z') = H'_{ur}(r',z')\vec{u}_{ur} + H'_{u\theta}(r',z')\vec{u}_\theta + H'_{uz}(r',z')\vec{u}_z \tag{1}$$

$$\vec{H}'_l(r',z') = H'_{lr}(r',z')\vec{u}_{ur} + H'_{l\theta}(r',z')\vec{u}_\theta + H'_{lz}(r',z')\vec{u}_z \tag{2}$$

where $H'_{ur}(r',z')$, $H'_{lr}(r',z')$, $H'_{u\theta}(r',z')$, $H'_{l\theta}(r',z')$, $H'_{uz}(r',z')$, $H'_{lz}(r',z')$ are components along the three directions $\vec{u}_r$, $\vec{u}_\theta$, $\vec{u}_z$.

$$H'_{ur}(r',z') = \frac{\sigma^*}{2\pi\mu_0} \frac{\sqrt{(r_{out} + r')^2 + (z' - h)^2}}{r'} \times ((1 - \frac{k_1^2}{2}))\mathbf{K}^*[k_1] - \mathbf{E}^*[k_1])$$

$$-\frac{\sigma^*}{2\pi\mu_0} \frac{\sqrt{(r_{in} + r')^2 + (z' - h)^2}}{r'} \times ((1 - \frac{k_2^2}{2}))\mathbf{K}^*[k_2] - \mathbf{E}^*[k_2]) \tag{3}$$

$$H'_{lr}(r',z') = \frac{-\sigma^*}{2\pi\mu_0} \frac{\sqrt{(r_{out} + r')^2 + (z')^2}}{r'} \times ((1 - \frac{k_3^2}{2}))\mathbf{K}^*[k_3] - \mathbf{E}^*[k_3])$$

$$-\frac{(-\sigma^*)}{2\pi\mu_0} \frac{\sqrt{(r_{in} + r')^2 + (z')^2}}{r'} \times ((1 - \frac{k_4^2}{2}))\mathbf{K}^*[k_4] - \mathbf{E}^*[k_4]) \tag{4}$$

Where u_0 is the air magnetic permeability (T.m/A). And

$$\mathbf{K}^*[k] = \mathbf{K}^*[\frac{\pi}{2}, k] = \int_0^{\phi=\frac{\pi}{2}} \frac{d\theta}{\sqrt{1 - k^2 \sin(\theta)^2}} \qquad \mathbf{E}^*[k] = \mathbf{E}^*[\frac{\pi}{2}, k] = \int_0^{\phi=\frac{\pi}{2}} \sqrt{1 - k^2 \sin(\theta)^2}\, d\theta$$

$$k_1 = \frac{2\sqrt{r_{out}r'}}{\sqrt{(r_{out} + r')^2 + (z' - h)^2}} \quad k_2 = \frac{2\sqrt{r_{in}r'}}{\sqrt{(r_{in} + r')^2 + (z' - h)^2}} \quad k_3 = \frac{2\sqrt{r_{out}r'}}{\sqrt{(r_{out} + r')^2 + z'^2}}$$

$$k_4 = \frac{2\sqrt{r_{in}r'}}{\sqrt{(r_{in} + r')^2 + z'^2}}$$

The top and bottom azimuthal components $H'_{u\theta}$ and $H'_{l\theta}$ are equal to zero due to the cylindrical symmetry. $H'_{uz}(r',z')$ and $H'_{lz}(r',z')$ contain imaginary number i, so only radial components $H'_{ur}(r',z')$ and $H'_{lr}(r',z')$ are used. The total radial component H'_r of magnet ring is given by Eq. (5).

$$H'_r = H'_{ur}(r',z') + H'_{lr}(r',z') \qquad (5)$$

2.2 Establishing localization model

The coordinate system in Figure 1 called Object Coordinate System (OCS) is actually moving with the capsule. So another stationary World Coordinate System (WCS) (Q, X, Y, Z) should be introduced to describe the position and orientation of the magnet ring. The two coordinate systems are shown as Figure 2. (r, z) and (r', z') are the coordinates of point P with regard to WCS and OCS, respectively. The origin of the OCS is regarded as the point that will be localized. The motion can be broken into translation and rotation. The extended translation matrix $\mathbf{T}$ is defined as Eq. (6). x_0, y_0, z_0 are the coordinates of the origin of OCS regarding WCS.

$$\mathbf{T} = \begin{bmatrix} 1 & 0 & 0 & 0 \\ 0 & 1 & 0 & 0 \\ 0 & 0 & 1 & 0 \\ -x_0 & -y_0 & -z_0 & 1 \end{bmatrix} \qquad (6)$$

Capsule's rotation can be broken into two subrotations (C. Hu, 2006). As shown by Figure 3, the rotation from initial pose to final pose can be broken into subrotation $\mathbf{R}_1$ and $\mathbf{R}_2$. Quaternion $\mathbf{q} = (q_0 q_x q_y q_z)^\mathrm{T}$ can be used to express the rotation. If the quaternion $\mathbf{q}$ is known, the angle α and the vector $\vec{r}_2$ can be also determined, so the task is to find the quaternion. The quaternion $\mathbf{q} = (q_0 q_x q_y q_z)^\mathrm{T}$ can be used to establish the extended rotation matrix $\mathbf{M}$.

$$\mathbf{M} = \begin{bmatrix} 1 - 2q_y^2 - 2q_z^2 & 2q_x q_y + 2q_0 q_z & 2q_x q_z - 2q_0 q_y & 0 \\ 2q_x q_y - 2q_0 q_z & 1 - 2q_x^2 - 2q_z^2 & 2q_y q_z + 2q_0 q_x & 0 \\ 2q_x q_z + 2q_0 q_y & 2q_y q_z - 2q_0 q_x & 1 - 2q_x^2 - 2q_y^2 & 0 \\ 0 & 0 & 0 & 1 \end{bmatrix} \qquad (7)$$

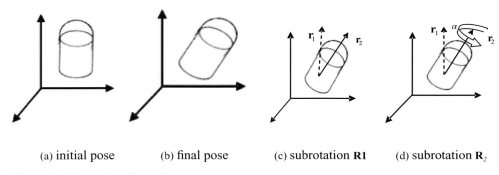

(a) initial pose   (b) final pose   (c) subrotation **R1**   (d) subrotation $\mathbf{R}_2$

Figure 3. The rotation of capsule.

The relation between the coordinate (x, y, z) of a point regarding WCS and the coordinate (x', y', z') of the same point regarding OCS satisfies Eq. (8). Extend Eq. (8), x', y', z' become functions of the parameters $x_0, y_0, z_0, q_0, q_x, q_y, q_z$, as shown by Eqs. (9)–(11). The parameters x, y, z, being the position of the magnetic sensor (evaluation point), are known in advance.

$$[x, y, z, 1].\mathbf{T}.\mathbf{M} = [x', y', z', 1] \tag{8}$$

$$x' = (x - x_0)(1 - 2q_y^2 - 2q_z^2) + (y - y_0)(2q_x q_y - 2q_0 q_z) + (z - z_0)(2q_x q_z + 2q_0 q_y) \tag{9}$$

$$y' = (x - x_0)(2q_x q_y + 2q_0 q_z) + (y - y_0)(1 - 2q_x^2 - 2q_z^2) + (z - z_0)(2q_y q_z - 2q_0 q_x) \tag{10}$$

$$z' = (x - x_0)(2q_x q_z - 2q_0 q_y) + (y - y_0)(2q_y q_z + 2q_0 q_x) + (z - z_0)(1 - 2q_x^2 - 2q_y^2) \tag{11}$$

Substitute x', y', and z' into (3), (4), (5), and (12), the theoretic values of radial component of magnetic field: H_r, being the function of unknown parameters $x_0, y_0, z_0, q_0, q_x, q_y, q_z$, are obtained. The components H_x and H_y respecting WCS can be measured by magnetic sensor. The measured value $\hat{H}_r$ is achieved.

$$[H_r, 1, 1, 1].\mathbf{M} = [H_r', 1, 1, 1] \tag{12}$$

$$\hat{H}_r = \sqrt{H_x^2 + H_y^2} \tag{13}$$

If there are N sensors, N measured $\hat{H}_r$ are obtained. With at least seven different measured values, seven unknown parameters can be calculated by minimizing E defined by Eq. (14).

$$E = \sum_{l=1}^{N} \left(\hat{H}_r - H_r \right)^2 \tag{14}$$

3 ALGORITHM AND EXPERIMENT RESULTS

To solve the localization model and evaluate the performance of algorithm, we define the localization error E_p and orientation error E_o. Where $x_c, y_c, z_c, q_{0c}, q_{xc}, q_{yc}, q_{zc}$ and $x_t, y_t, z_t, q_{0t}, q_{xt}, q_{yt}, q_{zt}$ are iterative and true values for $x_0, y_0, z_0, q_0, q_x, q_y, q_z$ respectively. Sample points are along a spiral locus that is on the surface of inverted cone. Sixteen magnetic sensors are simulated to sample magnetic field.

$$E_p = \sqrt{(x_c - x_t)^2 + (y_c - y_t)^2 + (z_c - z_t)^2} \tag{15}$$

$$E_o = \sqrt{(q_{0c} - q_{0t})^2 + (q_{xc} - q_{xt})^2 + (q_{yc} - q_{yt})^2 + (q_{zc} - q_{zt})^2} \tag{16}$$

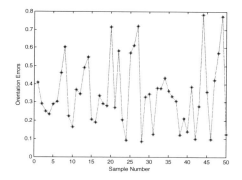

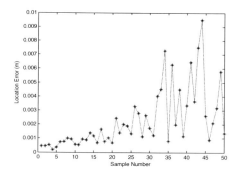

Figure 4. Localization errors with noise lever ±1.25%.

Figure 5. Orientation errors with noise lever ±1.25%.

The gradient decent algorithm often has higher speed than evolutionary algorithm, so the gradient decent algorithm is preferred. LM algorithm has better performance in magnetic localization system than other gradient decent algorithms mentioned above (C. Hu, 2006). Considering aspects of speed and precision, LM algorithm is selected finally. To simulate actual sampled data, some uniform rand noises with level ±1.25% were added to theoretical magnetic fields, which are regarded to the measured values. At the same time, to investigate initial guess error tolerance of algorithm, the position components (x_0, y_0, z_0) of every initial guess is 5 cm far from the true value, and (q_0, q_x, q_y, q_z) is 0.1 far from the true value.

Figure 4 shows the localization errors of fifty points, and average localization error is about 2.3 mm. We can see that the errors become larger. The reason is that the sample points are far from the sensor plane, which is in accordance with actual situation. Figure 5 shows the orientation errors of the fifty points, and the average orientation is about 0.33. The execution time of each point is about within 1 second, which reaches the real time speed.

4 CONCLUSIONS

There are only two expressions as orientation is expressed by quaternion. So, for possible decrease of local minimum, quaternion is selected to describe the orientation of capsule. Using the expression of magnetic fields of magnet ring, a localization model is established through translation transform matrix and rotation matrix consisted of quaternion. An appropriate algorithm is found to solve the model. Experiments show that LM algorithm has high speed, good precision, strong anti-noise ability and initial guess error tolerance.

ACKNOWLEDGEMENTS

This project is supported by the National Natural Science Foundation of China (Grant No. 61202196, 61273332, 61202195), The China Scholarship Council, Scientific Research Fund of SiChuan Provincial Education Department (Grant No.12ZA200), and also supported by Doctoral Fund of Yibin University (Grant No. 2011B06).

REFERENCES

A. Moglia, A. Menciassi, P. Dario, A. Cuschieri(2009) Capsule endoscopy: progress update and challenges ahead, Natural Reviews, Gastroenterology & Hepatology, 6(6), 353–362.

C. Hu (2006) Localization and Orientation System for Robotic Wireless Capsule Endoscope, University of Alberta.

C. Hu, M. Li, S. Song, W.A. Yang, R. Zhang, M. Q. H. Meng (2010) A Cubic 3-Axis Magnetic Sensor Array for Wirelessly Tracking Magnet Position and Orientation, *IEEE Sensors Journal*, 10(5), 903–913.

D. E. Fleischer (2010) Motion in the direction of making the video capsule our primary endoscope, *Gastrointestinal Endoscopy*, 72(2), 388–391.

Gavriel Iddan, Gavriel Meron, Arkady Glukhovsky, Paul Swain(2000) wireless capsule endoscope, *Nature*, 405, 417.

N. C. Atuegwu and R. L. Galloway(2008) Volumetric characterization of the Aurora magnetic tracker system for image-guided transorbital endoscopic procedures, *Physics in Medicine and Biology*, 53(16), 4355–4368.

R. Ravaud, G. Lemarquand, V. Lemarquand, C. Depollier(2008) Analytical calculation of the magnetic field created by permanent-magnet rings, *IEEE Transactions on Magnetics*, 44(8), 1982–1989.

Than T.D., G. Alici, H. Zhou , W.H. Li (2012) A review of localization systems for robotic endoscopic capsules, *IEEE Transactions on Biomedical Engineering*, 59(9), 2387–2399.

V. Schlageter, P. Drljaca, R. S. Popovic, Ku, P. Era(2002) A magnetic tracking system based on highly sensitive integrated hall sensors, *International Journal Series C*, 45(4), 967–973.

W. Weitschies, J. Wedemeyer, R. Stehr, L. Trahms(1994) Magnetic markers as a noninvasive tool to monitor gastrointestinal transit, *IEEE Transactions on Biomedical Engineering*, 41(2), 192–195.

Medicine Sciences and Bioengineering – Wang (Ed.)
© 2015 Taylor & Francis Group, London, ISBN: 978-1-138-02684-1

Establishment of an innovative personnel training platform by virtue of the laboratory built by central and local government together

He Li, Wei-jing Sun, Chun -mei Wang, Jing-hui Sun, Hao Jia, Hong-xia Sun,
Cheng-yi Zhang, Xin-tian Fan & Jian-guang Chen*
College of Pharmacy, Beihua University, Jilin City, China

ABSTRACT: In this study, the experience in the establishment of students' innovative personnel training platform by virtue of the Applied Pharmacological Laboratory, a central and local cooperation laboratory, sponsored by central and local governments together, is introduced.

1   INTRODUCTION

In order to support local colleges and universities, the state has set up a project built by central and local government together to improve the local higher education. Beihua University began to apply for the establishment of Applied Pharmacological Laboratory sponsored by the project in 2005. Through our hard work for 4 years, the application was approved by the central government and five million yuan was given to build the laboratory in 2009, which has provided a reliable material guarantee for further improving our laboratory to establish a creative personnel training platform. Nevertheless, a good material condition does not necessarily guarantee the success of a project, especially for a common undergraduate university such as our university. Successfully to improve our laboratory for establishing an ideal innovative personnel platform is a particularly difficult task (Li *et al.*, 2012, Fu *et al.*, 2011).

2   THE NEED FOR BUILDING THE INNOVATIVE PERSONNEL TRAINING PLATFORM

Innovation and personnel training is one of the important tasks of higher education, and many scholars committed to innovative students culture. To build a scientific culture platform for providing a good training environment for it is the premise of innovative personnel training. There are some reasons why the establishment of an innovative personnel training platform relying on the Applied Pharmacological Laboratory is necessary.

2.1   *Responsibility for the numerous students*

Teaching in numerous students at different levels, but mainly undergraduates. Annually, more than a thousand of undergraduates receive the experimental teaching in our laboratory. In addition, the laboratory is also responsible for the experimental teaching of graduate students, foreign students and adult education students. The establishment of the innovative personnel training platform in the Applied Pharmacological Laboratory has served for many students. The platform has provided a good experimental condition for them.

First Author: He Li, (1977-), E-mail: yitonglh@126.com
* Corresponding Author: Jianguang Chen (1962-), E-mail: Chenjg118@sohu.com

2.2 Promotion of the combination of teaching with research

The teachers in our laboratory has been responsible for a wide range of research projects for many years, including some national projects. In the above research projects, teachers, especially young teachers, have improved their academic levels and teaching abilities when their scientific research capacities have been improved. The research implementation in the laboratory has also provided a good condition for the establishment of an open laboratory to students.

2.3 Contribution to service for the local economy

To serve for the local economy is one of the university tasks. Our university is located in the Jilin region and the Applied Pharmacological Laboratory is a pharmacological laboratory with the best conditions in this region. The establishment of the innovative personnel training platform in the laboratory has contributed a lot to the local enterprises and institutions in personnel training, business consulting and achievements offering.

3 MEASURES TO ENSURE THE DEVELOPMENT OF AN INNOVATIVE TALENT TRAINING PLATFORM

3.1 Full scientific discussion and conception

After the Applied Pharmacological Laboratory project was approved to be founded, the construction scheme was drawn up organically by fully discussing and designing, and inviting some experts to evaluate it in various aspects repeatedly, such as the guiding ideology, goal, team formation, content, instrument allocation, perfection of rules and regulations, to ensure that the project would be carried out smoothly.

3.2 The content of the platform establishment included in the syllabus

In order to tie in with the establishment of innovative personnel training platform, the undergraduate experimental items implemented on the platform were written in the syllabus and most of them were designed as designed and integrated experiments intentionally. In this way, it would be ensured that the construction of the laboratory could be put into practice and follow the requirement that the Applied Pharmacological Laboratory should serve firstly for the personnel training of undergraduates, secondarily for that of graduates.

3.3 Opening and management of the experimental teaching demonstration centre

Since the Applied Pharmacological Laboratory was founded, the university-college two level management system was carried out, the laboratory was open to the students and shared by them both in experimental learning and research, the corresponding management regulations for the "open laboratory" were developed to achieve the implementation of all-day opening and ensure that the laboratory resources could be utilized fully and reasonably.

4 CONCLUSIONS

So far, in addition to the completion of the regular education in undergraduate, graduate, foreign students and adult education students, ten innovative projects of college students, basic skills training for pharmacy undergraduate before their graduation practice, more than 20 vertical and transverse research projects have been finished on the platform. The platform has provided a sufficient experimental space, useful laboratory equipment and techniques, and better laboratory personnel services for the students in the innovative training. The study should provide evidences in theory and practice for further improving the cultivation of students' creativity to ensure the teaching quality in colleges and universities.

REFERENCES

Fu L, Wu Y. & Xian F. H. (2011) Constructing interior medical teaching quality control system based on international medical teaching standard. *China Higher Medical Education* (2), 18–19.
Li T. J. , Zhang Y. F. & Rui Y. C. (2012) Exploration of the design and implementation of pharmacology experiment in undergraduate students. *Journal of Pharmaceutical Practice* (2), 154–155.

Medicine Sciences and Bioengineering – Wang (Ed.)
© *2015 Taylor & Francis Group, London, ISBN: 978-1-138-02684-1*

Extraction, isolation, purification and structure of a new polysaccharide from *Hypomesus olidus*

Xiu-yuan Guan & Xue-jun Liu*
College of Food Science and Engineering, Jilin Agricultural University, Changchun, Jilin Province, China

ABSTRACT: The polysaccharide was isolated from *Hypomesus olidus* using normal saline for extraction, the equivalence point to remove the protein and ethanol for deposition. The yield of polysaccharide from *Hypomesus olidus* under these conditions was 3.65%. Different polysaccharides (CZGY-1, CZGY-2, CZGY-3,) were obtained from the extract (i.e., crude polysaccharide) by diethylaminoethyl-52-cellulose column chromatography. The recovery rates of CZGY-1, CZGY-2 and CZGY-3 based on the amount of CZGY were 137.10 mg/g, 207.30 mg/g and 84.75 mg/g, respectively. CZGY-1 and CZGY-2 were polysaccharide substances and contained no proteins and nucleic acids from UV scanning spectrum. The polysaccharides obtained showed different structures by Fourier transform infrared there in the three elected.

1 INTRODUCTION

Polysaccharides are biologically active macromolecules, which were widely found in plants, microorganisms, animals and other organisms. Polysaccharide, which was isolated and purified, will play an important role on research on activity, the nature and structure of polysaccharides. A large number of researches on marine organisms show that glycosaminoglycans in marine bodies have antitumor (Takaya Y *et al*., 1994), anticoagulants (Mauro S G Pavao *et al*., 1998), antiproliferative (Yang W *et al*., 2012), immune function (Kozarski M *et al*., 2011) and other bioactives.

Due to coagulation factors leading to cardiovascular and cerebrovascular diseases have become common serious harm to public health. Currently anticoagulant drugs, which were used in the clinical treatment, primarily were heparin and coumarin. Heparin polysaccharide has played a very important role on the treatment of thrombotic diseases. But it is easy to cause bleeding, hyperkalemia side effects (Thomas D P *et al*., 1997). Polysaccharides, which were extracted in this paper, have anticoagulant effect (Xuejun Liu & Dongjiao Wang, 2012). It has an important significance in the development of new drug or functional food which has a preventive effect on thrombotic diseases.

2 MATERIALS AND METHODS

2.1 *Materials, reagents and instruments*

Hypomesus olidus were bought in aquatic product market in Changchun Jilin Province. After they were cleaned, heads were cut and placed in cold storage under low temperature ($-20°C$). Absolute ethanol(EtOH), 95% ethanol, phenol, sulfuric acid, glucose, NaCl, iodine et al. All chemicals and solvents were of analytical grade from China. Dialysis bag (MWCO 7000). Diethylaminoethyl (DEAE)-52-cellulose was from Sigma. The Fourier transform infrared (FT-IR) spectrophotometer

---

*Corresponding author: Tel:15304460733
Email address: liuxuejun63@163.com

was from Shimadzu, Japan. The instrument parameter was resolution 4.0, range 400–4000 cm^{-1}. 1900 UV spectrophotometer was from Beijing Purkinje general instrument co., LTD.

2.2 Extraction of polysaccharide

The head of *Hypomesus olidus*, which were cut, was homogenated with 2 vol of normal saline. After centrifugation by 3000 rpm for 10 min, supernatant 1 and precipitate were obtained. The precipitate was alkaline hydrolysis with 5 vol of 0.1 mol/L NaOH at 30°C for 8 h. The supernatant 2 was collected after centrifugation 3000 rpm for 10 min, which was mixed with supernatant 1. After concentrated, it was to remove the protein by the equivalence point method and exhaustively dialyzed against water for two days, the concentrated dialyzate was precipitated with 4 vol of 95% EtOH at 4°C for 12 h. The precipitate was washed with absolute ethanol, acetone and ether, respectively (Chi *et al.*, 2007). The washed precipitate was the crude polysaccharide, named as CZGY.

2.3 Isolation and purification of polysaccharide

The crude polysaccharide sample was dissolved in distilled water and forced through a filter (0.45 um), and the supernatant was loaded onto a DEAE-52-cellulose column (40 × 1.6 cm, internal diameter),which was eluted with distilled water and 0.1M –0.6M NaCl solution in order at a flow rate of 0.4 ml/min. The elution (4 ml/tube) was collected and carbohydrate content determined based on the phenol-sulfuric acid method at 490 nm absorbance (Jiang B et al., 2010). In this procedure, main fractions contained polysaccharides were obtained, which were then dialyzed concentrated, freeze-dried respectively.

2.4 The physical and chemical properties of polysaccharide

There were a series of tests: Molish test, phenol-sulfuric acid method to identify carbohydrates (Dongru Wu 1987), Fehling reagent to identify sugar (Longxiang et al., 1981), Iodine - potassium iodide reaction to identify starch (Qingyong Meng et al., 2004).

2.5 Identification of polysaccharide purity

The purified polysaccharide sample was dissolved in distilled water. Distilled water was used as a blank control museum. UV absorption spectra was recorded with 1900 UV spectrophotometer between 190 nm and 400 nm. It was used to determine characteristic absorption peak of polysaccharide samples and detect whether there were proteins and nuclear acid residues in the sample.

2.6 FT-IR spectra analysis of polysaccharide

The samples were incorporated into KBr and pressed into a pellet. Spectra were recorded at the absorbance mode from 4000 cm^{-1} to 400 cm^{-1} on a FT-IR spectrometer.

3 RESULTS AND DISCUSSION

3.1 Isolation and purification of polysaccharide

In the present study, CZGY was isolated from *Hypomesus olidus* and the yield was about 3.65%. Furthermore, the CZGY solution was separated through an anion-exchange chromatography of DEAE-52-cellulose, affording three independent elution peaks, which were obtained in 0.1M NaCl, 0.2 M NaCl and 0.4 M NaCl (Figure 1–3), as detected by the phenol–sulfuric acid assay. Then they were named as CZGY-1, CZGY-2, CZGY-3, respectively. The recovery rates of

CZGY- 1, CZGY-2 and CZGY-3 based on the amount of CZGY were 137.10 mg/g, 207.30 mg/g and 84.75 mg/g, respectively.

3.2 *Analysis of the physical and chemical properties of polysaccharide*

Between two layers of liquid formed a purple ring by Molish reaction, phenol – sulfuric acid reaction was orange, which were shown to contain carbohydrate. Fehling reagent was no brick-red precipitate, which proved no sugar. Iodine – potassium iodide reaction turned no blue, which proved no starch.

3.3 *FT-IR spectra analysis of polysaccharide*

The FT-IR spectrum of CZGY-1, CZGY-2, CZGY-3 (Figure 7–9) revealed a typical major broad stretching peak at 3600-3200 cm^{-1} for the hydroxyl group (O-H) and weak band at about 2900 cm^{-1} for the C-H stretching vibration. The absorption peak at 1600–1680 cm^{-1} was showed to contain Carboxyl group. The absorption peak at 1200–1000 cm^{-1} was the C-O-C and C-O-H. These were the absorption peaks of polysaccharides.

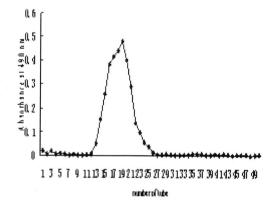

Figure 1.   Elution chromatogram of CZGY on DEAE-52-cellulose (for 0.1 M NaCl eluted).

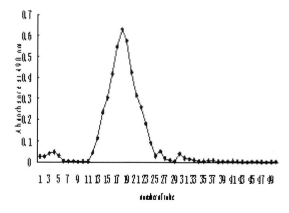

Figure 2.   Elution chromatogram of CZGY on DEAE-52-cellulose (for 0.2 M NaCl eluted).

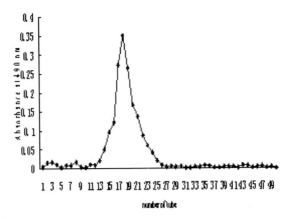

Figure 3.   Elution chromatogram of CZGY on DEAE-52-cellulose (for 0.4 M NaCl eluted).

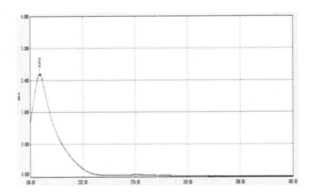

Figure 4.   UV scanning spectrum of CZGY-1 component.

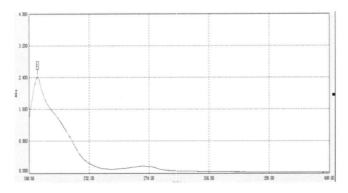

Figure 5.   UV scanning spectrum of CZGY-2 component.

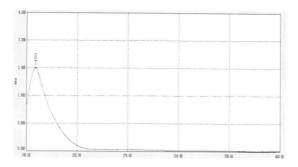

Figure 6.   UV scanning spectrum of CZGY-3 component.

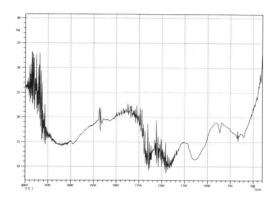

Figure 7.   Fourier transform infrared (FTIR) spectra of CZGY-1 with wave number.

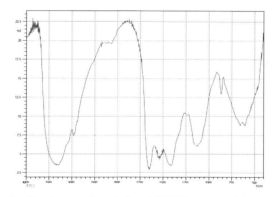

Figure 8.   Fourier transform infrared (FTIR) spectra of CZGY-2 with wave number.

In figure 9, the absorbance at 1730.15 cm^{-1} indicated the presence of carbonyl group, which showed to contain uronic acid. The polysaccharide was Acidic polysaccharides. The absorbance at 1606.70 cm^{-1} indicated the presence of amino group. This is consistent with the results of UV scanning of CZGY-3. The main absorptions of C-O and C=O stretching (1145.72 cm^{-1} and 1080.14 cm^{-1}) showed that the characteristics of sugar structures were pyranose configuration. The band at 864.11 cm^{-1} was ascribed to α-configuration in the CZYG-2 and CZGY-3 (J.W et al., 2011).

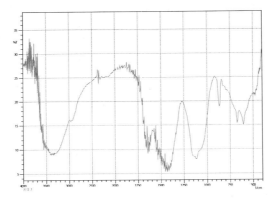

Figure 9. Fourier transform infrared (FTIR) spectra of CZGY-3 with wave number.

4 SUMMARY

The yield of polysaccharide, which was isolated from *Hypomesus olidus* using normal saline for extraction, the equivalence point to remove the protein and ethanol for deposition, was 3.65%. Polysaccharides obtained from the crude polysaccharide by DEAE-52-cellulose column chromatography showed different structures by FTIR. Our results indicated that the present extract seemed to be a good polysaccharide and could probably provide a basic reference for pharmacology research on new drugs and functional food.

ACKNOWLEDGEMENTS

This work was supported by the Key Project Science and Technology Department of Jilin Province (20130206061YY). The author is deeply grateful to Prof. Xunjun Liu for the support during the development of this scientific work.

REFERENCES

Chi, Z., Su, C.D., Lu, W.D.(2007). A new exopolysaccharide produced by marine Cyanothece sp. 113. Bioresour. Technol. 98, 1329–1332.

Dongru Wu,(1987)Carbohydrate biochemistry [M] Beijing: Higher Education Publishing.

Jiang B, Zhang HY, Liu CJ, et al.(2010) Extraction of water-soluble polysaccharide and the antioxidant activity from Ginkgo biloba leaves. Med Chem Res 19:262–70.

J.W. Li, L.P. Fan, S.D. Ding, Carbohydrate Polymers 83 (2011)477–482.

Kozarski M,Klaus A,Niksic M,et a1.(2011)Antioxidative and immunomodulating activities of polysaccharide extracts of the medicinal mushrooms Agaricus bisporus. Agaricus brasiliensis,Ganoderma lucidum and Phellinus linteus[J].Food Chemistry, 129(4):1667–1675.

Longxiang Zhang, Tingfang zhang, Lingyuan Li. Biochemical experimental methods and techniques [M] Beijing: Higher Education Publishing.6–9.

Mauro S G Pavao, Aiello K R M, Werneck C C, et al.. (1998)Highly sulfated dermat an sulfates from ascidiand:Structure versus anticoagulant activity of these glycosaminoglycans [J]. J BoilChem, 273(43):27848–27857.

Qingxiang Meng, Zhihui Liu, Meiyi Xu, et al.. (2004) Extraction and analysis of polysaccharides from Sargassum algae [J]. Spectroscopy and Spectral Analysis, 24 (12): 1560–1562.

Takaya Y,Uchisawa H,Matsue H,et al.(1994) An investigation of the antitum orpeptidoglycan fraction from Squid ink [J]. Biol Pharm Bull, 17(6):846–850.

Thomas D P.(1997)Does low molecular weight heparin cause less bleeding[J].Thromb Haemost,78:1422–1425.

Xuejun Liu,Dongjiao Wang.(2012)Experimental reseach on male fish anticoagulant. Food and Machinery. May, 28(3),21–23.

Yang W J, Pei F, Shi Y, et al.. (2012) Purification, characterization and anti-proliferation activity of polysac-charides from Flammulina velutpes [J].Carbohydrate Polymers,88(2):474–480.

Medicine Sciences and Bioengineering – Wang (Ed.)
© *2015 Taylor & Francis Group, London, ISBN: 978-1-138-02684-1*

Practice and reflection in the diagnostic bilingual teaching

Xing-xu Du
Affiliated Hospital of Beihua University, Jilin City, China

Wei-jing Sun & Chun-mei Wang*
College of Pharmacy, Beihua University, Jilin City, China

ABSTRACT: This paper discusses a practice in the diagnostic bilingual teaching and the reflection on it. The third-year clinical and nursing undergraduate students were selected as the objects of bilingual teaching, a method in which the traditional teaching method was combined with the modernized method that was used in the class, and the initial result was assessed. The results showed that the bilingual teaching could not significantly affect the learning of diagnostic specialized knowledge and most students should have a positive attitude to the learning of diagnostics with the bilingual teaching. It is believed that the bilingual teaching of diagnostics should be helpful in improving student's practical ability in the specialized foreign language to make them adapt the need in teaching, scientific research, and foreign exchange in the future, paraphrasing the same knowledge in a different thinking way and raising student's innovation ability. However, a considerable proportion of the students should be reluctant to be taught with the bilingual teaching. There are still some problems to be resolved due to the short practice.

1 INTRODUCTION

In "Certain Opinions on Strengthening Undergraduate Teaching Work in Higher Colleges and Universities to Improve the Quality of Teaching," a document of [2001]4, proposed by the National Ministry of Education in 2001, it was required that the teaching in English language and other foreign languages should be motivated positively. Since then, the bilingual teaching both in Chinese and English used in the teaching of undergraduate courses has become a tendency, and it has been believed that the bilingual teaching can perhaps become one of multistyle teaching methods. The aim of bilingual teaching is to put the higher education of our country in the background of economical globalization to reform and develop, set up an education platform with internationalization for students to enable them to have an opportunity to accept the advanced international education in discipline, and to be affected by the most advanced and outstanding things not only in knowledge and information but also in education idea and training mode in the world to cultivate them to become a new type of modernized talents. Since then, the bilingual teaching has entered a new stage and many scholars have conducted the research on the present situation, the mode, the question, the countermeasure, and so on in the bilingual teaching, but their viewpoints are conflicting, indicating that the bilingual teaching is still premature and in an exploration stage (Li Huixian, 2005, Han Qiu, 2009). The aim of this paper is to explore and establish the mode of the bilingual teaching in diagnostics, assess its effect and analyze its advantage and disadvantages to attempt to make it to meet the need of the undergraduate teaching in the discipline diagnostics.

*Miss Chunmei Wang is the corresponding author of this article, and her email address is 413437244@qq.com

2 TEACHING OBJECTS AND METHODS

2.1 *Teaching objects*

The third-year clinical and nursing undergraduate students were selected as the object of bilingual teaching. In the initial stage, the volunteer students from the identical grade were divided into bilingual teaching class (in both English and Chinese) and Chinese teaching class (only in Chinese) according to their desires; in the following stage, all students in the identical grade were taught in the bilingual language. Since 2005, there have been 515 clinical undergraduate students and 636 nursing undergraduate students taught in bilingual teaching in diagnostics.

2.2 *Recognizing and training of teacher qualifications*

At the beginning, teachers responsible for bilingual teaching in our university were selected and recognized by the experts of the university through inspecting their presentation in an interview in a way to give their lecture for 30 minutes. In the following stage, the teachers were determined by the experts in the department through various examining methods and the teacher had to be trained in the department through academic activities and teaching practices. Before the implementation of bilingual teaching, all teachers responsible for it had to be identified that they would have the ability to teach diagnostics not only in English and Chinese but also in their specialized knowledge. Fortunately, most teachers in our department were believed to be the qualified teachers and one of them was invited by the Teachers Training Center of Jilin Province to participate in the bilingual teaching symposium organized by the center, which provided an advantageous condition for the implementation of the bilingual teaching in our discipline.

2.3 *Teaching contents*

The teaching contents were determined according to the actual situation of our region and our university. The fundamental theories and skills described in Richard FL and Richard LD's Diagnostics as the main sources were selected. Simultaneously, more attention was paid to the introduction to different oversea thinking and learning ways.

2.4 *Teaching methods*

A method in which the traditional teaching method was combined with the modernized method was used in class. It included that the way of writing on the blackboard in English and speaking in English was taken as the primary method to avoid causing the students "not to remain" using course wares in a way to teach completely; most figures and tables were explained in a multimedia way to guarantee to give the students an enough amount of the information; the difficult and key points were introduced in Chinese as a auxiliary way, and the students were organized to discuss on them; the supplementary teaching materials were introduced to the students according to the teaching units further to widen their learning scope and the auxiliary network teaching was used.

2.5 *Assessment means*

The final written examination and the daily experimental result were unified to assess the students. The final examination paper was prepared by being written in English completely, the students were required to answer in English, and the result accounted for 80% of the final total score. The daily report was encouraged to be written in English, the performance of the student each time was evaluated to give the result and all experimental results accounted for 20% of final total score.

3 RESULTS

3.1 *Student performance appraisal*

The result showed that the average scores of students in the bilingual teaching class and Chinese teaching class were 75.6 ± 8.25 and 72.3 ± 7.36, respectively, and there was no significant difference between the two groups.

3.2 *Student questionnaire surveys*

The student questionnaire survey in 256 students showed that 83.7% students were interested in the learning of diagnostics with the bilingual teaching, the satisfied rate of the textbook was 82.8%, 87.0% students considered that the bilingual teaching could not influence the learning of specialized knowledge, and 98.8% students believed that the bilingual education could improve their English learning.

Although many colleges and universities have positively responded to the proposal of National Ministry of Education, and have started the bilingual teaching work widely since 2001, there have been many problems which remain to be solved, such as the teaching mode, teacher's training, teaching material selection, proportion of Chinese and English application, correct multimedia utilization, teaching content or amount in Chinese, setting questions by the end of terms and assessment means, and so on (Shi Yan, 2006, Xing Mengda, 2005, Zhang Mei, 2008). Especially, such a general college or university like ours is facing more challenge to the bilingual teaching. Therefore, the colleagues engaged in the teaching work should continue to work hard, accumulate experience, and conduct the long-term thorough research on the bilingual teaching to make it improved and meet the need in the undergraduate teaching.

We have been implementing repeatedly the diagnostic bilingual teaching for 7 years. During the practice, we have been trying to explore and establish an appropriate bilingual pattern for diagnostic teaching, assess effect, and inquire into its advantage and shortcoming to realize the goal of improving it.

4 DISCUSSION

The result showed that the average scores of students in the bilingual teaching class and Chinese teaching class were 75.6 ± 8.25 and 72.3 ± 7.36, respectively, and there was no significant difference between the two groups, indicating that the bilingual teaching could not significantly affect the learning of diagnostic specialized knowledge.

The student questionnaire survey in 256 students showed that 83.7% students were interested in the learning of diagnostics with the bilingual teaching, the satisfied rate of the textbook was 82.8%, 87.0% students considered that the bilingual teaching could not influence the learning of specialized knowledge, and 98.8% students believed that the bilingual teaching could improve their English learning. However, the students who were not interested in the bilingual teaching were 16.3%, who were not satisfied with the bilingual teaching material were 16.2%, and who thought that bilingual teaching could influence the learning of the specialized knowledge were 13%, demonstrating that a considerable proportion of the students should be reluctant to be taught with the bilingual teaching. What was found by us was similar to those reported by other scholars (Li Huixian, 2005, Shi Yan, 2006).

It is believed that the bilingual teaching of diagnostics should be helpful in improving student's practical ability in the specialized foreign language to make them adapt the need in teaching, scientific research, and foreign exchange in the future, paraphrasing the same knowledge in a different thinking way and raising student's innovation ability. However, there are no enough evidences to confirm the superiority of diagnostic bilingual teaching due to the short practice and other reasons.

On the contrary, there are still some problems to be resolved in the future, such as the teaching model, teaching material construction, students' interests, and specialized knowledge grasping.

5 CONCLUSIONS

The results indicate that the bilingual teaching could not significantly affect the learning of diagnostic specialized knowledge and most students should have a positive attitude to the learning of diagnostics with the bilingual teaching. It is believed that the bilingual teaching of diagnostics should be helpful in improving student's practical ability in the specialized foreign language to make them adapt the need in teaching, scientific research, and foreign exchange in the future, paraphrasing the same knowledge in a different thinking way and raising student's innovation ability. However, a considerable proportion of the students should be reluctant to be taught with the bilingual teaching. There are still some problems to be resolved in the future due to the short practice and other reasons.

REFERENCES

Li Huixian. (2005) *Journal Chinese Geological Education*, 3,118–119.
Han Qiu. (2009) *Journal Higher Education in China*, 19,37–38.
Shi Yan. (2006) *Journal of Chengdu University of Traditional Chinese Medicine: Educational Science Edition*, 6, 30–31.
Xing Mengda. (2005) *Journal Modern Education Science*, 2,74–75.
Zhang Mei. (2008) *Journal Researches in Education*, 11, 1173–1175.

Medicine Sciences and Bioengineering – Wang (Ed.)
© *2015 Taylor & Francis Group, London, ISBN: 978-1-138-02684-1*

Exploration of pharmacy graduation design quality assurance system

Jing-hui Sun[1], Guang-hong Wang & Guang-yu Xu[*]
Country College of Pharmacy, Beihua University, Jilin, Jilin, China

ABSTRACT: Graduation design is an important process in which undergraduate students can consolidate, comprehensively apply and practice the knowledge learned, and explore the knowledge in a new field. It can play a very important guiding role in the improvement of undergraduate overall capacity and quality training. In this study, 2014-class graduate students in our college were taken as the research subjects, and several survey methods such as the internship unit classification, the usual grade correlation analysis, and the questionnaire information feedback were used. Aiming at the problems of pharmacy graduation design quality in our college, the main research line of "the issues raised—analysis on the status quo study on the key questions—solution formation" was proposed by our research team. Finally, a relatively reasonable graduation design management system and a college–instructor–internship unit trinitarian graduation design management mode were established, which may provide a standardized guidance for the students to carry out the graduation design.

1   INTRODUCTION

Graduation design is the final link in the four-year undergraduate teaching in colleges and universities, a means to test the students' learning outcomes and comprehensive quality and an important content to evaluate the quality of teaching and efficiency in school management in colleges and universities (Zhang *et al.*, 2014). Therefore, it is necessary to explore the construction of a pharmacy graduate design pattern suitable for the current social situation and its quality assurance system, which should play a very important guiding role in improving the training of undergraduates' comprehensive capacity and quality, and has an urgent practical significance.

Although there have been some studies on graduate design, they are not suitable for the graduate design in our colleges and universities since there are significant differences in the content of graduation design, evaluation methods, and many other aspects between foreign countries and China (Boying *et al.*, 2012; He *et al.*, 2010). The domestic graduation design mainly takes its own profession as a starting point, rarely involving other professional fields, but foreign graduation designs pay more attention to the needs of the students and the selection of projects is primarily based on the students' interests, not restricted by their professions; in terms of quality assurance and evaluation, more attention is paid to the quantization, detail, and maneuverability of graduate design in our country, but more attention is paid to the students' self-perception and the evaluation of graduation units and colleagues. Overall, in our country, there are some exploratory studies on graduation design patterns and quality assurance, but mostly those on the common characters of graduation design and its management, and there is no relevant research on the pharmacy graduation design, especially on the pharmacy graduation design based on currently emergent new problems to our knowledge (Zeng, 2013; Luo et al., 2006). Through the survey and analysis of the current situation of pharmacy undergraduate graduation design in our college, the aim of our group was to establish a reasonable graduation design management system to provide a standardized guidance for the implementation of pharmacy students' graduation design.

---

[1] First Author: Jing-hui Sun, (1979-), E-mail: sunjinghui2008@126.com
[*] Corresponding Author: Guang-yu Xu, (1980-), E-mail: xuguangyu2005@163.com

2 INVESTIGATION OF THE CURRENT SITUATION OF GRADUATION DESIGN

2.1 Survey methods

2.1.1 Internship unit classification

The internship units where the graduates practiced from 2006 to 2013 were divided into six categories, such as pharmaceutical companies, drug inspection, drug development, clinical hospital, marketing company, and universities. Differences in the quality of thesis among the various categories of internship units were statistically analyzed to examine whether the differences in the quality of students' thesis would be caused by the difference in the internship units.

2.1.2 Usual grade correlation analysis

The correlation of quality of the students' thesis with the average of students' results on school days was analyzed to examine whether the graduation design would correlated with the usual grades.

2.1.3 Questionnaire information feedback

A questionnaire feedback method was applied. The questions included the difficulties encountered by graduates in internships, and views of graduates on the graduation design content and the internship units.

2.2 Survey results

The survey results showed that there was significant difference in the quality of graduation design among the various categories of internship units and no significant correlation between the usual grades and the quality of graduation design, indicating that the difference in thesis should be not caused by the division of students' internship units and the level of students' learning abilities. According to the survey results of the questionnaire, the students thought that the main reasons that could affect the quality of graduate design should be in three aspects as follows: (1) they rarely communicated with school teachers during the graduation practice so that they could not solve some problems in time when they faced them; (2) the learned theoretical knowledge was disjointed from the practical training and their internship was lack of theoretical guidance; (3) the school teachers responsible for the internship guidance could not give the students enough guidance because the students were far from the campus and the effective management of internship was insufficient. On the other hand, new problems arisen in the pharmacy graduation design also included the pressure from the severity of pharmacy graduate employment, the higher requirement of pharmacy practice, and other reasons. Most of the students out of the school could only finish their graduation design without the instruction of school teachers and those in the school had to run around looking for work or to participate in various trainings, which could result in less communication of them with the school teachers and bring some difficulties to the management of graduation design in college, severely impacting on the quality of pharmacy graduate design (thesis).

3 ESTABLISHMENT OF GRADUATION DESIGN MANAGEMENT SYSTEM

Based on the survey and analysis results, a corresponding graduation design management system was developed in our college.

3.1 Tutor's responsibility system

Based on the classification of students' graduation practice contents, the faculty was assigned to be responsible for the implementation of the tutor's responsibility system according to their majors. The graduation design of each graduate student was guided by a definite teacher in the school during the whole process to ensure the quality of all students' graduation design.

3.2 QQ groups and micro-letter group communication mechanism

With the support of QQ groups and micro-letter group, the communication mechanism of research instructors and students was established, involving information distribution, problem solution, data sharing, online review, online communication, and voice or video to hold the whole progress process of students' graduation design; a regular exchange interaction mechanism that QQ group and micro-letter group were taken as a link and the instructor was taken as a unit was established to solve the problems of graduation design in students, especially off-campus internship students, which could lay a foundation for the successful completion of graduation design work.

3.3 Graduation design management mode suitable for the current social situation

Because pharmacy is a subject with a strong experimental feature and the current employment situation is severe, it is necessary to study the establishment of a new management mode for the off-campus internship or training and the improvement of graduation management mechanisms in schools, and the construction of a reasonable graduation design management system, to provide a standardized guidance for the implementation of students' graduation design work. Due to the reasons described above, we tried to establish a graduation design management mode.

3.4 Construction of college–instructor–internship trinitarian graduation design management mode

To construct a college–instructor–internship trinitarian graduation design management mode, some attempts were made by us, including the perfection of graduation design workflow, the study on the guarantee mechanism of graduation design responsibility, process tracking and the information of whole process, the improvement of graduation design evaluation system, the coordination mechanism of college, instructor, and internship unit, and the exploration of quality guarantee system suitable for the features of pharmacy graduation design.

4 OPERATION OF GRADUATION DESIGN MANAGEMENT SYSTEM

The graduation design management system was used for the graduation design in 2014-grade students and evaluated the quality of graduation design, the evaluation internship units, and students' feedback. The results showed that "college–instructor–internship unit" tripartite coordination mechanism could effectively improve the quality of pharmacy graduation design, be well received by the students. The exchange interaction mechanism of instructors and students showed a good effect of questions and answers during the internship process, even beneficial to solving the students' psychological problems arisen during the transition from the school to the society to help them eliminate no sense of belonging during the internship.

5 PROSPECTS

Graduation design is an important link of practical teaching and a comprehensive reflection of higher education teaching quality. On the one hand, this study may guarantee the smooth implementation and the quality of graduation design (thesis), and on the other hand, improve the practical teaching system and quality of pharmacy professional training. Aiming at the problems of pharmacy graduation design quality in our college, the main research line of "the issues raised—analysis on the status quo study on the key questions—solution formation" was proposed by our research team. Finally, a relatively reasonable graduation design management system and a college–instructor–internship unit trinitarian graduation design management mode were established, which may provide a standardized guidance for the students to carry out the graduation design.

ACKNOWLEDGMENT

This research work was supported by research and teaching team of Beihua University (youth education project 2014035).

REFERENCES

Boying, G. Gregg, S. & Jon, T.N. (2012) Catalytic ring expansion of vinyl oxetanes: asymmetric synthesis of dihydropyrans using chiral counterion catalysis. *Angew. Chem., Int. Ed.* 124: 5773–5776.

He, W. Lu, L.H. Xin, C.Y. Cheng, S.K. & Sun, X.L. (2010) On how to improve graduation project of undergraduate pharmacy specialty. *Northwest Medical Education.* 18(1): 52–54.

Luo, X.H. Wu, C.F. & Bi, K.S. (2006) Establishment and implementation of the new practical teaching system for pharmaceutical specialities. *Pharmaceutical Education.* 22(5): 1–4.

Zeng, Q.B. (2013) Some thoughts on gradution project of pharmacy undergraduates. *Basic Medical Education.* 15(2): 160–162.

Zhang, B.L, Zhou, S.Y, Huan, M.L. & Cheng, Y. (2014) Research and practice of the graduation project for pharmacy specialty students. *Journal of Northwest Pharmaceutical.* 29 (2). 199–201.

Medicine Sciences and Bioengineering – Wang (Ed.)
© *2015 Taylor & Francis Group, London, ISBN: 978-1-138-02684-1*

Practice and reflection on the integration and optimization of general surgery teaching course system

Shu Jing
Affiliated Hospital of Beihua University, Jilin City, China

Wei-jing Sun
College of Pharmacy, Beihua University, Jilin City, China

Wei-hai Jiang*
Affiliated Hospital of Beihua University, Jilin City, China

ABSTRACT: At present, a prominent contradiction between the obvious reduction of teaching hour and the difficulty to guarantee the quality of medical teaching has brought us into a dilemma. The aim of this study is to deal with how to resolve the contradiction described above through integrating and optimizing the teaching course of general surgery teaching course system. The clinical medical undergraduates were selected as the investigation objects, the optimization of various teaching links was taken as the main line to carry on the practice of whole integration of general surgery course system, the feasibility of integration and optimization was evaluated by analyzing the teaching result. The integration and optimization of general surgery course teaching system may be a method to solve the problem, which would enhance the learning efficiency of students, improve their learning effect, save some time for the students to promote their multi-dimensional development and have more opportunity to choose what they like to do, and also enable the teachers to have more time to dedicate themselves to the scientific research and the teaching research. The study should provide a theoretical and practical basis for the next preparation of undergraduate student's training plan and syllabus.

1 INTRODUCTION

Higher education has its long history and always changes in its developing process. In different periods and different countries, the renovation of education idea and the reform of teaching method are eternal topics of higher education (Zhang *et al.*, 2010). Medical education also is so and always changes due to the development of society and the renewal of knowledge, and its traditional teaching system has been impacted by the trend of medical teaching reform. Many medical educators have made a great effort to reform the medical higher education to make it to meet the need of social development (Ma *et al.*, 2010). It is well known that the number of courses required for medical undergraduate students at present has increased greatly much more than that before, leading to a significant decrease in the teaching hour for each discipline. Therefore, a prominent contradiction between the obvious reduction of teaching hour and the difficulty to guarantee the quality of medical teaching has brought us into a dilemma in the medical higher education process (Zhao *et al.*, 2007). In this article, the aim is to deal with how to resolve the contradiction described above through integrating and optimizing the teaching pattern of general surgery teaching course system.

First Author: Shu Jing (1978-), E-mail: 10171812@qq.com
*Corresponding Author: Wei-hai Jiang (1979-), E-mail: 455066235@qq.com

2 INVESTIGATION OBJECTS AND METHODS

2.1 *Investigation objects*

150 Clinical medical undergraduates enrolled in the year of 2006 and 150 Clinical medical enrolled in the year of 2009 in our university were selected as the investigation objects. The 2006-grade students were taught using the traditional teaching method and the 2009-grade students were taught using the reformed method.

2.2 *Methods*

2.2.1 *The basis of the practice*
The cultivation aim established in the graduates' training plan and the teaching content written in the general surgery syllabus were taken as the basis to establish a basic and systemic knowledge point system which could be reasoned by analogy and did not limited only in the textbook.

2.2.2 *Transformation of the traditional teaching pattern to the reformed one*
The traditional teaching pattern and the reformed teaching pattern are shown in Figure 1 respectively.

2.2.3 *The integration and optimization process of general surgery teaching*
The implementation of this process needs the cooperation from the different departments of university besides the teachers and the students. To optimize the various general surgery teaching links was the principal line in this research which includes that ① according to the teaching units, the knowledge points in general surgery teaching theory and experiment were determined through fully discussing in a way of collective preparation by the teachers, in which the aim was to enable the students flexibly to grasp the elementary knowledge and basic skills of general surgery in a shorter period through learning the knowledge points; ② the traditional teaching method (the entire blackboard writing teaching) was reform to a new teaching method (the entire multimedia teaching) (Figure 1); ③ the paper was set up by taking the basic knowledge points as the key point; ④the analytical method of result analysis was the same as the former method.

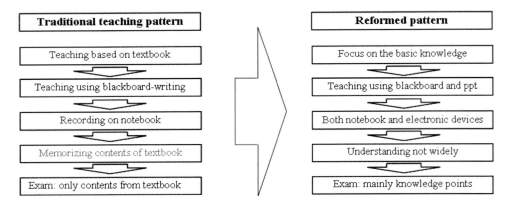

Figure 1.   Comparison of the two methods.

Table 1. Comparison of clinical medical students' scores before and after the integration and optimization.

Group	Average Scores
Before integration and optimization	78.59
After integration and optimization	71.38

3 RESULTS

3.1 *Comparison of clinical medical students' scores before and after the integration and optimization*

In this study, the clinical medical undergraduates were selected as the investigation objects, the optimization of various teaching links was taken as the main line to carry on the practice of whole integration of general surgery course system, the feasibility of integration and optimization was evaluated by analyzing the teaching result. The results are showed in Table 1.

4 DISCUSSION

In this study, the optimization of various teaching links was taken as the main line to carry on the practice of whole integration of general surgery course system, the feasibility of integration and optimization was evaluated by analyzing the teaching resultand the initial tentative plan was drawn up according to the summary of previous experiences to integrate and optimize the general surgery course system which would provide a theoretical and practical basis for the next preparation of undergraduate student's training plan and syllabus.

It is believed that the integration and optimization of general surgery teaching course could enhance the learning efficiency of students, improve their learning effect, which may solve the contradiction between the obvious reduction of teaching hour and the difficulty to guarantee the quality of medical teaching at present; it could save some time for the students to promote their multi-dimensional development and have more opportunity to choose what they like to do, and also enable the teachers to have more time to dedicate themselves to the scientific research and the teaching research. However, there are still some evidences to be confirrmed in the future because the practical time is not so long.

5 CONCLUSIONS

At present, a prominent contradiction between the obvious reduction of teaching hour and the difficulty to guarantee the quality of medical teaching has brought us into a dilemma. The integration and optimization of general surgery course teaching system may be a method to solve the problem, which would enhance the learning efficiency of students, improve their learning effect, save some time for the students to promote their multi-dimensional development and have more opportunity to choose what they like to do, and also enable the teachers to have more time to dedicate themselves to the scientific research and the teaching research. The study should provide a theoretical and practical basis for the next preparation of undergraduate student's training plan and syllabus.

REFERENCES

Ma, C.G. (2010) On training approaches and methods of college students' innovative ability. *Science and Technology Consulting Herald*, (09) 239–239.
Zhang, F.L. (2010) College students' innovative ability. *Theory Horizon*, (01), 179–180.
Zhao, Z.Ll. (2007) Discussion on relationship between research and teaching from university teaching level evaluation. *Technology and Innovation Management* (05) 62–63.

Medicine Sciences and Bioengineering – Wang (Ed.)
© 2015 Taylor & Francis Group, London, ISBN: 978-1-138-02684-1

Antibacterial property of silver nanoparticles with block copolymer shells

Xue-lian Li, Bing-guang Dai & Hong-xia Zhang*
The No.4 Hospital of Jinan, Jinan, People's Republic of China

Ran Wang, Shu-long Yuan & Xue Li*
School of Chemistry and Chemical Engineering, University of Jinan, Jinan, People's Republic of China

ABSTRACT: Silver nanoparticles (AgNPs) with the poly (2-vinyl pyridine)-*block*-poly (ethylene oxide) (P2VP-*b*-PEO) block copolymers shells was prepared by using UV irradiation method. The antibacterial activity of the prepared AgNPs was investigated. This kind of AgNPs exhibited excellent antimicrobial activity toward gram-negative Escherichia coli and Pseudomonas aeruginosa. The AgNPs with block copolymer shells may have potential for use as a long-term antibacterial agent.

1   INTRODUCTION

Silver nanoparticles (AgNPs) have been intensively investigated and widely used in consumer products such as textiles, personal care, and food storage containers for their potent antibacterial capacity (Dadosh, 2009, Xiu *et al.*, 2011). Recently, a number of studies of the antibacterial property of AgNPs have been reported. Xiu et al. demonstrated that AgNPs could kill E. coli by releasing Ag^+ ions from the oxidized surface (Xiu *et al.*, 2012). It was found that the antibacterial activity of nanosilver was dominated by Ag^+ ions when fine AgNPs (less than about 10 nm in average diameter) were employed that release high concentrations of Ag^+ ions. In contrast, when relatively larger AgNPs were used, the concentration of the released Ag^+ ions was lower (Sotiriou & Pratsinis, 2010). Song *et al.* reported the synthesis of silver/polyrhodaninecomposite-decorated silica nanoparticles and their antibacterial activity. The silver/polyrhodanine-nanocomposite-decorated silica nanoparticles exhibited excellent antimicrobial activity toward gram-negative Escherichia coli and gram-positive Staphylococcus aureus because of the antibacterial effects of the AgNPs and the polyrhodanine (Xiu *et al.*, 2011).

For applications, AgNPs must be stabilized by ligands or surfactants to prevent from their aggregation. Among the ligands or surfactants, polymer surfactants, which are stable in a variety of environments, including organic solvents and buffers, are attractive. Various block copolymers have been used for the synthesis of AgNPs (Zhang *et al.*, 2003, Wang *et al.*, 2008). We prepared pH-responsive AgNPs with P2VP-*b*-PEO shells by UV irradiation of the solutions of P2VP-b-PEO/AgNO$_3$ complexes (Yuan *et al.*, 2014). However, the effect of block copolymer shells on the antibacterial properties hasn't been investigated.

Here we first prepared water-soluble AgNPs with block copolymer shells by using diblock copolymer as protecting agent. Then the antibacterial property of the prepared AgNPs was investigated. To this end, P2VP-*b*-PEO and AgNO$_3$ precursors are dissolved together in water to make a solution of the PVP-*b*-PEO/AgNO$_3$ complexes, and the subsequent ultraviolet (UV) light irradiation led to the formation of AgNPs. The antibacterial performance of the resultant AgNPs were assayed by contacting with viable Gram-negative bacteria E. coli and Pseudomonas aeruginosa.

---

*Hong-xia Zhang and Xue Li, corresponding author.

2 EXPERIMENTAL

2.1 *Materials*

P2VP-*b*-PEO ($M_{w,P2VP}$ = 3000 g/mol, $M_{w,PEO}$ = 9000 g/mol, M_w/M_n = 1.06) were purchased from Polymer Source, Inc. Silver nitrate ($AgNO_3$) was purchased from Sinopharm Chemical Reagent Co., Ltd. 2,4-dihydroxy benzophenone (BPH, 99 %) was purchased from Alfa Aesar. Ultra pure water was used in all experiments. All chemicals were used as received without further purification.

2.2 *Sample preparation*

Given amounts of P2VP-*b*-PEO, AGNO₃ and BPH (2.0 wt% relative to P2VP-*b*-PEO block copolymers) were dissolved in water and stirred to make a homogeneous solution. The concentration of P2VP-*b*-PEO in water was 0.05 wt%. The molar ratio of $AgNO_3$/VP was changed from 0.1 to 1.0. The solution was irradiated with UV light for 14h in a reactor equipped with a 30 W lamp (Spectronics Co., USA) of wavelength 254 nm.

2.3 *Characterization*

UV-vis spectra of the prepared AgNPs were recorded on a TU1810 spectrometer (Beijing Purkinje General Instrument Co., China). Dilute solutions of the AgNPs were measured in quartz cuvettes, using pure solvent as a reference. Electron micrographs of the AgNPs were taken with an H-800 transmission electron microscope (Hitachi, Japan), operating at 100 kV. The samples were prepared by mounting a drop of the solutions on a carbon-coated Cu grid and allowing it to dry in air.

2.4 *Antibacterial activity of AgNPs*

Tripticaseine broth medium was used for growing and maintaining the bacterial cultures. A starter culture of each strain was inoculated with fresh colonies and incubated for 24 h in Tripticaseine medium. Then the fresh colonies were dispersed into saline to obtain 0.5 Maxwell unit (MU) microbial solution.

    0.1 ml of E. coli solution (0.5 MU) was added to the vials containing 1.0 ml, 2.0 ml and 3.0 ml AgNPs solution, respectively. After homogeneous mixing for 5 min, 0.2 ml of the above mixture was spread separately on the solid surface of the agar in Petri dishes. And then these discs were incubated at 37°C for 48 h in a bacterial incubator. As a control, a culture plate was inoculated without AgNPs solution. During all experiments with bacteria the material used was sterilized.

3 RESULTS AND DISCUSSION

3.1 *Preparation of AgNPs*

water is a selective solvent for the PEO blocks and a good solvent for $AgNO_3$. Complexation between Ag^+ and the pyridine units takes place when $AgNO_3$ is added to PVP-*b*-PEO solution. P2VP-*b*-PEO/Ag^+ complexes form micelles composed of P2VP/Ag^+ as a core and PEO as a corona. When a mixture solution of 0.05 wt% was irradiated with UV light for 14 h, the color of the solution turned from colorless to yellow, indicating the formation of AgNPs. Figure 1 is the UV-vis spectra of AgNPs. The UV–vis absorption band corresponding to the surface plasmon resonance (SPR) energy of the AgNPs is increased from 402 to 403, 426 and 430 nm when the molar ratio of Ag/VP changed from 0.1 to 0.3, 0.5 and 1.0, respectively. the results illustrate that the average diameter of AgNPs becomes larger when the molar ratio of Ag/VP was greater than 0.5. Figure 2 is the TEM images of AgNPs, the average diameter of the AgNPs calculated from the

TEM image is about 10.0 nm for Ag/VP =0.3 and 13 nm for Ag/VP=1.0. HRTEM image shown in Figure 2b illustrates that the AgNPs are covered by P2VP-b-PEO copolymer shells.

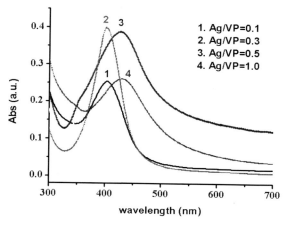

Figure 1.   UV-vis spectra of the obtained AgNPs.

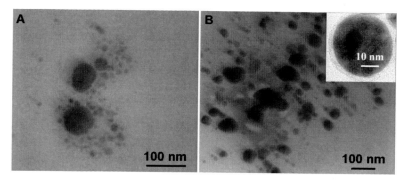

Figure 2.   TEM images of the AgNPs; (a) Ag/VP = 0.3, (b) Ag/VP = 1.0.

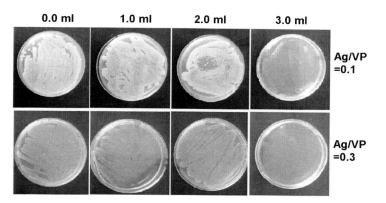

Figure 3.   Photographs of colonies of E. coli without AgNPs (0.0 ml) and with different content AgNPs (1.0, 2.0 and 3.0 ml).

3.2 Antibacterial activity of AGNPs

Antibacterium of AgNPs was assayed by contacting with viable Gram-negative bacteria E. coli. Figure 3 shows the digital photographs of agar plates incubated with bacteria for 48 h. Obviously, by addition of the produced AgNPs for 3.0 ml, nearly no colonies were developed on the plate incubated with bacteria, while the control plate was covered with significant bacterial colonies. The antibacterial assay with E. coli demonstrated that the AgNPs showed desirable antibacterial activity. When the molar ratio of Ag/VP is increased to 0.5 or more, the antibacterial activity is enhanced due to the increase of the Ag content (photographs not shown). The antibacterial activity of the AgNPs is attributed to silver ions. Recently, it was reported that the antibacterial activity of AgNPs depends not only on AgNPs also on the Ag^+ ions (Xiu et al., 2012). When Ag is exposed to oxygen, the surfaces are oxidized, and in aqueous solution the silver oxides are dissolved and Ag^+ ions are released (Sotiriou et al., 2012). The released Ag^+ ions can interact with negatively charged bacterial surfaces and induce cell death. When bacteria E. coli was replaced by Pseudomonas aeruginosa, similar results were obtained.

4 SUMMARY

AgNPs with PVP-b-PEO shells were prepared by UV irradiation of the solution of PVP-b-PEO/$AgNO_3$ complexes, and the average diameter of AgNPs increase with the increase of the molar ratio of Ag/VP. The obtained AgNPs with PVP-b-PEO shells exhibited antibacterial activity, which is enhanced with the increase of the molar ratio of Ag/VP. The antibacterial test on Pseudomonas aeruginosa, E. coli proved that AgNPs with block copolymer shells have a broad antibacterial property.

ACKNOWLEDGEMENTS

This work was funded by the National Natural Science Foundation of China (51173069) and Shandong Provincial Natural Science Foundation (ZR2010BM009).

REFERENCES

Dadosh, T. (2009) Synthesis of uniform silver nanoparticles with a controllable size. *Materials Letters*, 63(26), 2236–2238.

Sotiriou, G.A., Pratsinis, S.E. (2010) Antibacterial activity of nanosilver ions and particles. *Environ. Sci. Technol.*, 44, 5649–5654.

Sotiriou, G.A., Meyer, A., Knijnenburg, J.T.N., Panke, S., Pratsinis, S.E. (2012) Quantifying the origin of released Ag^+ ions from nanosilver. *Langmuir*, 28, 15929–15936.

Wang, H., Wang, X., Winnik, M.A., Manners, I. (2008) Redox-mediated synthesis and encapsulation of inorganic nanoparticles in shell-cross-Linked cylindrical polyferrocenylsilane block copolymer micelles. *Journal of the American Chemical Society*, 130(39), 12921–12930.

Xiu, Z.-M., Ma, J., Alvarez, P. J. J. (2011) Differential effect of common ligands and molecular oxygen on antimicrobial activity of silver nanoparticles versus silver ions. *Environ. Sci. Technol.*, 45, 9003–9008.

Xiu, Z., Zhang, Q., Puppala, H. L., Covin, V. L., Alvarez, P. J. J. (2012) Negligible particle-specific antibacterial activity of silver nanoparticles. *Nano Lett.*, 12, 4271–4275.

Yuan, S., Li, X., Zhang, X., Jia, Y. (2014) Fabrication of Au–Ag bimetallic nanostructures through the galvanic replacement reaction of block copolymer-stabilized Ag nanoparticles with $HAuCl_4$. *Science of Advanced Materials*, Available from: doi:10.1166/sam.2014.1909.

Zhang, L., Yu, J. C., Yip, H. Y., Li, Q., Kwong, K. W., Xu, A.-W., Po, K. W. (2003) Ambient light reduction strategy to synthesize silver nanoparticles and silver-coated TiO_2 with enhanced photocatalytic and bactericidal activities. *Langmuir*, 19(24), 10372–10380.

Medicine Sciences and Bioengineering – Wang (Ed.)
© *2015 Taylor & Francis Group, London, ISBN: 978-1-138-02684-1*

Effect of chiral *N*-isobutyryl-cysteine on PC12 cells response

Jing Mang, Jiao-qi Wang, Hong-yu Lui, Jin-ting He, Yan-kun Shao* & Zhong-xin Xu*
Department of Neurology, China-Japan Union Hospital, Jilin University, Changchun, Jilin Province, China

ABSTRACT: Surface property is a wide range of factors governing the biomaterial biocompatibility, which were taken into account seriously in the application of artificial implants. In the present research, the morphological changes of PC12 cells on N-isobutyryl-cysteine (NIBC) enantiomers modified gilded quartz plate were observed by laser scanning confocal microscope after MAP2 immunofluorescent staining. Results showed that cells on the L-NIBC modified surface extended more neurite-like branching, which confirms the differences of enantiomers in surface property.

1 INTRODUCTION

Surface properties such as surface topography, wettability, surface chemistry, and electrical surface charge could be pivotal for biomaterial biocompatibility by affecting the complex processes of cell adhesion, attachment and spreading onto biomaterials (Grinnell *et al*, 1972, Khorasani *et al*, 2005, and Khorasani *et al*, 2004). That determines the successful application of artificial implants and medical devices in body (Langer *et al*, 2004). Besides, recent studies have suggested that living systems including large numbers of biological macromolecules, show natural enantioselectivity due to chiral recognition (Maier *et al*, 2001). So chiral molecules applied on the surface of material could also play critical roles in biocompatibility (Hazen *et al*, 2003). N-isobutyryl-cysteine (NIBC) enantiomers, as one kind of the derivatives of cysteine, have been found to selectively recognize amino acids (Bückner *et al*, 1994). In this study, the attachment of PC12 cells on NIBC enantiomers modified gold surfaces has been studied by MAP2 staining and investigated by laser scanning confocal microscope. The results shown that cells planted on the L-NIBC modified gold surface extended more neurite-like branching than that on the D-NIBC modified gold surface.

2 EXPERIMENTAL

2.1 Cell culture

PC12 cells were cultured in high glucose DMEM medium with 10% (v/v) fetal bovine serum (FBS, GIBCO), 15% (v/v) horse serum (GIBCO) according to an instruction of the Cell Bank of the Chinese Academy of Sciences, at 37°C in a humidified atmosphere containing 5%CO2. They were passaged every 3–4 days with 0.25% trypsin (Sigma, New York, NY, USA).

*Author to whom correspondence should be addressed; Zhong-Xin Xu, E-Mail: xuzhongxin999@aliyun.com, Tel: +8613180802999 and Yan-Kun Shao, E-Mail: yankunshao@163.com

2.2 *The formation of chiral surface*

Quartz plate (D = 25.4 mm) gilded with gold were carefully washed with ultrasonic oscillator for 20 min before sterilized by autoclave treatment. Then the cleaned plates were immersed in filter sterilized N-isobutyryl-L(D)-cysteine (L- or D-NIBC, 0.02 mol/L diluted by 0.1M PBS), which were purchased from Sigma Chemical Co. (St. Louis, MO, USA). After 15 min at room temperature, the L- or D-NIBC modified chiral surfaces (L-/D-NIBC-Au) were obtained (Maier N.M. *et al*, 2001).

2.3 *Immunofluorescence*

Well growth PC12 cells were harvested and planted into 6-well plate with L- or D-NIBC modified plates in 1×10^{6}/ well. After 24 h, cells on the plates were washed with 0.01M PBS and fixed with 4% paraformaldehyde for 15 minutes. Then, they were treated with 0.3% Triton-100/PBS for 20 minutes, blocked in 2% BSA for 30 minutes at room temperature and incubated in rabbit anti-MAP2 (1:1,000; ab32454, Abcam) at 4°C overnight. Following washes, they were incubated in FITC marked goat anti-rabbit IgG (Boster, Wu Han, BA1032, China) for 1 h and stained with DAPI (1 μg/ml) for 15 minutes at 37°C avoiding light. After washes with PBS, they were dehydrated by 85%, 95% and 100% alcohol by turns and observed by laser scanning confocal microscope at 520 nm.

3 RESULTS AND DISCUSSION

Chiral recognition is one of the most fundamental characteristics of natural systems, which plays a critical role in understanding the surface properties and the interactions of biological molecules. Due to that natural enantioselectivity, chiral molecules provide a new clue in exploring biomaterial or artificial implant. In this work, the morphological changes of PC12 cells were observed by laser scanning confocal microscope after MAP2 staining. As shown in Fig.1, cells attached on L-NIBC modified gold partly extended neurite-like branching with an oblong nucleus, while those cells on D-NIBC were still round. Similar stereospecific interaction has also been found between immune cell and NIBC enantiomers, that D-NIBC modified gold can decrease the macrophage adhesion, while the L-NIBC has the opposite effect (Sun *et al*, 2007). These results suggest that L-NIBC modified surface has special biological effects in promoting cellular adhesion and tractility. Besides, studies showed that L-NIBC modified surface had stronger interaction with human serum albumin molecules than D-NIBC modified surface (Chen *et al*, 2012). Taken together, the surface chirality has great influence on the cell interactions and biocompatibility in artificial implant, which could provide new clue in the future study of biomaterial biocompatibility.

4 SUMMARY

In this study, we investigate the morphological changes of PC12 cells after 24 h of L-/D-NIBC-Au adhesion by laser scanning confocal microscope after MAP2 staining. Cells on the L-NIBC modified gold surface extended more neurite-like branching than that on the D-NIBC. Further study will focus on the mechanisms and applications of L-NIBC induced cellular responses, which may provide us a reference for surface properties and give us a new clue in the application of artificial implants.

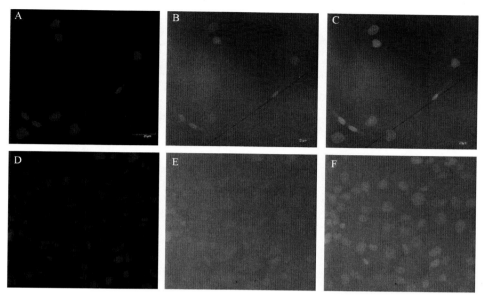

Figure 1. Cells on N-isobutyryl-L(D)-cysteine(NIBC) modified gilt quartz plate (a–c) PC12 cells on L-NIBC gold (d–f) PC12 cells on D-NIBC gold.

REFERENCES

Bückner H., Haasmann S., Langer M., et al. (1994) Liquid chromatographic determination of d- and l-amino acids by derivatization with o-phthaldialdehyde and chiral thiols: applications with reference to biosciences, J. Chromatogr. A 666: 259–273.

Chen Qiao, Zhou Juan, Han Qian, et al. (2012)The selective adsorption of human serum albumin on N-isobutyryl-cysteine enantiomers modified chiral surfaces.69:155–158

Grinnell F, Milam M, Srere PA. (1972) Studies on cell adhesion. II. Adhesion of cells to surfaces of diverse chemical composition and inhibition of adhesion by sulfhydryl binding reagents. Arch Biochem Biophys. 153(1):193–8.

Hazen R M, Sholl D S. (2003) Chiral selection on inorganic crystalline surfaces[J]. Nature Materials, 2(6): 367–374.

Khorasani M.T., Mirzadeh H. (2004) Colloid Surf B Biointerfaces. 35(1):67–71.

Khorasani M.T., Mirzadeh H., Kermani Z. (2005) Applied Surface Science. 242:339–345.

Langer R, Tirrell D A. (2004) Designing materials for biology and medicine[J]. Nature, 428(6982): 487–492.

Maier N.M., Franco P., Lindner W. (2001) Separation of enantiomers: needs, challenges, perspectives, J. Chromatogr. A 906: 30–33.

Sun T, Han D, Riehemann K, et al. (2007) Stereospecific interaction between immune cells and chiral surfaces. J Am Chem Soc. 129(6):1496–7.

Medicine Sciences and Bioengineering – Wang (Ed.)
© *2015 Taylor & Francis Group, London, ISBN: 978-1-138-02684-1*

Induction of Programmed Cell Death through mitochondria-dependent pathways in Tamba black soybean (*Glycine max*)

Jin-Jin Li, Lei Zhang, Jing-Jing Zhang, Ping Wang, Li-Mei Chen & Hong-Juan Nian*
Biotechnology Research Center, Kunming University of Science and Technology, Kunming, China

ABSTRACT: Programmed Cell Death (PCD) is not only essential for plant normal development and reproduction but also induced by various biotic or abiotic stresses. Many studies have suggested that aluminum (Al) induces PCD in plants. To investigate possible mechanisms of PCD, biochemical and physiological features of root tip cells of *Tamba* black soybean were examined after Al treatment. DAPI (4′, 6-diamidino-2-phenylindole) results showed a nucleus aggregation in the cell edge, displaying a semicircular shape. A burst of Reactive Oxygen Species (ROS) and increased mitochondrial malondialdehyde (MDA) content were observed in Al-treated soybean root tip cells. Mitochondrial membrane potential ($\Delta\Psi$m) was decreased in Al-treated cells when compared with control cells. These results suggest that mitochondrial MDA and ROS accumulation play important roles in Al-induced PCD.

1 INTRODUCTION

Programmed Cell Death (PCD) plays crucial roles in plant development and reproduction. PCD process is able to be triggered by different environmental stimuli (Darehshouri *et al.*, 2008; Efthimios *et al.*, 2010; Liu *et al.*, 2013; Moharikar *et al.*, 2006; Panda *et al.*, 2008). The main morphological and biochemical features of apoptosis in animals include membrane depolarization, release of cytochrome *c* (Cyt c) from mitochondria, increase activity of caspase-like proteases, and nuclear fragmentation by endonucleases. Animal-like PCD hallmarks were also found in plants undergoing stresses.

Aluminum (Al) is one of the major factors limiting crop productivity in acid soil. Recent researches have reported some apoptosis-like characters under Al treatment. Reactive oxygen species (ROS) burst and mitochondrial dysfunction are considered to be the crucial events in Al phytotoxicity (Boscolo *et al.*, 2003; Keith *et al.*, 1998; Panda *et al*, 2008; Yamamoto *et al.*, 2002; Yin *et al.*, 2010). Mitochondrial transmembrane potential (MTP) loss and mitochondrial swelling were subsequently induced by the ROS burst, and then caspase-3-like enzyme was activated which resulted in the execution of PCD (Li & Xing, 2010). Mitochondria and Cyt c play important roles in caspase activation and cell death in tobacco cells stressed by Al (Panda *et al*, 2008). However, whether and how Al induces the soybean root tip cell PCD are still not very clear. In this study, the aim was to evaluate how Al treatment affect soybean root tip cell survival by assessing several typical apoptosis features and whether mitochondria participate in Al stress–induced cell PCD.

---

*Nian Hong-Juan was Corresponding author. E-mail: hjnian@163.com

2 MATERIALS AND METHODS

2.1 Al stress treatments

The uniform growth of soybean seedlings were selected and pregrown overnight in a 0.5 mM $CaCl_2$ solution (pH 4.2) at 25° under constant light (100 $\mu mol \cdot m^{-2} \cdot s^{-1}$). Then, seedlings were transferred into a 0.5 mM $CaCl_2$ solution containing different concentrations of $AlCl_3$ (pH 4.2) for appropriate time. Seedlings grown in a 0.5 mM $CaCl_2$ solution without Al treatment were used as a control. Primary and lateral roots of soybean were then collected for further research.

2.2 Isolation of mitochondria

Isolation of mitochondria was done according to the method described previously (Tang, 2007).

2.3 DAPI (4', 6-diamidino-2-phenylindole) staining

The soybean root tip cells were stained using the KeyGEN cell apoptosis DAPI detection kit according to the manufacturer's instructions (KeyGEN, Nanjing, China). For each experiment 50 cells were analyzed per concentration and time point. Each experiment was performed three times in total.

2.4 Mitochondrial malondialdehyde (MDA) content assay

The MDA content was assayed with the thiobarbituric acid (TBA) method. In brief, 0.2 ml of mitochondria was added in 1 ml of 0.6% (w/v) TBA. The mixtures were incubated in a water bath at 100°C for 15 min with occasional shaking. The reaction was stopped by placing the reaction tubes into an ice bath. After centrifugation at 4,000 g (4°C) for 10 min, the absorbance of the supernatant was measured at 532 nm and 450 nm.

2.5 Detection of ROS production

Soybean root tip was treated with 0, 50, 100, 200 μM $AlCl_3$ for 46 h, then stained with 100 μM 2', 7'-dichlorofluorescin diacetate (H_2DCFDA) (Invitrogen, Eugene, USA) for 30 min at room temperature. The stained soybean root tips were observed in an epifluorescence microscope (LEICA DMR) using an excitation wavelength of 480 nm.

2.6 Measurement of mitochondrial membrane potential ($\Delta\Psi m$)

Measurement of $\Delta\Psi m$ was according to the method described previously (Fu et al., 2007).

3 RESULTS

3.1 Al stress–induced PCD

Chromatin condensation was analyzed by costaining cells with DAPI. Results of DAPI stain showed that the nuclear morphology of control cells (cells without Al treatment) was round and dyeing uniformity. Nuclear condensation was observed in Al-treated cells. Some of the nuclei of these cells were semicircular in shape. After 48 h treatment with 50 μM Al, some of soybean root tip cells appeared nuclear shrinkage and slight chromatin condensation were observed in all cells investigated. More and more cells undergo apoptosis with increase of concentration of Al. Most of the cells began to apoptosis after 200 μM Al treatment (Figure 1).

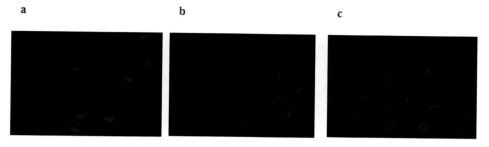

Figure 1. DAPI staining of soybean root tip cells exposed to different Al concentrations: 0 μM (a), 50 μM (b), and 200 μM (c).

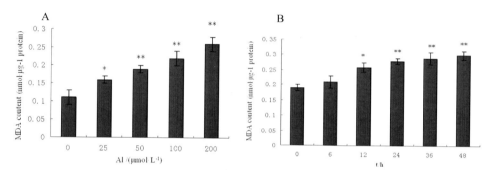

Figure 2. Mitochondrial MDA content of soybean root tip cells under Al stress.

Note: A: Soybean root tip cells treated with different concentrations of Al for 48 h; B: Soybean root tip cells treated with 50 μM Al for different times. Data are means of three replicates + SE; *indicates significantly different from the control ($P < 0.05$); **indicates highly significantly different from the control ($P < 0.01$).

3.2 *Mitochondrial MDA content increased after Al treatment*

MDA is a final product of lipid peroxidation. As shown in Figure 2, the mitochondrial MDA content of soybean root tip cells was raised with the increase of Al concentration. The content of MDA increased by 45.5% after 25 μM Al treatment and 136.4% after 200 μM Al treatment when compared with the control, which showing significant differences ($P < 0.05$) (Figure 2A). When 50 μM Al stress root tip cells, the content of mitochondrial MDA was elevated along with the increase of Al treatment time. MDA content of mitochondria compared with control rose 36.8% when treated for 12 h and rose 57.9% when treated for 24 h (Figure 2B). These results suggest that Al stress causes strong oxidative damage to membrane lipids of mitochondria.

3.3 *Al stress increased ROS production*

H$_2$DCFDA can move across cell membranes and is converted into a highly fluorescent compound after oxidation by ROS, most notably H$_2$O$_2$. To determine whether Al stress induced the production of ROS in soybean root tip cells, H$_2$DCFDA was used as a probe to monitor the intracellular ROS level. As shown in Figure 3, ROS levels increased significantly in a concentration-dependent manner during Al stress. Moreover, the higher the Al concentration, the more soybean root tip cells accumulated ROS.

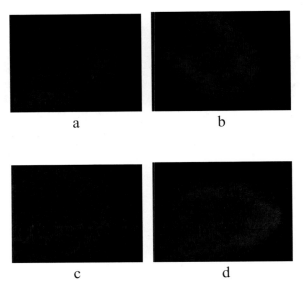

Figure 3. Intracellular reactive oxygen species (ROS) production of soybean root tip cells exposed to different Al concentrations: 0 μM (a), 50 μM (b), 100 μM (c), and 200 μM (d).

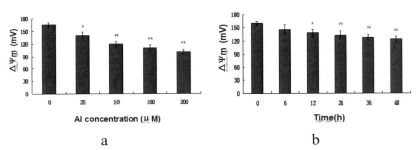

Figure 4. Mitochondrion membrane potential ($\Delta\Psi$m) of soybean root tip cells treated with 0, 25, 50, 100, 200 μM Al for 48 h (a) or treated with 50 μM Al for 0, 6, 12, 24, 36, 48 h (b). Data are means of three replicates + SE. *indicates that the value is significantly different from the control ($P < 0.05$). **indicates highly significantly different from the control ($P < 0.01$).

3.4 *Al stress led to decreased mitochondrial membrane potential ($\Delta\Psi$m)*

$\Delta\Psi$m is an important parameter for mitochondrial function and was measured using UV spectro-photometry method in this study. $\Delta\Psi$m decreased significantly when compared with the control after exposure to Al stress for 48 h. As shown in Figure 4, $\Delta\Psi$m of cells 48 h after treatment with 25 μM Al decreased 15.2%, while treatment with 200 μM Al reduced 39.4%, when compared to the controls (Figure 4a). Similar results were observed when cells were treated with 50 μM Al for different time. The longer the treatment time, the lower the $\Delta\Psi$m. As shown in Figure 4b, $\Delta\Psi$m of cells treated by Al for 12 h and 48 h were decreased 13.8% and 23.1%, respectively, when compared to the control level. However, mitochondria staining suggested that cells with a lower $\Delta\Psi$m maintained mitochondria membrane integrity (data not shown).

4 SUMMARY

Morphological and biochemical features of apoptosis in root tip cells of *Tamba* black soybean after Al stress were observed, including a nucleus aggregation, a burst of ROS, increased mitochondrial MDA, and decrease in $\Delta\Psi$m. These results help understand the physiological mechanisms of Al toxicity to plants.

ACKNOWLEDGMENT

This work was supported by the National Natural Science Foundation of China (31160020).

REFERENCES

Boscolo, P. R., Menossi, M., & Jorge, R. A. (2003) Aluminum Induced Oxidative Stress in Maize. *Phytochemistry*, 62: 181–189.

Darehshouri, A., Affenzeller, M., & Lütz-Meindl, U. (2008) Cell Death upon H_2O_2 Induction in the Unicellular Green Alga *Micrasterias*. *Plant Biol (Stuttg)*, 10: 732–745.

Efthimios, A., Andronis·Kalliopi, A., & Roubelakis-Angelakis, K. A. (2010) Short-term Salinity Stress in Tobacco Plants Leads to the Onset of Animal-like PCD Hallmarks in Planta in Contrast to Long-term Stress. *Planta*, 231: 437–448.

Fu, X. Y., Liu, X. K., & Yu, T. (2007) Effects of Pinacidil-induced Hyperpolarized Arrest on Myocardial Mitochondrial Injury during Ischemia-reperfusion in Rats. *Chinese Journal of Anesthesiology*, 10: 881–885 (In Chinese).

Keith, D. R., Eric, J. S., Yogesh, K. S., Keith, R. D., & Richard, C. G. (1998) Aluminum Induces Oxidative Stress Genes in *Arabidopsis thaliana*. *Plant Physiol*, 116: 409–18.

Li, Z., & Xing, D. (2010) Mechanistic Study of Mitochondria-dependent Programmed Cell Death Induced by Aluminum Phytotoxicity using Fluorescence Techniques. *J Exp Bot*, 62: 331–43.

Liu, D., Yang, J., Li, Y., Zhang, M., & Wang, L. (2013) Cd-induced Apoptosis through the Mitochondrial Pathway in the Hepatopancreas of the Freshwater Crab *Sinopotamon henanense*. *PLoS One*, 8, e68770.

Moharikar, S., D'Souza, J. S., Kulkarni, A. B., & Rao, B. J. (2006) Apoptoticlike Cell Death Pathway is Induced in Unicellular Chlorophyte *Chlamydomonas reinhardtii* (Chlorophyceae) Cells Following UV Irradiation: Detection and Functional Analyses. *J Phycol*, 42: 423–433.

Panda, S. K., Yamamoto, Y., Kondo, H., & Matsumoto, H. (2008) Mitochondrial Alterations Related to Programmed Cell Death in Tobacco Cells under Aluminum Stress. *C R Biol*, 2008, 311: 597–610.

Tang, C. D. (2007) A Simple Method for Extraction of Plant Mitochondria. *Journal of Guan Dong Industry Techincal College*, 6: 26–29 (In Chinese).

Tonshin, A. A., Saprunova, V. B., Solodovnikova, I. M., Bakeeva, L. E., & Yaguzhinsky, L. S. (2003) Functional Activity and Ultrastructure of Mitochondria Isolated from Myocardial Apoptotic Tissue. *Biochemistry (Moscow)*, 68: 875–881.

Yamamoto, Y., Kobayashi, Y., Rama, D. S., Sanae, R., & Matsumoto, H. (2002) Aluminum Toxicity is Associated with Mitochondrial Dysfunction and the Production of Reactive Oxygen Species in Plant Cells. *Plant Physiol*, 128: 63–72.

Yin, L. N., Mano, J. C., Wang, S. W., Tsuji, W., & Tanaka, K. (2010) The Involvement of Lipid Peroxide-derived Aldehydes in Aluminum Toxicity of Tobacco Roots. *Plant Physiol*, 152: 1406–17.

Zhang, J. T. (1998) *Method of Modern Pharmacology Experiment*. Beijing: Medical University.

Medicine Sciences and Bioengineering – Wang (Ed.)
© 2015 Taylor & Francis Group, London, ISBN: 978-1-138-02684-1

Considering geometric transformations in noninvasive ultrasonic measurement of arterial elasticity

LLi-li Niu, Ming Qian, Long Meng & Yang Xiao
Paul C. Lauterbur Research Center for Biomedical Imaging Shenzhen Institutes of Advanced Technology, Chinese Academy of Sciences Shenzhen, China

Xiao-wei Huang
School of Biomedical Engineering, Southern Medical University, Guangzhou, China

Hai-rong Zheng*
Paul C. Lauterbur Research Center for Biomedical Imaging Shenzhen Institutes of Advanced Technology, Chinese Academy of Sciences Shenzhen, China

ABSTRACT: Measurement of arterial elasticity has been proposed as one way to detect and evaluate early asymptomatic atherosclerosis. Conventional correlation-based methods for measuring arterial wall movements consider only the translation, ignoring the rotation and deformation, which limits the accuracy of measurement of arterial displacement and its biomechanical properties. This study presents a texture matching method based on ultrasonic B-mode image considering geometric transformations to accurately measure arterial displacement and acquire arterial elasticity noninvasively. Feasibility of the method was validated by in vitro arterial phantom made of polyvinyl alcohol cryogel. Results show that the elastic modulus of the arterial phantom agrees well with the results obtained from mechanical tests, deviating only 4.1%. The texture matching method was shown to be able to measure the displacement and elasticity of the arterial wall with complex geometric transformations and may have broad clinical applications for evaluating early stage atherosclerosis.

1   INTRODUCTION

The steady increase in the incidence of cerebrovascular and cardiovascular diseases mainly caused by atherosclerosis is becoming a more and more serious problem (J. Steinberger *et al.*, 2009). Therefore, it is crucial to diagnose atherosclerosis in the early stages. Clinical ultrasound examination mainly relies on changes in hemodynamics (C. Cheng *et al.*, 2006) and intima-media thickness (J. Polak *et al.*, 2010) to characterize plaque and stenosis for patients with overt symptoms, and routinely neglects arterial elasticity as an important diagnostic criterion. However, it is worth noting that changes in arterial elasticity may occur early in the atherosclerotic process, even before the anatomical changes of intima-media thickening become perceptible (R. Selzer *et al.*, 2001). Therefore, evaluation of arterial elasticity may serve as a valuable clinical tool for early detection and monitoring of atherosclerosis in individuals before the event of clinical symptoms.

Most conventional methods for non-invasive evaluation of arterial elasticity included using the Moens-Korteweg equation from measured pulse wave velocity (V. Marque *et al.*, 2000) and using local arterial stiffness from the change in geometric shape (S. Laurent *et al.*, 2006). However, the elasticity evaluated by these methods is only a single value for the whole arterial wall, which may not be sufficient for understanding of changes in the arterial wall.

This paper proposes a novel texture matching method to accurately measure the displacements of the arterial wall, thereby improving the measurement accuracy of arterial elasticity. The accuracy of the method to measure the displacements and elasticity of the arterial wall is demonstrated

---

*Author for Correspondence: ZHENG Hairong, Ph.D. Email: hr.zheng@siat.ac.cn

by an in vitro arterial phantom made of polyvinyl alcohol (PVA) cryogel, using a Sonix RP (10 MHz) ultrasound imaging system.

2 METHODS

2.1 The texture matching method

The procedure of the texture matching method is illustrated in Figure 1. Let $f^{(1)}(x,y), \ldots, f^{(N)}(x,y)$ denote a cineloop consisting of N images, where (x,y) correspond to the coordinates of a pixel in the image plane. In each image $f^{(n)}(x,y)$, a region of interest (ROI), $g^{(n)}(x,y)$, is selected. Each ROI is divided into a grid of small sections known as interrogation windows. Given an interrogation window in an image, matching consists in finding the most similar texture in the next image. The normalized cross-correlation (NCC) technique, which combines the sub-pixel method and the filter and interpolation method, is used to calculate the translational displacements of the texture of each interrogation window. Then, a multiple iterative algorithm uses the gradient of displacement to estimate rotation and deformation. Finally, the 2D normalized cross-correlation technique is applied with a reduced interrogation window to obtain higher spatial resolution, and a spurious vector elimination algorithm is used to obtain more accurate displacement estimates. A detailed description of these algorithms can be found in (L. Niu et al., 2010). The texture matching method starts when n = 1 and is repeated with the same ROI until n = N-1. The lateral and axial components of all displacement vectors are stored in 3D arrays, where the three dimensions are lateral and axial positions within an image and frame number.

From the estimated displacement, the elastic modulus, $E(x, y)$, is approximately given by H. Hasegawa et al. (2004):

$$E(x,y) = \frac{1}{2}\left(\frac{R_i}{h_0 \cdot L} + \frac{L-x+1}{L} \right) \frac{\Delta P}{\Delta \varepsilon_{max}(x,y)} \qquad (1)$$

where L and R_i are the number of layers and the inner radius of the artery, respectively. ΔP is pulse pressure measured at the brachial artery. $\Delta \varepsilon_{max}$ is the maximum strain of each layer during one cardiac cycle.

2.2 In vitro study for arterial phantom mode

A closed-loop compression system was designed to pressurize an artery phantom while simultaneously scanning with an ultrasound system (Sonix RP). The pulse pressure was generated by Harvard Apparatus® pulsatile pump (Model 55-3305). A pressure transducer was placed between

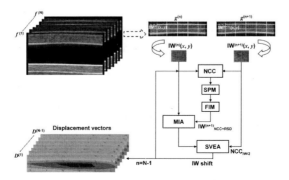

Figure 1.   Block diagram of the texture matching method.

the pump and the phantom to measure intraluminal pressure. The general schematic of the system is shown in Figure 2.

An aqueous solution of PVA undergoes a series of freeze-thaw cycles, and the final product is referred to as PVA cryogel. The number of freeze-thaw cycles controls properties of PVA cryogel, including speed of sound and elasticity. Manufacture of an arterial phantom using PVA cryogel was described by (J. Dineley *et al.*, 2006). An arterial PVA phantom (6 freeze-thaw cycles; Wall thickness: 3 mm; Inner radius: 3 mm) was placed in a water tank connected to the flow path filled with degassed water. Pulsatile flow which simulates the ventricular action of the heart was produced from the pump at a heart rate of 70 beats/min. A L14-5W/60 linear array transducer (10 MHz) was connected to the Sonix RP system to image the longitudinal section of the arterial PVA phantom. A sequence of 2D ultrasound B-mode images were acquired at a frame rate of 223 Hz using 128 ultrasound beams with a focal depth of 17 mm and field of view (FOV) of 30 mm (depth) by 32 mm (width).

3 RESULT

Figure 3(a) shows the B-mode image of the PVA phantom and the rectangle indicates the ROI. Figure 3(b) and (c) show the axial and lateral strain as a function of time. It can be seen that the axial and lateral strain profiles exhibit a periodic pattern, following the pulse cycle of 70 beats/min. The elastic modulus of the arterial PVA phantom was calculated as 343 kPa by Eq. (1). The elastic modulus of the PVA phantom was also tested on an electronic universal material testing machine (Model CMT6104) to validate the calculated elastic modulus using the texture matching method. Five cylindrical PVA samples were tested on the CMT6104. The mean elastic modulus of five samples is 328.8 kPa, suggesting that there is a difference of 4.1% between the calculated value and the measured value.

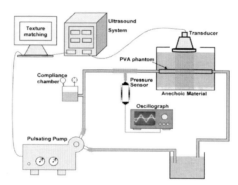

Figure 2.   General schematic of the in vitro phantom study.

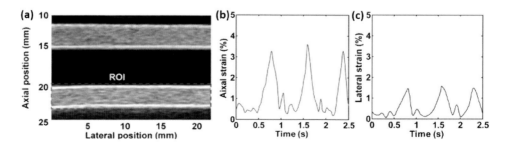

Figure 3.   (a) B-mode image of the arterial PVA phantom and the rectangle indicates the ROI; (b) axial strain and (c) lateral strain computed over the ROI of the PVA phantom as a function of time.

4   SUMMARY

A novel texture matching method based on B-mode image has been developed for accurately measurement of the displacements and elasticity of the arterial wall in this study. In this method, geometric transformations are considered to improve the measurement accuracy. The ability of the method has been demonstrated by an in vitro PVA phantom. The results show a difference of 4.1% between the calculated and measured value of the elastic modulus of the PVA phantom. The texture matching method may be appropriate for clinical studies and may offer a valuable tool for detecting changes in arterial elasticity and identifying patients with atherosclerosis at the early stage.

ACKNOWLEDGMENTS

The work was supported by National Research Program (973 Grant Nos. 2011CB707903 and 2013CB733800) from Ministry of Science and Technology, China, and National Science Foundation Grants (NSFC Grant Nos. 11325420, 11302239, 11304341, 61020106008, 11002152, 11272329, 61002001, and S2013040014610).

REFERENCES

C. Cheng, D. Tempel, R. van Haperen, A. van der Baan, F. Grosveld, M. Daemen, R. Krams, R. de Crom, (2006) Atherosclerotic lesion size and vulnerability are determined by patterns of fluid shear stress, Circulation, 113(23):2744–2753.

H. Hasegawa, H. Kanai, N. Hoshimiya, Y. Koiwa, (2004) Evaluating the regional elastic modulus of a cylindrical shell with nonuniform wall thickness, J Med Ultrasonics, 31(2): 81–90.

J. Dineley, S. Meagher, T. Poepping, W. McDicken, P. Hoskins, (2006) Design and characterisation of a wall motion phantom, Ultrasound Med Biol, 32(9):1349–1357.

J. Polak, S. Person, G. Wei, A. Godreau, D. Jacobs Jr, A. Harrington, S. Sidney, D. O'Leary, (2010) Segment-specific associations of carotid intima-media thickness with cardiovascular risk factors: the Coronary Artery Risk Development in Young Adults (CARDIA) Study, Stroke, 41(1): 9–15.

J. Steinberger, S. Daniels, R. Eckel, L. Hayman, R. Lustig, B. McCrindle, M. Mietus-Snyder, (2009) Progress and challenges in metabolic syndrome in children and adolescents, Circulation, 119(4): 628–647.

L. Niu, M. Qian, K. Wan, W. Yu, Q. Jin, T. Ling, S. Gao, H. Zheng, (2010) Ultrasonic particle image velocimetry for improved flow gradient imaging: algorithms, methodology and validation, Phys Med Biol, 55(7):2103–2120.

R. Selzer, W. Mack, P. Lee, H. Kwong-Fu, H. Hodis, (2001) Improved common carotid elasticity and intima-media thickness measurements from computer analysis of sequential ultrasound frames, Atherosclerosis, 154(1): 185–193.

S. Laurent, J. Cockcroft, L. Van Bortel, P. Boutouyrie, C. Giannattasio, D. Hayoz, B. Pannier, C. Vlachopoulos, I. Wilkinson, H. Struijker-Boudier, (2006) Expert consensus document on arterial stiffness: methodological issues and clinical applications, Eur Heart, 27(21):2588–2605.

V. Marque, H. Van Essen, H. Struijker-Boudier, J. Atkinson, I. Lartaud-Idjouadiene, (2000) Determination of aortic elastic modulus by pulse wave velocity and wall tracking in a rat model of aortic stiffness, J Vasc Res, 38(6):546–550.

Medicine Sciences and Bioengineering – Wang (Ed.)
© 2015 Taylor & Francis Group, London, ISBN: 978-1-138-02684-1

The improved mosaic algorithm for spine medical image based on the SUFR

Hui-min Liu*, Jun-hua Zhang & Jun-hui Gong
School of Information Science and Engineering, Yunnan University, Kunming, China

ABSTRACT: An improved Speeded-Up Robust Features (SURF) algorithm is proposed to accelerate the feature points' detection and improve the mosaic accuracy in the spine medical image mosaic. The algorithm comprises three steps: first, the Sobel operator is used to detect the edges to acquire the edge information of an image. Second, a large number of feature points are detected in the edge regions. Finally, images are spliced with the feature points obtained. Compared with the traditional SURF algorithm, the experimental results show that the precision and speed of splicing are improved by using the proposed method.

1 INTRODUCTION

Image mosaic is the technique that combines a number of pieces of overlap images into a seamless image. This technique is widely used in the fields of biomedical, aerospace, navigation, and 3D image reconstruction, especially in medical image field (Zitova & Flusser, 2003). Researchers have presented some image mosaic methods. Among them, the method based on the feature detection has achieved rapid development in recent years. It has the advantages of simple calculation and high precision. Lowe developed the Scale Invariant Feature Transform (SIFT) algorithm (Lowe, 1999). Mikolajczyk and others developed the Harris–Laplace and Hessian–Laplace algorithms (Mikolajczyk et al., 2001). These methods have the characteristics of scale invariance and robustness. The Speeded-Up Robust Features (SURF) algorithm was developed and improved by Herbert Bay (Herbert et al., 2006). It has a scale invariant in the extracting feature points and the advantages of partial invariance for illumination, affine, and perspective transformation. However, the speed is still slow and precision of calculation is low.

This paper extends the method based on the SURF algorithm and the structure of this paper is shown as follows: first, the SURF algorithm is introduced in Section 2. In Section 3, the improved method is described. It includes the Sobel edge detection and feature points replacement, as well as the image mosaic with new points. Finally, the conclusions and future works are given.

2 THE SURF ALGORITHM

The SURF algorithm is developed for the SIFT algorithm and it mainly includes feature points' detection, feature description, and feature matching.

2.1 *Feature points' detection*

Feature points' detection generally contains three steps: constructing the integral image, establishing the scale space, and obtaining locations of feature points.

---

*Hui-min Liu: Corresponding author, Email: tongxinlhm@163.com

2.1.1 Constructing the integral image

For a point $p(x, y)$ in the integral image, the size of the integral image is the area of starting from the origin to the point p. It is represented by the mathematical formula (Viola & Jones, 2001):

$$I_{\Sigma}(P) = \sum_{i=0}^{i<x} \sum_{j=0}^{j<y} I(i, j) \tag{1}$$

Where $I(i, j)$ is the pixel value of (i, j) in the original image and $I_{\Sigma}(p)$ is the corresponding coordinates. If the rectangular region is constituted by four points of A, B, C, and D, the gray value of the sum in the rectangular window is $\Sigma = A - B - C + D$.

2.1.2 Establishing the scale space

Establishing the scale space with the SURF algorithm is based on maintaining the original image size unchanged and filtering the original integral image by changing the box type filter. The SURF algorithm greatly improves efficiency of the algorithm by adopting the box type filter to approximate the Gaussian kernel function.

2.1.3 Obtaining locations of feature points

After establishing the scale space, the fast Hessian matrix is used to detect extreme points on each layer of the image scale space. Gaussian scale space is the only linear scale space, and the SURF algorithm approximate calculates the scale space of image with the Hessian matrix (Viola & Jones, 2001), as follows:

$$H((x, y), \sigma) = \begin{bmatrix} L_{xx}((x, y), \sigma) & L_{xy}((x, y), \sigma) \\ L_{yx}((x, y), \sigma) & L_{yy}((x, y), \sigma) \end{bmatrix} \tag{2}$$

Where L_{xx}, L_{xy}, L_{yy} are the results of convolution between the image points and the second-order partial derivatives $\dfrac{\partial^2 g(\sigma)}{\partial x^2}, \dfrac{\partial^2 g(\sigma)}{\partial y^2}, \dfrac{\partial^2 g(\sigma)}{\partial xy}$ of the Gauss filter. The definition of the 2-dimensional Gaussian function is $g(\sigma) = \dfrac{1}{2\pi\sigma^2} e^{-(x^2+y^2)/2\sigma^2}$.

For the Hessian matrix, when parameter σ is larger than a certain threshold, it enters into the next step. The SURF algorithm can get the images with different scales by changing the scale of the Gaussian kernel function. After the image scale space is established, the extremal point algorithm is used to detect feature points. Each pixel value is compared with surrounding six pixel points and eight pixel points in the vertically adjacent scale spaces and it is denoted as a feature point if its gray value is greater or smaller than the other pixel values.

2.2 Descriptor of feature points

The descriptor of feature points includes determining the main direction and generating descriptors.

2.2.1 Determining the main direction

The points are in the domain which is a circle with the center of the feature point and the radius of $6s$ (s as the feature point scale value) and calculated the Harr's wavelet transform. The transformation is in the X and Y directions with the square area of $4s \times 4s$ (Ping Sha & Luming Yang, 2006). The obtained responsive values are given a certain weight coefficient, according to their distance, and then the weighted responsive values are computed by histogram. It begins from the X axis and a new vector will be obtained by counting the Harr's wavelet response within a circular area of 60 degrees range.

The vectors are calculated with the same method every 5 degrees. Traversing the entire circular area can obtain 72 new vectors, and the main direction of the feature point is the direction of the longest vector.

2.2.2 Generating the descriptor

The detected feature point is treated as a center. The region of $20s \times 20s$ in the neighborhood is selected out. The main directions of the area are rotated to the direction of the main directions of feature points. To make the most use of spatial information of images, the region is divided into 4×4 subregions and each subregion is $5s \times 5s$. The feature point is described by counting the Harr's wavelet responsive value of pixels. In each subregion, each pixel is separately calculated by counting the Harr's wavelet responsive values in X and Y directions, which are denoted as d_x, d_y. Centering on the feature point, the d_x and d_y are weighted by the Gaussian function ($\sigma = 3.3s$). All values in the subregion are summed and they are denoted as Σd_x and Σd_y. The absolute value of area is respectively summed to reflect the Harr's wavelet responsive values changing in X and Y directions, which are $\Sigma|d_x|, \Sigma|d_y|$ in mathematical expression. For each region, four results of Σd_x, Σd_y, $\Sigma|d_x|$, $\Sigma|d_y|$ are used to establish a 3-dimensional feature vector:

$$S = (\Sigma d_x, \Sigma d_y, \Sigma|d_x|, \Sigma|d_y|) \tag{3}$$

Vectors in subregion are added to feature vectors to form a feature vector of 64 dimensions. Then, descriptors are normalized so that they have the advantages of brightness and scale invariance.

2.3 Feature matching

After feature descriptors is generated, initial judgment is made by the trace of the Hessian matrix to speed up registration. Then, two feature vectors are matched by the Euclidean distance.

2.3.1 The initial judgment by the Hessian matrix

In the process of feature point detection, the Hessian matrix trace is calculated. If the brightness of feature points and small neighborhood are brighter than that of the background area, the Hessian matrix trace is positive, otherwise it is negative. Two Hessian trajectories of feature points are compared. Two feature points have the same values if they have the same contrast. If the value is different, it indicates that the contrast of two different feature points is different and the similarity measures between the feature points are given up.

2.3.2 Euclidean distance of the similarity measure

A distance set can be got by calculating the Euclidean distance from the feature point to all feature points on the reference image. The minimum and the near-minimum Euclidean distance are obtained by comparing distance sets and a threshold is set (typically 0.7). When the ratio of the minimum Euclidean distance and the near-minimum Euclidean distance is less than the threshold, the feature point and the corresponding minimum Euclidean distance is matching, otherwise there are no matched points. The smaller threshold set, the less matched points, but registration more stable. The similarity measure between two feature descriptors is computed by the Euclidean distance:

$$D = \left[\sum_{k=0}^{k=n} (X_{ik} - X_{jk})^2 \right]^{1/2} \tag{4}$$

In the above equation, X_{ik} is represented the kth element of the feature descriptor i in the registered figure, and X_{jk} is the kth element of the j feature descriptor. The symbol n represents the dimension of the feature vector.

3 THE IMPROVED ALGORITHM

Characteristics extracted from the image have a great influence on image registration. Generally, good characteristics that can make mosaic images have the peculiarity of repeatability, uniqueness, and robustness.

The description of the feature point is counting the Harr's wavelet response of pixel values in the X and Y directions within the feature point's neighborhood. Gradient changes of point in image edge surrounding are relatively large that the detected feature points have better robustness and it can inhibit mismatching due to some information of the feature point is not obvious. Using the Euclidean distance to match feature points will produce mismatching, especially for images with noise. The mismatch images will have great effects on the following action. In this paper, firstly the feature points is extracted by detecting the edges of the image to get the peripheral areas of the image using the Sobel operator, then feature points are found in those area.

3.1 The Sobel edge detection

The edge is the pixel set that the pixel values in the image are sharply changing. The variation of brightness near the edge is so apparent that the point's gray level exceeds a certain value in the neighborhood can be regarded as an edge point. The center pixel is gray weighted by the Sobel operator in four directions. According to the maximum principle, the edge points are detected. This method not only can smooth the noises to get better detective results but also can provide more correct edge information. Usually, the operator (Harris and Stephens, 1988) is expressed by:

$$f_x'(x,y) = f(x-1,y+1) + 2f(x,y+1) + f(x+1,y+1) - f(x-1,y-1) - 2f(x,y-1) - f(x+1,y-1)$$

$$f_y'(x,y) = f(x-1,y-1) + 2f(x-1,y) + f(x-1,y+1) - f(x+1,y-1) - 2f(x+1,y) - f(x+1,y+1) \quad (5)$$

$$G(f(x,y)) = \left| f_x'(x,y) \right| + \left| f_y'(x,y) \right|$$

In the formulae (5), $f_x'(x,y)$ and $f_y'(x,y)$ are the first-order differentiation on the X and Y directions, $G(f(x,y))$ is the value of the gradient by the Sobel operator, and $f(x,y)$ is the total value of the coordinates of pixels for input images. Set a constant T, when $G(f(x,y)) > T$ edge points are marked and values of pixel are set to 0, otherwise 255. The T is properly adjusted to achieve the best result. The direction of gradient is given by:

$$\Theta = \arctan\left(\frac{f_x'(x,y)}{f_y'(x,y)} \right) \quad (6)$$

The Sobel operator is introduced in the average factor that can smooth random noise in images. Different segmentation in rows and columns can enhance edge pixels to make edge information more prominent.

3.2 Replacing feature points

Fewer points can be found by the original SURF algorithm so that images cannot be spliced and fused. More feature points and match points can be detected after applying the Sobel edge detection. What is more, those points mainly focus on the edge regions, which make the detection and mosaic process faster and more accurate.

However, the obtained images are binary images after the edge detection and splicing, which cannot display more specific information. For convenient observation and study, binary images should be recovered to the format that is the same of original images. Therefore, the improved method comprises following steps: first, original images are detected by the Sobel detection and spliced with the SURF algorithm. Second, the data of feature points and match points in above step are saved. Finally, original images are spliced with the SURF algorithm using the data obtained in the second step.

4 THE EXPERIMENTAL RESULTS

The results of the improved method are compared with the original SURF algorithm. All experiments use the Matlab 2012b software under the Win7 operating system. Figure 1(a) shows two divided and mosaic spine images, and images in the (b) is the results of images in (a) by the Sobel detection. The feature points and match points are found seeing in Figure 2. Figure 2 (c) shows that it can find the number of feature points are 120 and 146, respectively, then 32 match points. However, that of the numbers are 1436, 1152, and 297, in Figure 2 (d). Extracted feature points, namely match points, are used to registrant, given in Fig 3(e) and (f). Finally, the mosaic results with different methods are shown in Figure 4 (g) and (h), and they are compared with the original image (o):

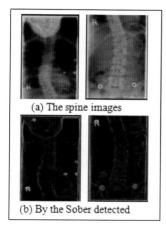

(a) The spine images

(b) By the Sober detected

Figure 1.   Mosaic images.

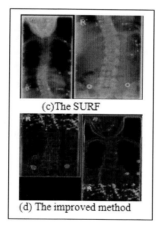

(c)The SURF

(d) The improved method

Figure 2.   Extracted feature points.

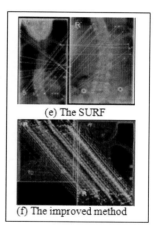

(e) The SURF

(f) The improved method

Figure 3.   Image registration.

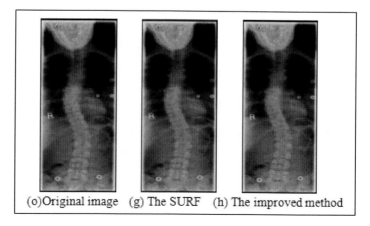

(o)Original image   (g) The SURF   (h) The improved method

Figure 4.   All results and the original image.

The SURF algorithm and the improved method of image mosaic are based on the SIFT algorithm. From figures above, the feature points after the Sobel edge detection mainly focus on edge areas that the experimental process for feature points are on the edge areas, too. So more feature points can be found easily and the overall splicing is faster and more accurate. While for some spine medicinal images with the SURF algorithm, fewer feature points can be detected so that images cannot be spliced and fused. And then many points can be found for mosaic images with the improved method.

Figure 5 shows feature points found with the two spine images by different methods. In the (a) with the SURF algorithm there exist 31 and 33 feature points respectively with only two match points, which are not enough for mosaic images. But enough feature points can be obtained by using the Sobel detection to get edge information before the SURF algorithm. As shown in the (b), the improved method, we can find the numbers of the feature points are 502 and 614 in the two images, then 71 match points. The results of the improved method for splicing and fusion with the same spine images are seen in Figure 6:

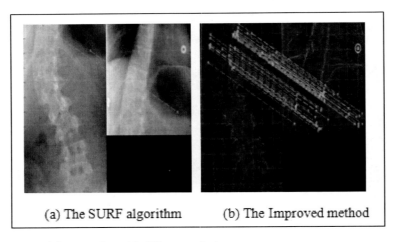

(a) The SURF algorithm   (b) The Improved method

Figure 5.   Extracted feature points with different methods.

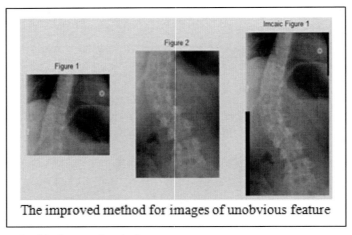

The improved method for images of unobvious feature

Figure 6.   The result of the improved method.

From results above, characteristics of mosaic images are not obvious that are not enough to match feature points and splicing by the SURF algorithm. However, the improved method makes the edge important information so outstanding that can find enough feature points for splicing. Moreover, this method not only realizes splicing but also achieves better results.

To further consolidate the reliability of the improved method, 9 points are chosen randomly and recorded in Figure 4 (o), (g), and (h). Table 1 shows their coordinates. The mark of No. represents different points. In Table 1, two points are randomly selected to get a distance among those 9 points and then the coordinate distance and the Mean Squared Error (MSE) of the two points are calculated in mosaic image of Figure 4. MSE1 shows the distances of the same corresponding points in Figures 4 (a) and (b). MSE2 is the results of different distances of the same corresponding points in (a) and (c). Among those results, the data of 22 groups are chosen and shown in Table 2. The Grope No. is the number of the group, and the Random points represent the distance of two different points, the two tables are as following:

Table 1. Different coordinates of the same points in different images.

No.	Coordinates in (o)	Coordinates in (g)	Coordinates in (h)
1	(171, 136)	(170, 135)	(171, 138)
2	(216, 337)	(215, 334)	(217, 337)
3	(359, 512)	(358, 508)	(359, 513)
4	(289, 513)	(288, 508)	(288, 513)
5	(91, 1066)	(90, 1061)	(90, 1065)
6	(299, 1053)	(298, 1048)	(298, 1054)
7	(357, 408)	(357, 404)	(358, 408)
8	(67, 664)	(67, 659)	(67, 664)
9	(38, 631)	(38, 626)	(38, 631)

Note: This will be used to introduce the random coordinates of the points in the Table 2.

Table 2. The MSE of different points' distance.

Grope No.	Random point	MSE1	MSE2	Grope No.	Random point	MSE1	MSE2
1	1-2	1.9036	1.4936	12	2-7	0.1008	0
2	1-3	6.3931	1.6000	13	2-8	2.4967	0.0864
3	1-6	7.8464	0.6365	14	2-9	2.4836	0.1347
4	1-7	1.8092	0.5839	15	3-8	0.3942	0
5	1-8	8.4782	1.9250	16	3-9	0.4403	0
6	1-9	8.4974	1.8648	17	4-8	0.3414	0.3414
7	2-3	1.1992	0.1980	18	4-9	0.4092	0.4092
8	2-4	1.7036	0.2867	19	5-7	0.1519	0.0151
9	2-5	1.9427	0.2077	20	6-8	0.1308	0.0608
10	2-6	1.9734	0.2935	21	6-9	0.1380	0.0533
11	8-9	0	0	22	7-8	0.2185	0.2814

As shown in Table 1 and Table 2, compared with the SURF algorithm, the MSE of the random two points' distance is smaller and more precise with the improved method. Therefore, the improved method is better than the traditional method.

5 CONCLUSION AND FUTURE WORK

A new method is proposed in this paper for the actual needs of image mosaic. It is based on the SURF algorithm, but images are detected by the Sobel edge detection before the SURF algorithm, which makes feature points focus on edge areas. The experimental results show that the improved method not only reduces the computing time but also improves the accuracy.

The method proposed in this paper is used for spine medical images without noise, and the result of the SURF algorithm for image mosaic with the change of perspective and brightness is not ideal. The next work will further study and improve current method, which can adaptively detect the perspectives and brightness changing and realize all kinds of splicing.

REFERENCES

Harris and Stephens. *A combined corner and edge detector* [J]. In Alvey Vision Conference, 1988, pp:147–152.

Herbert Bay, Ess A, Tuytelaars. *SURF: Speeded-Up Robust Features* [C]. GRAZ: The 9th European Conference on Computer Vision, 2006.

Herbert Bay, Ess A, Tuytelaars. *Speeded-Up Robust Features (SURF)* [J]. Computer Vision and Image Understanding, 2008, 110 (3), pp: 346–359.

Lowe D G. *Object recognition from local scale-invariant features* [C]. Los Alalllitos: The 7th IEEE International Conference on Computer Vision, 1999.

Lowe D G. *Distinctive image features from scale-invariant key points* [J]. International Journal of Computer Vision, 2004, 60(2), pp: 91–110.

Mikolajczyk K, Schmid C. *Indexing based on scale invariant interest points* [C]. Vancouver: The 8th IEEE International Conference on Computer Vision, 2001.

Ping Sha, Luming Yang. Yaorong Zeng. *The improved integral image algorithm of rotating type Haar features improvement* [J]. Computer Technology and Development, 2006(16).

Viola, Jones. *Rapid object detection using a boosted cascade of simple feature.* In: CVPR (1), 2001, pp: 511–518.

Zitova Barbara, Flusser Jan. Image Registration Methods: A Survey [J]. *Image and Vision Computing*, 2003, 21 (11), pp: 77–1000.

Medicine Sciences and Bioengineering – Wang (Ed.)
© 2015 Taylor & Francis Group, London, ISBN 978-1-138-02684-1

Interaction of IVIG and camptothecin

Yong-chun Liu*, Xiao-xia Wei & Xiu-ying Xu
College of Chemistry and Chemical Engineering, Qibo College of Medicine, Cooperative Innovation Center of Industrial Surfactant, Longdong University, Qingyang, Gansu, China

Xiao-jun Yao
College of Chemistry and Chemical Engineering, State Key Laboratory of Applied Organic Chemistry, Lanzhou University, Lanzhou, China

Rui-xia Lei, Xu-dong Zheng & Jian-ning Liu
College of Chemistry and Chemical Engineering, Qibo College of Medicine, Cooperative Innovation Center of Industrial Surfactant, Longdong University, Qingyang, Gansu, China

ABSTRACT: The interaction of camptothecin (CPT) with intravenous immunoglobulin (IVIG) was studied *in vitro* by fluorescence spectra, Fourier Transformation Infrared (FT-IR) spectra and molecular docking. The binding parameters calculated according to the Sips equation suggested that the binding of IVIG to CPT was a spontaneous entropy driven, non-specific and weak drug-protein interaction, characterized by two binding sites with the average affinity constant K_o of 9.683×10^3 L·mol^{-1} at pH 4.0 and 310 K. The contents of secondary structural composition of free IVIG and its CPT complex were calculated by FT-IR difference spectra, self-deconvolution, second derivative resolution enhancement and the curve-fitting procedure of amide I band, respectively. The observed spectral changes indicated a partial unfolding of the typical β structure of protein. Molecular docking was used to calculate the interaction mode between CPT with human IgG and the docking result of ΔG^o (-22.11 KJ·mol^{-1}) was consistent with that of Sips method. IVIG can serve as a transport protein (carrier) for CPT.

1   INTRODUCTION

In early 1980s, the mechanism of antitumor activity of camptothecin (CPT) was identified as inhibition of topoisomerase I (Top I) (Hsiang & Liu, 1988). Recently parts of CPT analogues have been registered for using in patients with cervical, ovarian, gastric, breast, skin, small cell or non-small cell lung cancer and melanoma in the USA, several Asian and European countries, and some are at the eve of registration (Herben *et al.*, 1998). Typical chemical features are the planar aromatic five-ring system with a lactone moiety and *S*-configuration at C-20. The chemically unstable *E*-ring lactone of CPT is conserved for all active derivatives and derivatives with more stable *E*-rings (21-*S*-lactam and 20-deoxy-camptothecin) are inactive (Herben *et al.*, 1998). This lactone moiety is chemically unstable and undergoes pH-dependent reversible hydrolysis to a hydroxyl carboxylate form, which is devoid of topoisomerase I inhibitory activity (Jaxel *et al.*, 1989). Under acidic conditions (pH < 4) the lactone structure predominates, whereas at pH values > 10 the open-ring form is exclusively present (Underberg *et al.*, 1990; Fassberg & Stella, 1992). *In vivo* the equilibrium also depends on the binding to albumin. However, the lactone levels for CPTs are lower at equilibriums either in PBS, HSA or in whole human blood conditions at pH 7.4 (Mi & Burke 1994). DNA topoisomerases are the targets of antimicrobial and anticancer drugs, and mammalian Top I is the selective target of CPTs (Kohn, 1996; Liu, 1989). Although CPTs have proven to be effective, drug resistance is still a critical clinical problem. Several groups have shown that ATP-binding cassette (ABC) proteins are involved in efflux and cellular resistance

---

*Corresponding author. E-mail: ychliu001@163.com

to CPTs in yeast and mammalian cells. The mechanism for multidrug resistance in these cells involves overexpression of the BCRP gene (also known as MXR, ABCP, or ABCG2), an ABC half-transporter, which is associated with high levels of resistance to a variety of anticancer agents, including anthracyclines, mitoxantrone, and the CPTs, by enhancing drug efflux (Mao, 2005). 5D3, a monoclonal antibody, can recognize this protein on the cell surface. In ABCG2-expressing cells 5D3 antibody showed a saturable labeling and inhibited ABCG2 transport and ATPase function (Özvegy-Laczka, et al., 2005).

Recently, great attention has been paid to IVIG potential use as adjuvant anti-neoplastic agent (Shoenfeld & Fishman, 2001; Phuphanich & Brock, 2007). Studies revealed that IVIG may stimulate the production of IL-12, enhanced NK cell activity, and can decrease the level of matrix metalloproteinase-9 (MMP-9) expression in the U937 monocyte line with a decrease in the m-RNA level of MMP-9, a vital step in the invasion of metastatic cancer cells. In addition, the commercial IVIG (IgG ≥ 95%, pH 4), containing 10^7 types of specific molecules of IgG and traces of IgM and IgA, has widely specific types of antibodies and presents natural and intact function of biology, which will present superiorities in binding to genetic variants of ABCG2 between interindividual or colony variability in drug response (Shen, 2001). By the formation of IVIG and CPTs at pH 4.0, especially the preparation of an intravenous anti-tumor aqueous emulsion of long-circulating IVIG nanoparticles containing CPTs (pH 4.0), IVIG will prospectively maintain the lactone moiety of CPTs, but also avoid being devoured by the reticuloendothelial system (RES) (Moghimi, et al., 2001).

In this study, the interaction of IVIG and CPT will be studied in vitro. It is anticipated that more complete understanding of IVIG interacting with CPT analogs will lead to the rational targeted drug therapy.

2 EXPERIMENTAL

2.1 Materials

Intravenous immunoglobulin (IVIG, Medical name: Lyophilized Human Immunoglobulin (pH 4) for Intravenous Injection, a component of IgG ≥ 95%) was obtained from Chengdu Rongsheng Pharmaceutical Co., Ltd., China. CPT (purity ≥ 98%) was obtained from Sichuan Ruibo Tech. Co., Ltd., China. Citric acid−Na_2HPO_4 buffers were selected to keep the pH of the solution at 4.0 or 7.4, respectively. CPT ($1.0 \, \text{mmol·L}^{-1}$) solution was prepared by dissolving CPT in DMF solution.

2.2 Methods

Fluorescence spectra were recorded using RF−7000 spectrofluorophotometer (Hitachi) with a 1 cm quartz cell. Both the excitation and emission bandwidths were 5 nm. The binding parameters were calculated by the data of fluorescent intensity and Sips procedure, which is based on the following equation (Liu et al., 2008):

$$\lg \frac{r}{n-r} = \alpha \lg c + \alpha \lg K_o \tag{1}$$

Quenching data were also analyzed according to Stern−Volmer equation, which could be used to determine the fluorescent quenching mechanism (Yang et al., 1994):

$$F_o/F = 1 + K_q \tau_o [Q] = 1 + K_{SV} [Q] \tag{2}$$

Based on the temperature dependence of the average affinity constant, thermodynamic parameters were calculated for CPT-IVIG binding by Gibbs-Helmholtz equation, and the free energy change ($\Delta G°$) was estimated from the following relationship:

$$\ln K_o = -\Delta H°/RT + \Delta S°/R \tag{3}$$

552

$$\Delta G^{\circ} = \Delta H^{\circ} - T \Delta S^{\circ} \tag{4}$$

FT-IR measurements were carried out at a constant room temperature (296 K) on a Nicolet Nexus 670 FTIR spectrometer (America) equipped with a Germanium attenuated total reflection (ATR) accessory, a DTGS KBr detector and a KBr beam splitter. Spectra processing conformed with the literatures (Dong *et al.*, 1990; Purcell *et al.*, 2000).

The structure of the drug was constructed with the Maestro (Maestro, 2009.) building tools. The build structure was then preprocessed by the LigPrep (LigPrep, 2009) which uses OPLS-2005 force field (Kaminski *et al.*, 2001) and gave the corresponding low energy 3D conformers of the drug. The ionized state was assigned by using Epik (Epik, 2009) at a target pH value of 7.0 ± 2.0. The 3D crystal structure of the human IgG for molecular docking was retrieved from the Protein Data Bank (PDB ID code 1AJ7) (Wedemayer et al., 1997). The drug was docked into the 5-(paranitrophenylphosphonate)-pentanoic acid binding site of the human IgG using the Glide (Glide, 2009) with the standard precision (SP) scoring mode.

3   RESULTS AND DISCUSSION

3.1   *Analysis of fluorescence quenching of IVIG by CPT*

When exited at 281 nm, pH 4.0 and 289 K, IVIG solution shows a characteristic emission maximum at 335 nm mainly due to its tryptophan (Trp) residues. The addition of CPT to IVIG solution causes a decrease in the emission at 335 nm with the binding of IVIG to CPT, while an increase in the emission at 432 nm is due to the inner structure of CPT as shown in Fig. 1. Additionally, a slight blue shift of the emission maximum wavelength of IVIG takes place in that the chromophores of protein may be placed in a more hydrophobic environment (Yuan *et al.*, 1998). Stern–Volmer dynamic quenching constant K_{SV} ($4.988 \sim 14.67 \times 10^3$ L·mol^{-1}) was calculated from the good linear relationship between F_o / F and the concentration of quencher $[Q]$, then K_q ($4.988 \sim 14.67 \times 10^{11}$ L·mol^{-1}·s^{-1}) was calculated when τ_o was taken as 10^{-8} (s^{-1}) (Yang *et al.*, 1994). The current value of K_q shown in Table 1 is much greater than that of the maximum $K_{q(max)}$ (2.0×10^{10} L·mol^{-1}·s^{-1}), indicating that there is indicative of a static type of quenching mechanism arisen from the formation of dark complex between the fluorophore and quenching agent.

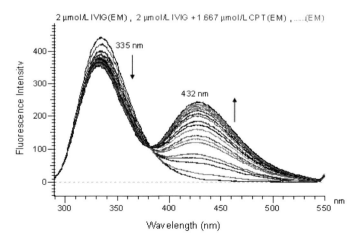

Figure 1.   Fluorescence spectra of IVIG binding to CPT at pH 4.0 and 289 K. The concentration of IVIG is 2.0 μmol·L−1. IVIG is titrated by successive addition of CPT solution to give a final concentration of 33.33 μmol·L−1.

The binding parameters for the IVIG-CPT interaction were estimated by Sips plots and data were summarized in Table 1. Sips plots displayed better linear correlations whether the number of binding sites (n) were taken as 2 or 4, and the affinity constants present $0.2636\sim9.683 \times 10^3$ L·mol^{-1} ($n = 2$) and $0.04152\sim5.341 \times 10^3$ L·mol^{-1} ($n = 4$), indicating that CPT are probably located in the regions of F(ab)$_2$ and Fc of IgG, and that the binding of IVIG to CPT is of non-specific and weak interaction with respect to the other strong ligand-protein complexes with the binding constants ranging from $10^6 \sim 10^8$ L·mol^{-1} (Ouameur, et al., 2005). However, the average affinity constants (K_o) are higher when $n = 2$ than those when $n = 4$, indicating that F(ab)$_2$ region appear stronger affinities than Fc region of IgG. Hence, the main binding sites of IgG to CPT are the CDRs of F(ab)$_2$. Moreover, the value of the affinity heterogeneity index (α) is closer to 1 (theoretic value) when $n = 2$ than those when $n = 4$, indicating that the difference of affinity heterogeneity between the F(ab)$_2$ region is slighter than that of Fc region, however, there may exist cooperative effects.

On the other hand, experiment of a fluorimetric titration at pH 7.4 was carried out as the same method of pH 4.0. It is found that the drug can quench the fluorescence of IVIG, however, both Sips method and Stern−Volmer equation are unfit to the system, in which the lactone and carboxylate moieties of CPT exist simultaneously and the binding modes may be different between lactone and carboxylate moieties with IVIG.

3.2   Binding mode

The thermodynamic parameters of IVIG binding to CPT at pH 4.0 were calculated from the linear relationship between lnK_o and the reciprocal absolute temperature and data were collected in Table 2.

There is a negative linear dependence of lnK_o on $1/T$ that is consistent with an endothermic molecular reaction. The binding of IVIG to CPT involves typical hydrophobic interaction (Liu et al., 2008) at pH 4.0 either $n = 2$ or $n = 4$. Moreover, the major contribution to ΔG° arises from ΔS° term, so the binding process is entropy driven. Furthermore, it is predicted that at pH 7.4 and with the shifting of lactone-carboxylate equilibria to the right, electrostatic interaction may play a role in the binding process.

Table 1.   Parameters of IVIG binding to CPT at pH 4.0.

Temperature /K	$K_o \times 10^3$ /L·mol^{-1}	α	$K_o \times 10^3$ /L·mol^{-1}	α	$K_{SV} \times 10^3$ /L·mol^{-1}	$K_q \times 10^{11}$ /L·mol^{-1}·s^{-1}
	$n = 2$		$n = 4$		$n = 2, n = 4$	
289	0.2636	0.4529	0.04152	0.4391	4.988	4.988
296	0.8933	0.5784	0.1968	0.5544	6.737	6.737
303	4.135	0.9097	1.645	0.8830	11.74	11.74
310	9.683	1.373	5.341	1.343	14.67	14.67

Table 2.   Thermodynamic parameters of interaction of IVIG and CPT at pH 4.0.

Temperature/K	ΔG° /KJ·mol^{-1}	ΔH° /KJ·mol^{-1}	ΔS° /J·mol^{-1}·K^{-1}	ΔG° /KJ·mol^{-1}	ΔH° /KJ·mol^{-1}	ΔS° /J·mol^{-1}·K^{-1}
	$n = 2$			$n = 4$		
289	−13.39			−8.953		
296	−16.72			−13.00		
303	−20.98	131.5	501.4	−18.66	177.8	645.9
310	−23.66			−22.12		

3.3 FT-IR spectra

The FT-IR spectra of the amide I band were carried out to investigate the change of secondary structure of the protein in the presence and in the absence of CPT. Fig. 2 shows the FT-IR spectra of free IVIG at pH 4.0 and 296 K, including the difference spectra, self-deconvolution, second derivative resolution enhancement (A) and the curve-fitting procedures (B) of amide I band (FT-IR spectra of IVIG after addition of CPT not shown). Then the contents of secondary structural composition of free IVIG and its CPT complex were estimated as shown in Table 3.

It is found that the contents of b—sheet composition of IVIG have decreased while the contents of remainders including α—helix and random coil increased after addition of CPT. Especially, the contents of β—sheet composition of IVIG have decreased to a little in the larger amount of addition of the drug. This indicates that the interaction of IVIG and CPT takes place and a partial unfolding of the typical β structure of protein does.

3.4 Molecular docking

Figure 3 shows the molecular docking plot of CPT and human IgG. As shown, the drug molecule is located in CDR of F(ab)$_2$ of IgG, closing to amino acid residues of Tyr-91, Tyr-94, Tyr-98, Tyr-99, Trp-103, and may exchange energy with transfer and quench the fluorescence of the chromophores of IVIG. Moreover, the docking result of ΔG° is -22.11 KJ·mol^{-1}, which is consistent with the result of Sips method.

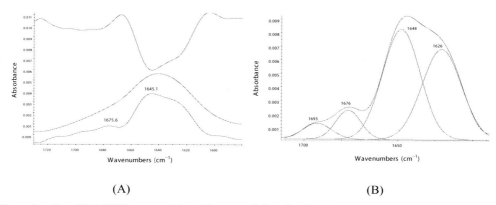

Figure 2.   Free IVIG FT-IR spectra (A) and the curve-fitting plot (B) of amide I band at pH 4.0 and 296 K.

Table 3.   Contents of secondary structural composition of IVIG and its CPT complex at 296 K. The concentration of IVIG is 2.0 μmol·L^{-1}.

Amide I components	pH 4.0			pH 7.4		
	IVIG	IVIG + 4.0 mol·L^{-1} CPT	IVIG + 8.0 μmol·L^{-1} CPT	IVIG	IVIG + 4.0 μmol·L^{-1} CPT	IVIG + 8.0 μmol·L^{-1} CPT
β—anti (%)	5.10	2.79	10.24	3.61	6.16	4.85
Turn (%)	8.28	13.72	3.46	24.88	3.68	10.46
β—sheet (%)	40.04	11.09	a little	39.49	23.73	a little
Remainders (%)	46.58	72.40	~86.30	32.04	66.43	~84.69

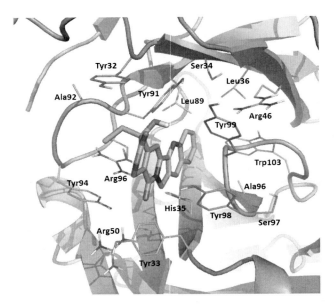

Figure 3.   Molecular docking plot of CPT and human IgG.

4   SUMMARY

The interaction of CPT with IVIG was studied *in vitro* by FT-IR spectra and molecular docking. The binding was spontaneous entropy driven, non-specific and weak drug–protein interaction with a partial unfolding of the typical β structure of protein. IVIG can serve as a transport protein (carrier) for CPT. Future research efforts will focus on achieving an intravenous anti-tumor aqueous emulsion of long-circulating IVIG nanoparticles containing CPT derivatives at pH 4.0, which will prospectively maintain not only the lactone moiety of CPTs, but also probably reverse cellular resistance to CPTs.

ACKNOWLEDGMENTS

This study was supported by Gansu Applied Chemistry Key Subject Fund (No. GSACKS20130113) and Longdong University Doctor Fund.

REFERENCES

Dong, A.C., Huang, P. & Caughey, W.S. (1990) Protein secondary structure in water from second-derivative amide I infrared spectra. *Biochemistry*, 29, 3303–3306.
Epik, version 2.0, Schrödinger, LLC, New York, NY, 2009.
Fassberg, J. & Stella, V.J. (1992) A kinetic and mechanistic study of the hydrolysis of camptothecin and some analogues. *J Pharm Sc*, 81, 676–684.
Glide, version 5.5, Schrödinger, LLC, New York, NY, 2009.
Herben, V.M.M., Ten Bokkel Huinink, W.W., Schellens, J.H. & Beijnen, J.H. (1998) Clinical pharmacokinetics of camptothecin topoisomerase I inhibitors. *Pharm World Sci*, 20(4), 161–172.
Hsiang, Y.H. & Liu, L.F. (1988) Identification of mammalian DNA topisomerase I as an intracellular target of the anticancer durg camptothecin. *Cancer Res*, 48, 1722–1726.

Jaxel, C., Kohn, K.W., Wani, M.C., Wall, M.E. & Pommier, Y. (1989) Structure-activity study of the actions of camptothecin derivatives on mammalian topoisomerase I. Evidence of a specific receptor site and for a relation to antitumor activity. *Cancer Res*, 49, 1465–1469.

Kaminski, G.A., Friesner, R.A., Tirado-Rives, J. & Jorgensen, W.L. (2001) Evaluation and reparametrization of the OPLS-AA force field for proteins via comparison with accurate quantumchemical calculations on peptides. *J Phys Chem B*, 105, 6474–6487.

Kohn, K.W. (1996) DNA filter elution: a window on DNA damage in mammalian cells. *Bioessays*, 18, 505–513.

LigPrep, version 2.3, Schrödinger, LLC, New York, NY, 2009.

Liu, L.F. (1989) DNA topoisomerase poisons as antitumor drug. *Annu Rev Biochem*, 58, 351–375.

Liu, Y.C., Yang, Z.Y., Du, J., Yao, X.J., Lei, R.X., Zheng, X.D., Liu, J.N., Hu, H.S. & Li, H. (2008) Interaction of curcumin with intravenous immunoglobulin: A fluorescence quenching and Fourier transformation infrared spectroscopy study. *Immunobiology*, 213, 651–661.

Maestro, version 9.0, Schrödinger, LLC, New York, NY, 2009.

Mao, Q.C. (2005) Role of the breast cancer resistance protein (ABCG2) in drug transport. *AAPS J*, 7, E118–E133.

Mi, Z. & Burke, T.G. (1994) Marked interspecies variations concerning the interactions of camptothecin with serum albumins: a frequency-domain fluorescence spectroscopic study. *Biochemistry*, 33, 12540–12545.

Moghimi, S.M., Hunter, A.C. & Murray, J.C. (2001) Long-circulating and target-specific nanoparticles: theory to practice. *Pharmacol Rev*, 53, 283–318.

Ouameur, A.A., Marty, R. & Tajmir-Riahi, H.A. (2005) Human Serum Albumin Complexes with Chlorophyll and Chlorophyllin. *Biopolymers*, 77, 129–136.

Özvegy-Laczka, C., Várady, G., Köblös, G., Ujhelly, O., Cervenak, J., Schuetz, J.D., Sorrentino, B.P., Koomen, G.J., Váradi, A., Német, K. & Sarkadi, B. (2005) Membrane Transport, Structure, Function, and Biogenesis. *J Biol Chem*, 280, 4219–4227.

Phuphanich, S. & Brock, C. (2007) Neurologic improvement after high-dose intravenous immunoglobulin therapy in patients with paraneoplastic cerebellar degeneration associated with anti-Purkinje cell antibody. *J Neurooncol*, 81, 67–69.

Purcell, M., Neault, J.F. & Tajimir-Riahi, H.A. (2000) Interaction of taxol with human serum albumin. *Biochimica et Biophysica Acta*, 1478, 61–68.

Shen, M.C. (2001) Pharmacological and immunological mechanism of the third generation IVIG. *Chin J Blood T Transfusion*, 14, 325–327.

Shoenfeld, Y., Levy, Y. & Fishman, P. (2001) Shrinkage of melanoma metastases following high dose intravenous immunoglobulin treatment. *Isr Med Ass J*, 3, 698–699.

Underberg, W.J.M., Goossen, R.M.J. & Smith, B.R. (1990) Equilibrium kinetics of the new experimental anti-tumor compound SK&F 104864-A in aqueous solution. *J Pharm Biomed Aanl*, 8, 681–6833.

Wedemayer, G.J., Patten, P.A., Wang, L.H., Schultz, P.G. & Stevens, R.C. (1997) Structural Insights into the Evolution of an Antibody Combining Site. *Science*, 276, 1665–1669.

Yang, M.M., Yang, P. & Zhang, L.W. (1994) Study on Interaction of Caffeic Acid Series Medicine and Albumin by Fluorescence Method. *Chinese Science Bulletin*, 9, 31–36.

Yuan, T., Weljie, A.M. & Vogel, H.J. (1998) Tryptophan fluorescence quenching by methionine and selenomethionine residues of calmodulin: orientation of peptide and protein binding. *Biochemistry*, 37, 3187–3195.

Medicine Sciences and Bioengineering – Wang (Ed.)
© *2015 Taylor & Francis Group, London, ISBN: 978-1-138-02684-1*

Reduction of dopamine increases methylglyoxal-induced mitochondrial dysfunction in SH-SY5Y cells

Bing-jie Xie, Fan-kai Lin, Kaleem Ullah, Lei Peng, Hong Qing & Yu-lin Deng*
School of Life Science and Technology, Beijing Institute of Technology, Beijing, China

ABSTRACT: As evidence for the roles of methylglyoxal in the development of diabetic neuropathy, oxidative stress and mitochondrial dysfunction play a key role in the mechanism of methylglyoxal-induced cell apoptosis. In this study, the results showed that dopamine can reduce the methylglyoxal-induced the oxidative stress and mitochondrial dysfunction in the SH-SY5Y cells. a-Methyl Tyrosine (MT) can inhibit the synthesis of dopamine, if SH-SY5Y cells was pre-incubated in the (MT), methylglyoxal-induced the oxidative stress and mitochondrial dysfunction was increased. One of PD symptoms is the reduction of the striatal DA content. In addition, the oxidative stress involving lipid peroxidation and mitochondrial dysfunction contributes to the pathogenesis of Parkinson's Disease (PD). The results give one suggestion that methylglyoxal could enhance the processing the PD.

1 INTRODUCTION

Parkinson's Disease (PD) is the most common neurodegenerative movement disorder produced in aged people. Several studies show that oxidative stress involving lipid peroxidation may contribute to the pathogenesis of PD (Yoshikawa, 1993). Recent studies have shown that diabetic patients with insulin resistant type 2 diabetes have a 23–180% increased risk for the development of PD (Hu *et al.*, 2007). In individuals with short duration older-onset diabetes without complications have increased PD risk 103–617% (Driver *et al.*, 2008). Methylglyoxal is known to be a toxic compound, and it is interesting that the toxicity of methylglyoxal is widely implicated in cell apoptosis. Diabetic neuropathy is a neurodegenerative condition comparable to Alzheimer's disease. It includes many physiological mechanisms such as mitochondrial dysfunction, abnormal protein aggregation and inflammation (Picklo *et al.*, 2002). Oxidative stress and mitochondrial dysfunction play a key role in the mechanism of methylglyoxal-induced cell apoptosis, which serves as an evidence for the roles of methylglyoxal and high glucose in the development of diabetic neuropathy (Di Loreto *et al.*, 2008). Both the mitochondrial dysfunction and oxidative stress, either by increased production of ROS or impairments in the mechanism for scavenging ROS, could contribute to cell death in PD (Dawson and Dawson, 2003). In our study, the result showed that methylglyoxal increased the lipid peroxidation caused by oxidative stress and decreased the mitochondrial membrane potential in the SH-SY5Y cells. a-methyl tyrosine (MT) is a tyrosine hydroxylase inhibitor, inhibited the synthesis of dopamine. In our study, we show that if the SH-SY5Y cells was pre-incubated in MT for 24 h, methylglyoxal-induced the oxidative stress and mitochondrial dysfunction was increased, it was decreased by adding the dopamine. Our result suggests that results give one suggestion that methylglyoxal could enhance the processing the PD.

2 MATERIALS AND METHODS

2.1 *Chemicals and substrates*

The following drugs and chemicals were used: Dulbecco's modified Eagle's medium (DMEM), trypsin-EDTA (GIBCO, Karlsruhe, Germany), fetal calf serum (Seromed, Berlin, Germany), CCCP, methylglyoxal, dopamine, MTT (Sigma), malondialdehyde (MDA) concentration assay kit, (Jiancheng, Nanjing), detection of mitochondrial membrane potential (JC-1) kit.

2.2 *Cell culture and cell viability assay*

SH-SY5Y was maintained in Dulbecco's modified Eagle's Medium (DMEM) supplemented with 10% fetal calf serum, penicillin/streptomycin (100 U/ml; 100 μg/ml), and 2 mM l-glutamine at 37 °C in a humidified atmosphere containing 5% CO2/95% air. Cell viability was determined by the MTT assays. Cells were seeded into 96-well culture plates (180 μl vol.) at a density of 1×10^4 cells. The cells were inoculated with different concentrations of the drug. After treatment, adding 20μL of MTT solution (5mg/mL) every hole, 37 ô incubation for 4 hours, and then, add 200μL DMSO, In the end, measured absorbance in 570 nm and calculated cell survival.

2.3 *Measurement of Mitochondrial Membrane Potential (MMP) and intracellular reactive oxygen species production assay*

Cells seeded in confocal confluence on a small dish. The MMP was assessed using JC-1 kit. Choose moderate cell density, staining a clear vision, collecting green and red fluorescence images at 488 nm and 514 nm excitation light. In one experiment, all green or red fluorescent image used the same conditions. The light intensity ratio of green/red represented the mitochondrial damage. The intracellular reactive oxygen species production was checked by the MDA concentration. MDA concentrations were measured by using the kit. For the preparation of sample, cells were collected by centrifugation, resuspended the cells in PBS containing protease inhibitor solution. Breaking cells 40 s using the sonication apparatus (2s on, 1s off), and then determined the protein concentration using the Bradford and concentrations of MDA.

2.4 *Statistics*

Fluorescence results are presented as a percentage of the fluorescence measured in untreated (control) cells. The data presented in this study are the mean (±S.D.) of 2–5 different experiments, performed in duplicate, triplicate, or quadruplicate. Statistical analysis of the results was carried out by Student's *t*-test (single comparison) or post hoc ANOVA (multiple comparisons). Statistical significance was established at a *p*-value <0.05 (*) or <0.01 (**), respectively.

3 RESULTS

3.1 *Effect of reduction of dopamine on cell viability in methylglyoxal-induced SH-SY5Y cells*

In our previous study, a-methyl tyrosine (MT), at a dose of 1 mM significantly reduced the synthesis of dopamine, and decreased the content of dopamine in the SH-SY5Y cells. After pre-incubated with a-methyl-tyrosine for 24 h and further 24 h in the presence of methylglyoxal (0-1 mM) SH-SY5 cells showed an increase of cell apoptosis (Figure 1). When the concentration of methylglyoxal increased up to 800 μM, the result showed significant differences.

3.2 Effect of dopamine on cell viability in methylglyoxal-induced SH-SY5Y cells

A-methyl tyrosine (MT) decreased the content of dopamine in the SH-SY5Y cells and increased methylglyoxal-induced cell apoptosis. So, in this study, cells were co-cultured with methylglyoxal and dopamine (100 μM) for 48h. Cytotoxicity of methylglyoxal was decreased with increasing content of dopamine.

3.3 Effect of dopamine on mitochondrial membrane potential in methylglyoxal-induced SH-SY5Y cells

The MMP was measured using (JC-1) kit. The result provides evidence that increased levels of methylglyoxal may seriously decrease the mitochondrial membrane potential (MMP) and affect mitochondrial function ($p < 0.05$, $n = 3$, Fig. 5.), and the Cells were pre-treated a-methyl-tyrosine, the MMP decreased 25% compared with methylglyoxal-induced SH-SY5Y cells. Cells were co-cultured with methylglyoxal (600 μM) and dopamine (100 μM), the MMP increased compared with methylglyoxal-induced SH-SY5Y cells.

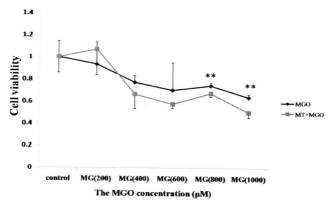

Figure 1. Effect of reduction of Dopamine on cell viability in methylglyoxal-induced SH-SY5Y cells. Cells were pre-incubated with 1 mM a-methyl-tyrosine for 24 h and further for 24h in the presence of methylglyoxal (0–1 mM).

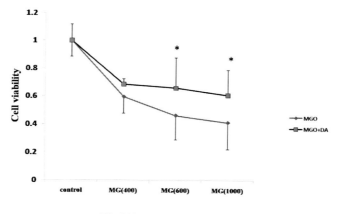

Figure 2. Effect of dopamine on cell viability in methylglyoxal-induced SH-SY5Y cells. Cells were co-cultured with dopamine (100 μM) and methylglyoxal(0–1 mM) for 48 h.

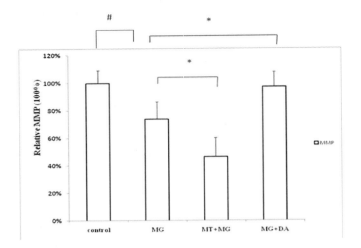

Figure 3. Effect of dopamine on mitochondrial membrane potential in methylglyoxal-induced SH-SY5Y cells.Cells were pre-treated a-methyl-tyrosine (1 mM) for 1 h and then exposed to methylglyoxal (600μM) for 24 h, and co-cultured with methylglyoxal (600 μM) and dopamine (100 μM) for 24 h.

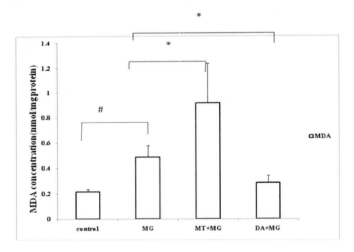

Figure 4. Effect of dopamine on ROS production in methylglyoxal-induced SH-SY5Y cells. Cells were pre-treated a-methyl-tyrosine (1 mM) for 1 h and then exposed to methylglyoxal (600 μM) for 24 h, and co-cultured with methylglyoxal (600μM) and dopamine (100 μM) for 24 h.

3.4 *Effect of dopamine on ROS production in methylglyoxal-induced SH-SY5Y cells*

MDA concentrations respond indirectly the level of oxidative stress. The result showed that Methylglyoxal can increase the level of intracellular oxidative stress to produce cytotoxicity, the cells were pre-treated a-methyl-tyrosine(1 mM) enhance methylglyoxal-induced oxidative stress in the SH-SY5Y cells were co-cultured with methylglyoxal (600 μM) and dopamine (100 μM), can reduce the MDA content in methylglyoxal-induced SH-SY5Y cells.

4 SUMMARY

In the diabetic patient's brain, the glucose metabolism become abnormal leading to more reactive carbonyl compounds such as methylglyoxal or glyoxal and unsaturated carbonyls such as hydroxynonenal or acrolein (de Arriba *et al.*, 2007). Protein structure and functions are modified due to MG which is a cytotoxic metabolite, and it modify tissue proteins through the maillard reaction resulting in advanced glycation end products (AGEs; Vlassara and Palace, 2002). The toxicity of methylglyoxal is widely implicated in cell apoptosis. But its function for increased risk of developing PD along with its role in dopamine neurons apoptosis in diabetic patients is unclear. According to other studies, it is found that lack of dopamine was one of the main causes of dopaminergic neurons degeneration and death. A-methyl tyrosine (MT) is a tyrosine hydroxylase inhibitor, inhibited the synthesis of dopamine. The result showed that if the SH-SY5Y cells were pre-incubated in the A-methyl tyrosine (MT) for 1 h, cytotoxicity of methylglyoxal will be increased and will be decreased by adding the dopamine. In this study, Cytotoxicity of methylglyoxal increased the formation of intracellular reactive oxygen species, decreases mitochondrial membrane potential, and caused the SH-SY5Y cell apoptosis. Our study suggests that the dopamine level was decreased, which increased the cytotoxicity of methylglyoxal. This study will be helpful to understand the diabetes risk in connection with PD and its increased occurrence. Our study first time tells the relationship between the diabetic and PD, give the advice that the reason of the diabetic - PD was due to the cytotoxicity of methylglyoxal.

REFERENCES

Dawson, T.M., and Dawson, V.L. (2003). Molecular pathways of neurodegeneration in Parkinson's disease. *Science,* 302 (5646), 819–822.

de Arriba, S.G., Stuchbury, G., Yarin, J., Burnell, J., Loske, C., and Munch, G. (2007). Methylglyoxal impairs glucose metabolism and leads to energy depletion in neuronal cells–protection by carbonyl scavengers. *Neurobiol Aging,* 28 (7), 1044–1050.

Di Loreto, S., Zimmitti, V., Sebastiani, P., Cervelli, C., Falone, S., and Amicarelli, F. (2008). Methylglyoxal causes strong weakening of detoxifying capacity and apoptotic cell death in rat hippocampal neurons. *The international journal of biochemistry & cell biology,* 40 (2), 245–257.

Driver, J.A., Smith, A., Buring, J.E., Gaziano, J.M., Kurth, T., and Logroscino, G. (2008). Prospective cohort study of type 2 diabetes and the risk of Parkinson's disease. *Diabetes Care,* 31, 2003–2005.

Hu, G., Jousilahti, P., Bidel, S., Antikainen, R., and Tuomilehto, J. (2007). Type 2 diabetes and the risk of Parkinson's disease. *Diabetes Care,* 30 (10), 842–847.

Picklo, M.J., Montine, T.J., Amarnath, V., and Neely, M.D. (2002). Carbonyl toxicology and Alzheimer's disease. *Toxicol Appl Pharmacol,* 184 (3), 187–197.

Vlassara, H., and Palace, M.R. (2002). Diabetes and advanced glycation endproducts. *Journal of internal medicine,* 251 (11), 87–101.

Yoshikawa, T. (1993). Free radicals and their scavengers in Parkinson's disease. *European neurology,* 33 Suppl 1, 60–68.

Medicine Sciences and Bioengineering – Wang (Ed.)
© *2015 Taylor & Francis Group, London, ISBN: 978-1-138-02684-1*

A sensitive determination of 1-acetyl-6,7-dihydroxyl-1,2,3,4-tetrahydroisoquinoline (ADTIQ) in rat substantia nigra by Multiple Reaction Monitoring (MRM)

Bing-jie Xie, Han-yan Wu, Kaleem Ullah, Lei Peng, Hong Qing & Yu-lin Deng*
School of Life Science and Technology, Beijing Institute of Technology, Beijing, China

ABSTRACT: It was considered that 1-acetyl-6,7-dihydroxyl-1,2,3,4-Tetrahydroisoquinoline (ADTIQ), and its precursor methylglyoxal were closely related to glucose metabolism. ADTIQ was similar in structure with catecholamine isoquinolines (CAIQs). Therefore, ADTIQ was thought to be related to diabetes and Parkinson's Disease (PD). The quantitation of ADTIQ in a biological sample could play an important role in detection of diabetic-PD. Herein, a sensitive and precise method was established to quantify ADTIQ by LC/MS/MS in Multiple Reaction Monitoring (MRM) mode. The [M + H] + precursor/ product ions were 208.1/190.1. The linear range of calibration curve was from 0.01–2 nM, and the lower limit of ADTIQ quantitation is 0.002 nM. Recoveries for biological sample were 137–162% with acceptable inter-day, intra-day precision and accuracy. Furthermore, the assay method was used for the determination of ADTIQ in rat substantia nigra.

1 INTRODUCTION

Parkinson's Disease (PD) is an age-related neurodegenerative disorder with a prevalence of 1–2% in people over 50 (Shastry, 2001). The prospective epidemiological studies have identified type 2 diabetes patients have a 23–180% increased risk for developing PD (Driver et al., 2008; Hu et al., 2007). 1-acetyl-6,7-dihydroxyl-1,2,3,4-Tetrahydroisoquinoline (ADTIQ), a dopamine (DA)-derived tetrahydroisoquinolines (TIQs), is a compound that could be a bridge between hyperglycemic and Parkinson's disease. ADTIQ was first discovered in frozen PD human brain tissues (Deng *et al.*, 2012), and the structure is similar to 1-methyl-4–phenyl -1, 2, 3, 6-tetrahydropyridine (MPTP). ADTIQ as a novel endogenous neurotoxins was considered to be related to Parkinson's disease (PD) (Deng *et al.*, 2012). Moreover, methylglyoxal as the precursor of ADTIQ was formed during glycolysis and has received considerable attention as a risk factor for diabetic complications (Lu *et al.*, 2011). Therefore, it seemed important and necessary to determine ADTIQ in vitro /in vivo, which might give hint for pathogenesis of diabetic-PD. There were kinds of methods for determination of catecholamine isoquinolines (CAIQs), including gas chromatography mass spectrometry (GC-MS), HPLC coupled with electrochemical detection (HPLC-ECD) (Wu *et al.*, 2011). However, these assay methods were limited due to their own drawbacks: Samples need to be aderivatized under GC-MS (Rojkovicova *et al.*, 2008). Measurement by HPLC-ECD was interfered by coeluting compounds in complex biological samples (Wang *et al.*, 2008). With respect to accuracy, simplicity and selectivity, a liquid chromatography electrospray ionization triple quadrupole (HPLC-ESI-QQQ) mass spectrometry assay was used to quantify ADTIQ level in rat substantia nigra, which has been applied in determination of salsolinol (Sal) and *N*-methylsalsolinol (NMSal). Multiple Reaction Monitoring (MRM) was one of high sensitivity, high accuracy and high reproducibility assay methods for complex biological samples[14]. As shown in Scheme 1, in the multiple-reaction-monitoring mode (MRM), where a precursor ion is fragmented in the second quadruple (Q2), and the resulting fragments are detected in the third quadruple (Q3). In the end, the ion-pair of precursor-product ion was used to measure the compound level. Pairs of precursor and product ions are selected in MRM, excluding a large number of interfering ions, which greatly reduce the background of interferent and significantly improve signal-to-noise ratio. Herein, the method of detection of ADTIQ using HPLC-MS/MS (MRM) was established, and this method was used to measure the level of ADTIQ in rat substantia nigra.

2 MATERIALS AND METHODS

2.1 *Chemicals and substrates*

ADTIQ was synthesized in our lab and molecular weight was detected by HPLC-MS. HPLC-grade formic acid and acetonitrile were purchased from Fisher Scientific Canada (Edmonton, Canada). Water was obtained from a Milli-Q Water Plus purification system (Bedford, MA, USA). All other chemicals and HS-F5column (3µm, 150 mm × 2.1 mm,) were from Sigma (St. Louis, MO, USA).

2.2 *Sample preparation and HPLC-ESI-MS/MS*

Sprague Dawley (SD) rats were obtained from the Experimental Animal Institute of the Medical Science Academy (Beijing, China), and animal experiments were performed in accordance with the guidelines. The brain substantia nigra tissues of rats ($n = 5$) were first homogenized in 5 mM PBS (Phosphate Buffer Solution, pH 7.4). And then the homogenate was added with 2 M perchloricacid (PCA) containing 10 mM sodium metabisulfite and 10 mM ethylene diamine tetra acetic acid (EDTA) at the ratio of 4:1(v/v), following with centrifugation at 17000g (gravity) for 20 min at 4°C, and the supernatant was removed through a Millipore HV filter (poresize 0.22 mm) before HPLC-MS/MS analysis. The sample was maintained at 4°C in a thermostatic autosampler. Detection of ADTIQ was under the Agilgent 1100 series HPLC combined with an electrospray ionization triple quadrupole mass spectrometer (Agilent 6460, USA). Samples were analysed on a Discovery® HS F5 (2.1 × 150 mm, 3 µm) column maintained at 30 °C. The mobile phase was composed of methanol–water (25/75 v/v) with 10 mM ammonium formate (NH_4COOH, pH 3.5) at a flow rate of 0.15 ml/min. The injection volume was 20 µl. The data were collected at the multiple-reaction-monitoring mode (MRM) mode. The $[M+H]^+$ precursor ions were used for isoproterenol (m/z 212.1) and ADTIQ (m/z 208.1). The product ions selected for the MRM scans were m/z 107.1 for isoproterenol (ISOP) and m/z 190.1 for ADTIQ.

2.3 *Preparation of standard curves and Quality Control (QC) samples*

The concentration with water and generate working solutions stored at −80°C. The internal standard (ISOP) was prepared at 100 nmol/mL and diluted to 10 nmol/mL with water during sample analysis. To prepare the standard curve, 90 µL of water were spiked with 10 µL of the internal standard solution (10 nmol/mL) and 10 µL of ADTIQ working solutions to generate calibration levels covering a range of 0.01–2 nM.

2.4 *Statistics*

The data were expressed as mean ± SD from at least three independent experiments with triplicate wells. Statistical significance was evaluated using t-test analysis. The differences were considered statistically significant at a p-value < 0.05 (*) or < 0.01 (**).

3 RESULTS

3.1 *Optimization of LC-ESI-QQQ conditions*

As the structure of ADTIQ is similar to Sal and NMSal, the chromatographic conditions optimized before were also used for ADTIQ. In addition, the $[M + H]^+$ precursor/ product ions pair (m/z 208.1/190.1) was chosen for ADTIQ as shown in Figure 1 in the MS/MS scan spectrum, which was the same with previous results. Moreover, fragmentor and collision energy for ADTIQ were set at 135V and 22eV, respectively, in order to gain relative high precise and sensitivity.

3.2 *Calibration Curve of HPLC-ESI-MS analysis for ADTIQ*

The linearity of ADTIQ was shown in Table 1. The regression analysis resulted in the equations $y = 2.53x + 0.27$ with the concentration of ADTIQ from 0.01 to 2 nM and correlation coefficient r values > 0.999, where y represents the ratio of ADTIQ peak area to that of isoproterenol and x represents the concentration of ADTIQ. The limit of detection (LOD) and limit of quantification (LOQ) was 0.002 nM and 0.01 nM, which were determined at signal-to-noise ratios (S/N) of 5 and 15, respectively.

3.3 *Precision and accuracy of HPLC-ESI-MS analysis for ADTIQ*

The stability of ADTIQ was performed for 3 days. Quality control (QC) samples with low, medium, and high concentrations of standard ADTIQ in water (pH = 7) were used to evaluate the accuracy and precision of the assay. Intra-day precision was demonstrated by the assay of three replicates on each of three concentrations of QC samples. Inter-day precision was assessed by the assay of six replicate QC samples on three different days by the same analyst and using the same equipment. The ADTIQ concentrations of QC samples were 0.01, 0.25 and 2 nM. As shown in Table 2, the intra-day precision ranged from 0.48% to 3.41% RSD, and the inter-day precision ranged from 4.91%, 2.79%, and 5.78% RSD. Meanwhile, the accuracy ranged from 96.7% to 97.2%. These results indicate that the method is accurate and precise, meeting the standards for biological sample. For recovery detection, QC samples were added to biological matrix which derived from the mixture of the substantia nigra of rats (n = 5). And the endogenous ADTIQ in biological matrix was determined first, which was subtracted from the quantity of ADTIQ in QC samples in order to eliminate endogenous interference to evaluate recovery. As shown in the Table 2, recoveries. For QC samples were 147%, 162% and 137%.

As shown in the Table 2, the recoveries of QC samples were 147%, 162% and 137%.

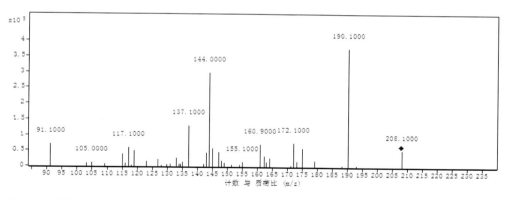

Figure 1.   MS/MS spectrum of the parent ion at m/z 208.1 of ADTIQ in positive mode

Table 1.   Calibration curve of ADTIQ

QC	Transition	Equation	Line Arrange	R^2	LOD	LOQ
ADTIQ	208.1/190.1	$y = 2.53x + 0.27$	0.01~2	0.9999	0.002	0.01

Table 2. Precision and accuracy of HPLC-ESI-QQQ analysis for ADTIQ

QC Sample	Accuracy (%)	Recoveries (%)	Intra-day precision (%)	Inter-day precision (%)
0.01	96.7	147	3.41	4.91
0.25	101.3	162	0.48	2.79
2	97.1	137	2.1	5.78

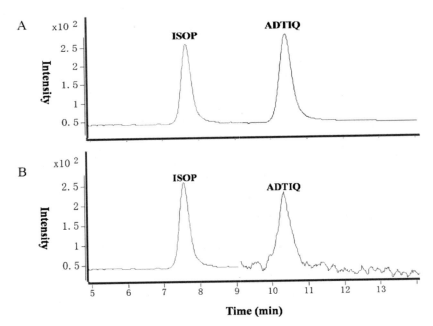

Figure 2. The extracted ion chromatograms of ADTIQ and ISOP. (A) Standard isoproterenol and ADTIQ (B) ADTIQ in rat substantia nigra.

3.4 Quantification of ADTIQ in substantia nigra

The assay method was applied for the determination of the amount of ADTIQ in rat substantia nigra ($n = 5$). As shown in Figure 2a, the standard ADTIQ and ISOP reached a baseline separation under the optimized chromatographic conditions, and endogenous ADTIQ in rat substantia nigra is shown in Figure 2b. The results show that the ADTIQ concentrations were 0.012 ± 0.009 nM/mg protein in rat substantia nigra.

4 SUMMARY

In conclusion, determination of ADTIQ by HPLC-ESI-QQQ with good precision, accuracy, and sensitivity was established, and the validated method was applied to quantify the amount of ADTIQ in rat substantia nigra. It may also be utilized to quantify ADTIQ in other biological samples in the future, could be helpful for disease diagnosis.

REFERENCES

Deng, Y., Zhang, Y., Li, Y., Xiao, S., Song, D., Qing, H., Li, Q., and Rajput, A.H. (2012). Occurrence and distribution of salsolinol-like compound, 1-acetyl-6,7-dihydroxy-1,2,3,4-tetrahydroisoquinoline (ADTIQ) in parkinsonian brains. *J Neural Transm,* 119 (4), 435–441.

Driver, J.A., Smith, A., Buring, J.E., Gaziano, J.M., Kurth, T., and Logroscino, G. (2008). Prospective cohort study of type 2 diabetes and the risk of Parkinson's disease. *Diabetes Care,* 31 (10), 2003–2005.

Hu, G., Jousilahti, P., Bidel, S., Antikainen, R., and Tuomilehto, J. (2007). Type 2 diabetes and the risk of Parkinson's disease. *Diabetes Care,* 30, 842–847.

Lu, J., Randell, E., Han, Y., Adeli, K., Krahn, J., and Meng, Q.H. (2011). Increased plasma methylglyoxal level, inflammation, and vascular endothelial dysfunction in diabetic nephropathy. *Clin Biochem.* 44 (4), 307–311.

Rojkovicova, T., Mechref, Y., Starkey, J.A., Wu, G., Bell, R.L., McBride, W.J., and Novotny, M.V. (2008). Quantitative chiral analysis of salsolinol in different brain regions of rats genetically predisposed to alcoholism. *J Chromatogr B Analyt Technol Biomed Life Sci,* 863 (2), 206–214.

Shastry, B.S. (2001). Parkinson disease: etiology, pathogenesis and future of gene therapy. *Neurosci Res,* 41 (1), 5–12.

Wang, R., Qing, H., Liu, X.Q., Zheng, X.L., and Deng, Y.L. (2008). Iron contributes to the formation of catechol isoquinolines and oxidative toxicity induced by overdose dopamine in dopaminergic SH-SY5Y cells. *Neurosci Bull,* 24 (3), 125–132.

Wu, H., Yuan, B., and Liu, Y.M. (2011). Chiral capillary electrophoresis-mass spectrometry of tetrahydroisoquinoline-derived neurotoxins: observation of complex stereoisomerism. *J Chromatogr A,* 1218 (20), 3118–3123.

Medicine Sciences and Bioengineering – Wang (Ed.)
© 2015 Taylor & Francis Group, London, ISBN: 978-1-138-02684-1

Effect of unitary, binary and ternary carboxylates on crystal phase selection in the process of calcium oxalate crystallization

Yu-bao Li, Qiong-zhi Gan & Jian-ming Ouyang[1]
Institute of Biomineralization and Lithiasis Research, Jinan University, Guangzhou, Guangdong, China

ABSTRACT: The effect of three kinds of carboxylates on formation of different crystal phases of calcium oxalate (CaOx) was comparatively studied in physiological saline and in artificial urine. These carboxylates were sodium glycinate (NaGlu, monocarboxylate), sodium tartrate (Na$_2$Tart, dicarboxylate), sodium citrate (Na$_3$Cit, tricarboxylate), respectively. In artificial urine, the percentage of the formed Calcium Oxalate Dehydrate (COD) increased with the increase of the number of carboxyl groups (–COOH) of carboxylate, and calcium phosphate and CaHPO$_4$·2H$_2$O were also formed. However, only Na$_2$Tart could induce the formation of Calcium Oxalate Trihydrate (COT) and COD in saline. The causes of formation of different crystal phases were discussed from the structures of carboxylates and the components of the system.

1 INTRODUCTION

As the most common component of urinary calculi, calcium oxalate (CaOx) included three hydrates: monoclinic monohydrate (COM), tetragonal dihydrate (COD) and triclinic trihydrate (COT). COM is the most stable phase in thermodynamics (Langdon *et al.*, 2009). Since there is difference of crystal phases and surface charge density among COM, COD and COT, the affinity of COM crystals to renal tubule cells was larger than that of COD and COT. Namely COD and COT are easily excreted from human body along with the urine compared with COM. Moreover, COT can be a precursor in CaOx stone formation (Bretherton *et al.*, 1998).

It was shown that the formation of COM, COD and COT was closely related to the concentration ratio of Ca^{2+} and Ox^{2-}, the coexisting ions, as well as the types and concentrations of inhibitors (Kirboğa *et al.*, 2009). For example, the presence of citrate, pyrophosphate, and metal ions can affect the nucleation and growth rates of different kinds of CaOx hydrates, finally affect their formation. Vieira *et al.* (Vieira *et al.*, 2004) studied the relationship between CaOx crystal morphology, crystal habit and [Ca^{2+}]/[Ox^{2-}] ratio as well as the relative supersaturation degree (*RS*) of CaOx solution. The results indicated that [Ca^{2+}]/[Ox^{2-}] ratio was a key factor to decide the morphology of crystals. When *RS* <10 and [Ca^{2+}]/[Ox^{2-}]<1, CaOx crystals were not found. When $10 \leq RS \leq 30$ and [Ca^{2+}]/[Ox^{2-}]>1, COM and COD were formed in the solution. When the initial concentration of CaOx solution was greater than 0.1 mol/L and [Ca^{2+}]/[Ox^{2-}] approached 1, COD was formed as a main crystal phase. When [Ca^{2+}]/[Ox^{2-}] was deviated from 1, COM was formed as a main crystal phase. When the initial concentration of CaOx solutions was much less than 0.01 mol/L, COT was formed (Ouyang *et al.*, 2005).

The addition of SiO$_2$ or sugar in CaOx crystallization system selectively promoted the formation of COT and COD, respectively (Yu *et al.*, 2004). At an initial CaOx concentration of 44 ppm, a mixture of hexagonal platelets of COM and needles of COT was formed. At an initial CaOx concentration of 130 ppm, COD was the major crystalline phase formed with small amounts of COM and COT crystals. Such transitions were attributed to adsorptive capabilities (Γ) of

---

[1]Corresponding authors. E-mail address: toyjm@jnu.edu.cn

polymeric molecules by three hydrate forms, which followed a sequence of $\Gamma(COM)> \Gamma(COT)> \Gamma(COD)$. Therefore, the polymeric molecules would be strongly adsorbed on the surface of COM, and then prevented the nucleation and growth of COM, making COD and COT stable in the solution. Khan *et al.* (Khan *et al.*, 1997) studied the crystal phases formed in CaOx solution with $RS = 10$ with or without COM seeds at 37°C in artificial urine by constant composition. The results show that a mixture of COM and COT crystals was produced without COM seeds in CaOx solution with $RS = 10$. Th ddition of COM seeds produced more COM crystals and a small amount of COT. In general, only single crystal phase was formed in a seed system. However, COT was formed in the system with COM as seeds. It was because the nucleation free energy (ΔG) of the COT was lower than that of COM. Moreover, in artificial urine with $RS = 10$, the overlap in the ΔG for heterogeneous nucleation of COM and COT phases leaded to the coexistence of COM with COT.

In this article, the effect of sodium glycinate (NaGlu), sodium tartrate (Na$_2$Tart) and sodium citrate (Na$_3$Cit) on formation of COM, COD and COT was studied in saline and artificial urine. The cause of the formation of different crystal phases was discussed from the structures of carboxylates and the components of system.

2 EXPERIMENTAL SECTION

2.1 *Reagents and apparatus*

Sodium glycinate (NaGlu), sodium tartrate (Na$_2$Tart), sodium citrate (Na$_3$Cit) and other reagents were all in analytical purity. X-ray diffraction (XRD) results were recorded on a D/max 2400 X-ray diffractometer (Rigaku, Japan). A Fourier-transform infrared (FT-IR) spectrometer (Nicolet Company, USA) was also used. The preparation of artificial urine: 0.106 mol/L NaCl, 0.064 mol/L KCl, 0.0032 mol/L NaH$_2$PO$_4$, 0.017 mol/L Na$_2$SO$_4$, 0.0038 mol/L MgSO$_4$, 0.0032 mol/L Na$_3$Cit. The pH of the solution was adjusted to 6.0 with 0.5 mol/L trihydroxymethyl aminomethane (Tris).

2.2 *XRD detection and quantitative calculation of COM, COD, and COT*

CaOx supersaturated solution with the initial concentration of 0.8 mmol/L was prepared in saline and artificial urine. After different carboxylates (NaGlu, Na$_2$Tart and Na$_3$Cit) was respectively added, these solutions were placed into 6-well culture plates with clean 12 mm × 12 mm hydrophilic quartz substrates at the bottom. After crystallization for 1 h, the quartz substrates were taken out and washed by distilled water and dried in a vacuum desiccator for 24 h, then these substrates were characterized by means of XRD and FT-IR. The percentage of COM, COD and COT was quantitatively calculated according to the literature (Lacmann *et al.*, 1999). For example, the percentage of COM was calculated as follows: $COM\% = \dfrac{I_{COM}}{I_{COM} + I_{COD} + I_{COT}}$, where I_{COM}, I_{COD} and I_{COT} were corresponding to the intensity of the strongest diffraction peak of COM, COD and COT, respectively.

3 RESULTS AND DISCUSSION

3.1 *In physiological saline*

Figure 1 shows the XRD patterns of the crystal precipitated from CaOx supersaturated solution with an initial concentration of 0.8 mmol/L in saline in the presence of 2.0 mmol/L different kinds of carboxylates, respectively. Only COM crystals were detected in control subjects (Figure1a) and after adding monocarboxylate NaGlu (Figure1b). The interplanar spacings of $d = 5.96, 3.65, 2.96, 2.35$ and 1.98 Å were detected, which were assigned to the ($\bar{1}01$), (020), ($\bar{2}02$), (130) and ($\bar{3}03$) planes of COM, respectively (PDF card number: 20-0231).

After dicarboxylate (Na₂Tart) was added (Figure 1c), we detected the diffraction peaks of COT and COD besides COM. The peaks at d = 6.64, 5.46, 5.25 and 2.64 Å were assigned to the (100), (110), ($0\bar{1}1$) and ($0\bar{2}2$) planes of COT (PDF card number: 20-0232), and those d = 3.34, 2.85 and 2.78Å were assigned to the (112), (222) and (411) planes of COD. Quantitative analysis showed that the composition ratio was follows: COM: COD: COT = 12: 19: 69 (Table 1). No precipitate was detected after tricarboxylate (Na₃Cit) was added, it was due to the strong coordination of Na₃Cit, with Ca^{2+} ions, which inhibited the formation of CaOx precipitate.

3.2   In artificial urine

Figure 2 shows the XRD patterns of the crystals precipitated from CaOx supersaturated solution in artificial urine. The percentages of COD and COM were 26% and 12% in control subjects, respectively. The diffraction peak of d = 2.98 Å was assigned to the ($\bar{2}02$) plane of COM (Figure 2a). The diffraction peaks at d = 6.05, 3.16 and 2.78 Å were assigned to the (200), (202) and (411) planes of COD, respectively.

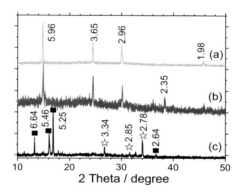

Figure 1.   XRD patterns of the crystals precipitated from CaOx supersaturated solution in saline with different inhibitors. (a) Blank; (b) NaGlu; (c) Na2Tart. c(Ca2+) = c(Ox2−) = 0.8 mmol/L. The peaks with ■ represent COT, ☆ represent COD, and without mark represent

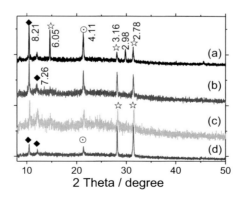

Figure 2.   XRD patterns of the crystals precipitated from CaOx supersaturated solution in artificial urine with different inhibitors. (a) Blank; (b) NaGlu; (c) Na2Tart; (d) Na3Cit. c(Ca2+) = c(Ox2−) = 0.8 mmol/L. ☆: COD, ◆: CaP, ⊙: CaHPO4·2H2O, and without mark: COM.

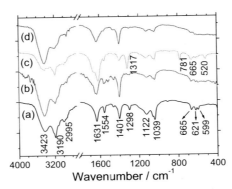

Figure 3. FT-IR spectra of the crystals precipitated from CaOx supersaturated solution in artificial urine with different inhibitors. (a) Blank; (b) NaGlu; (c) Na2Tart; (d) Na3Cit. $c(Ca2+) = c(Ox2-) = 0.8$ mmol/L.

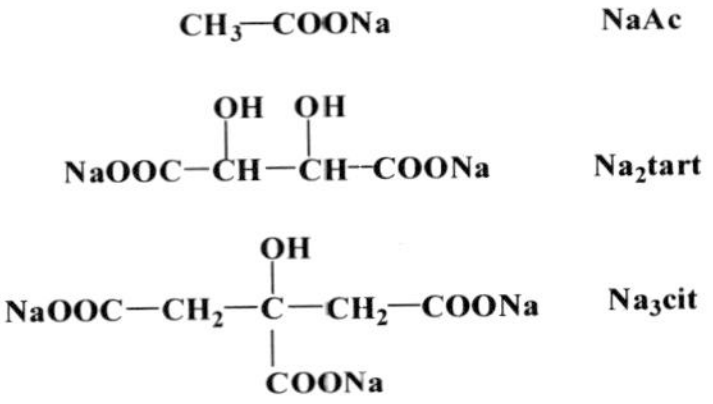

CH$_3$—COONa   NaAc

$$\begin{matrix} & \text{OH} & \text{OH} \\ & | & | \\ \text{NaOOC}-&\text{CH}-&\text{CH}-\text{COONa} \end{matrix}$$ Na$_2$tart

$$\begin{matrix} & & \text{OH} & & \\ & & | & & \\ \text{NaOOC}-&\text{CH}_2-&\text{C}-&\text{CH}_2-&\text{COONa} \\ & & | & & \\ & & \text{COONa} & & \end{matrix}$$ Na$_3$cit

Scheme 1: Molecular structures of the sodium carboxylates used in this study.

We detected the presence of COD, calcium phosphate (CaP) and CaHPO$_4$·2H$_2$O in artificial urine after NaGlu, Na$_2$Tart and Na$_3$Cit was added, respectively, whereas COM was not detected (Figure 2b-d). The diffraction peaks at d = 8.21, 7.26 Å were assigned to the (012), (111) planes of CaP (PDF card number: 09-0169). The peak at d = 4.11Å was assigned to the (021) plane of CaHPO$_4$·2H$_2$O (PDF card number: 09-0077). The results suggested that NaGlu, Na$_2$Tart and Na$_3$Cit could inhibit the formation of COM and promote the formation of COD. The percentages of the various components were listed in Table 1. Furthermore, the presence of CaP and CaHPO$_4$·2H$_2$O in artificial urine was confirmed by FT-IR detection (Figure 3). The characteristic absorption peaks at 1298 and 1401cm^{-1} were assigned to HPO$_4$$^{2-}$, the peaks at 2994, 1038 and 1122 cm^{-1} were assigned to PO$_4$$^{3-}$, and the peaks at 3423 and 3192 cm^{-1} were assigned to O-H stretching vibration absorption of crystal water (Lacmann $et\ al.$, 1999).

The causes for NaGlu, Na$_2$Tart and Na$_3$Cit to affect the crystal phase selection in the crystallization process of CaOx were as follows: Carboxylates can adsorb on the surface of the three hydrates of CaOx crystals (COM, COD and COT). For example, a computer model shows that citrate (cit^{3-}) can find eight possible adsorption sites on COM, five on COT, and only three on COD in 16 Å × 16 Å areas of crystal surface models (Cody $et\ al.$, 1994). Therefore, COM has the most strongly adsorbing ability. Since COD and COT contain fewer adsorption sites, the probability of cit^{3-} adsorbed on them can be increased only by increasing inhibitor concentration. Therefore, a small amount of Na$_3$Cit could inhibit COM nucleation, but promote the formation of COT and COD. When the concentration of Na$_3$Cit was higher than a certain threshold, Na$_3$Cit could adsorb on COD, the crystal phase with the weakest adsorption capacity, thereby inhibited the transformation of COD to COM, making COD stable in the solutions (Arvaniti $et\ al.$, 2010). There are many kinds of inhibitors in artificial urine, whereas no inhibitor in saline. When 2.0 mmol/L NaGlu, Na$_2$Tart or Na$_3$Cit was added, all these molecules could bind to the adsorption sites of COD and reduce its dissolution rate, namely the stability of COD increased in artificial urine. Therefore, the percentage of COD in artificial urine was higher than that in saline.

Table 1. Crystal components formed from CaOx supersaturated solution in the presence of 2.0 mmol/L different carboxylates in artificial urine and in saline. $c(Ca^{2+}) = c(Ox^{2-}) = 0.8$ mmol/L.

Inhibitor	In artificial urine					In saline		
	COM / %	COD / %	COT / %	CaP /%	CaHPO$_4$·2H$_2$O /%	COM / %	COD / %	COT / %
Blank	12	26	–	34	28	100	–	–
NaGlu	–	28	–	43	29	100	–	–
Na$_2$Tart	–	32	–	39	29	12	19	69
Na$_3$cit	–	57	–	23	20	–	–	–

4 CONCLUSIONS

NaGlu, Na$_2$Tart, and Na$_3$Cit have significant effects on the formation of different components in CaOx supersaturated solution. Only Na$_2$Tart induced the formation of COT and COD in saline. The percentage of COD increased with the increase of the number of carboxyl group (–COOH) of inhibitors in artificial urine, and calcium phosphate and CaHPO$_4$·2H$_2$O were also formed in this system. The cause of the formation of different crystal phases was discussed from the structure of carboxylates and the components of the system.

ACKNOWLEDGEMENT

This research work was supported by the Natural Science Foundation of China (81170649).

REFERENCES

Arvaniti, E.C., Lioliou, M.G., Paraskeva, C.A., Payatakes, A.C., Østvold, T., & Koutsoukos, P.G. (2010) Calcium oxalate crystallization on concrete heterogeneities. *Chemical Engineering Research and Design*, 88(1): 1455–1460.

Bretherton, T. & Rodgers, A. (1998) Crystallization of calcium oxalate in minimally diluted urine. *Journal of Crystal Growth*, 192(3–4): 448–455.

Carvalho, M. & Vieira, M.A. (2004) Changes in calcium oxalate crystal morphology as a function of super-saturation. *International Brazil Journal of Urology*, 30(3): 205–208.

Cody, A.M. & Cody, R.D. (1994) Calcium oxalate trihydrate phase control by structurally-specific carboxylic acids. *Journal of Crystal Growth*, 135: 235–245.

Kirboğa, S. & Öner, M. (2009) Inhibition of calcium oxalate crystallization by graft copolymers. *Crystal Growth & Design*, 9(5): 2159–2167.

Lacmann, R., Herden, A. & Mayer, C. (1999) Kinetics of nucleation and crystal growth. *Chemical Engineering and Technology*, 22(4): 279–289.

Langdon, A., Wignall, G.R., Rogers, K., Sørensen, E.S., Denstedt, J., Grohe, B., Goldberg, H.A. & Hunter, G.K. (2009) Kinetics of calcium oxalate crystal growth in the presence of osteopontin isoforms. *Calcified Tissue International*, 84(3): 240–248.

Opalko, F.J., Adair, J.H. & Khan, S.R. (1997) Heterogeneous nucleation of calcium oxalate trihydrate in artificial urine by constant composition. *Journal of Crystal Growth*, 181(4): 410–417.

Ouyang, J.M., Deng, F., & Duan, L. (2005) Effect of concentrations of lecithin, calcium and oxalate on crystal growth of calcium oxalate in vesicles. *Colloids and Surfaces A*, 257–258: 215–220.

Yu, H., Sheikholeslami, R. & Doherty, W.O.S. (2004) The effects of silica and sugar on the crystallographic and morphological properties of calcium oxalate. *Journal of Crystal Growth*, 265(3–4): 592–603.

Medicine Sciences and Bioengineering – Wang (Ed.)
© *2015 Taylor & Francis Group, London, ISBN: 978-1-138-02684-1*

On-chip microbubble destruction by surface acoustic waves

Long Meng, Fei-yan Cai, Fei Li, Li-li Niu & Hai-rong Zheng*
*Paul C. Lauterbur Research Center for Biomedical Imaging, Shenzhen Institutes of Advanced Technology,
Chinese Academy of Sciences, Shenzhen, China*

ABSTRACT: We present a microfluidic device that applies the surface acoustic wave to destroy individual microbubbles. Furthermore, the microbubble cluster in a two dimensional standing waves also can be destroyed. This technique has been proven to be simple, accurate, effective and ideal for a lab-on-a-chip system.

1 INTRODUCTION

Improvement of the cell's membrane permeability transiently in a control fashion enabling transport of foreign substance into the cells without causing the irreversible cell damage is critically important in various applications, such as the gene therapy, pharmaceutics and stem cell research (Y. Qiu *et al.*, 2010). Sonoporation employs acoustic inertial cavitation of microbubbles to induce transient cell-pores in the membranes allowing some impermeable molecules to be transferred into cells (Wu & Nyborg, 2008). The collapse of a microbubble under excitation of ultrasound may produce a variety of mechanical phenomena, such as high fluid streaming velocity, shear stress at the membrane, shock waves and jetting, which are considered to be the primary causes of sonoporation. The cavitation activity appears to be a random process, which makes it difficult to realize the targeted sonoporation on a single-cell.

To manipulate the position and control the severity-level of cavitation, various methods have been developed to facilitate a single cell sonoporation, including the biochemial method (Z. Fan *et al.*, 2012), laser-induced cavitation (Sankin *et al.*, 2010), and optical tweezers (Prentice *et al.*, 2005). Biochemical method uses the surface-modified microbubbles attached to the membrane of the targeted cells by specific ligand-receptor binding. This method is only applicable to certain types of cells. For the laser-induced cavitation method, the microbubble is generated via laser-induced breakdown in water, and the collapse position of microbubbles can be adjusted mechanically by changing the laser focus point. Optical tweezers provide precisely positioning microbubbles by a focused laser beam; however, it is difficult to transport microbubbles over a large working distance due to the tight optical focusing requirements. Moreover, it uses complicated optical systems, which would not allow it to easily integrate the sonoporation into a microfluidic device.

Ultrasound is a high frequency mechanical wave which can effectively transfer momentum and energy to the micro-objects in a liquid medium. The bioparticles suspended in the medium can be aggregated (Vanherberghen *et al.* 2010), positioned (Bernassau *et al.* 2013) and separated (Lenshof *et al.* 2012) by the acoustic radiation force or acoustic streaming. The acoustic technique provides us a noninvasive, contactless versatile method. Recently, the surface acoustic wave (SAW) based microfluidic device has been demonstrated to precisely manipulate droplet, particles, microbubbles, and cells. In this study, we introduce a microfluidic SAW device that makes the destruction of microbubbles reality. The advantage of using the microfluidic SAW device is its capability to achieve both spatial manipulation of microbubbles and excite them to go through inertial cavitation. The level of single cell membrane permeability can be altered easily.

---

* Author for Correspondence: ZHENG Hairong, Ph.D. Email: hr.zheng@siat.ac.cn.

2 METHODS

Fig. 1(a) shows the schematic of the destruction of microbubbles on a microfluidic device. The microbubbles can be positioned toward the targeted cell and initiate inertial cavitation on site. The SAW-based device used in the experiment consists a SAW device and a cylindrical PDMS microchannel, as shown in Fig. 1 (b). The SAW device was fabricated by depositing a periodic array of interdigital transducers (IDTs) on the surface of a 128°Y-X LiNbO3 substrate using standard UV photolithography. Two pairs of IDTs having the same finger width and spacing of 40 μm were oriented in two mutually perpendicular directions, corresponding to X and Y directions. The propagation velocities of SAW in the X and Y directions were previously measured to be 3900 m/s and 3640 m/s, respectively, their corresponding resonance frequencies of the SAW in each direction are 24.39 MHz and 22.96 MHz, respectively. The depth and radius of cylindrical PDMS microchannel are 30 μm and 600 μm. The PDMS microchannel was bonded to LiNbO3 substrate by plasma treatment (150 W, 1 min). Four series of independent signals were produced by two dual-channel arbitrary signal generators (Tektronix AFG 3102). The continuous sinusoidal signal with the amplitude of 3 Vp-p was utilized to transport and position microbubbles while a short acoustic pulse which will be described later amplified by a power amplifier (Amplifier Research 150A100B) to fragment microbubbles. The process to transport microbubbles to the targeted cell and initiate the inertial cavitation immediately afterwards was monitored using an inverted fluorescence microscope system (Leica DMI 3000B) with a CCD camera (Mikrotron MC1310). The microbubbles containing cores of octafluoropropane (C_3F_8) gas surrounded by phospholipid shells were prepared in house by the agitating method. The mean diameter of the microbubbles was 0.91 μm and about 99% microbubbles were smaller than 2.33 μm in diameter measured by an automatic particle size analyzer (AccuSizer 780A). The lipid-coated microbubble was chosen because the elastic behavior of the bubble shell is likely to generate significant high amplitude of radial pulsations in response to ultrasound according to computer-simulation. Our previous study has shown that SAW could not affect the integrity of microbubbles significantly at a relatively low-input power.

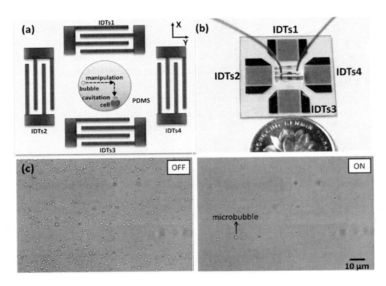

Figure 1.   (a) The schematic of the targeted single cell sonoporation on a SAW device. (b) A picture of the SAW-based microfluidic sonoporation device: It has two orthogonal pairs of IDTs with the resonance frequency of 24.39 MHz and 22.98 MHz in the X and Y direction, respectively. (c)The lipid microbubbles were injected into the PDMS channel and distributed uniformly.

3 RESULTS

To demonstrate the ability to induce cavitation, the aqueous suspension of microbubbles was introduced acting as inertial cavitation nuclei. The microbubbles were injected into the micro-channel by a syringe pump (Harvard pump model 44) and distributed uniformly. When a single-shot pulsed radio-frequency (RF) signal (24.39 MHz frequency, 41 µs pulse duration, 100V amplitude) was applied to IDTs1 in the X direction, more than 99% microbubbles exposed to SAW in the microchannel collapsed rapidly, resulting from the strong acoustic field (Fig.1(c)). Meanwhile, the microbubbles, located outside the IDTs1 aperture without the direct SAW irradiations, still remained intact, suggesting the SAW could induce microbubbles' inertial cavitation at 24.39 MHz, which is much greater than the megahertz resonance frequencies of micro-size bubbles. The non-focusing plane-wave nature of SAW produced by single IDT made the inertial cavitation reproducible anywhere in the channel if there are microbubbles there.

To achieve controllable spatial manipulation of microbubbles, an acoustic standing SAW wave (SSAW) was established to trap individual microbubbles into an acoustic radiation force potential well, where an acoustic pressure node of the standing wave is. In a standing wave, the microbubbles can be forced to aggregate at acoustic pressure nodes or antinodes by the Bjerknes force, depending on the relationship between the resonance frequency of microbubble and acoustic frequency. In our experiment, the SAW frequencies (24.39 MHz and 22.96 MHz) are much larger than the resonance frequency of microbubble (about 0.8 MHz-8 MHz), thus the microbubbles will be forced to move to the near-by pressure nodes. When we applied continuous electric voltages to each IDTs in the X and Y directions, the two dimensional SSAWs were formed in the microchannel and the microbubbles aggregated into acoustic nodes immediately. Then, a series of RF electric pulses (24.39 MHz frequency, 41µs pulse duration, 100 Hz pulse repetition frequency, 190V amplitude) were applied to the IDTs1 in the X direction, the high acoustic pressure in the fluid caused the microbubble to violently collapse resulting in fragmentation of a microbubble cluster, as shown in Fig. 2. In the process of fragmentation, the diameter of the microbubble cluster decreased dramatically with time; the accompanying translational and rotational motions of the cluster were also observed. It was noted that when the diameter of the microbubble cluster was larger than 10 µm, it was difficult to fragment microbubble cluster completely by using the same acoustic SAW pulses. This may attribute to dissipative loss of SAW energy due to the absorption of the microbubble cluster, thus the acoustic pressure imposed on a single microbubble of the

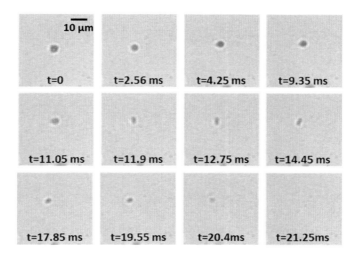

Figure 2.   The cavitation process of the microbubble cluster recorded at 1170 frames/s.

cluster was insufficient to cause inertial cavitation. Thus, the diameter of the microbubble cluster for the experiment was limited to less than 5 μm to achieve optimized acoustic inertial cavitation.

4 SUMMARY

In conclusion, we have shown that a microfluidic device can be used to manipulate microbubbles' positions and induce microbubble cavitation at the desired time. Furthermore, the ability to use a SAW microfluidic device to precisely control the position of microbubbles and initiate inertial cavitation near a single cell has the potential to efficiently deliver the microorganism or drug into a targeted cell.

ACKNOWLEDGMENTS

The work was supported by National Science Foundation (Grant Nos. 11304341, 11302239, 11274008, 61020106008, and 11325420), Shenzhen Basic Research Program (No. JCYJ20130402113127516).

REFERENCES

A. L. Bernassau, C. R. P. Courtney, J. Beeley, B. W. Drinkwater and D. R. S. Cumming, (2013) Interactive manipulation of microparticles in an octagonal sonotweezer, Appl Phys Lett 102: 164101.

A. Lenshof, C. Magnusson and T. Laurell, (2012) Acoustofluidics 8: Applications of acoustophoresis in continuous flow microsystems, Lab Chip12(7): 1210–1223.

B. Vanherberghen, O. Manneberg, A. Christakou, T. Frisk, M. Ohlin, H. M. Hertz, B. Önfelt and M. Wiklund, (2010) Ultrasound-controlled cell aggregation in a multi-well chip, Lab Chip 10: 2727.

G. N. Sankin, F. Yuan and P. Zhong, (2010) Pulsating tandem microbubble for localized and directional single-cell membrane poration, Phys Rev Lett 105: 078101.

J. Wu and W. L. Nyborg, (2008) Ultrasound, cavitation bubbles and their interaction with cells, Adv Drug Delivery Rev 60(10):1103–1116.

P. Prentice, A. Cuschieri, K. Dholakia, M. Prausnitz and P. Campbell, (2005) Membrane disruption by optically controlled microbubble cavitation, Nature Phys1: 107–110.

Y. Qiu, Y. Luo, Y. Zhang, W. Cui, D. Zhang, J. Wu, J. Zhang, and J. Tu, (2010) The correlation between acoustic cavitation and sonoporation involved in ultrasound-mediated DNA transfection with polyethylenimine (pei) in vitro, J Controlled Release 145 (1): 40–48.

Z. Fan, H. Liu, M. Mayer and C. X. Deng, (2012) Spatiotemporally controlled single cell sonoporation, Proc Nat Acad Sci U.S.A 109: 16486–16491.

Medicine Sciences and Bioengineering – Wang (Ed.)
© *2015 Taylor & Francis Group, London, ISBN: 978-1-138-02684-1*

Assessing Cerebral Auto-regulation using Least angle regression

Xue-cong Wu[a]

Guangdong Provincial Key Laboratory of Robotics and Intelligent System, Shenzhen Institutes of Advanced Technology, Chinese Academy of Sciences, Shenzhen, China
Harbin Institute of Technology Shenzhen Graduate School, Shenzhen, China

Jia Liu[a,*] & Pan-deng Zhang[a]

Guangdong Provincial Key Laboratory of Robotics and Intelligent System, Shenzhen Institutes of Advanced Technology, Chinese Academy of Sciences, Shenzhen, China

Xiao-ping Yang[b,*]

Harbin Institute of Technology Shenzhen Graduate School, Shenzhen, China

ABSTRACT: In this paper, we propose a Multiple-Input-Single-Output (MISO) model to study the Cerebral Auto-regulation (CA) system. Traditional identification algorithm cannot effectively reduce or eliminate the impact from the unrelated items of impulse response sequence of CA system, and it fails to identify the desired effect. Therefore, in this paper, by using and comparing two different identification algorithms that consist of the Least Square (LS), and Least angle regression (Lars) of L1-norm, under the condition of noise or no noise, the impulse response sequence of CA system is obtained, which is made use of to gain the size of phase at the specific frequency band.

1 INTRODUCTION

Cerebral Auto-regulation (CA) is the mechanism that maintains blood flow relatively constant in spite of blood pressure changes within a certain range (50~150 mmHg in general) in the brain. CA acts through vasomotor effectors which control cerebrovascular resistance (CVR) (Aaslid & Rune, 1989). With this mechanism, the brain obtains enough oxygen and nutrition continuously, which maintains normal physiological function. In order to quantify CA, Tiecks proposed a model using ABP and CBF signals and assigned an autoregulatory index (ARI) ranging from 0 to 9 (Tiecks, Frank P, 1995). However, partial arterial CO2 pressure can also affect the effectiveness of CA.

Transfer function analysis may be able to identify different components of CA and also provide a deeper understanding of recent findings by other investigators (Panerai, R. B, 1998). From a certain extent, the gain, phase and relevance of transfer function at specific frequencies reflect the strength of the regulating ability, and brain signal energy mainly concentrates in low-frequency (Zhang & Rong, 1998; Xu & Ren, 2012).

Among them, the bigger phase, the greater adjustment ability. Frequency in the 0.1 HZ possesses physiological significance, and the system has the maximum phase (Diehl & Rolf, 1995).

The least squares (LS) solution is the classic system identification algorithm, and it gets the weight coefficients of CA system which makes the cost function minimum. Least angle regression (Lars), a useful and less greedy version of traditional forward selection methods, can reduce some weight coefficients to 0, with the function of the variable selection, which can receive a set of sparse impulse response sequence (Efron, Bradley, 2004). The essence of Lars is that on the basis of the LS cost function, it increases the sums of squares of residuals plus an L1-norm penalty on the weight coefficients (Hesterberg, Tim, 2008).

[a] {xc.wu, jia.liu, pd.zhang}@siat.ac.cn
[b] xpyang8@126.com

This article that focus on analysis and comparison of two different identification algorithms can obtain the impulse response sequence of CA system with noise or no noise, then gain the size of phase o the specific frequency band.

2 METHODS

We set up multiple input single output (MISO) model that consider both the ETCO2 and ABP as input signals to produce a corresponding CBF output signal. Then, based on the model, LS and Lars algorithm are made use of to identify the CA systems. Before the systematic identification, we carry out filter processing of the collected signals to make sure that the signal frequency concentrates near the 0.1HZ, closer to the physiological frequency of the body.

System identification is based on the established model, using the key identification algorithm, to achieve estimates of weight coefficients with the minimum cost function. Then the impulse response sequence of CA system is as follows:

$$J_{min} = 0 \rightarrow \beta = [\beta_0, \beta_1, \ldots \ldots, \beta_{M-1}]^T \tag{1}$$

LS method is the classic system identification algorithm, and its cost function is: $J = \| Y - X\beta \|_2^2$, To achieve estimates of weight coefficients with the minimum cost function, there is:

$$\beta^{LS} = \arg\min \| Y - X\beta \|_2^2 \tag{2}$$

Lars algorithm is a residual fitting process, when subtracting the influence of the variable having been selected, the result obtained is residual. Then on the basis of the residual new features will be chosen. Lars algorithm uses mathematical formulas to accelerate the computations. Rather than taking many tiny steps with the first variable, the appropriate number of steps is determined algebraically, until the second variable begins to enter the model. So the fitting process is also a process of residual decreases. The cost function is: $J = \| Y - X\beta \|_2^2 + t \| \beta \|_1^1$. Lars minimizes the residual sum of squares, subject to a constraint on the sum of absolute values of the weight coefficients:

$$\beta^{L1\text{-}Lars} = \arg\min \| Y - X\beta \|_{2, \, s\,t:}^2 \| \beta \|_1^1 \leq t \tag{3}$$

3 RESULT

In order to establish the corresponding MISO model, we simulate the ABP, ETCO2 and CBF signals. In the process of simulation, we set up three different sections of 200 seconds, and add certain random signal as noise into the ABP signal, with corresponding to the ARI at 1, 7 and 3 from the classical Tiecks model, and then there will produce the corresponding CBF signal respectively, also with certain random signal as noise. Finally, its simulation flow chart is as Fig. 1:

The special processing including Gaussian filter for signal processing and the Hilbert transform, is to get analytical signal closer to the physiological frequency at 0.1HZ; Special processing/double refers to process the collected signals two times with the way of special processing, namely that after Special Processing, we will process the gauss filter and Hilbert transform once again, to get more accurate signal components.

The (a) in Fig. 2 which adopts the special processing, gets the results of phase identification based on LS and Lars algorithms. We can see from the graph, that the phase curve, which gets from Lars algorithm has a lot of volatility, while that of LS algorithm is relatively smoother, and the error is very small. But in (b) from Fig. 2, through the special processing/double, namely to produce special processing once again, the early large fluctuation of Lars algorithm improves a

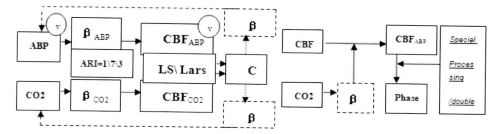

Figure 1.　Flow chart of MISO model

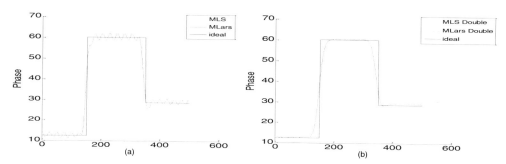

Figure 2.　The result of phase identification based on the simulation signal without noise. (a) LS and Lars in Special Processing (b) LS and Lars in Special Processing/double

great lot, and on the contrary the curve is very smoother than that of LS. At the same time, when ARI = 1 or ARI = 7, the identification results are basically identical with LS algorithm, but when ARI = 3, the curve is a little closer to the ideal value than LS, with smaller error.

However, in the process of collecting physiological signal, it is inevitable to mix noise signal. Noise affects the result of system identification, making that there occur some unrelated items with the disruptive impact of the impulse sequence. Therefore, in the process of analysis of the function of CA, noise signal must be taken into account.

In (a) from Fig. 3, when joining a certain amount of random noise into the simulation signal, the identification result is much more different from that of (a) in Fig. 2 without noise. For the LS algorithm, when ARI = 1 or ARI = 3, namely in recognition of the front part and the back part, phase swings near the ideal value up and down, and the range is very large. While in Lars algorithm, volatility is small, and the error is also small.

By comparing (a) from Fig. 3 and (a) from Fig. 2, we can see that when the physiological signal is mixed with random noise, the curve of phase identification result from Lars algorithm is much smoother than that of LS algorithm, and its value is much closer to the ideal value. Therefore Lars algorithm can effectively eliminate noise interference, reduce the influence of unrelated items, and make the identification result tend to be more practical. And the LS algorithm can't well damp noise interference, so that the identification result deviates from the actual.

In (b) from Fig. 3, through Special Processing/double, signals receive special processing. Eventually it can be found that the fluctuating range of the curve, which is caused by noise interference weakens a lot, and the curve is much smoother.

Then, through comparing (b) and (a) in Fig. 3, we can see that special processing/double makes the margin fluctuation, caused by noise, of curve result from LS algorithm significantly reduce, and makes curve result from Lars algorithm much smoother. And more importantly, in (a) Lars algorithm has effectively damped the noise interference, while in (b) the influence of noise gets the further inhibition, eventually with the result of a much smaller fluctuation, and a much smoother curve.

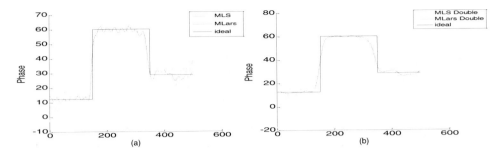

Figure 3. The result of phase identification based on the simulation signal with random noise. (a) LS and Lars in Special Processing (b) LS and Lars in Special Processing/double

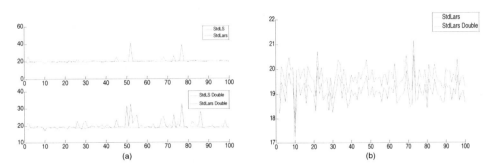

Figure 4. Comparison of Std curves with random noise (a) LS and Lars (b) Special Processing and Special Processing/double in Lars

In order to prove that the result of phase identification is not accidental under the condition of random noise signal, we carry out the simulation operation a total of 100 times in a row. So in this process it will produce 100 groups of random noise signals without regularity, finally through calculating the standard deviation to evaluate the smoothness of the curve (i.e., the size of the fluctuation of the curve), and the bias with the ideal value to evaluate the accuracy of the curve.

It can be found from (a) in Fig. 4, that whether in Special Processing or in Special Processing/double, Std value under Lars algorithm, is much smaller than that of LS, and almost no large fluctuation in a curve. So even when physiological signal is mixed with noise, the process of identification under Lars algorithm is still very stable. Seen from (b) in Fig. 4, in Special Processing and Special Processing/double identification, the Std curves are not the same under Lars algorithm. Standard value which gets from Special Processing/double is always less than that of the special processing.

4 CONCLUSION

For sensitive physiological signal such as ABP or CBF, by the analysis of the process of phase identification we can know, the LS can be effective to identify phase when there isn't noise in the input signal. But to the physiological signal, it is inevitable to be mixed with some random noise, and it will have a negative effect on the process of phase identification. Under the restriction of L1-norm punishment function, Lars algorithm makes the impulse response sequence of CA system multiple variable selection, and eventually can effectively eliminate the impact of unrelated items of an impulse response sequence, and make a more accurate identification of CA system than LS algorithm. Hence, Lars may have relatively higher sensitivity to signal and lower sensitivity to noise than LS.

ACKNOWLEDGMENTS

The work described in this paper is partially supported by the Project of Chinese Academy of Sciences and Foshan City Collaborative Platform (2013HT100051), and Shenzhen Fundamental Research Program (JC201005280481A), and a grant from Shenzhen Science and Technology Project [Reference No. ZDS Y20120617113312191], and Guangdong Innovative Research Team Program (201001D0104648280).

REFERENCES

Aaslid, Rune. (1989) Cerebral auto-regulation dynamics in humans. *Stroke* 20.1: 45–52.

Tiecks, Frank P. (1995) Comparison of static and dynamic cerebral auto-regulation measurements. *Stroke* 26.6: 1014–1019.

Panerai, R. B. (1998) Frequency-domain analysis of cerebral autoregulation from spontaneous fluctuations in arterial blood pressure. *Medical and Biological Engineering and Computing* 36.3: 315–322.

Zhang, Rong. (1998) Transfer function analysis of dynamic cerebral auto-regulation in humans. *American Journal of Physiology-Heart and Circulatory Physiology* 274.1: H233–H241.

Xu, Ren, and Jia Liu. (2012) Optimal time-frequency distribution of arterial blood pressure for assessing cerebral auto-regulation. *Biomedical and Health Informatics (BHI)*, 2012 IEEE-EMBS International Conference on. IEEE.

Diehl, Rolf R. (1995) Phase Relationship Between Cerebral Blood Flow Velocity and Blood Pressure A Clinical Test of Auto-regulation. *Stroke* 26.10: 1801–1804.

Efron, Bradley. (2004) Least angle regression. *The Annals of statistics* 32.2: 407–499.

Hesterberg, Tim. (2008) Least angle and ℓ1 penalized regression: A review. *Statistics Surveys* 2: 61–93.

Medicine Sciences and Bioengineering – Wang (Ed.)
© *2015 Taylor & Francis Group, London, ISBN: 978-1-138-02684-1*

Importance of bioinformatics in modernization of Traditional Chinese Medicine

Yu Bai
College of Pharmacy, Jilin Medical College, Jilin city, Jilin, China

Zhuo-yuan Xin
Key Laboratory of Zoonosis, Ministry of Education, Norman Bethune College of Medicine, Jilin University, Changchun, Jilin, China

Gui-hua Cui, Chun-hong Sui, Wen-liang Li, Shun-fu Dong, Li-qin Han & Wen-xiu Zhao
College of Pharmacy, Jilin Medical College, Jilin city, Jilin, China

Guang-yu Xu*
College of Pharmacy, Beihua university, Jilin city, Jilin, China

ABSTRACT: Traditional Chinese Medicine (TCM) is an important component of medical science. However, it is difficult for the international market to accept this precious treasure of China, because of the confusing therapeutic targets and the unclear mechanism. Bioinformatics is a novel inter discipline based on the mathematics, computer science and life science. Bioinformatics provides us a new technology to deal with the biological problems, which has a wide range of applications. So, it has great significance to study the mechanism of TCM utilizing bioinformatics. In this study, we collected the articles published in recent years, to analysis the usage of bioinformatics in the research of TCM resource, identification and functional gene selection. We wish that bioinformatics would provide new hope for the development of TCM.

1 INTRODUCTION

The Traditional Chinese Medicine (TCM) is one of the precious treasures in China, with a history over 2000 years. However, the international market, still can not accept TCM, because of the lacking of an efficient appraisal system for TCM, in the new era. The modernization of TCM is an innovatory progress to make TCM be approved by the whole world, in which the study of the effect of TCM is the most important.

Bioinformatics is a novel field of intersectional research based on mathematics, computer science and life science, which provide new ways to deal with the biological problems via the analysis of massive omics data (Brent, 2006). Nowadays, this burgeoning method has been applied in several field of research, especially in the study of medicine, including the selection of new genes related to disease (Read, 2002), identification of new targets for therapy (Giacomelli, 2010), examination of cancer metastasis degree and prediction of the clinical curative effect (Chen CN, 2005), etc. Hence, it is significant to utilize bioinformatics in the modernization of TCM.

In this study, articles published in recent years were collected to summarize the usage of bioinformatics in the research of TCM, including the study of TCM resource, the identification of TCM and the selection of TCM functional genes, etc. And we deemed that the introduction of bioinformatics would bring new opportunities for the development of TCM.

First Author: Yu Bai, (1980-), E-mail: baiyu218@163.com
*Corresponding Author: Guangyu Xu, (1980-), E-mail: xuguangyu2005@163.com

2 APPLICATION OF BIOINFORMATICS IN TCM RESOURCE RESEARCH

With the improvement of living standards, it has become a popular topic that TCMs are used to maintain health. At present, many varieties are far from demand as a result of the increasing dosage. And together with the excessive mining, several species are becoming extinct. So, the research on TCM resource is extremely urgent now. Fortunately, the rapid developments of bioinformatics bring us an efficient technology.

2.1 Bio-cloud computing

Along with the evolution of Next Generation Sequencing (NGS), the studies have turned into a large data era. A more complex algorithm and higher computing efficiency are required to process the huge amount of data produced from NGS. Bio-cloud computing is such a technology that has the capacity to deal with the demand for the large scale of calculation, which can simplify the processing of big-dataset and mobile data. And we have benefited a lot from the platform construction based on cloud computing, the software designing for data storage, and the perfection of workflow framework. In recent years, several cloud-computing platforms have been built, including TTRSIS for rice functional omics research and iPlant Atmosphere for plant science. Facing the challenge of omics data, the utilization of bio-cloud computing in TCM resource research will be an inevitable tendency.

2.2 Genome comparison

Genome comparison, also known as comparative genomics, brings us more accurate information about intraspecific differences. Since ancient time, there are wide varieties of TCMs, many of which have a close genetic relationship. For instance, Panax ginseng C. A. Mey and Panax pseudoginseng Wall. var. notoginseng (Burkill) Hoo et Tseng have a different efficacy, although both of them belong to Araliaceae. And the locations of a species have a strong relation with the quality, which can be illustrated clearly by the differences between authentic ingredients and general ingredients. Genome comparison would help us to demonstrate these discrepancies via the analysis of evolutionary relationships. The genomic variances among the different individuals of the same species, may be the genetic basis for the various TCM efficacies.

3 APPLICATION OF BIOINFORMATICS IN TCM IDENTIFICATION RESEARCH

TCM identification by the sources, trait, microscopy and physicochemical properties are used all the time. Following the post-genomics era, bioinformatics would be a powerful tool in the research of TCM identification.

3.1 Bio-microarray

Like an electronic chip, bio-microarray is a kind of solid supporter, on which high-density labeled probes are set up. Characteristics of the specimens are analyzed simultaneously in a large scale and quantity, through the hybridization and the detection of the signal strengths. Nowadays, the hotspots including electron beam direct writing, digital microfluidics-based bio-microarrays, three-dimensional bio-microarrays and disposable plastic bio-microarrays, has been widely used in many fields of research, especially in the identification of TCMs. In the exploration, we have benefited a lot from the utilization of bio-microarray based on the DNA sequencing.

3.2 DNA barcode

DNA barcode is easy to find in our daily life, which gives us great convenience and efficiency, although, many people are still unfamiliar with it. Hebert, a Canadian scientist, formally presented the definition of plant DNA barcode in 2003 that the plant DNA barcode was a technology to study the base change rules based on the amplification and sequencing for the specific genes in plant genomes. In recent years, Medicinal Materials DNA Barcode Database, the first database aimed at TCMs in the world, which provides the basic information and photos of TCMs, has been built, that has great reference values for TCM identification. What is more, together with DNA barcode, several databases including Nucleotide database (http://www.ncbi.nlm.nih.gov/nuccore) in the USA, EMBL-EBI database (http://www.ebi.ac.uk) in Europe and DDBJ (http://www.ddbj.nig.ac.jp) in Japan, are also needed in TCM identification.

3.3 Phylogenetic dendrogram

Phylogenetic dendrogram is an important branch of bioinformatics, which has been used widely in the study of the evolutionary relationship among species. On the basis of molecular data differences, phylogenetic dendrogram help us a lot in the study of the formation process and evolutionary mechanism of species. Following the increasing genome data, this technology becomes more and more popular.

4 APPLICATION OF BIOINFORMATICS IN TCM FUNCTIONAL GENES SCREENING

Screening of the TCM functional genes has contributed to the further study of diseases, which laid the foundation of the prevention, treatment and diagnosis of diseases. In recent years, it has become the central point that if the functional genes of medicinal plants can be used as therapeutic targets.

4.1 SAGE

SAGE (system analysis of genes expression) is used to detect the genes that cannot be tested by bio-microarray, which is no matter if these genes are known or not. Then, SAGE can also be used to analyze the whole transcriptome data of a cell, and on the other hand, SAGE is a useful tool for the qualitative and quantitative analysis of the desired genes. In the field of the medicine, biology, and pharmacology, SAGE has been wildly selected. But, nowadays, the usage of SAGE in TCM functional gene screening is relatively less.

4.2 Expressed Sequence Tag

Expressed Sequence Tag (EST) is utilized firstly in the regions of seeking of new human genes, construction of human genome map and identification of the coding regions in genome . For TCMs, Many pharmaceutical plant databases have been established using EST, such as a cDNA library database for Catharanthus roseus (L.) G. Don leaves and roots, which provides a wonderful resource for the transcriptome data analysis and functional gene finding, and databases for many other TCMs. Hence, EST has created favorable conditions for the screening and utilization of TCM functional genes.

5 PROSPECT

The TCM is a priceless treasure of China, which has summarized the abundant experiences of Chinese people's long struggle with diseases, and contributes a lot to the prosperity of the China. Since the era of "Shen Nong's Herbal Classic", blossoming of TCM has experienced a long period of glory. But, after nearly a century years of unrest, the development of TCM was grinding to a halt, which was a disgrace. With the improvement of living standard, the TCM is highlighted by the domestic and overseas scientists. And through the wide-ranging and frequent communication around the world, TCM will continue the brilliant achievements.

ACKNOWLEDGMENTS

This work was supported by the Wu Jieping Medical Foundation (320.6750.13229), Wu Jieping Medical Foundation (320.6750.13216), Jilin Education Foundation (Ji Education Science [2014]505)

REFERENCES

Brent R, Bruck J. 2020 computing: can help to explain biology [J]. Nature, 2006;440(7083): 416–417.

Chen CN, Lin JJ, Chen JJ, et al.2005.Gene expression profile predicts patient survival of gastric cancer after surgical resection [J]. J. Clin. Oncol, 2005, 23: 7286–7295.

Giacomelli L, Covani U. Bioinformatics and data mining Studies in oral genomics and proteomics : New trends and Challenges [J]. Open Dent J. 2010.4: 67–71.

Read TD ,Sal z berg S L ,Pop M, et, al. Comparative genome Sequencing for discovery of novel polymorphisms in Bacillus anthracis [J]. science, 2002, 296 (5575): 2028–2033.

Medicine Sciences and Bioengineering – Wang (Ed.)
© *2015 Taylor & Francis Group, London, ISBN: 978-1-138-02684-1*

Application of case-based learning model in the clinical practice of orthopedic graduates

Wei-hai Jiang[1] & Wei Sun[*]
Affiliated Hospital, Beihua University, Jilin, Jilin 132001, China

ABSTRACT: Clinical practice of medicine is a bridge to combine the medical theory with the practice. Interests play an essential role in their future sustainable development in clinical work. To mobilize the students' initiative and stimulate their interests, improve their abilities in their professional work and the enthusiasm in their profession during the clinical practice, the authors recently adopted a case-based learning mode in our practical teaching work and have achieved a good teaching result. In this paper, the methods, process and roles of case-based learning model in the orthopedic practice of graduates are discussed. Effects of case-based learning on realizing the objective to culture the comprehensive ability in the clinical practical teaching of orthopedic graduates should be more pronounced. By using the case-based learning model, the independent thinking, problem-solving skills of students can be trained well, and the students' learning initiative and enthusiasm can be mobilized.

1   INTRODUCTION

The clinical practice of medicine is a bridge to combine the medical theory with the practice, a preliminary practice of the theoretical knowledge learned by medical students and a critical stage in which medical students are trained in the clinical thinking, clinical awareness, clinical skills and other capabilities. Training objectives of orthopedic graduates include to fully understand the fundamental expertise and skill in orthopedics, have the capability of diagnosis and treatment of common diseases, become a qualified orthopedic doctor, and complete the transition from a medical student to an orthopedic doctor, so that how to mobilize the students' initiative and stimulate their interests plays an essential role in their future sustainable development in the clinical work, which is also one of problems worthy to be deeply thought by the clinical teachers during the practical period. In recent years, the authors adopted a case-based learning mode in our practical teaching work and have achieved a good teaching result. In this paper, the significance, methods, process and roles of case-based learning model in the orthopedic practice of graduates are introduced and discussed.

2   INTRODUCTION TO CASE-BASED LEARNING

Case-based learning model is a teaching model based on fully mobilizing the enthusiasm both teaching and learning, to give play to bilateral activities of teacher-led and student-centered, to take the improvement of students' abilities in the clinical practice as the target, and to realize the learning objectives by taking a typical case determined through selecting, systemizing and processing as a teaching unit to ask the students to preview, present succinctly and discuss (Dochy *et al.*, 2003).

---

[1] First Author: Jiang Weihai (1979-)
[*]Corresponding Author: Sun Wei (1979-), E-mail: 50598236@qq.com

Case-based model began at Medical School, Harvard University, in The United States in 1910. In 1958, a "case analysis course" was first set up in Capital Medical University in our country. The main difference between case-based learning model and general case teaching is that case-based learning model requires the teacher to make a thorough tutorial design; In addition, the typical cases in case-based learning model can complement and improve the atypical insufficiency inward cases to ensure the quality of teaching content.

During this process, the role of teachers is crucial. The teachers should select some representative clinical cases, then systemize and process them to find the typical characteristics and display in a most appropriate way, design some clinical problems with high quality, organize the students to analyze and discuss the problems, and adopt a diversified teaching mode (such as living examples, multimedia, etc.) to improve the degree of participation and interest in the teaching. Therefore, teachers must not only recognize the characteristics and significance of case-based learning model, seriously prepare the lessons before class and know very well contents of the typical cases as well as case content-related basic medical knowledge, such as anatomy, but also have the rich clinical experience; they are required to master the development and the current understanding of typical diseases; they have not only an ability in both theoretical knowledge and clinical skills, but also are able to organize the students to discuss, guide and inspire them to improve their clinical thinking and analytical ability, which may put forward a higher requirement to the teachers. For students, through the reflection and discussion on the issues, their initiative and thinking can be tremendously simulated, so that the initiative of students can be better mobilized and an output pathway of the knowledge to the students will appear (Eshach & Bitterman, 2003).

3 PROCESS OF CASE-BASED LEARNING

The teaching procedure of the implementation process of case-based learning included several links, such as cases displaying asking questions, discussing questions, evaluating and presenting briefly and succinctly.

3.1 Case preparation and display

Selection criteria: common and typical cases suitable for students to learn and think of cases that the content was complete in various forms and displayed in a way of multimedia, writing or electronic documents, etc., questions based on the teaching objectives focused on the clinical diagnosis, differential diagnosis and treatment, appropriately involving the anatomical and other basic knowledge, in various forms, and paid more attention to the vividness and lead function of questions and easiness to the improvement of the students' interests.

3.2 Putting forward the questions

The questions put forward included those design by the teachers and those discovered by the students. Those designed by the teachers should conform to the logical clinical thinking, so that through the in-depth discussion, the students could understand the clinical diagnosis and treatment of diseases and the clinical thinking. Before the teaching, teachers showed the outline and questions of cases to the students to facilitate them to preview and look up the information, which might able to train the students to consult literatures in an independent thinking way, master-related basic concepts and theories, give full play to their initiative when they were encouraged to learn the guidance learning materials, be brave to identify problems, and put forward the difficult points perceived by themselves. The students were encouraged to pre-contact with patients to increase the perception of diseases, and find problems and put forward their own views through comparing the specific cases with textbooks or related literatures.

3.3 *Discussion and questioning*

Discussion is not only the main form of this teaching model, but also the core of it. Through the discussion, questioning, expressing their respective views and brainstorming, the learning activity was in depth. The discussion could be divided into several stages and carried out under the guidance of teachers. Firstly, the difficult points and key problems raised by the students were discussed. Everyone had his own opinions and expressed his ideas as far as possible, in which the students explained the feeling of preview and the experience on the earlier contact with patients, elaborated problems found by them, and listed some analytical key points summarized through combined cases for the implementation of seminars. Secondly, the teachers raised the questions designed by them. According to the logic of clinical thinking, the teachers inspired and coached the students, pointed out the key to solving the problems, and encouraged to debate students with different opinions. Finally, the students were asked to have a try to organize to discuss and summarize the numerous views and interpretations for the preliminary conclusion.

3.4 *Evaluation of the succinct presentation*

Based on the above discussion, the students were guided by teacher to discuss aim at the targeted problems. Focuses were on how to analyze cases and how to make the diagnosis and differential diagnosis, replied the representational problems in the discussion reasonably.

4 ROLE OF CASE-BASED LEARNING IN THE GRADUATE PRACTICE IN ORTHOPEDECS

The application of case-based learning model in the graduate practice in orthopedics can greatly improve the initiative of students and significantly elevate the students craving for the knowledge, so that the students' active learning ability was significantly enhanced. The teaching model requires students to take the initiative to ask questions and find their own answers, learn how to use various pathways to learn, such as internet and library. By finding the answers and group discussion, the students' abilities in analyzing and problem-solving can be improved significantly. The teaching model encourages the students to learn through the discussion and the exchange among them, so that they can develop a sense of good communication skills and cooperation with others. In the teaching process with this teaching mode, the participation degree of students was high and their sense of accomplishment can be met greatly.

5 SUMMARY

In summary, the effect of case-based learning on realizing the objective to culture the comprehensive ability in the clinical practical teaching of orthopedic graduates should be more pronounced. By using the case-based learning model, the independent thinking, problem-solving skills of students can be trained well, so that the students' learning initiative and enthusiasm can be mobilized. In this way, they can understand the reasoning steps of clinical diagnosis, improve their abilities to deal with the practical problems in clinic independently, and be full of interest in orthopedics.

REFERENCES

Dochy F, Segers M, Van den Bossche P, et al. (2003) Effects of problem-based learning: am eta-analysis [J]. *Learn Instruct, 13: 533.*
Eshach H, Bitterm an H. (2003) From case-based reasoning to problem-based learning [J]. *A cadMed, 78 (5): 4916.*

Medicine Sciences and Bioengineering – Wang (Ed.)
© *2015 Taylor & Francis Group, London, ISBN: 978-1-138-02684-1*

The effect of 1800 MHz electromagnetic radiation on telomerase expression in NIH/3T3 cells

Yan Li, Ming-lian Wang*, Qiao-li Liu, Qing-xia Hou & Huan Liu
College of Life Sciences and Bioengineering, Beijing University of Technology, Beijing, China

ABSTRACT: We detected the expression of telomerase in NIH/3T3 cells to investigate the potential adverse effects of long-term 1800 MHz electromagnetic radiation (EMR). NIH/3T3 cells were intermittently (5 min on/10 min off) exposed to 1800 MHz radiation at an average specific absorption rate (SAR) of 2 W/kg by simulating GSM (Talk mode). The telomerase expression was detected by ELISA. These results showed that the telomerase expression in group exposed for 60 days had no significant difference compared to the sham group, however, its expression in the 138 days exposed group significantly increased ($p < 0.05$) compared to the sham group. These results indicate that telomerase expression might increase after 138 days exposure to 1800 MHz electromagnetic radiation (EMR) in NIH/3T3 cells.

1 INTRODUCTION

With the gradually mature of mobile communications, electromagnetic radiation had arisen widely attention as one of the environmental problems. The electromagnetic radiation of 1800 MHz has been applied in the Global System for Mobile Communication (GSM). Mobile phone technology replays radiofrequency electromagnetic radiation (Mailankot *et al.*, 2009). The world's two major mobile phone radiation standard setters-Institute of Electrical and Electronics Engineers (IEEE) and the International Commission on Non-Ionizing Radiation Protection (ICNIRP) of organisms (including humans) allowed per unit of absorbed radiation kilogram SAR standards for a unified, 2.0 watts per kilogram of peak radiation standards are adopted by most countries. SAR standard of mobile phone electromagnetic radiation should be limited in the international health organization certification license, European standard limit of SAR is 2.0 W/kg. Radiofrequency electromagnetic fields (EMF) issued cellular phones ranging from 800 to 2,000 MHz (Hardell L *et al.*, 2008; Health Protection Agency 2013). Some epidemiological studies have shown that mobile phone EMR may cause the risk of developing certain forms of cancers as or acoustic neuroma (Hardell *et al.*, 2004) eye cancer (Stang *et al.*, 2001). Researches did not indicate the obvious influence about a mouse in retinal ganglion cell responses with the 1800 MHz EMR (Ahlers, MT *et al.*, 2013). Previous studies found that 1800 MHz EMR gave rise to reactive oxygen species and DNA damage, induced cell apoptosis to some extent (Qingxia Hou *et al.*, 2014). The World Health Organization (WHO) has classified electromagnetic radiation pollution as the fourth pollutant listing after water, gas, and sound pollution. The point about whether EMR will lead to the occurrence of tumors is still controversial, so the International Agency for Research on Cancer (IARC) classifies EMR as possibly carcinogen to humans (2B) (IARC, 2012). 1800 MHz has become the most frequently occupied band in CDMA, GSM and GSM1X dual-mode 3G phones currently.

Telomerase plays an important role in cell growth and development, the main biological function is through reverse transcriptase activity replication and extension of the telomere DNA to stabilize the chromosome length of telomere DNA. In normal somatic cells, telomerase activity

---

*Wang Minglian is the corresponding author for this study (E-mail: mlw@bjut.edu.cn).

was quite strict regulation, the active control is closely related to cancer and aging. Findings established a functional link between Endoplasmic Reticulum stress and telomerase both of which have important implications in the pathologies associated with aging and cancer (Junzhi Zhou et al., 2014).

Telomere and telomerase interplay plays a key role involved in genomic stability and cellular replication potential, and its dysfunction feature in the oncogenetic process (Roberta Bertorelle et al., 2014). Telomere fusion may lead to general genomic instability (Raynaud CM et al., 2008). Telomere shortening incolorectal polyps was recently correlated with large-scale genomic rearrangements (Roger L et al., 2013).

Therefore, this study will examine 1800 MHz electromagnetic radiation on telomerase expression in cells, and is expected to provide the basis for health assessment and improvement of the standard of mobile phone radiation dose of electromagnetic radiation (SAR 2.0 W/kg around).

2 MATERIALS AND METHODS

2.1 Cell culture

NIH/3T3 cells (purchased from China Union Medical University Center for Basic Medical Cell) are mouse embryonic fibroblasts. NIH/3T3 cells are sensitive to the environmental factors, they are frequently used to prepare potential carcinogens. Cells were cultured in Dulbecco's Modified EAGLE's Medium (DMEM, Gibco, USA), mixed with 10% fetal bovine serum (FBS, Hyclone, USA) in an incubator at 37°C with 5% CO_2 (Thermo Scientific, USA), and continued cell culture every 3–4 days.

2.2 Exposure system

The sXc (System for Exposure of Cells, IT'IS Company) 1800 MHz exposure system was composed of a narrow band amplifier, an arbitrary function generator, a signal generator, and two rectangular waveguide chambers. One for exposure and another for sham-exposure about two waveguides. The probes and fans were linked to a computer controlling and exposure parameters containing SAR, exposure pattern automatically and exposure time. In order to entire duration of exposure, the temperature was kept at 37 ± 0.1 and the temperature in the exposed and the sham-exposed are different and cultures never exceeded 0.1. Therefore, under constant temperature conditions to obtain the data.

Exposures were carried out by adapting a pulse modulated 1800 MHz GSM (Talk) signal at a repetitive rate of 217 Hz. Exposed NIH/3T3 cells intermittently (field on for 5 min, field off for 10 min) or sham-exposed to 1800 MHz EMR at an average SAR of 2 W/kg, which is defined as safety limit to mobile phone emission radiation by the ICNIRP recently.

2.3 Telomerase detection

Collected all cells for the extraction of intracellular proteins. The concentration of cells should reach 1 million/ml, dilute cells suspension with PBS 2000 rpm, 5 min, repeated three times, collected cells, repeated freeze-thaw cycles, smudge cells and release of inclusions, centrifugation with the speed of 12000 rpm, 20 min, remove supernatant.

Diluted standard substance and added sample which diluted five times, incubate 30 min at 37°C, configurate liquid, washing (add washing buffer to every well, still for 30 s then drain, repeated 5 times, pated to dry), add enzyme except blank, incubate, washing five times, color. Add chromogen solution A 50 µl then add B 50 µl to each well, evade the light preservation for 15 min at 37°C, add stop solution to stop the reaction, take blank well as zero to assay.

3 STATISTICAL ANALYSIS

Each experiment was repeated six times. Take the standard density as horizontal, draw the standard ordinate for OD value, calculated the straight line regression equation of the standard, then calculated the sample density, multiplied by the dilution ratio. While the sample actual density. Using PerkinElmer Victor [3] to determine standard curve, SPSS statistical software for significance test analysis.

4 RESULTS

The effect of 1800 MHz electromagnetic radiation on telomerase expression presented in Table 1. The results show that long-term electromagnetic radiation effected intracellular telomerase content, and the telomerase increasing effect turned obvious after 138 days exposure.

Table 1. The telomerase content in cells after 1800 MHz EMR [$(x \pm s)$, U/L].

Group	n	Telomerase content (U/L)
60 days sham	6	7.41 ± 0.04
60 days exposure	6	7.57 ± 0.19
138 days sham	6	7.41 ± 0.04
138 days exposure	6	7.87 ± 0.19

$n = 6$: each experiment was repeated 6 times.

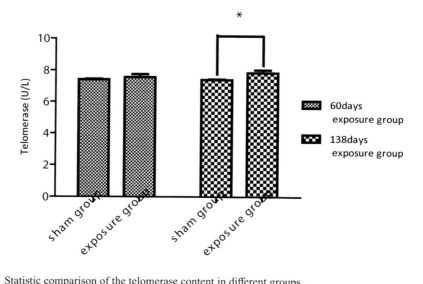

Figure 1. Statistic comparison of the telomerase content in different groups.

5 DISCUSSION

The experiment results show that 1800 MHz EMF have an effect on the expression of telomerase in NIH/3T3 cells. While there have many factors apply to telomerase, only a few studies report that telomeres in late stage cancer compared to in preneoplastic lesions and early neoplastic stages are longer, the activation of telomerase or highest expression of telomerase may explain the augment in telomere length accompany disease progression (Gertler, R et al., 2004; Garcia-Aranda C et al., 2006). It has been advanced that short telomeres may also impact genome-wide DNA methylation recently, which may modulate oncosuppressor and oncogene gene expression (Pucci F et al., 2013). 1800 MHZ EMF exposure affect the expression of telomerase, from the analysis we can infer that the long term exposure have a significant difference in the expression of telomerase.

ACKNOWLEDGEMENTS

This research was supported by the National Key Basic Research Project (2011CB503705) and Beijing Municipal Education Commission Science and Technology Project (KM201310005029).

REFERENCES

Ahlers MT, Ammermüller J. (2013). No influence of acute RF exposure (GSM-900, GSM-1800, and UMTS) on mouse retinal ganglion cell responses under constant temperature conditions. Bioelectromagnetics 10, 21811.

Gertler, R., Rosenberg, R., Stricker, D., Friederichs, J., Hoos, A., & Werner, M., et al. (2004). Telomere length and human telomerase reverse transcriptase expression as markers for progression and prognosis of colorectal carcinoma. J Clin Oncol, 22(10), 1807–1814.

Garcia-Aranda C, de Juan C, Diaz-Lopez A, Sanchez-Pernaute A, Torres AJ, Diaz-Rubio E, Balibrea JL, Benito M, Iniesta P.C. (2006). Correlations of telomere length, telomerase activity, and telomeric-repeat binding factor 1 expression in colorectal carcinoma. 106: 541–551.

Hardell, L., Hallquist, A., Hansson Mild, K., et al. (2004). No association between the use of cellular or cordless telephones and salivary gland tumours. Occup Environ Med 61, 675–679.

Hardell L, Sage C. (2008) Biological effects from electromagnetic field exposure and public exposure standards. Biomed Pharmacother, 62:104–109.

Health Protection Agency. (2013) Radiation: Mobiletelephony and health background information. [Online] Availablefrom: http://www.hpa.org.uk/webw/HPAweb&HPAwebStandard/HPAweb_C/11957338525 58p–115893460778.

Junzhi Zhou Beibei Mao, Qi Zhou, Deqiang Ding, Miao Wang, Peng Guo Yuhao Gao, (2014). Endoplasmic reticulum stress activates telomerase. Aging Cell 13, pp 197–200.

Mailankot M, Kunnath AP, I Jayalekshmi H, Koduru B, Valsalan R. (2009) Radio frequency electromagnetic radiation (RF-EMR) from gsm (0.9/1.8 ghz) mobile phones induces oxidative stress and reduces sperm motility in rats. Clinics, 64(6):561–5.

Pucci F, Gardano L, Harrington L. (2013) Short telomeres in ESCs lead to unstable differentiation. Cell Stem Cell; 12:479–486.

Qingxia Hou, Minglian Wang, Shuicai Wu, Xuemei Ma, Guangzhou An, Huan Liu, and Fei Xie (2014) Oxidative changes and apoptosis induced by 1800-MHz electromagnetic radiation in NIH/3T3 cells. Electromagn Biol Med. ISSN: 1536–8378.

Roger L, Jones RE, Heppel NH, Williams GT, Sampson JR,Baird DM. (2013). Extensive telomere erosion in the initiation of colorectal adenomas and its association with chromosomal instability. J Natl Cancer Inst; 105: 1202–1211.

Roberta Bertorelle, Enrica Rampazzo, Salvatore Pucciarelli, Donato Nitti, Anita De Rossi (2014).Telomeres, telomerase and colorectal cancer. World J 20(8): 1940–1950.

Raynaud CM, Jang SJ, Nuciforo P, Lantuejoul S, Brambilla E, Mounier N, Olaussen KA, André F, Morat L, Sabatier L, Soria JC. (2008). Telomere shortening is correlated with the DNA damage response and telomeric protein down-regulation in colorectal preneoplastic lesions. Ann Oncol; 19:1875–1881.

Stang, A., Anastassiou, G., Ahrens, W., et al. (2001). The possible role of radiofrequency radiation in the development of uveal melanoma. Epidemiology 12, 7–12.

Medicine Sciences and Bioengineering – Wang (Ed.)
© 2015 Taylor & Francis Group, London, ISBN: 978-1-138-02684-1

A reliable method for cloud data storage security

Fan Yang & Yu-tai Rao*

Department of Electronics and Information Engineering, Hubei Radio & TV University, Wuhan, Hubei, China

ABSTRACT: The intelligent health monitoring system based on the internet technology and wireless communication technology can effectively help the patients to master their physical signs, and can effectively forecast their diseases, and can also sound the alarm and position for patients in case of emergency. This is based on the system's accurate collection of patients' data and scientific and reasonable analysis. It is the key to success that how to collect data accurately. The research of this paper is to add a trusted third party between the patient and the system, to ensure the system that the safety and integrity of uploading after collecting the patients' data, to ensure the system that the safety and integrity of sounding the alarm.

1   RESEARCH CONTENT

With the rapid development of the Internet technology and the wireless communication technology, the research and application of the intelligent health monitoring system have been vigorously developing, the intelligent health monitoring system can help the patients to collect real-time vital signs, and to understand their physical index, it can also help the doctors monitor the patient's condition, if there is an emergency the system will alarm. The intelligent health monitoring system is divided into patient client, hospital client, cloud server and so on, the patient client includes body sensor, identification, data collection, upload and download terminal, the hospital client includes data collection, upload and download terminal, cloud server is responsible for the data storage and data analysis results. The key of the intelligent health monitoring system can work properly is to upload and download data accurately.

The massive data security is the key to the cloud properties, cloud data can be divided into static and dynamic storage data according to the storage mode, static memory data refer to the data stored in the cloud server already, and dynamic storage data refers to the data sent through the communications network to the user or sent through the network to the cloud. Obviously, the static and the dynamic in fact can be understood as the data in two different states in different periods. Static data security depends mainly on the cloud server, storing static data in the remote server by network security technology after years of development has been very mature, for the cloud dynamic data security will be challenging. Dynamic data are affected by outside influence and communication equipment at the time of transmission, which may cause the receiver never received the data, or the receiver receives part of the data, or the receiver receive the data which has been illegally tampered. Especially in the massive data transmission, data security and integrity are particularly difficult to ensure.

---

* The paper's author for correspondence, his email is 2079406@qq.com

2 ALGORITHM

2.1 *Introduction*

Ateniese has proposed that the model that the data have proved to have, when the data is storing, the data is marked in order to verify that the data has been stored (Ateniese *et al.*, 2008). The model can not verify publicly the dynamic stored data. Wang has proposed that protocol that can verify publicly the dynamic stored data, there are random processes corresponding to arbitrary data file modification, and will always be passed on, which will seriously affect the efficiency of verification (Wang *et al.*, 2009). Aiming at the shortages of these methods, this paper proposed a dynamic data validation method based on third party certification. Every time when depositing or modifying data, the third party which was common has the right certification, users have the legitimacy to the subsequent operation. The third party can obtain the user's time and address of storing data to verify whether the data has the legal deposit, and then uses the Merkle hash algorithm to verify that the data integrity. This method not only can effectively protect the privacy and security, but also can be publicly verified whether the dynamic and static data have been stored in completely.

2.2 *Algorithm*

The dynamic data validation method based on third party certification is as follows:

1. When patients or doctors want to upload the data, the third party embedded in the patient's terminal and the hospital terminal starts authentication. Third party asks the user to confirm the time and the place, and the third party verification agreement, then allows uploading.
2. After the data are uploaded or downloaded, the data will be verified by the Merkle Hash algorithm whether to be complete, and the integrity verification is to verify the patient and doctor.
3. To establish the Merkle Hash tree for the patients' terminal, the data of every N terminal of the patients' terminals in one geographical area are looked as a leaf node. Suppose there are M leaf nodes. The patient tree consists of Log_2M+1 layer.
4. To establish the Merkle Hash tree for the hospital terminal, the data of the same department doctor terminal are looked as a leaf node. Suppose there are P leaf nodes. The doctor tree consists of Log_2P+1 layer.
5. Every leaf node of the third party's Hash tree sets a user interface corresponding to each terminal, which makes the verification more efficient.
6. When a patient or a hospital terminal has uploaded or downloaded data, the third party will query the Merkle Hash trees in their own cache. The third party begins to query from the leaf node from the point of initiation of the query terminal, then queries to the hash tree top progressive, if the hash tree path agrees with the cloud server's, the data transmission is correct.

3 SIMULATION EXPERIMENT

The simulation experiment is designed to validate whether this proposed method is a reliable method of safe cloud storage; it can effectively play a role in the massive data transmission. The cloud server architecture in Baidu cloud, the database uses Oracle, the client program is the Android program based on My Eclipse platform, the third party is in the cloud server, the client program can trigger it. Each computer uses the program enable more than 50 terminals' program run at the same time, and each computer accesses Internet from different gateway, respectively, through 3G network, the experiment used a total of 66 computers. Assuming that each terminal transceiver data whose length is 2M every time, the experiment in the mail every terminal's mean time and data integrity of sending and receiving, made a comparison of the methods in Q.Wang and the method in this paper (Tables 1 and 2).

Table 1. Q.Wang's method.

The number of terminals of every computer	The average transmission time (Second)	Data integrity
50	0.01	100%
400	0.01	100%
1600	0.015	99%
12,800	0.02	97%
102,400	0.031	95%
1,638,400	0.078	91%

Table 2. This paper's method.

The number of terminals of every computer	The average transmission time (Second)	Data integrity
50	0.011	100%
400	0.011	100%
1600	0.013	100%
12,800	0.018	99.6%
102,400	0.023	99.6%
1,638,400	0.048	99%

4 SUMMARY

Under the same conditions, with larger scale, the stability of the paper's method about the data integrity is higher; time consumption growth will be slower. The method proposed in this paper is a reliable, safe cloud storage. This method is suitable for the intelligent health monitoring system.

ACKNOWLEDGEMENTS

My heartfelt thanks should go first to my supervisor, Associate Professor Yutai Rao of Hubei Radio & TV University forhis many enlightening suggestions for improving the quality of this paper. I should also thank Science and Technology Research Program of Hubei Provincial Department of Education under Grant No.B2014187 for the financial support of this project.

REFERENCES

C. Erway, A. Kupcu, C. Papamanthou, and R. Tamassia(2009) Dynamic provable data possession. *In Proceedings of the 16th ACM conference on Computer and communications security (CCS'09),* Chicago, Illinois, USA, November 9–13, 2009.

G. Ateniese, R. Di Pietro, L.V. Mancini, and G. Tsudik(2008) Scalable and efficient provable data possession. *In Proceedings of the 4th international conference on Security and privacy in communication networks*, Istanbul, Turkey, September 22–26, 2008.

Lakshman A,Malik P(2010)Cassandra:A decentralized structured storage system.*ACM SIGOPS Operating Systems Review,*44(2):35–40.

Q. Wang, C. Wang, J. Li, K. Ren, and W. Lou(2009) Enabling public verifiability and data dynamics for storage security in cloud computing. *In 14th European Symposium on Research in Computer Security (ESORICS'09)*, Saint Malo, France, September 21–23, 2009.

U.S.Department of Commerce(2011)*The NIST definition of cloud computing,National Institute of Standards and Technology.*

Wang L,Laszewski G V(2010)Cloud computing:a perspective study.*Journal of New Generation Computing*, 28(2):137–146.

Medicine Sciences and Bioengineering – Wang (Ed.)
© 2015 Taylor & Francis Group, London, ISBN: 978-1-138-02684-1

Thinking on strengthening university library health information service model innovation in the age of big data

Jian-yu Lu, Ju-zhi Zhou & Huan-li Ruan
Library Information Center, Ningbo College of Health Sciences, Ningbo city, China

Gui-chai Luo
Chinese Maternal and Child Care Service Centre, Jiangdong District, Ningbo City, Zhejiang, China

ABSTRACT: This paper analyzed the problems existing in the health information service and discussed the strengthening the importance and urgency of strengthening the health information services to the community. In addition, this paper elaborated that it should strengthen the health information services based on the innovative way of the whole life cycle of innovation, health information service resource library building based on a network share-based, part-time team building and other health information services to build university library health information service innovation model in the age of big data.

1 INTRODUCTION

In recent years, due to the lack of health information literacy, communication barriers in health information, the sense conflicts between doctors and patients, lack of knowledge of disease self-management, high medical costs and other issues have become important factors that had a serious impact on public health. Establishing and improving the information service innovation based on the health of the whole life cycle for improving the literacy of community health information had important practical significance.

2 THE URGENCY OF STRENGTHENING HEALTH INFORMATION SERVICES

Recently, people are more concerned the health problem as the continuous improvement of our living standards, and the focus also changed from the center for the treatment of disease to disease prevention and health care management. Accordingly, the request of health information such as medical treatment, disease prevention, health care, rehabilitation etc., is increasing day by day. This led to form a pattern with complicated, personalized and diversified characteristics, and has become the fastest-growing information needs (Li, *et al.*, 2012). For example, Our citizens are most interested in medical and health information about science and technology, and the Interest rates as high as 82.7% (China Association for Science and Technology, 2010). According to the investigate of Jindan Cao to the public library readers, about 87% of the readers have the requirement for health information, 93.4% concerning the health information, and the readers wish to obtain health information from public library can account for 78.5% (Cao et al. 2010). However, the whole level of our people's health literacy is only 6.48%, it is normally lower in the skill of how to obtain the health information and knowledge on matter in the city or village person, especially serious for rural people (The Ministry of Health, 2009). It is urgent and important to promote residents' health information literacy activities for personal health and the public health of the economy and national decisions.

3 THE RESEARCH ADVANCE OF HEALTH INFORMATION SERVICE AT HOME AND ABROAD

Since 2003, the Medical Library Association (MLA) is proposed in the United States for the first time, it caused high attention at home and abroad, and gradually become a research focus in recent years. Health information literacy (HIL) is regarded as one of the key factors for residents health promotion, and its importance is increasingly protruding (Zhang & Du, 2010).

The United States, Britain, and Australia and some other countries attach great importance to the education and service of the public health information literacy research, and they regard the health information literacy as a long-term priority education research for health promotion, with the aim of giving different education contents to different objects. Since the 1990s, The U.S. national library of medicine has completed the transformation of the information to the public health service, which provided professional services not only for medical staff, but also to the public through residents electronic health records and health information services health information, and regard it as a long-term priority in the public health information services and assistance (Shen, 2010). More and more MLAs set up the Consumer Health Librarian (CHL) to develop the public health information consulting services between the patients and the public, to provide health information prescription. It improved the fairness and accessibility of health services better (Hammond, 2005).

Research on the health information literacy in China is still in infancy and research program in the patients and the public health information literacy is still rare (Zhang & Du, 2010). Now, with the popularity of construction of the regional health information platform on the basis of the residents of electronic health records, and the connectivity, business cooperation and information sharing between all kinds of medical institutions at all levels can make people easily to get access to the real-time understanding of people from birth to death of the entire life cycle of health information, such as medical diagnosis and treatment, however, the Internet can not meet the demand of the user's health information completely, and due to the swelling number of health information, health information disordering situation is becoming more and more serious. For general community residents, it is difficult to accurately extract relevant health information in the face of vast amounts of health information data due to the lack of professional retrieval skills. Also, the public is difficult to judge the quality of health information by retrieving (Yuan & Fan, 2012).

The teaching form of our current residents' health information literacy is single, and separate from professional disciplinary education phase. Generally, the low health information consciousness, information ability, information moral and information problems such as lack of legal consciousness is ubiquitous, which cannot meet the demand of comprehensive training residents health information literacy and effectively improve the disease prevention and control ability and the level of public health management. Reflecting the above problems, the poor readability of residents in our country health information, the health information source of fuzzy reliability, and the lack of the evaluation of health information capacity are mainly due to the unclear orientation of information literacy education goals, the misunderstanding of teaching contents and methods, the ignorance of cultivation and training of health information services and information ability to the public, and the lack of effective evaluation system and so on, this have serious influence on the effect and efficiency of promoting public health literacy. To change such status, the professional service person of the field of library and information science must be involved in. In the current wave of big data such as electronic health records, electronic medical records, digital and networking, making our health information concept, system, mechanism and emergency ability face unprecedented challenges. The new growth point of health information demand not only challenges the college library information service, but also takes the opportunity of service innovation at the same time.

4 PRACTICING ACTIVELY AND BUILDING INNOVATION MODEL OF HEALTH INFORMATION SERVICE BASED ON THE WHOLE LIFE CYCLE

At present, the systematic research and practice of the university library information service mode is still very rare, and the systemic health information service mode has not formed. This obviously can't satisfy the requirement of current rapid healthy university library information service development. How to reform the information service mode of university libraries in the era of big data, to meet the users' demand of the growing health information, to provide targeted, diversified and personalized information service, to improve citizen's health information literacy and the ability to obtain and make use of health information has become an important research topic of university libraries. Therefore, we need to learn advanced foreign experience actively, to explore and construct the university library service innovation patterns based on the whole life cycle of health information.

4.1 *To strengthen service mode innovation based on the whole life cycle of health information*

It should follow the requirements of the whole life cycle health management goal, focus on the residents of electronic health records, and take the service health influence factor of the whole process in life as the breakthrough point, to strengthen the innovative construction of the provide and retrieve of library collection in health information, literature information reference service, health service and health information network services, health prescription, health publicity information service, characteristic information service innovation of service methods and other service mode. It also should push the health information service actively into the hospital, into the community, into the family, and into the residents, and it must reflect the trend of integration of professional disciplines in the service content. Finally, to realize the organic unification between the health information service innovation and the ascension of disease prevention skills.

4.2 *To strengthen the construction of sharing health information service based on network database*

The sharing health information service repository should aim at sharing health services information, focusing on creating high-quality goods service resources, facing the vast resource processing, which is an integration of health information resource management platform that storing distributed resources, managing resources, evaluating resources, and managing knowledge. It should combine the regional medical construction goals and objectives, strengthen the construction of synergy innovation mechanism among university library and relevant government departments, industry enterprises (such as medical institutions, health agencies, etc.), integrate the resource in medical and health industry and high quality health information literacy at home and abroad, construct and improve the health information service system that with large capacity, open, interactive, and adapt to the big data network, build the health information service database module with targets and standards, service guide, service evaluation, to achieve the health resource sharing among university library, the government, and the industry, to obtain the latest information from real-time access to health information service, to promote the innovation of information service, to improve health information services level for the community residents for disease control and prevention.

4.3 *To strengthen the construction of health information service team*

The combination of health information services team between full-time and part-time is the key and a concrete guarantee for the implementation of health information service. It should continuously optimize the structure of health information service team, strengthen the training work for professional information services librarian, enlarge the proportion of professional service person, and hire a rich practical experience of frontline positions of medical librarians as part-time health information service librarian to formulate the service plan, progress, and evaluation jointly. It also should research the reform of action-oriented health information service methods and modern ways of service positively, and construct the model teaching methods of interactive health information service that problem-centric (PBL), heuristic, discussion-based, and scenario analysis. According to different stages, different period, different types of service groups and individual services, interactive and health information service for different stages, different period, different types of service groups and individuals, selecting the optimization of service methods and modern ways of service to carry out the corresponding health information push service and service support.

ACKNOWLEDGEMENT

This study was supported by a grant from the Scientific Research Project in the year of 2014 of the Department of Education, Zhejiang province, China (Project number: Y201432688).

REFERENCES

China Association for Science and Technology. The eighth Chinese citizens scientific literacy survey released [EB/OL]. November 25, 2010. http://www.cast.org.cn/n35081/n35473/n35518/12451858.html

Hammond PA. (2005). Consumer health librarian, Reference Services Review, 33(1):38–43.

Jindan Cao, Yan Song, Gang Cao. (2010). Public library consumer health information demand investigation. A medical and social, (11):20 to 22.

Lining Shen. (2010). The present state of health information services in foreign countries scanning and revelation. *Medical information magazine*, 31(6):38–40.

Shijing Zhang, Jian Du. (2010). Health information literacy should be the key point of China council for the promotion of public health literacy. *Medical information magazine*, 31(2):45–49.

The Ministry of Health held the first Chinese residents' health literacy survey conference [EB/OL]. 2014-03-26. http://www.gov.cn/xwfb/2009-12/18/content_1490659.htm

XilinYuan, YingyingFan. (2012). New field information literacy: research and practice of health literacy. *Medical information magazine*, 33(6):2–6.

Yan Li, Jindan Cao, Yuling li, et al. (2102).The public library of diversified health information service mode under the driven of demand. Library science research, (23):57–61.

Yongying Xiao, Lanman He. (2012). Public library health information service research progress abroad. The library construction, (2):54–58.

Medicine Sciences and Bioengineering – Wang (Ed.)
© *2015 Taylor & Francis Group, London, ISBN: 978-1-138-02684-1*

Application of synthetic index method in the evaluation of rational drug use in primary health institutions

Sheng Wang
School of Public Health, Soochow University, Suzhou, China
School of Medical, Hangzhou Normal University, Hangzhou, China

Ge Gao*
School of Public Health, Soochow University, Suzhou, China

ABSTRACT: Objective: To study the application effect of synthetic index method in the evaluation of rational drug use in primary health institutions. Methods Based on random sampling, the prescription of 150 primary health institutions in 15 counties is checked, and the rational drug use in primary health institutions is evaluated with synthetic index method. Results The synthetic indexes of rational drug use in primary health institutions of 15 counties are calculated, then are sorted and stratified according to advantages and disadvantages. Conclusions Synthetic index method is simple, practical and reliable, and can reflect the levels of rational drug use in primary health institutions.

1 INTRODUCTION

World Health Organization (WTO) proposed the concept of rational drug use in 1985. Rational drug use requires that "patients receive medications appropriate to their clinical needs, in doses that meet their own individual requirements, for an adequate period of time, and at the lowest cost to them and their community". The survey of WTO shows the 1/3 of the global patients died of irrational drug use, rather than the disease itself (Geneva, 1993). Irrational drug use has become a global issues that seriously impact on public health, and arouses widespread concern. Rational drug use has extensive content, it relates to variety of drugs, dosage, route of administration, price and other aspects (LI Xintai & WANG Wenhua, 2011). The traditional scoring method is difficult to fully and fairly evaluate the rational drug use in primary health institutions, so the synthetic index method is empirically applied in this paper. The method calculates the synthetic index of rational drug use of different institutions or areas with several core indicators, with a view to a more scientific and reasonable evaluation of the rational drug use performance in different institutions or areas.

2 DATA AND METHODS

2.1 *Data source*

The Multi-stage stratified sampling is used in the survey. 15 counties of Zhejiang Province and 10 primary health institutions of each county are randomly sampled. The 6 days' outpatient prescriptions of the sample institutions are collected, that come from the first Monday of odd months in 2012. 20 prescriptions a day per institution is checked. 18000 prescriptions of 150 primary health institutions in 15 counties are analyzed.

---

*WANG Sheng (1978-), Ph.D. candidate, mainly engaged in epidemiology and health statistics.
 E-mail: wangsheng0925@163.com.
 Correspondence to: Gao Ge; E-mail: gaoge01@suda.edu.cn.

2.2 Research methods

Data are entried and corrected with epidata3.1, analyzed with SPSS13.0. The rational drug use of primary health institutions in 15 counties is evaluated and sorted with the synthetic index method.

3 RESULTS AND ANALYSIS

3.1 The evaluation index system and index value

The core evaluation indicator of rational drug use that developed by WHO and INRUD in 1993, and the domestic and international research results are referenced (FU Wei & SUN Yi, 2004). In this study, the indicator system includes the mean of drug varieties per prescription, the proportion of antibiotic prescriptions, the proportion of hormones prescription, the proportion of injections prescription, the mean of the national essential drugs varieties per prescription, and the average amount of prescription (ZHANG Xinping & YANG Chunyan, 2005). The indicator values of 6 evaluation indexes can be found in Table 1.

3.2 The standardization of the indicator value

The mean of each indicator value of rational drug use in primary health institutions of 15 counties are as a reference value. The means can be found in table 1. In six indicators, the mean of the national essential drugs varieties per prescription is a positive indicator, the other five indicators are negative indicators. The positive indicator according to the formula $Y=X/M$, the negative indicators according to the formula $Y=M/X$ (Y is the standardized value, X is the indicator value, M is the reference value), the standardized indicator values (Y) of each county are calculated and scheduled rank (R). The result can be found in Table 2.

Table 1. The indicator values of evaluation indicators for rational drug use.

County	The mean of drug varieties per prescription	The proportion of antibiotic prescriptions(%)	The proportion of hormones prescription(%)	The proportion of injections prescription(%)	The mean of the national essential drugs varieties per prescription	The average amount of prescription
A	2.97	45.83	5.42	34.86	1.97	66.01
B	2.64	43.83	6.75	33.42	1.51	74.45
C	3.45	59.54	8.89	45.83	2.74	62.57
D	4.45	63.42	11.00	59.17	3.50	40.76
E	2.83	53.37	11.91	48.88	2.19	67.59
F	4.29	64.50	13.83	50.75	3.17	81.65
G	3.46	62.00	21.92	42.50	2.30	56.76
H	3.87	62.80	22.28	41.97	2.37	43.99
I	3.88	59.22	16.67	30.38	2.13	61.67
J	3.08	45.08	11.58	30.92	1.78	93.54
K	3.60	61.33	16.67	38.50	2.13	47.70
L	3.59	64.67	12.75	52.33	2.41	37.25
M	2.85	39.50	7.92	39.42	1.97	46.15
N	3.01	48.17	11.17	32.67	2.43	69.22
O	3.29	59.08	13.25	41.42	2.47	44.35
Mean	3.42	55.49	12.80	41.53	2.34	59.58

Table 2. The standardized values (Y) and ranks (R) of evaluation indicators for rational drug use.

County		The mean of drug varieties per prescription	The proportion of antibiotic prescriptions	The proportion of hormones prescription	The proportion of injections prescription	The mean of the national essential drugs varieties per prescription	The average amount of prescription
A	Y	1.1515	1.2108	2.3616	1.1913	0.8419	0.9059
	R	3	5	6	4	1	2
B	Y	1.2955	1.2660	1.8963	1.2427	0.6453	0.8032
	R	5	4	6	3	1	2
C	Y	0.9913	0.9320	1.4398	0.9062	1.1709	0.9557
	R	4	2	6	1	5	3
D	Y	0.7685	0.8750	1.1636	0.7019	1.4957	1.4671
	R	2	3	4	1	6	5
E	Y	1.2085	1.0397	1.0747	0.8496	0.9359	0.8847
	R	6	4	5	1	3	2
F	Y	0.7972	0.8603	0.9255	0.8183	1.3547	0.7324
	R	2	4	5	3	6	1
G	Y	0.9884	0.8950	0.5839	0.9772	0.9829	1.0536
	R	5	2	1	3	4	6
H	Y	0.8837	0.8836	0.5745	0.9895	1.0128	1.3594
	R	3	2	1	4	5	6
I	Y	0.8814	0.9370	0.7678	1.3670	0.9103	0.9697
	R	2	4	1	6	3	5
J	Y	1.1104	1.2309	1.1054	1.3431	0.7607	0.6393
	R	4	5	3	6	2	1
K	Y	0.9500	0.9048	0.7678	1.0787	0.9103	1.2537
	R	4	2	1	5	3	6
L	Y	0.9526	0.8580	1.0039	0.7936	1.0299	1.6054
	R	3	2	4	1	5	6
M	Y	1.2000	1.4048	1.6162	1.0535	0.8419	1.2958
	R	3	5	6	2	1	4
N	Y	1.1362	1.1520	1.1459	1.2712	1.0385	0.8639
	R	3	5	4	6	2	1
O	Y	1.0395	0.9392	0.9660	1.0027	1.0556	1.3484
	R	4	1	2	3	5	6

3.3 The calculation of weight coefficient

Delphi method and RSR method are used in the calculation. First, the sum of ranks of the indicator value ($\sum$R) are calculated, and according to the formula $RSR = \dfrac{\sum R}{mn}$ (m is the number of indexes, n is the number of institutions) and $SR = \dfrac{RSR}{\sum RSR}$, the rank-sum ratio (RSR) and subtraction ratio(SR) of the evaluation indicators are calculated. Second, 10 experts give their weight to each indicator value, and the arithmetic average are calculated as the experience weights (W'), then according to the formula $W = (SR \cdot W') / \sum(SR \cdot W')$, the weight coefficient of each evaluation indicator (W) is calculated. The result can be found in Table 3.

Table 3. The rank-sum, rank-sum ratio, subtraction ratio, experience weight, weight coefficient of evaluation indicator.

Evaluation indicator	Rank-sum ($\sum R$)	Rank-sum ratio(RSR)	Subtraction ratio(SR)	Experience weight(W')	$SR \cdot W'$	Weight coefficient(W)
the mean of drug varieties per prescription	53	0.5889	0.1683	0.12	0.0202	0.1218
the proportion of antibiotic prescriptions	50	0.5556	0.1587	0.22	0.0349	0.2104
the proportion of hormones prescription	55	0.6111	0.1746	0.16	0.0279	0.1682
the proportion of injections prescription	49	0.5444	0.1555	0.20	0.0311	0.1875
the mean of the national essential drugs varieties per prescription	52	0.5778	0.1651	0.12	0.0198	0.1193
the average amount of prescription	56	0.6222	0.1778	0.18	0.0320	0.1929
total	315	3.5000	1.0000	1.00	0.1659	1.0000

Table 4. The synthetic index of each evaluation indicator, the synthetic index for rational drug use, the results of comprehensive evaluation.

County	The synthetic index of each evaluation indicator (I)						The synthetic index for rational drug use (G)	sort
	The mean of drug varieties per prescription	The proportion of antibiotic prescriptions	The proportion of hormones prescription	The proportion of injections prescription	The mean of the national essential drugs varieties per prescription	The average amount of prescription		
A	0.1403	0.2548	0.3972	0.2234	0.1004	0.1747	1.2908	1
M	0.1462	0.2956	0.2718	0.1975	0.1004	0.2500	1.2615	2
B	0.1578	0.2664	0.3190	0.2330	0.0770	0.1549	1.2081	3
N	0.1384	0.2424	0.1927	0.2384	0.1239	0.1666	1.1024	4
D	0.0936	0.1841	0.1957	0.1316	0.1784	0.2830	1.0664	5
O	0.1266	0.1976	0.1625	0.1880	0.1259	0.2601	1.0607	6
C	0.1207	0.1961	0.2422	0.1699	0.1397	0.1844	1.0530	7
L	0.1160	0.1805	0.1689	0.1488	0.1229	0.3097	1.0468	8
J	0.1352	0.2590	0.1859	0.2518	0.0908	0.1233	1.0460	9
E	0.1472	0.2188	0.1808	0.1593	0.1117	0.1707	0.9885	10
K	0.1157	0.1904	0.1291	0.2023	0.1086	0.2418	0.9879	11
I	0.1074	0.1971	0.1291	0.2563	0.1086	0.1871	0.9856	12
H	0.1076	0.1859	0.0966	0.1855	0.1208	0.2622	0.9586	13
G	0.1204	0.1883	0.0982	0.1832	0.1173	0.2032	0.9106	14
F	0.0971	0.1810	0.1557	0.1534	0.1616	0.1413	0.8901	15

3.4 The results of comprehensive evaluation

According to the formula $I = WY$, the synthetic index (I) of each evaluation indicator is calculated, and according to the formula $G = \sum I$, the synthetic index (G) of each county for rational drug use is calculated. According to the synthetic index (G), 15 counties are sorted for the level of rational drug use. The result can be found in Table 4.

Table 5. The distribution of G and corresponding probit value.

Groups(G)	Median(G)	Frequency	Cumulative frequency	Rank R (R)	Average rank ($\overline{R}$)	$\overline{R}/n$ (%)	Probit Y
0.8901~	0.9226	2	2	1~2	1.5	10.00	3.72
0.9551~	0.9876	4	6	3~6	4.5	30.00	4.48
1.0201~	1.0526	5	11	7~11	9	60.00	5.25
1.0851~	1.1176	1	12	12	12	80.00	5.84
1.1501~	1.1826	1	13	13	13	86.67	6.11
1.2151~	1.2476	1	14	14	14	93.33	6.50
1.2801~	1.3126	1	15	15	15	98.33*	7.13

*Estimated by $\left(1 - \dfrac{1}{4n}\right) \times 100\%$

Table 6. The stratification of 15 counties for rational drug use.

Level	Percentile(P_X)	Probit	Theoretical value of G	Sort results
The good	< P15.866	< 4	<0.929	G, F
The general	P15.866~	4~	0.929~	N, D, O, C, L, J, E, K, I, H
The poor	P84.134~	6~	1.157~	A, M, B

3.5 Reasonable stratification with RSR method

The value of G is divided into several groups by size. The median, frequency, scope of rank, and the average rank of each group are obtained, then the rank-sum ratio ($\overline{R}/n$) and its corresponding probit value (Y) are calculated. To make Y as the independent variable and G as the dependent variable, a regression equation is formed. The equation is $G = 0.114Y + 0.473$. The test proves that the value of G is normal distribution. F = 398.322, P = 0.000 < 0.001, the regression equation is significant. The result can be found in Table 5.

With the stratification requirements of RSR, the level is divided into the good, the general and the poor. Putting the probit value into the regression equation, the theoretical value of G is calculated. With the comparison of theoretical and actual values, the 15 counties are stratified. The result can be find in Table 6. The analysis of variance shows the stratification is effective (F = 45.236, P = 0.000 < 0.001) .

4 DISCUSSION

The synthetic index is a composite indicator with no units of measurement, that can reflect the relative level of things. It is made by a number of indicators with different nature, different types, different levels and even different units of measurement (SU Qiling, 2004). The synthetic index method is to use the synthetic index to fully reflect the comprehensive level of things with different nature and units, and it is an evaluation method that can compare and analyze the different aspects of quality (SUN Zhenqiu, 2006).

In this study rational drug use of primary health institutions in 15 counties are evaluated and sorted with the synthetic index method. The results show, the weight coefficient is determined by Delphi method combined with the RSR method, and give full consideration to the importance of different indicators. The index be calculated can reflect overall level of rational drug use of primary health institutions, and avoid the one-sidedness of different indicators.

The synthetic index method have the advantage of simple, intuitive and effective, as a quantitative assessment tool to evaluate rational drug use of primary health institutions. As long as we can properly grasp two key points in the application, that is establish appropriate indicators system and reasonable weight coefficient, research findings will be intuitive and convincing. This method changes the practice of scoring for areas or institutions based on the subjective impression. It can be horizontal comparison between regions or institutions, point out the weaknesses of them, that will improve rational drug use levels of primary health institutions.

ACKNOWLEDGEMENTS

Supported by the humanities and social science research projects, the Ministry of education of China (11YJC630196).

REFERENCES

FU Wei, SUN Yi & SUN Junan. (2004) Analysis on rational drug use and management measures of rural township hospitals. Chinese Health Economics, 23 (6) : 25–27.
Geneva. (1993) How to investigate drug use in health facilities: Selected drug use indicators. WHO.
LI Xintai, WANG Wenhua & YIN Aitian. (2011) Study on the impact of essential medicine system on rational drug use in township hospitals of Shandong province. Chinese Health Economics, 30 (4) : 22–23.
SUN Zhenqiu. (2006) Medical evaluation method and its application. Beijing,Chemical industry press.
SU Qiling. (2004) The volume of statistics management and health statistics. Beijing, People's Health Publishing House.
ZHANG Xinping & YANG Chunyan. (2005) The research on evaluation indicators of medicines use in rural areas in China. Chinese Primary Health Care, 19 (12) : 12–14.

Medicine Sciences and Bioengineering – Wang (Ed.)
© 2015 Taylor & Francis Group, London, ISBN: 978-1-138-02684-1

Study on near infrared spectroscopy to detect cerebral blood oxygen parameter in computing task

Chuan-jun Guo*

Department of Computer, Harbin Finance University, Harbin, China

ABSTRACT: In order to detect the haemodynamic parameters in the brain, a set of multichannel and dual wavelength system is designed and implemented based on near infrared spectroscopy. The system adopted the array probe and it can be applied for different objects because the measured area and the detecting spacing can be adjusted according to the actual requirement. The software Lab Windows/CVI is selected as the development platform and it has the advantages of good compatibility and real-time performance. The program has a friendly interface between hardware and software. The time resolution of the system is 100 ms and the system can rapidly reflect the change trend of hemodynamic parameters of the brain tissue. Through the *in vivo* monitoring of cerebral hemodynamic parameters in the mathematical logic operation task, the trend of haemoglobin changes is in line with the theory. The experimental results demonstrate that the blood oxygen detection technology based on near infrared spectroscopy can accurately provide haemodynamic information for the research of brain function.

1 INTRODUCTION

With the development of cognitive neuroscience, many novel technologies have been explored to study the neural basis of creativity so as to analyze the mechanism of the brain activity (Karl *et al.*, 2010). The burgeoning technologies for brain activity detection mainly include electroencephalogram (EEG), event-related potential (ERP), positron emission tomography (PET), functional magnetic resonance imaging (fMRI). Functional near infrared spectroscopy (fNIRS) is one of the brain activity measurement technologies and it has many advantages such as noninvasive, small volume, low power consumption and low cost. fNIRS has now been gradually becoming one of the research hotspots in biomedical fields (Saager, 2008). At present, near infrared spectroscopy has been utilized to monitor the oxygenation state of the brain tissue and the skeletal muscle, evaluate the cerebral function by detecting human cerebral blood oxygenation in cognition, and assess the drug therapeutic effect, and estimate the blood flow and blood oxygen in a plastic surgery procedure.

The neural activity in the brain can convert into the blood flow and the cerebral metabolism information. Near infrared spectroscopy can be used to measure the haemodynamic information and then indirectly assess the cerebral cortical activity (Robertson *et al.*, 2010). Near infrared spectroscopy has presented the potential in neurology area and clinical diagnosis of the nervous system diseases. In the present study, a set of multichannel dual-wavelength NIRS system has been designed based on the modified Lambert-Beer Law and the relevant blood oxygen detection theory. The system is then implemented to study the change of the haemodynamic information during the computing task.

---

*The corresponding email is guochuanjun82@126.com.

2 FIRST HEADING

The near infrared possessing 650–1000 nm range is defined as "optical window". In this NIR region, the absorption coefficient of biological tissue is limited in the range of 0.01-1 mm⁻¹. The NIR light can penetrate skin and skull, and can reach several centimeters' depth in the cerebral tissue (Luu & Chau, 2009). The diffuse reflection will occur due to scatter effect and the light density will be detected by photoelectric sensor. By detecting the diffused light, the very useful information like tissue parameter can be acquired (Ren et al., 2010).

In Physiology, Optical density (OD) refers to the absorption stage of light. According to Lambert-Beer law, the intensity of incident light is I_{input}, the intensity of output light is I_{output}, then the relation of the incident light and the output light (Zhang et al., 2012) can be expressed as formula (1):

$$OD = \lg \frac{1}{T} = \lg \frac{I_{input}}{I_{output}} \tag{1}$$

Lambert-Beer Law cannot accurately describe the relation in biological tissue since the biological tissue is a highly scattering turbid. Taking into diffusion scatter, the photons have a longer transmission path and this increase the probability to be absorbed. Some researchers considered the multiple scattering and attenuation into the highly scattering medium. They described the light path in biological tissue with the average differential optical path. Thus there is the following equation:

$$OD = \log(\frac{I_{input}}{I_{output}}) = DPF \cdot d \sum_i \varepsilon_i \cdot c_i + G \tag{2}$$

where DPF is differential path-length factor and it is correlated with the light wavelength, absorption coefficient, scattering coefficient and scattering phase. DPF shows the increment of the light path caused by scattering effect; ε_i is the molar absorptivity, determined by wavelength and light absorbing property of medium, its unit can be $mM^{-1} \cdot cm^{-1}$ or $mM^{-1} \cdot mm^{-1}$ (M is molarity), c_i is the molarity of the medium; G is the attenuation factor about the effect of the uppermost tissue layer, including its optical properties and physical structure. The change of the optical density was considered, and the expression for blood oxygen change was calculated with the actual wavelength of 760 nm and 850 nm:

$$\begin{bmatrix} \Delta C_{HbO_2} \\ \Delta C_{Hb} \end{bmatrix} = \begin{bmatrix} -0.0552 & 0.0979 \\ 0.0815 & -0.0351 \end{bmatrix} \begin{bmatrix} \Delta OD^{760nm} \\ \Delta OD^{850nm} \end{bmatrix} \tag{3}$$

where ΔC_{HbO2} and ΔC_{Hb} are the change in the concentration of oxyhaemoglobin and deoxyhaemoglobin, respectively.

3 DESIGN OF THE NIRS SYSTEM

The NIR system includes the optical probe, the upper computer and the detection circuit. The detection circuit is the main part of the system and it is used to obtain the electronic signal from the probe and filter out high frequency interference. The circuit can also amplify the analog signal, realize analog-to-digital conversion and communicate data between upper computer and the circuit. The optical probe consisting of LEDs and photoelectric sensors can be used to obtain optical signal from specified tissue. The upper computer can process optical signal, store data and display the waveform.

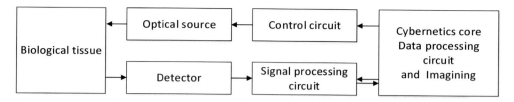

Figure 1.　Schematic of the NIRS system.

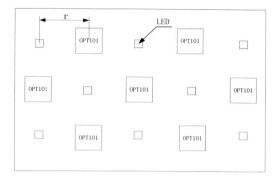

Figure 2.　Sensor distribution of the probe.

The hardware of the system is shown in Figure 1. In this system, TB62726, an application specific integrated circuit, is used as the driving circuit of the dual-wavelength LEDs (760 nm and 850 nm). The photodiodes OPT101 is produced by BURR-BROWN. It can receive the optical signal and also change the optical signal into electrical information. Then the signal is amplified and filtered by analog circuit, which is designed to limit the signal to meet the threshold condition of A/D. C8051F020, an on-chip module, generates and sends digital signal to upper computer. The data are processed in upper computer. The results are analyzed and displayed with the software Labwindow/CVI. The distribution of LEDs and detectors in the probe is shown in Figure 2. The small boxes represent the LEDs and the big boxes represent the detectors. According to different individuals and measured sites, probe can be used to measure different area by controlling the sequence of the electric current.

The software possesses two functions: controlling main circuit and collecting signals in lower computer software; imagining the blood oxygen and blood volume by calculating in upper computer. The software includes the following module: (1) drive modular; (2) A/D conversion module; (3) data processing module; (4) data storing module; (5) data display module. Lower computer software directs the hardware initialization, constant current driving, data collecting, A/D conversion, data processing and serial communication. Upper software is developed in LabWindows/CVI, and its program editing bases on biologically measuring principal. Thus the change of hemoglobin concentration can be monitored. Figure 3 shows the software design of upper computer.

4　RESULTS

The human brain can be divided into different areas, such as the processing center for thought, langue, memory, sensory information, and movement. The functions of different centers vary from each other. By using the brain-monitoring technology, the specific brain functionality for different cerebral area can be known more intuitively. Cerebral blood volume would change during physical activity and the change will represent the cerebral activity intensity. The cerebral activity could therefore be analyzed.

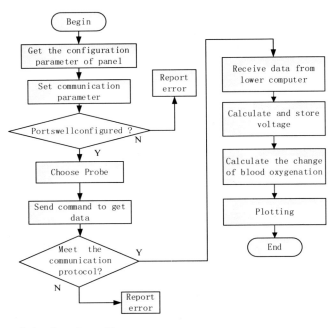

Figure 3.   Software design flow chart of lower computer.

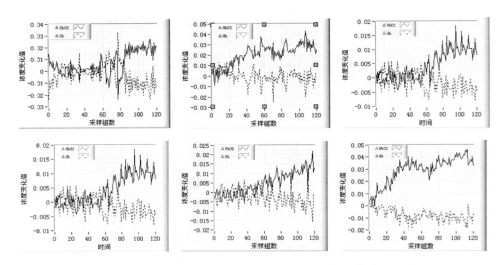

Figure 4.   The change of hemodynamic parameters during logical-mathematical computing.

In this study, each volunteer was arranged complex computing task and kept computing during a full experimental period. During the test, volunteers should keep relaxed posture and focus on computing in quiet and low-light space at room temperatures. Because the irrelevant stimulation should be weakened to avoid that averted vision brings about false reaction. And Mental Arithmetic is used as training software.

Figure 4 shows the real-time information of hemodynamic parameters in six channels. The full line is the oxyhaemoglobin and dotted line is deoxyhaemoglobin. From the figure it can be known that total hemoglobin and oxyhaemoglobin increases, but deoxyhaemoglobin decreases when the brain is activated. With the text last, the activated cerebral area will have stronger movement. The results of study match the reasoning about hemodynamic parameters on physiology. Now there is no any research achievement have been got inland. But some existing literature indicates that the activated area in brain will be different from the people with various mother tongue. There is more studies in this field should be scheduled. In a word, the results of this study correspond the theory on the metabolic tendency of hemodynamic parameters. So that, this NIR system in study can be used to monitor cerebral movement.

5 DISCUSSION

The present study here bases on the modified Lambert-Beer Law. The continuous wave spectroscopy was adopted and a set of multichannel and dual wavelength system is designed and implemented. Through the in vivo monitoring of cerebral hemodynamic parameters in the mathematical logic operation task, the blood-oxygen detection system can be evaluated. The experiment demonstrated that the system can provide the haemodynamic information with a relatively high time resolution. In the further research, more relevant physiological stimulation can be studied according specific cognitive demand, and this could help monitoring the cerebral function in clinical psychological research.

ACKNOWLEDGMENTS

The authors are grateful for the support from the Science and Technique Key Project of Heilongjiang province (No. GC12C108) and the project from Science and Technology Department of Heilongjiang Province (No. GZ13A005).

REFERENCES

Karl F, Ashburner J, Stefan Kiebel. (2010) Statistical Parametric Mapping: The Analysis of Functional Brain Images, 3–10.
Luu S, T. (2009) Decoding subjective preference from single-trial near-infrared spectroscopy signals. Journal of neural engineering, 2009, 6:016003.
Ren N, Liang J, Qu X, Li J, Lu B, Tian J. (2010) GPU-based Monte Carlo simulation for light propagation in complex heterogeneous tissues. OPTICS EXPRESS, 18(7):6811–6823.
Robertson F C, Douglas T S, Meintjes E M. (2010) Motion Artifact Removal for Functional Near Infrared Spectroscopy: A Comparison of Methods. IEEE Transactions on Biomedical Engineering, 57(6):1377–1387.
Saager R. (2008) Corrected near-infrared Spectroscopy C-NIRS: An optical system for extracting hemodynamic signatures unique to the brain. Ph.D Dissertion of University of Rochester, 96–160.
Zhang Y, Sun J, Rolfe P. (2012) RLS adaptive filtering for physiological interference reduction in NIRS brain activity measurement: a Monte Carlo study. Physiological Measurement, 33(6):925–942.

Medicine Sciences and Bioengineering – Wang (Ed.)
© *2015 Taylor & Francis Group, London, ISBN: 978-1-138-02684-1*

Differences in medical education teaching between China and Japan

Shu Jing
Affiliated Hospital of Beihua University, Jilin City, China

Wei-jing Sun, Jian-guang Chen[1] & He Li[2]
College of Pharmacy, Beihua University, Jilin City, China

ABSTRACT: There are some differences in history, culture, custom, social background and so on among different nationalities. The differences in the concrete process of some teaching links, such as teaching management, teaching syllabus, lecture, setting paper and test, in Chinese and Japanese medicine colleges and universities are compared and analyzed.

1   INTRODUCTION

There are some differences in history, culture, custom, social background and so on among different nationalities. It leads to differences in the educational system, education pattern as well as course contents among them (Wu *et al.*, 2011, Zhang *et al.*, 2011, Zhang et al., 2012). In this paper, we tried to compare and study the differences in the concrete process of some teaching links, such as teaching management, teaching syllabus, lecture, setting paper and test, in Chinese and Japanese medicine colleges and universities, and find out its positives and negatives so as to abandon its disadvantage and profit from its advantage. Our observation, several proposals and viewpoints are put forward here.

2   SYLLABUS AND TEXTBOOK

In our country, each specialty has the uniform syllabus and textbook, and teachers have to follow the syllabus for teaching, and students have to read the textbook during the lecture. In Japan, there is no uniform syllabus and textbook, and in general, teachers recommend several textbooks to their students, but not mandatory to read the uniform textbook and even not any textbook during the lecture; teachers select teaching materials from different textbooks including the textbook used in some foreign countries such as the United States; copy the selected material, especially some related figures and tables, and distribute the materials for reference to the students who attend a lecture time just before each lecture; generally, teachers do not carry on the explanation from the beginning to the end only by virtue of a set of teaching materials. Compared to those described above in China, we think that there are some merits and also some demerits in those in Japan. The merit includes: (1) it is advantageous for the student to expand their visions and understand different academic style from different teaching material and (2) it is advantageous for the student to develop a self-study habit to study independently since they have to read these teaching materials from different sources in order to prepare for the test; the shortcoming includes: (1) what the student learn is not insufficiently systematized and normalized, and (2) the elementary knowledge of the students is not comprehensive and solid enough.

---

[1] Mr Jianguang Chen is the corresponding author of this article, and His email address is 644257703@qq.com.
[2] Miss He Li is the corresponding author of this article, and Her email address is yitonglh@126.com.

3 EXPERIMENTAL TEACHING

What we have done in experimental teaching includes: (1) the content is formulated in the syllabus; (2) the experimental item is approximate in the same major; (3) in general, the experimental preparation is carried out by the teacher; (4) most of students have no opportunity to do experiments except the experimental content formulated in the syllabus. However, in Japan, the experimental teaching is quite different from us, what they have done is: (1) the experimental content is not restricted and is determined by the teachers in individual department; (2) the experimental item is not approximate in the same major and the teacher determines it based on the research work or the experimental methods having established in his laboratory; (3) the experimental preparation is performed by students themselves, which means the students finish their experiments independently from the beginning to the end.

4 PRACTICE OUTSIDE CLASSROOM TEACHING

In Japan, the students after completing the theoretical and experimental learning of each course in the classroom, they must enter the faculty working office and laboratory for several months. Under the instruction of the teachers, each student can independently select a research thesis based on the research work in the department, design the experimental protocol, conduct the operation, analyze and summarize the result, write the paper and publish in a magazine or in a paper collection. However, most of medical students in our country have no such training process except the graduation practice. The reason why Chinese medical students have no such opportunity to be trained well is, in part, that some objective conditions restrict us to do so, such as too many medical students received in medical colleges and universities. The objective reason certainly can confine us to give the students opportunity to practice in a laboratory, but there are also some subjective reasons affect us to do so. We can also try our best to overcome the objective restriction positively to create some conditions for our students. For example, the similar method like Japanese may be adopted to train the students from the specialties in which there are a few students, and the students from other specialties can be trained in turn by stages in departments and laboratories; the establishment of a open laboratory is a good way to make up our deficiency; the students should be encouraged to take part in the research work of graduates and teachers during spare time. In any case, a teacher' duty is to teach his students well and perhaps he can achieve his goal if he tries his best enough.

5 CONCLUSION

The differences in the concrete process of some teaching links, such as teaching management, teaching syllabus, lecture, setting paper and test, in Chinese and Japanese medicine colleges and universities are compared and analyzed. We try to find out its positives and negatives so as to abandon its disadvantages and profit from its advantages. There are some points which are worth us profiting from Japan in the experimental teaching. The Japanese medical students have more time to practice in the scientific thinking, selection of research thesis, designing thesis, experimental performance, analysis of experimental data, summarizing the result and writing paper, suggesting that in this way, they can be trained well in scientific thinking, innovative and skilled abilities, and it is beneficial to the education of students, especially medical students. It is believed that we cannot mimic all aspects in the teaching management in foreign countries because there are many differences between China and any other foreign countries, but we can profit from them by imitating their good methods having been verified.

REFERENCES

Wu B, Wang S & Yu X. S.(2011) Present State of Education and Medical Services of General Practice in Japan.*Chinease general practice* 14(04):1115–1116.

Zhang F. Q., Wang C. Y, Su Y, & Wang N(2011) Comparison of oral medical education between Japan and China. *Beijing Journal of Stomatology* 19(06):349–350.

Zhang Y. Q. &Yu S. C.(2012) Analysis and enlightenment of medical undergraduate curriculum planning in Japan. *China higher medical education* (01):123–125.

Medicine Sciences and Bioengineering – Wang (Ed.)
© *2015 Taylor & Francis Group, London, ISBN: 978-1-138-02684-1*

Improvement of medical students' cultivation in international exchange

Xu-dong Qiu
Affiliated Hospital of Beihua University, Jilin City, China

Wei-jing Sun
College of Pharmacy, Beihua University, Jilin City, China

Wei-yan Zhao, Xing-xu Du & Shi-wei Zhao*
Affiliated Hospital of Beihua University, Jilin City, China

ABSTRACT: In the present study, the experience in the exchange of our university with Crimea State Medical University in Ukraine is summarized and discussed, including the medical teaching procedures and the examining and assessing system. The internationalization of higher education has been a current tendency and has been developed in many countries and areas, and the internationalization level of their own education has been improved through the different way now. What they have done in medical teaching in Ukraine should give us some enlightenment on our medical teaching. It is concluded that the emphasis in the practical teaching on the basis of understanding of some basic theoretical knowledge, the great attention paid to the assessment on the students' performance in the normal days and the implementation of a strict teaching procedure, and an strict examining and assessing system are beneficial in cultivating more outstanding medical students and outstanding doctors in the future, and medical students could further improve in the internationalization consciousness, English proficiency, knowing of the academic trend in medicine as well as the distinct learning way through the international exchange since it is advocated no longer to work quietly and diligently oneself alone and an effective exchange could let conducive to each other.

1 INTRODUCTION

The internationalization of higher education is a current tendency. Many countries and areas have vigorously developed the internationalization level of their own education through the different way now. The international status of colleges or universities may be enhanced, their works may be brought in line with the international practice and more new international information may be achieved by them (Yin Hao, 1995). Medicine is a practical science, and the cultivation of the students' abilities in research and creativity can promote the development in medicine (Zhang Dan & Ding Meiping, 2010). Strengthening the international exchange is supposed to be able to widen the field of students' vision and improve the practical ability of the students. In our university, the exchange with Crimea State Medical University in Ukraine has been developed in recent years, in which the students in our university and in Crimea State Medical University have been able to exchange visits and practice in clinic for a short term. The improvement of international exchange in the medical students has played a positive role in elevating the medical teaching level, improving the comprehensive quality of the medical students, and raising the students' communicative

---

*Shiwei Zhao is the corresponding author of this article, and his email address is 413437244@qq.com.

and innovative abilities in our university. In the present study, the experience in the exchange of our university with Crimea State Medical University in Ukraine is summarized.

2 THE NEED FOR BUILDING THE INNOVATIVE PERSONNEL TRAINING PLATFORM

2.1 *Focus on practical teaching*

One of the distinguishing features of medical education in Ukraine is to pay great attention to the students' cultivation in practice particularly. For example, it was found by us during the exchange that the specimen was often made by the students themselves in the anatomical teaching, suggesting that the students trained in this way could have a strong ability in practice, their fundamental skills should be reliable and the operation should play a solid foundation for their scientific research work in the future to make them quickly get involved in the clinical work as soon as they begin their clinical practice.

In Ukraine, the students in medical colleges or universities began to study clinical courses from the third year and the place for teaching them clinical specialized knowledge (for example, internal medicine department, surgery and so on) was arranged at the teaching hospital, in which first teachers taught their students in the classroom and then led them to observe patients, including asking them about their illness and making a physical examination on them and so on. In this way, the students could achieve the training in the combination of specialized knowledge with the clinical practice on the same day. Moreover, in the operating room of a teaching hospital, the operation procedure was designed to be easily seen by the students since the ceiling over the operating table and the wall surrounding the operating room were made of glass, and were transparent. Just from the beginning of their learning surgery, their students had the opportunity to watch the surgery process and the aseptic performance and so on, even the opportunity to attend a surgery. There were regular related seminars there every week, in which the theory was explained in combination with the clinical practice to make the students' applied ability become strong and achieve the goal to study for uses. The students were asked to practice in clinic for a certain time during each winter vacation and summer vacation and the practical content was from the easy to the deep. It is believed that such an access to the clinical practice as what happened in Ukraine and a learning of it at the very beginning should help the students to understand the characteristics of various clinical departments.

2.2 *Teaching in a small class and emphasizing in the communication*

When we visited the classrooms in Crimea State Medical University in Ukraine, we found that all students were taught by the teachers in a small class. There were only 7–10 students in each class in the university. In this way, the teachers could know each student well and have more opportunities to communicate with, indicating that the teachers and classmates might have more time to exchange in the study. Especially during the discussion class, the students were permitted to freely ask any questions to the teacher, express their own viewpoints, even to query what the teacher said, and the students were given a certain score according to its performance each time during the class and recorded as the regular grade. The regular grade was considered to be a very important inspection standard for a student in a college or university in Ukraine so that most students were generally willing to preparing for the communication in the class positively and earnestly. We can know from what we have seen in Ukraine that in a classroom with a natural and vivid atmosphere, and supplemented by the corresponding test, the students may be able to read, investigate and explore what they consider to be important, and gradually develop a learning method and habit to observe, think and judge independently.

The students' application ability in English was generally strong in Ukraine since a teaching environment was created, and they were encouraged positively and warmly to exchange with the students from foreign countries or other place in English in order to achieve the teaching of internationalization truly. The students from India and African countries enrolled in Crimea brought some overseas cultural atmosphere. The foreign students studied with Ukraine students together, discussed questions, communicate each other very well in the clinical practice and some of them stayed for the further graduate study after they graduated as undergraduate students in the university. It is concluded that an excellent medical teaching system and the atmosphere should be very important to the internationalization of a college or university according to our exchange experience in Crimea State Medical University in Ukraine.

2.3 *Examination system: emphasizing in the presence and the multiformity in the examination and evaluation*

In Ukraine, the roll-call was a convention in each class. Any student's absence from class must be reasonably explained, and the student was permitted to leave by showing the application for leave, and he or she had to go to see the department head to receive a bill in which he or she was required to pay for the making-up for the missed lesson list because the university required that all students should not miss any class absolutely. If a student missed class many times, the university was authorized not to arrange the student to participate in the terminal examination even if he or she had made up for the missed lessons in time, and the reason was that the student had no sense of responsibility and was not serious in the study. Otherwise, the students who were always extremely diligent would be given a very high score and a good comprehensive evaluation even if their intelligences were average and their theory test results were somewhat low. In each class, some review questions were put to students and the result of asking questions was considered when the final result by the end of the term was given, indicating that this way could help the students not only better understand the key content but also supervise the student to review what they had learned after class. There was a test for each unit after it was finished and its result was also considered when the final result by the end of the term was given. The five-grade marking system was implemented in the universities of Ukraine, regardless of a required course examination or a selected course examination, two ways, namely the written examination and the oral examination, were carried out to examine the students, which was believed to reflect the situation accurately in which how the student understood the specialized knowledge. There were two national unification examinations for medical undergraduates and those who failed in three make-up tests would be expelled from school. We found that students' test scores were displayed in public on a bulletin board outside the department. It can be deduced that a doctor with a high quality may be raised through carrying out the strict examining and assessing system in the medical schools in Ukraine.

3 DIFFERENCES IN MEDICAL TEACHING IN CHINA FROM THOSE IN UKRAINE

In contrast to those in Ukraine, the students have no enough opportunities to practice in the teaching of basic medicine. For example, the students learn anatomy by observing the specimen, but rarely participate in the specimen preparation; The clinical medicine course is completed in class, and the break practice time is limited and the test content is not strictly close to the practice relation, leading to the poor performance in the combination of the theoretical knowledge with the practice although they can grasp the medical theory very well. In recent years, foreign students from different countries have been enrolled in colleges and universities in our country so that the perfection of the teaching process and the examining and assessment system is important. We should adopt both a strict teaching procedure, and an examining and assessing system to cultivate more outstanding doctors.

4 CONCLUSIONS

The internationalization of higher education is a current tendency. Many countries and areas all have vigorously developed the internationalization level of their own education through the different way now. What they have done in medical teaching in Ukraine should give us some enlightenment on our medical teaching. It is concluded that the emphasis in the practical teaching on the basis of understanding of some basic theoretical knowledge, the great attention paid to the assessment on the students' performance in the normal days and the implementation of a strict teaching procedure, and an strict examining and assessing system are beneficial to cultivating more outstanding doctors, and medical students could be further improved in the internationalization consciousness, English proficiency, knowing of the academic trend in medicine as well as the distinct learning way through the international exchange since it is advocated no longer to work quietly and diligently oneself alone and an effective exchange could let each other win-win (Zhang Meng & Sun Fuchuan, 2006).

REFERENCES

Yin Hao. (1995). International exchange system of medical students. *Foreign Mdical Sciences (Medical Education)*, 16(3), 44–48.
Zhang Dan, Ding Meiping. (2010) Survey-based analysis of the international exchange programs on medical students' international medical education. *Northwest Medical Education*, 18(2), 221–223.
Zhang Meng, Sun Fuchuan. (2006) Higher education internationalization with medical student's education for all-round development. *Chinese Medical Ethics*, 19: 59–60.

Medicine Sciences and Bioengineering – Wang (Ed.)
© 2015 Taylor & Francis Group, London, ISBN: 978-1-138-02684-1

Optimization for fundus molecular imaging

Yu-Hong Liu
Chengdu Medical University, Chengdu, Sichuan, China

Ping Zhang
Chongqing Medical University, Chongqing, China

Dan-mei Xie
Shanghai Dianji University, Shanghai, China

Ti-chun Wang & Zheng-xiang Xie*
Chongqing Medical University, Chongqing, China

ABSTRACT: Fundus molecular imaging is an imaging modus under a special environment. Generally, there are two types of an autoflourescence imaging excited by Blue laser (488nm) and infrared laser (787nm), briefly called B-AFI and IR-AFI. An optimization method for the two types of images was reported in this text.

1 INTRODUCTION

Fundus molecular imaging is an imaging modus under a special environment. Generally, there are two types of the special imaging modi, which are an autoflourescence imaging (emission > 500 nm which belong to visible light) excited by Blue laser (488nm) and an autoflourescence imaging (emission > 800 nm which belong to invisible-near infrared light) stimulated by infrared laser (787nm) (Kellner, *et al.*, 2010; Keilhauer, *et al.*, 2006; Schmitz-Valckenberg, *et al.*, 2008), briefly called B-AFI and IR-AFI. These two imaging modi are not a simultaneous imaging for whole field but a raster scan imaging. This is not a reflection imaging like fundus color photo but an emission imaging. Due to imaging under a lower liuminance therefore making the noise higher, the noise has to be removed by means of frame superposition before the resulting image is completed.

It is well known that the autoflourescence possesses visible wide-band spectrum in B-AFI modus and the image corresponds to lipofuscin concentration in B-AFI. Paper (Keilhauer, et al., 2006) pointed out that the image reflects to melanin concentration in the IR-AFI. Whereas fundus color photo corresponds to the fundus retinal reflection coefficient. Therefore B-AFI and IR-AFI are called fundus molecular imaging or retina molecular imaging.

Since the imaging environment is worse and the imaging light is weaker, the visual quality of resulting image is lower so that the image had to finish an optimal processing to make human vision comfortable. We will describe the optimization of retina molecular imaging and assessment for its quality in the next.

2 BASIC TOOLS

2.1 *Zadeh-X transformation*

We called the following adaptive-optimal transformation used to optimized image the adaptive Zadeh-X transformation (Xie et al 2007; Xie *et al.*, 2013, Xie *et al.*, 2010).

---

*The corresponding author is ZX Xie and his Email is bmezxxie@163.com.

$$T_{Opt}(i,x,y) = k \frac{O_{Std}(i,x,y) - Theta}{Delta_{Opt}} + Theta, \quad i = 0,1,2 \tag{1}$$

The constraint condition is as follows.

$$T_{Opt}(i,x,y) = \begin{cases} 255, & T_{Opt}(i,x,y) > 255 \\ \\ 0, & T_{Opt}(i,x,y) < 0 \end{cases} \quad i = 0,1,2 \tag{2}$$

where k is called an expansion or a contraction factor, here let $k = 255$. $i = 0,1,2$ represents three color channels of the red, the green and the blue in an image, respectively(the same below). O_{Std} (i, x, y) and $T_{Std}(i, x, y)$ represent chromatic value of a pixel point (x,y) before and after transformation at i^{th} channel of an iamge, respectively. $Theta \in [0,255]$ and $Delta_{Opt \in}[1,255]$ are called transformation parameters. The transformed image is just the original image when $Theta = 0$, $Delta_{Opt} = 255$. When $Delta = 1$, formula (1) with (2) denotes a binarization transform.

The $Delta_{Opt}$ is called the optimal transformation parameter and defined as follows.

$$Delta_{Opt} = 4 * Abs(Theta - AL_{Std})^{0.857} \begin{cases} AL_{Std} > 127.5, & Theta = 255 \\ AL_{Std} \leq 127.5, & Theta = 0 \end{cases} \tag{3}$$

where subscript "Std" means standardization. AL_{Std} presents the averaging liuminance of a standardized image. An image with full bandwidth gray/chromatic spectrum (see below) is called a standardization image.

2.2 *No reference image quality assessment function*

We proposed a universal no reference image quality assessment function, *UNAF*, that possesses the convex characteristics and whose maximum corresponds to the most optimal quality image as follows (Xie *et al.*, 2013, Xie *et al.*, 2010).

$$UNAF = AIE * AC^{1/2} * NNF * AHF * ABWF \tag{4}$$

Where *AIE, AC, NNF, AHF* and *ABWF* were called averaging information entropy, averaging contrast, normalized neighboring function, averaging hierarchical factor and averaging bandwidth factor of an image. They were called the visual quality parameters of an image. Their weighted exponents were determined by sample trials with great number. About the detailed information of the five parameters, please refer to the references at the paper end.

3 RESULTS FOR OPTIMIZING IMAGES

The results for optimized images of fundus molecular imaging were described in figure 1. The main visual parameters and UCAF value of all images of fundus molecular imaging are listed from 1 to 10 columns in table 1. The major feature parameters of gray spectra of all mages of fundus molecular imaging are listed form 10 to 12 columns in table 1. All gray spectra are with 4th flattening order. Fig. a) and c) are a normal B-AFI image with non full band gray spectrum and an optimized image of a) with full band gray spectrum, respectively. Fig. e) and g) are a normal IR-AFI image with non full band gray spectrum and an optimized image of e) with full band gray spectrum, respectively. Fig. i) and k) are an abnormal B-AFI image with non full band gray spectrum and an optimized image of e) with full band gray spectrum, respectively. Fig. n) and q) are an abnormal IR-AFI

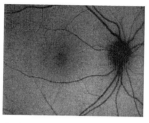

a) Normal B-AFI(chen-OS)

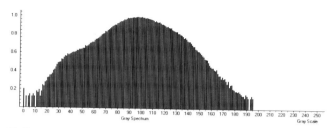

b) Gray spectrum with non full band and 4th flattening order of a)

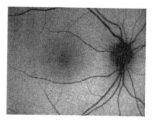

c) Optimized image of a)

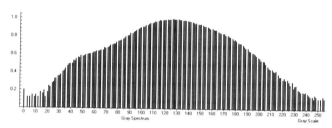

d) Gray spectrum with full band and 4th flattening order of c)

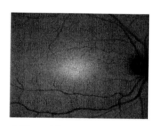

e) Normal IR-AFI (Kellner, *et al.*, 2010)

f) Gray spectrum with non full band and 4th flattening order of e)

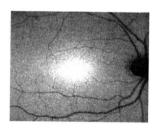

g) Optimized image of e)

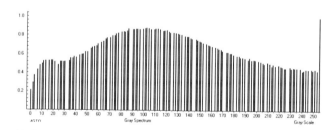

h) Gray spectrum with full band and 4th flattening order of g)

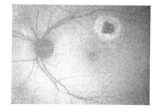

i) Abnormal B-AFI of a man 76 years old

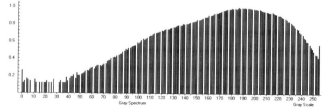

j) Gray spectrum with full band and 4th flattening order of i)

Figure 1.   Images of fundus molecular imaging and their gray spectra with 4th flattening order (*Continued*)

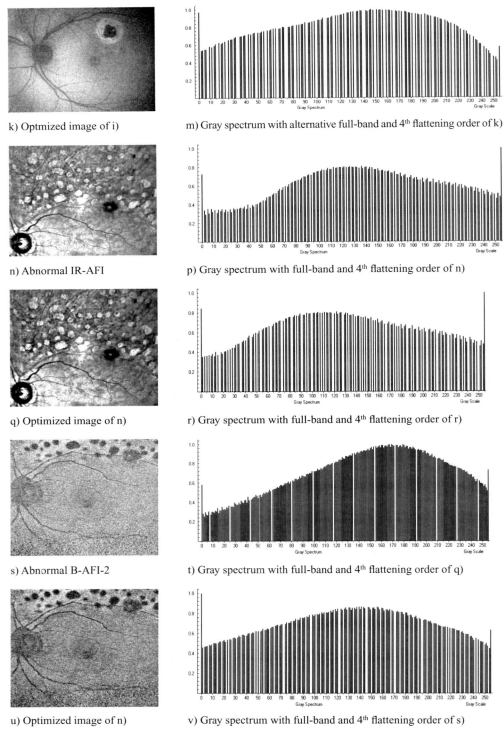

k) Optmized image of i)

m) Gray spectrum with alternative full-band and 4th flattening order of k)

n) Abnormal IR-AFI

p) Gray spectrum with full-band and 4th flattening order of n)

q) Optimized image of n)

r) Gray spectrum with full-band and 4th flattening order of r)

s) Abnormal B-AFI-2

t) Gray spectrum with full-band and 4th flattening order of q)

u) Optimized image of n)

v) Gray spectrum with full-band and 4th flattening order of s)

Figure 1.   Images of fundus molecular imaging and their gray spectra with 4th flattening order. (*Continued*)

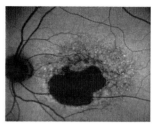

w)Abnormal B-AFI-2(Schmitz, et al. 2008)

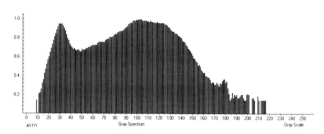

x) Gray spectrum with non full-band and 4ᵗʰ flattening order of u)

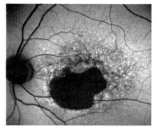

y) Optimized image of u)

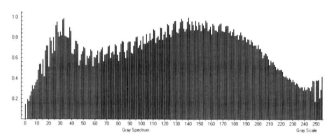

z) Gray spectrum with full-band and 4ᵗʰ flattening order of w)

Figure 1.   Images of fundus molecular imaging and their gray spectra with 4ᵗʰ flattening order.

Table 1.   Main visual parameters and UNAF values and spectral parameters.

| Visual parameters of an image | | | | | | | | | | spectral parameters | |
Im	AIE	AC	AL	AHF	ABWF	NNF	AIE*AC$^{1/2}$	UNAF	Note	Im	Peak value	Peak position.
a)	6.7535	9.4565	97.6696	0.7461	0.7656	0.7660	20.7680	9.0877	Ori	b)	253205	96,3975
c)	6.7535	12.3654	127.7212	0.7461	1.0000	0.9983	23.7484	17.6877	Op	d)	253205	126,3975
e)	6.7277	10.1399	62.0140	0.8203	0.8281	0.4864	21.4105	7.0743	Or	f)	114244	54,2185
g)	6.5455	18.7614	116.7516	0.5195	1.0000	0.9157	28.3515	13.4877	Op	h)	114244	255,3586
i)	6.8508	10.0685	179.9085	0.7734	1.0000	0.5890	21.7383	9.9022	Or	j)	306774	186,4417
k)	6.7884	15.5804	137.0410	0.5195	1.0000	0.9157	26.7953	12.8792	Op	m)	306774	146,4417
n)	6.8880	8.3094	143.1955	0.6367	1.0000	0.8796	19.8553	11.0859	Or	p)	313311	255,10043
q)	6.8419	9.2216	130.2479	0.5703	1.0000	0.9784	20.7768	11.5938	Op	r)	313311	255,10043
s)	7.3486	25.4707	162.8491	0.9453	1.0000	0.7228	37.0871	25.3388	Or	t)	272000	179,2955
u)	7.2435	32.8559	133.8220	0.7188	1.0000	0.9504	41.5201	28.3628	Op	v)	272000	0,5209
w)	6.9510	5.2045	92.5259	0.8633	1.0000	0.7257	15.9941	7.8858	Or	x)	172966	103,2400
y)	6.9466	7.9413	123.9505	0.6667	1.0000	0.9722	19.5758	12.6872	Op	z)	172966	140,2052

Note Im: Image number; Or: Original image; Op: Optimized image.

image with full band gray spectrum and an optimized image of e) with full band gray spectrum, respectively. The others are the abnormal images and the corresponding optimized images.

After optimization, there are such variations as that the contrast, NNF, UNAF of each optimized image are bigger than its corresponding original image, AL tends to 127.5, and gray spectra are more flattening. Increase of UNAF demonstrates that the visual quality of the optimized image is better than the original.

ACKNOWLEDGEMENTS

Authors thank national natural science foundation committee of china for supporting this work (Grant No. 60975008). We thank Miss XY Xue for her image manipulations and thank Miss MM Chen for her help.

REFERENCES

Kellner, U, Kellner S, Weinitz S. Fundus Autofluorescence (488 nm) and Near-Infrared Auto-fluorescence (787 nm) Visualize Different Retinal Pigment Epithelium Alterations in Patients with Age-Related Macular Degeneration. *Retina, 2010; 30(1):6–15.*

Keilhauer, C N and Delori, F C. Near-Infrared Autofluorescence Imaging of the Fundus: Visualization of Ocular Melanin. *Investigative Ophthalmology & Vision Science (IOVS), 2006; 47(8): 3556–3564.*

Schmitz-Valckenberg, S, Holz, F G, Alan C. Bird, A C and Spade,R F. Fundus Autofluorescence Imaging, Review and Perspectives. *Retina, 2008; 28(3):385–409.*

Xie, Z X, Wang, Y, Peng, Z Y, Wang, Z F, Liu, Y H, Li, H. An image hiding and mining technique based on the Zadeh-X transformation. Chinese Journal of Medical Physics, 2007, 24(1): 9–13.

Xie, Z X, Chen, M M and Xiong, X L. Existence verification and adaptive acquirement of optimal quality image. Journal of pattern recognition and image processing. *2013; 4(1):101–109.*

Xie, Z X, Wang, Z F, Lv, X F. Single Image Quality Assessment and Creation of the Best Quality Image. 2nd International Conference on Information Science and Engineering, ICISE2010 – Proceedings. PP. 4022–4025, 2010.

Medicine Sciences and Bioengineering – Wang (Ed.)
© *2015 Taylor & Francis Group, London, ISBN: 978-1-138-02684-1*

BDNF of the hippocampal CA3 relates to the spatial memory in rats exposed to music

Ying-shou Xing, Yang Xia & De-zhong Yao
Key Laboratory for NeuroInformation of Ministry of Education, School of Life Science and Technology, University of Electronic Science and Technology of China, Chengdu, China
School of Electronic Information Engineering, Yangtze Normal University, Fuling, China

ABSTRACT: Objective: To explore the effects of music on the spatial memory and the expression of Brain-Derived Neurotrophic Factor (BDNF) in the hippocampal CA3 region of developing rats. Methods: Postnatal rats were randomly divided into an experimental group and control group. The rats of experimental group were exposed to music from the first day after birth, and continued through postnatal day (PND) 28, then the spatial memory was detected by the Morris water maze and BDNF expression was detected by immunohistochemisty in the CA3 region of the hippocampus. Results: The escape latencies of rat were decreased obviously after music exposure for 28 days and the expression of BDNF in the hippocampal CA3 region was increased obviously compared with the control group. Conclusion: Early auditory enrichment with music enhances the developing rats' spatial memory and the expression of BDNF in the CA3 region of the hippocampus.

1 INTRODUCTION

Several studies indicated that music exposure can enhance people's learning and memory (Rauscher, 1993). Meanwhile, Hong *et al.* demonstrated that prenatal music caused the increase of neurogenesis in the hippocampus and enhanced spatial learning ability in young rats, but some researches considered that exposure to the music in utero would have been ineffective because rats are deaf as newborns (Steele, 2003). It is well known that CA3 is an important structure in the hippocampus, and it is closely related to the spatial learning and memory (Handelman *et al.*, 1981). In the present study, we explored the effect of postnatal music on the spatial memory by Morris water maze, and measured the expression of BDNF in rat CA3 region, which plays an important role in memory formation.

2 MATERIALS AND METHODS

2.1 *Animals and treatments*

All experiments were performed according to the experimental guidelines at the University of Electronic Science and Technology of China, and the experimental protocol was approved by the ethics committee of the University of Electronic Science and Technology of China. In the experiment, 30 SD rats born from time-mated dams (Animal Research Institute of Sichuan Province, China) at the University of Electronic Science and Technology of China. The subjects were randomly assigned to three groups ($n = 15$ in each group; 8 males and 7 females). Rats were maintained on a 12-h-light/12-h-dark cycle (light on at 08:00h) at a controlled ambient temperature ($22 \pm 2°C$). Food and water were made available *ad libitum*.

The behavioral assessment was done at PND28 during development, and after learning test, five rats from the Mozart's music group and the control group were decapitated, which performed immunohistochemical experiments.

Musical stimuli were the Mozart's piano sonata, K.448, which is usually used in studies on the "Mozart effect". The sound level of the control group was 55dB (ambient noise), and the musical group was 65–75dB. The musical stimuli were played repeatedly for 12h starting from 8.00 p.m. to 8.00 a.m. so that the rats would not be disturbed in their sleep. All acoustic interventions began on PND1 and continued through PND28.

2.2 Morris water maze test

The hidden platform water maze task (Gallagher et al 1993) was used to study the learning and memory of the three groups rats. The training apparatus was a circular, galvanized steel pool, 120 cm in diameter and 60 cm deep. The pool was filled with water (26 ± 1°C temperature) made opaque with a mixture of white, thick and non-toxic milk. On the first day of testing, the rats were given a pretraining session. Each animal was placed in the water and allowed to swim for 2 min. It was then allowed to climb onto the platform where it rested for 20 s. This procedure was repeated three times, and then the latencies (time taken to find the platform) were recorded for 4 days, with the max permitted exploring time of 60 s (named acquisition trial). The rats were allowed to rest on the platform for 20 s before being given another trial. Each subject was given four trials before being placed in a holding cage while the other rats were trained.

On the morning of the fifth day after acquisition training, the platform was removed, and the rats were permitted to explore in the pool for 60 s (named probe trial), and spatial specificity was measured by duration of time spent in the target quadrant (% of total time, chance level = 25%).

2.3 Immunohistochemistry

At the end of behavior experiment, subjects were anesthetized and transcardially perfused with fixative (4% paraformaldehyde). The brains were then removed and placed in the same fixative for 24 h, and transferred into a 30% sucrose solution for cryoprotection. Serially sectioned in the coronal plane at 30 μm, which were made using a freezing microtome (Leica, Nussloch, Germany). The tissue was processed free floating for immunohistochemistry (IHC) as previously described (Lemaire et al 2000). Briefly, for antigen retrieval, sections were incubated with 0.25% Trypsin in Phosphate-buffered saline (PBS) for 5min. Following extensive washin in PBS, sections were blocked with 10% goat serum solution for 1 h. Primary antibodies were applied overnight at 4°C. The sections were then washed three times with PBS and incubated for1 h with a species-specific secondary antibody. Subsequently, the sections were washed extensively again and placed on Superfrost Plus slides. After mounting, sections were observed and photo-documentation was realized under a Leica microscope equipped with a Spot® digital camera.

2.4 Statistical analysis

For behavioral tests, the escape latency of hidden-platform acquisition training uses repeated measures and multivariate analysis of variance (ANOVA) process of the general linear model. Group differences in the duration of time spent in quadrants were analyzed with two-way analyses of variance (ANOVA).

For the IHC, the area in the selected region was measured using Image-Pro Plus software (Media Cybernetics, Silver Spring, MD). The mean density of protein expressed in the areas was measured hemilaterally. Statistical analysis was performed by two-way ANOVA.

All values are expressed as mean ± S.E.M., and the statistical analyses were performed using SPSS (version 16.0). The post hoc comparison using the LSD method was used where applicable to provide more detail about the differences among groups. The level of statistical significance was set at $P < 0.05$.

3 RESULTS

3.1 *Behaviour test*

There are statistically significant differences between two groups in learning tests for 4 days. It was readily apparent that Mozart's music group showed good task acquisition and searched accurately for the platform after it was removed from the pool (Figure 1). On the acquisition trial (Figure 1A), although the two groups showed a decrease in escape latency to find the hidden platform, the analysis of acquisition trials revealed a large group difference in maze acquisition. *Post hoc* tests of the differences showed that acquisition performances were significantly better in the Mozart's music group than in the control group ($P < 0.05$). On the probe trial (Figure 1B), which was performed one day after the acquisition trial, the group differences persisted when the rats were tested for the probe trials. In a two-way ANOVA, the Mozart's music group showed a longer-time spent in the target quadrant than the control group ($P < 0.05$), and the Mozart's music group exhibited less time in the opposite quadrant than the control group.

3.2 *The level of BDNF*

To explore the molecular effect of different experimental conditions, BDNF levels in the selected brain regions were measured (Figure 2). In the hippocampal CA3 of the Mozart's music group, the BDNF protein level was increased significantly compared with that of the age-matched control rats (ANOVA, $P < 0.05$).

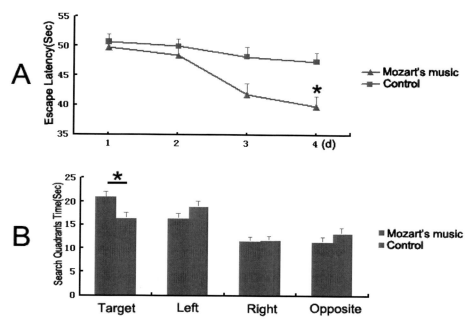

Figure 1. Enhanced performance of the rats exposed to Mozart's music in learning capability as measured by the Morris water maze on PND28. (A) The acquisition trial. (B) The probe trial. Although two types of rats showed a decrease in escape latency to find the hidden platform, rats exposed to Mozart's music exhibited a faster learning curve than the control rats. And the time spent to search the target in the target quadrant in Mozart's music group was significantly higher than that in the control group. In addition, The time spent in the opposite quadrant in Mozart's music group rats was lower than that in the control group (*$P < 0.05$).

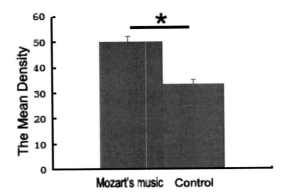

Figure 2. BDNF protein levels in the hippocampal CA3 region of music-exposed for 28 consecutive days and control rats. The data represent mean ± S.E.M. Asterisks denote significant differences among groups (*P < 0.05).

4 DISCUSSION

Water maze is one of the most commonly used tools to detect the rat's ability of the hippocampus-based learning and memory by means of spatial positions. Rats' training in Morris water maze, each laboratory is slightly different according to the number of training and frequency, but they need three to six days to learn the spatial localization. Although there have been putative effect of music on learning and memory, more and more evidence have proved that spatial learning and working memory acquisition and retention in mouse, rat or human are improved by exposure to music (Meng, 2009). In our learning test, which were consistent with previous research results, the rats of Mozart's music group had a faster learning capability and prolonged memory on the target quadrant than the control group rats.

It is generally recognized that environmental enrichment (such as music) has a major, long-lasting impact on adult brain perception. Also, an enriched environment affects neurogenesis and neurotrophin levels in the rat brain. The neurotrophin, brained-derived neurotrophinic factor (BDNF), which play a critical role in mediating enduring changes in central synaptic structure and function and dendritic structures of neurons (Tolwani *et al.* 2002). Numerous *in vivo* studies reported that exposure to music caused an increase in hipppocampal neurogenesis in animals (Angelucci *et al.* 2007) and induced long-lasting changes in BDNF/TrkB signaling in the hippocampus and learning performance in mice (Chikahisa *et al.* 2006).

Learning memory structural basis is the brain limbic system, especially the hippocampal CA3 area, is the animal forming the important structure of spatial learning and memory process (Mahanam *et al.* 2011), involved in long-term memory. Thus, in our study, rats exposed to Mozart's music enhances the spatial memory, the mechanism which may be related to BDNF increased on the expression of hippocampal CA3 region.

REFERENCES

Angelucci, F., et al., (2007) Investigating the neurobiology of music: brain-derived neurotrophic factor modulation in the hippocampus of young adult mice. *Behavioural pharmacology*, 18(5–6): 491.
Chikahisa S, Sei H, Morishima M, Sano A, Kitaoka K, Nakaya Y, Morita Y. (2006) Exposure to music in the perinatal period enhances learning performance and alters BDNF/TrkB signaling in mice as adults. *Behav Brain Res*.169:312–319.
Frances H. Rauscher.(1993) Music and spatial task performanc. *Nature*, 365:611–611.

Gallagher, M., R. Burwell, and M.R. Burchinal. (1993) Severity of spatial learning impairment in aging: development of a learning index for performance in the Morris water maze. *Behavioral neuroscience,* 107(4): 618

Handelman GF, Olton DA. (1981) Spacial memory following damage to hippocamal CA3 pyr amidal cells with kainic acid: Impairment and recover y with preoperative training. *Brain Res,* 217: 41.

Lemaire, V., et al.,. (2000) Prenatal stress produces learning deficits associated with an inhibition of neurogenesis in the hippocampus. *Proceedings of the National Academy of Sciences,* 97(20): 11032–11037.

Mahanam T, Sangdee A, Govitrapong P, Tongjaroenbuangam W. (2011) Effect of melatonin on hippocampal CA3 pyramidal cells following dexamethasone treatment in mice.

Meng, B., et al., (2009) Global view of the mechanisms of improved learning and memory capability in mice with music-exposure by microarray. *Brain research bulletin,* 80(1): 36–44.

Steele KM. (2003) Do rats show a Mozart effect?

Tolwani RJ, Buckmaster PS, Varma S, Cosgaya JM, Wu Y, Suri C, et al. (2002) BDNF overexpression increases dendrite complexity in hippocampal dentate gyrus. *Neuroscience* 114:795–805.

Ecology, Environment and Chemistry

Medicine Sciences and Bioengineering – Wang (Ed.)
© 2015 Taylor & Francis Group, London, ISBN: 978-1-138-02684-1

Differential microbial community complexity levels between different locations in the GuJingGong pits

Kai-qiang Li[†], Hui-min Zhang[†]
School of Marine Science and Technology, Harbin Institute of Technology, Weihai, China

An-jun Li, Hong-kui He & Qing-wu Zhou
The GuJing Group Co., Ltd., Bozhou, Anhui, China

Zhi-zhou Zhang[*]
School of Marine Science and Technology, Harbin Institute of Technology, Weihai, China

ABSTRACT: It is essential to decipher the structure and dynamics of microbial communities in the different locations of a liquor-making pit in order to understand the relationship between aimed fermentation efficiency and the environmental pit conditions. In this study, two GuJing-Gong factories (West and Quarter) were analyzed in the context of microbial community complexity of pit bottoms and sidewalls. It was found that the two factories have very similar microbial community complexity in depth samples while the surface samples were different significantly. The dominant species in all samples were uncultured bacteria.[1]

1 INTRODUCTION

A series of research have been undertaken over molecular dissection of microbial community structures for Chinese brand liquors. Knowing the microbial community components is the first step to tackle the relationship between fermentation parameters and microbial community dynamics. Besides, liquor fermentation factories often need to set up new plants in order to increase production, and it is expected the new pits can acquire the same fermentation quality as the old pits as soon as possible. Rapidly tracking and modulating the microbial community structure is a wanted technology in several industry fields, such as fermentation, environment protection, agriculture, and medical clinics, where a natural microbial community plays important roles.

Xiaoran et al studied bacterial and fungal diversity in the traditional Chinese liquor (Fen) fermentation process, and they found the most abundant OTU (operational taxonomic unit) which contributed to 51% of the total 16S rRNA gene sequences was affiliated with Lactobacillus acetotolerans, while sixty percent of the fungal ITS1 region sequences were affiliated with the family Saccharomycetaceae (Li, 2011). In the past 28 years, similar studies reported significant progress in this field (Xiao-Ran, 2013 and therein;all other references).

In this study, a molecular approach based on 16s rDNA library amplification /TA-cloning / sequencing was employed to decipher the compositional structure of GuJingGong liquor -making microbial communities at different pit locations. The main result of this study is that the dominant microbial species in pit bottom and sidewall (both surface and depth samples) are large-proportion uncultured bacteria.

---

[*]Contact by emailing zhangzzbiox@hitwh.edu.cn
[†]Equal contribution

2 MATERIALS AND METHODS

2.1 Sampling

Two freshly depleted pits in two liquor-making factories, West and Quarter, were chosen for sampling. In each pit, four 2 cm × 2 cm × (0–2) cm-depth pit mud samples were picked in the middle point of four sidewalls and mixed well as one sidewall surface sample; at the same four middle points of the sidewalls, four 2 cm × 2 cm × (2–4) cm-depth pit mud samples were picked and mixed well as one sidewall depth sample. Meanwhile, the middle point and four corner points were chosen for bottom samples. Five 2 cm × 2 cm × (0–2) cm-depth bottom samples were picked up and mixed well as one bottom surface sample, while five 2 cm × 2 cm × (2–4) cm-depth bottom samples were picked up and mixed well as one bottom depth sample. So, total eight samples were prepared and stored at -80 degree for further analysis.

2.2 TA cloning

Genomic DNA was extracted from 8 GuJingGong pit mud samples (S10-S17) using Solarbio D2600 kit for soil genome purification. 16s rDNA amplification was undertaken using universal primers 27F (5′- AGA GTT TGA TCC TGG CTC AG-3′) and 1492R (5′TAC GGY TAC CTT GTT ACG ACT T3′). Amplified target bands (about 1500 bp) were gel-purified using Sangon SanPrep kit (Cat#: SK8132). For TA cloning, 4 ul purified 16 s rDNA (about 20 ng) for each genome sample was ligated with 0.5 ul pMD19-T vector (50ng/ul, TaKaRa) for 4 hours at room temperature, then transformed into 60 ul competent DH5a cells. Cells were selected on LB plates with 100 ug/ml ampicillin and X-gal/IPTG according to standard protocols.

2.3 DNA sequencing and sequence analysis

About 130 white colonies from each of the 12 transformations were randomly picked for DNA sequencing using both 27F and 1492R. About 1299 effectively sequenced 16s rDNA fragments were subjected to Basic Local Alignment Search Tool (BLAST) analysis at the National Center for Biotechnology Information (NCBI) database (www.ncbi.nlm.nih.gov).

3 RESULTS AND DISCUSSION

3.1 Diversity of bacteria

Effectively sequenced colonies in 8 samples were summarized in Table 1 (Detailed information is requestable). The total number of successfully sequenced TA clones for each sample (S10 to S17) is 111, 125, 117, 124, 92, 108, 128 and 113, respectively. Rarefaction curve analysis on the colony numbers and OTUs indicated that the sampling libraries of S10-S17 were statistically big enough (data not shown), as highlighted by the fact that many OTUs have only one clone in the sequenced community. Interestingly, depth samples (bottom depth and sidewall depth) had the very similar OTUs between the two factories, suggesting that the two factories possessed the similar microbial community complexity, though with apparently different compositional structures (Table 1); The surface sample OTUs showed apparent difference between the two factories (Figure 1). This may be due to the vulnerability to rapid degradation after exposed to the air for some anaerobic bacteria in the pit mud.

3.2 Richness of uncultured species

It is amazing that almost all eight samples were occupied with unknown uncultured species as the major components (Table 1). From the lists of the four most abundant species in each sample, it is undoubted that uncultured (name known or unknown) species play dominant roles in the process

Table 1. Pit samples and the main species in them.

Factory	Pit Location (Effective clone)	OTU	Main Species (TA clone number)
West	Bottom Depth (S10) (111)	30	unknown uncultured bacterium (61)
			firmicutes (cultured and uncultured) (8)
			uncultured clostridia (5)
			uncultured porphyromonadaceae (3)
	Bottom Surface (S11) (125)	12	unknown uncultured bacterium (55)
			uncultured lactobacillus (39)
			uncultured firmicutes (6)
			uncultured clostridia (4)
	Sidewall Surface (S12) (117)	19	unknown uncultured bacterium (69)
			clostridia (cultured and uncultured) (16)
			uncultured firmicutes (12)
			uncultured tissierella sp (2)
	Sidewall Depth (S13) (124)	23	unknown uncultured bacterium (85)
			uncultured clostridium (6)
			syntrophomonas wolfei (3)
			uncultured porphyromonadaceae (3)
Quarter	Bottom Surface (S14) (92)	21	unknown uncultured bacterium (28)
			uncultured firmicutes (8)
			enterobacter sp (4)
			uncultured lysobacter sp (4)
	Bottom Depth (S15) (108)	30	unknown uncultured bacterium (37)
			clostridia (cultured and uncultured) (16)
			rumen bacterium (5)
			Moorella sp (4)
	Sidewall Depth (S16) (128)	24	unknown uncultured bacterium (64)
			uncultured clostridia (9)
			uncultured firmicutes (7)
			syntrophomonas bacterium (6)
	Sidewall Surface (S17) (113)	13	uncultured lactobacillus (32)
			unknown uncultured bacterium (22)
			stenotrophomonas maltophilia (5)
			dyella sp (2)

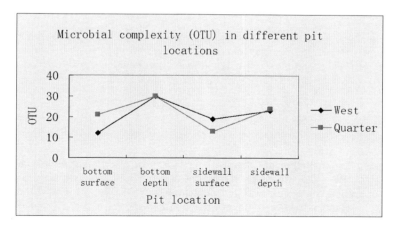

Figure 1. OTU number as a quantification parameter of microbial community complexity.

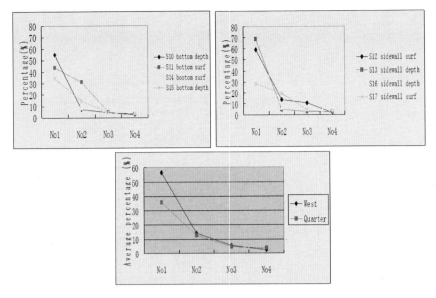

Figure 2.   The relative abundance of the four most dominant species (taxa) in each sample.

of GuJingGong liquor fermentation. It posed a situation that a lot of work has to be done for those uncultured species before good knowledge is acquired at cellular and molecular levels. From S10 to S17, the unknown uncultured species occupied 61/111, 55/125, 69/117, 85/124, 28/92, 37/108, 64/128, and 22/113, respectively. If the known uncultured species are counted, the total uncultured species constituted 50-70% in the whole microbial community.

The abundance is represented as the percentage over the total number of effective clones in each sample. It is evident that the most abundant uncultured species in West factory is more than that in Quarter, both in the bottom samples and in the sidewall samples. The difference of the average abundance of the four most dominant species between two factories mainly lies in the No.1 dominant species, as shown in the Figure 2 bottom, suggesting that the pit mud of Quarter factory is less mature than that of West (which is older) factory.

3.3   *The common microbial species*

For bottom samples, uncultured firmicutes and uncultured clostridia are common species; for sidewall samples, the common species are also uncultured firmicutes and uncultured clostridia. Looking at all four depth samples, it was found that all of them have uncultured clostridia, while sidewall surface sample had dominant species significantly different from other three surface samples.

4   SUMMARY

GuJingGong is a famous liquor in China with an 1800-year history, but molecular level studies on its microbial community structure and dynamics are far from enough. One striking feature of the pit mud microbial community for GongJingGong liquor is the richness of unknown uncultured species. The general fraction of unknown uncultured species is over 50% of all successfully sequenced TA clones. Other "known" uncultured species also has a large proportion in most samples. This highlights a situation that there is a long way to go before we understand the relationship between the liquor quality/flavor and the sub-structures of the microbial community. Twenty-four years ago, Ward et al first reported that 16S rDNA sequencing revealed a large proportion of uncultured species in a natural microbial community (Ward,1990), suggesting that it is not easy to get understood how to purposely manipulate different species in any natural microbial community. By now, it is still a big challenge to decipher the physiological roles of each type of microorganism in a natural community.

ACKNOWLEDGEMENTS

This work was funded by GREDBIO fund, HIT (hitwh200904), HIT-NSRIF (2011101), 985 fund and Weihai (2011DXGJ13, 2012DXGJ02).

REFERENCES

Han, S., Lei, Z.H., Li, Q., Lu, L.H., and Zhao, L.Q. (2009) Study on the cultured microbial community and the metabolism regulation during the brewing process of the Fen liquor. *Food Fermentation Industries* 35, 9–13.

Jung, M.-J., Nam, Y.-D., Roh, S.W., and Bae, J.-W (2012) Unexpected convergence of fungal and bacterial communities during fermentation of traditional Korean alcoholic beverages inoculated with various natural starters. *Food Microbiol.* 30, 112–123.

Li, X.R., Ma, E.B., Yan, L.Z., Meng, H., Du, X.W., Zhang, S.W., and Quan, Z.X. (2011) Bacterial and fungal diversity in the traditional chinese liquor fermentation process. *Food Microbiol.*146, 31–37.

Shi AH. (1986) Analysis on microorganisms in liquor pit of strong aroma style during fermentation. *Liquor Mak* (4):24–29.

Shi, J.H., Xiao, Y.P., Li, X.R., Ma, E.B., Du, X.W., and Quan, Z.X. (2009) Analyses of microbial consortia in the starter of fen liquor.. Lett. *Appl. Microbiol.* 48, 478–485.

Ward DM, Weller R, Bateson MM. (1990) 16S rRNA sequences reveal numerous uncultured microorganisms in a natural community. *Nature*, 345:63–65.

Xiao-Ran Li, En-Bo Ma, Liang-Zhen Yan, Han Meng, Xiao-Wei Du, and Zhe-Xue Quan. (2013) Bacterial and Fungal Diversity in the Starter Production Process of Fen Liquor, a Traditional Chinese Liquor. *Journal of Microbiology* Vol. 51, No. 4, pp. 430–438.

Yao, W.C., Tang, Y.M., Ren, D.Q., Liao, J.M., Shen, F.H., Xu, D.F., Ying, H. and Fan, L. (2005) Study on the differences of microbes in the different layers of Guojiao Daqu. *Liquor Making.* 32, 35–37.

Zhang WX, Qiao ZW, Shigematsu T, Tang YQ, Hu C, Morimura S, Kida K. (2005) Analysis of the bacterial community in Zaopei during production of Chinese Luzhou-flavor liquor. *J Inst Brew* 111(2):215–222.

Zhang, W.X., Qiao, Z.W., Tang, Y.Q., Hu, C., Sun, Q., Morimura, S. and Kida, K. (2007) Analysis of the fungal community in Zaopei during the production of Chinese Luzhou-flavour liquor. *J Inst Brew.* 113, 21–27.

Medicine Sciences and Bioengineering – Wang (Ed.)
© 2015 Taylor & Francis Group, London, ISBN: 978-1-138-02684-1

Effect of ultrasonic pretreatment on the oil removal of ASP flooding produced water

Fu-jun Xia

Oilfield Construction Design and Research Institute, Daqing, China

ABSTRACT: The effect of oil removal rate of ASP flooding produced water with pretreatment in an ultrasound cleaning tank was investigated in this study. Experiments were carried out with 28 kHz and 40 kHz ultrasonic irradiation at different treating times. The results showed that the emulsification of ASP flooding produced water pretreated by ultrasonic would decrease. The optimum condition of ultrasonic pretreatment was as following: voltage 220V, ultrasonic frequency 28 kHz, duty cycle 50%. A reduction of 90% of oil content could be reached after ultrasound irradiation. It can also be concluded that 2–4 h standing time after treated by ultrasound could enhance the oily water deoiling.

1 INTRODUCTION

At present, oil displacement by adding agents with different ingredient has been carried out in the test areas, both of different geological structures and oil horizons in the Daqing oil field. Because the oily water obtained by the dehydration of ASP flooding produced liquid contained surfactants, alkali and polymer (polyacrylamide), which nature is different from that of the wastewater from water flooding and polymer flooding. ASP flooding produced water was of high emulsifying and strong stability, and it was difficult to remove the suspended solid (SS) after filtering (Zhang *et al.*, 2007). In recent years, although treatment technology of produced water, such as ultrasonic (Sun & Fu, 1999; Xia *et al.*, 2001), supercritical water oxidation (Wang *et al.*, 2006), photocatalysis-ultrasonic technology (Li *et al.*, 2007), electrochemical method (Sun *et al.*, 2007), both in the study of laboratory experiment and oilfield application have obtained a preliminary progress (Liu *et al.*, 2005; Jing *et al.*, 2004; Wang *et al.*, 2006), these techniques have many problems in practical use according to the operating experimental station. Much addition of agents could lead to more sludge and higher cost. The water quality, after treatment, is still difficult to attain to the standard of recycling and reusing water. Therefore, oily wastewater is not being disposed of properly. However, the nature of the ASP flooding produced water which is of high viscosity, small oil droplet, high degree of emulsification and re-emulsification is different from that of general oily water (Zhang *et al.*, 2007; Liu *et al.*, 2005; Jing *et al.*, 2004; Tang *et al.*, 2010). Ultrasonic oily wastewater treatment, which is fast and effective, has recently garnered much attention.

The objective of this work is to investigate the process of ASP-flooding produced water treated by ultrasound and examine the oil contents of oily sludge as well as the determination of the effects of ultrasound irradiation and frequency.

2 MATERIALS AND METHODS

2.1 *The characteristics of produced water by ASP flooding*

The characteristics of the water produced by ASP flooding in the Daqing oil field were investigated, and the results were shown in Table 1.

Table 1. The characteristics of ASP flooding-produced water.

Analysis Program	Total Alkalinity	Surfactants	Polymer Content	Water Viscosity	Drop Diameter	Experiment Temperature
Test Results	4200 mg/L	42 mg/L	640 mg/L	4.29 mpa.s	less than 10 μm > 50%	21~23°C

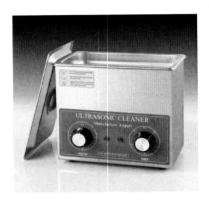

Figure 1. Experimental prototype of an ultrasonic cleaner.

2.2 Experiment equipment and methods

2.2.1 Experiment equipment

The experiment was carried out in an experimental prototype of an ultrasonic cleaner (model VGT-1840QT, China) (Figure 1).

2.2.2 Experimental methods

Oily wastewater was sampled with five 250 mL jars, then placed in the ultrasonic instrument under the operation condition of frequency 55 kHZ, power 100%. 50 mL water samples were extracted from the bottom with a syringe at regular intervals from the bottle of jars, followed by the measurement of their oil content. After that, also 50 mL water samples were extracted from the bottom of jars with a syringe when the jars were placed into the incubation in 40°C water bath for 4h. While, 1000 mL water was sampled into a 1000 mL jar, and did the same things as above for control.

In order to determinate the optimum condition of ultrasonic treatment of ASP flooding produced water, following experiments were carried out: 250 mL water samples were taken into six 250 mL jars, which were then placed in the ultrasonic instrument, and the instrument was operated with different conditions. These jars were removed into the 40°C water bath to stand for 4h at regular intervals, and also 50 mL water samples were extracted from the bottom with a syringe to determinate their oil contents.

2.3 Analysis methods

The oil contents of the samples were analyzed by IR spectroscopy analyzer (Model JDS-106). In this method, carbon tetrachloride was used to extract oil from the samples firstly, then the absorbance was measured at IR wavelengths of 3030 cm^{-1}, 2960 cm^{-1}, and 2930 cm^{-1}, and the total oil contents were obtained from the calibration curve. The instrument was calibrated for the standard oil supplied by the manufacturer.

3 RESULTS AND DISCUSSION

3.1 *Effect of ultrasonic time on the residual oil content of ASP flooding produced water*

There are many factors that affect the ultrasonic treatment, among which, such as the ultrasonic treatment voltage, ultrasonic time, operation style and ultrasonic frequency are more important. The effects of ultrasonic time on the removal rate of the ASP flooding produced water were shown in Figure 2. It could be seen that the residual oil content of ASP flooding produced water with the initial oil content of 132.01 mg/L decreased gradually along with the increasing of ultrasonic time. But the effect of removing oil by sedimentation was better than ultrasound. Moreover, with the pretreatment of ultrasound, the residual oil content of wastewater was lower than that without ultrasound pretreatment after placement for 4h.

It could be concluded from Figure 2 that ultrasound can promote the coalescence of the droplet, and it has no removing oil's effect only if added by a sedimentation device. In addition, when the ultrasonic time was greater than 5min, the residual oil content did not change obviously. So the ultrasonic time of 5min was chosen for the optimum operation condition at the following experiments.

3.2 *Optimization of ultrasonic treatment condition of oily water*

The experimental results of the above showed that ultrasonic can play a promoting role for oil water separation, and in order to determinate the optimum operation condition of ultrasonic treatment, the effects of different operating conditions of ultrasonic on the oil removal were investigated.

It could be seen from Figure 3 that the oil removal rates of ASP flooding produced water were greatly improved with the different ultrasonic operation conditions. However, the oil content

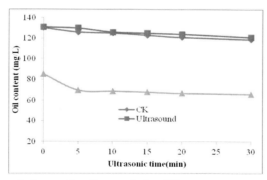

Figure 2.   Effect of ultrasonic time on the oil removal after different treatments.

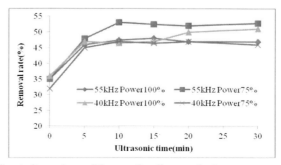

Figure 3.   Effect of different ultrasonic conditions on the oil removal rate.

decreased sharply in the first 5 min of the operating period, subsequently, it maintained a stable state. Oil content was reduced from 122.14mg/L to 56.04mg/L with the ultrasonic condition of frequency 55 kHz, power 75% and the time 10 min following by the sedimentation for 4h, and the oil removal rate could reach 54.12%. However, oil content was reduced from 122.14mg/L to 79.03mg/L without ultrasonic pretreatment in the application of sedimentation for 4h, and the oil removal rate was only 35.30%. So it could be concluded that the oil removal rate would increase nearly by 20% after pretreatment by ultrasonic, and the ultrasonic condition of frequency 55kHz, power 75% and the time 10min following by the sedimentation for 4h was chosen as the optimal condition.

Promotion of oil removal from ASP flooding produced water by ultrasonic was through the role of changing the particle surface characteristics of water, and as a result, the ability of oil droplet coalescence with each other was greatly improved leading to the change of particle size distribution of oil droplet in ASP flooding produced water during the settlement process. In addition, the oil bead diameter increased as well as the separation speed, so the effect of sedimentation separation on ASP flooding produced water enhanced greatly. But, it was demonstrated from above experimental results that ultrasonic has no effect of removing oil by itself, and the action time was very short, only for 5min, so it must be followed by the settling equipment.

3.2.1 *Effect of static sedimentation on the oil removing after ultrasonic demulsification pretreatment*

After the optimization of ultrasonic pretreatment, optimization of the static sedimentation experiment was carried out, and the operation conditions were shown in Table 2.

The removal rate of oil from ASP flooding produced water was not so obviously improved with the ultrasonic pretreatment at the operation condition 1 as shown in Table 2 (Figure 4a). Moreover, the residual oil content did not increase significantly after sedimentation for over 2h both with and without the pretreatment of ultrasonic. The reason was that crude oil emulsification degree was too high because of the high ultrasonic frequency or the strong sound intensity, So that the oil removal rate is lower.

Therefore, the lower ultrasonic frequency experiment was carried out at the operating condition 2 as shown in table 2. The results were shown in Figure 4b. It could be stated that in the first 4h sedimentation time, the oil removal rate was nearly the same of the ASP flooding produced water both with and without the pretreatment of lower frequency ultrasonic. The oil removal rate of ASP flooding produced water after ultrasonic pretreatment was obviously better than without ultrasound with the settling time. Furthermore, the oil removal rate of ASP flooding produced water could reach 90% with the pretreatment of ultrasonic after sedimentation for 12h. On the contrary, the oil removal rate was only about 80% without the pretreatment of ultrasonic at condition 2.

In order to optimize the condition of ultrasound furthermore, lower input voltage was taken to carry out the experiment, and the results were shown in Figure 4c. It could be seen that there

Table 2. Ultrasonic demulsification operation conditions.

Condition	Voltage	Frequency	Time	Duty ratio
1	220 V	40 KHz	10 min	50%
2	220 V	28 KHz	10 min	50%
3	195 V	28 KHz	10 min	50%
4	220 V	28 KHz	10 min	100%
5	175 V	28/40 KHz	10 min	50%

Foot note: Duty ratio 50%: ultrasonic signal emission time and rest time were the same, Intermittent ultrasound; Duty ratio 100%: Continuous ultrasound.

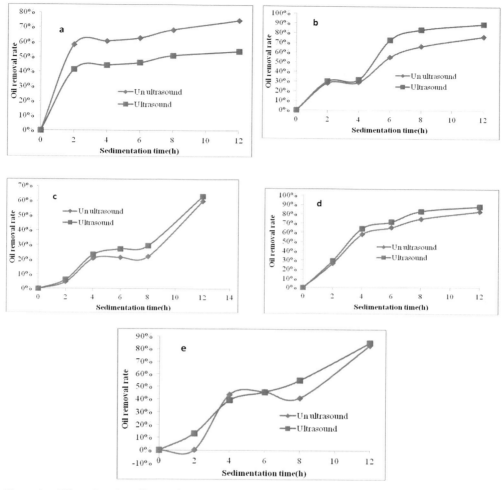

Figure 4. Effect of static sedimentation on the oil removing by ultrasonic pretreatment. (a: at condition 1; b: at condition 2; c: at condition 3; d: at condition 4; e: at condition 5).

was no obvious improvement of oil removal rate of ASP flooding produced water with ultrasonic pretreatment of oily wastewater compared to that without it in further reducing of the ultrasonic sound intensity. According to the above experimental results, the input voltage of 220kV was considered as the optimal.

The continuous signal generator of ultrasound was carried out in order to investigate the oil removal rate, which is the duty ratio was 100%. A specific operation conditions were shown in Table 2 (condition 4). The results showed that it has no obvious differences between oil removal rate of continuous and intermittent ultrasound on ASP flooding produced water. The addition of ultrasonic time has no significant improvement of oil removal rate. However, the total oil removal rate was a little lower. The effect of ultrasonic pulse processing on the oil removal rate of oil water is better than that of the continuous ultrasonic treatment (Figure 4a and Figure 4d). The reason was that the intermittent ultrasonic could damage the reticular structure of the emulsion more effectively, and smaller oil droplets were merged into a large oil droplets leading to the separation of the oil from sewage.

The ultrasonic frequencies of 40 kHz and 28 kHz were chosen for the operation condition 5 as shown in Table 2. The results were shown in Figure 4e. It could be seen that the oil removal rate had not improved significantly with ultrasonic pretreatment compared to that without ultrasonic pretreatment in the use of two joint ultrasonic frequencies (Figure 4e). As a result, the effect of two ultrasonic frequencies join action on the oil removal was not good.

It could be concluded that the emulsification of ASP flooding produced water pretreated by ultrasonic would decrease, and the oil removal rate could improve greatly following by further coalescence settling separation with settlement processing device. The condition of ultrasonic pretreatment in the voltage of 220V, 28 kHz ultrasonic frequency, duty cycle 50% was the optimum condition.

4   SUMMARY

The oil contents of ASP flooding produced water after deoiling by ultrasonic generator were tested for different ultrasonic operation conditions. After ultrasound irradiation, it is a reduction of 90% of oil content. The emulsification of ASP flooding produced water pretreated by ultrasonic would decrease, and the oil removal rate could improve greatly following by further coalescence settling separation with settlement processing device. The condition of ultrasonic pretreatment in the voltage of 220V, 28 kHz ultrasonic frequency, duty cycle 50% was the optimum condition. The oil contents of ASP flooding produced water after pretreatment with or without ultrasonic standing for different times were also investigated. The optimum standing time was between 2h and 4h.

REFERENCES

Jing, G., Yu, S., Han, Q. (2004) Progress research on produced water treatment technology of polymer flooding. Industrial Water and Wastewater, 35, 16–18.
Liu, S., Zhao, X., Dong, X., et al., (2005) Treatment of produced water from polymer flooding process using a new type of air sparged hydrocyclone. SPE Asia Pacific Health, Safety and Environment Conference and Exhibition-Proceedings, 49–52.
Li, S. Z., Wang, L., Li, L. (2007) Kinetics model of degradation by photocatalysis-ultrasonic technology on oil refinery waste water. Journal of Anhui Normal University (Natural Science), 30, 142–145.
Sun, B. J. & Fu, J. (1999) Ultrasonic separation experiment of the oil wastewater in the three oil production. Journal of the Univer sity of Petroleum, China, 23, 115–117.
Sun, H. Y., Yang, Y., Chen, B. N. (2007) Study on the treatment of oil-bearing wastewater by electric floating methods. Technology research papers: Chemistry and Chemical Technology, 362–363.
Tang, X., Zhang, B., Höök, M., etc., (2010) Forecast of oil reserves and production in Daqing oilfield of China. Energy, 35, 3097–310.
Wang, F., Zhu, N., Xia, F., Wu, D. (2006) Experimental study on ASP flooding produced water. Industrial Water Treatment, 26, 17–19.
Wang, L., Wang, S. Z., Zhang, Q. M., Shen, L. H., Duan, B. Q. (2006) Reaction mechanism and kinetics of oil-bearing sewage disposal by supercritical water oxidation. Journal of xi'an jiao tong university, 40, 115–119.
Xia, F. J., Zhang, B. L., and Deng, S. B. (2001) Flooding oily wastewater by ultrasonic method for processing polymer. Oil-gas field surface engineering, 20, 34.
Zhang, L., Xiao, H., Zhang, H., etc., (2007) Optimal design of a novel oil–water separator for raw oil produced from ASP flooding. *Journal of Petroleum Science and Engineering* , 59, 213–218.

Medicine Sciences and Bioengineering – Wang (Ed.)
© *2015 Taylor & Francis Group, London, ISBN: 978-1-138-02684-1*

Antibiotics-resistant profiles of airborne *enterococcus faecalis* in an enclosed-type chicken shed

Zeng-min Miao*, Song Li*, Yu-jing Tang & Rong-mei Wang
Department of Life Sciences, Taishan Medical University, Taian, Shandong, China
Department of Sports Medicine, Taishan Medical University, Taian, Shandong, China
Department of Basic Medicine, Taishan Medical University, Taian, Shandong, China

ABSTRACT: This study was carried out to examine the drug-resistant characteristics of airborne *Enterococcus faecalis* (*E. faecalis*) isolated from an enclosed-type chicken shed in Qingdao, China. An anderden-6 stage air sampler was employed to collect air samples inside the chicken shed continuously for 1 week. From these sampling media, we identified 80 non-repetitive airborne *E. faecalis* isolates. The resistance of the airborne *E. faecalis* isolates to 7 commonly prescribed antibiotics was then analyzed. The resistance rates of isolates to 7 antibiotics (gentamicin, streptomycin, tetracycline, erythromycin, penicillin, amoxicillin, and vancomycin) were respectively 85% (68/80), 82.5% (66/80), 81.3% (65/80), 62.5% (50/80), 60% (48/80), 56.3% (45/80), and 10.0% (8/80). These results showed that the resistance airborne *E. faecalis* of chicken house is of high prevalence.

1 INTRODUCTION

Enterococci are the opportunistic pathogen and regarded as a bio-indicator of fecal contamination and antibiotic resistance among animals and waters (Sapkota et al., 2007). They are widely distributed in nature, and commonly reside in the intestines of humans and animals. They can cause infection in multiple organ systems, including infections of the urinary tract, skin, soft tissue, pelvic cavity, abdominal cavity, and existing surgical sites, as well as causing blood-borne infections such as bacteremia, endocarditis, and meningitis. *Enterococci* are inherently resistant to many antibiotics due to the presence of a tough cell wall. Furthermore, new resistance phenotypes can be induced by means of plasmids, transposons, or by spontaneous mutation. This high use of antibiotics in livestock industry has generated a selection pressure, which has led to the emergence of multidrug-resistant strains of *Enterococcus* (Magiorakos et al., 2012).

Recently, there have been an increasing number of reports regarding *Enterococcus* infection in animals, and the risk associated with *Enterococcus* infection is increasing. *Enterococcus* infection in animals may be fatal, and the clinical management of infection is made more difficult by the strong and wide-spectrum of antibiotic resistance in pathogenic *enterococci* (Braga et al., 2012) *Enterococcus* is one of the most common airborne microorganisms in an animal shed environment, and it can be transmitted through air exchange. But little information about the resistance profiles of airborne *Enterococcus* in animal sheds is available. To fill the literature gap, airborne *E. faecalis*, the commonly collected bacteria in the air of chicken house, was chosen as the indicator strain. An Andersen-6 stage microbial sampler was employed to collect air samples from one enclosed-type chicken shed continuously for 1 week, and then the resistance profiles of the identified *E. faecalis* were analyzed.

---

* Co-corresponding authors of this manuscript are Z.M. Miao (zengminmiao@126.com) and S. Li (sli@tsmc.edu.cn).

2 MATERIALS AND METHODS

2.1 Sampling site and strategy

An enclosed-type chicken shed in Qingdao, China was chosen as the sampling site. There were two rows of chicken cages, and each row was two stories high. The length, width, and height of the shed were 40 m, 4 m, and 3 m, respectively. The temperature inside the shed was maintained at 22 ± 3°C, with a relative humidity of 66 ± 5%. Feces were cleared once daily. Three thousand adult egg-laying hens were housed in the shed. Ventilation was carried out by mechanical fans.

From 1–7 August 2013, an andersen-6 stage microbial sampler was used to collect air samples per day. *Enterococcus* chromogenic culture medium was used as the sampling medium. During the sampling process, the air sampler was placed in the middle of the shed, 1.5 m above the floor. Air flow velocity was 28.3 L/min, and the operation time per sampling was 1 min.

2.2 Isolation and identification of airborne Enterococcus faecalis

Samples collected on the *Enterococcus* chromogenic culture medium were incubated at 37°C for 24 h. Colonies that were suspected to be enterococci were picked and then identified by the API system according to the previous reference.

2.3 Antibiotic susceptibility test

The susceptibility of *E. faecalis* isolates to seven commonly used antibiotics (penicillin, amoxicillin, erythromycin, gentamicin, streptomycin, tetracycline, and vancomycin) was analyzed by the Kirby-Bauer disc diffusion method recommended by the Clinical and Laboratory Standards Institute. *E. faecalis* ATCC 29212 and *Staphylococcus aureus* ATCC 29213 were used as control strains. Interpretation of results and quality control were conducted according to the CLSI guidelines (2010).

3 RESULTS

3.1 Collection and identification of airborne E. faecalis

80 non-repetitive airborne *E. faecalis* isolates were collected in 1 week. They were mainly concentrated on stage D of the andersen-6 stage sampler, with an average concentration of 10^2 colony forming units per cubic meter (CFU/m^3).

3.2 Antibiotic susceptibility test

The resistance rates of airborne *E. faecalis* strains to gentamicin, streptomycin, tetracycline, erythromycin, penicillin, amoxicillin, and vancomycin were 85% (68/80), 82.5% (66/80), 81.3% (65/80), 62.5% (50/80), 60% (48/80), 56.3% (45/80) and 10.0%, respectively (Figure 1).

4 DISCUSSION

Enterococcus species mainly reside in the intestinal tracts of humans and animals, where they are part of the normal commensal microbial flora. With the widespread use of broad-spectrum antibiotics, the number of clinical isolates exhibiting antibiotic resistance has been rising. Because *enterococci* possess both inherent and acquired antibiotic resistance, infection caused by *Enterococcus* species has become a clinically challenging problem. In veterinary clinical practice, there have been increasing reports of animal infection caused by *Enterococcus* species, which pose a significant threat to the animal husbandry industry. The antibiotic susceptibility tests carried out in the

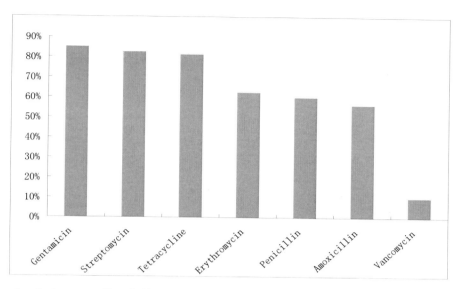

Figure 1.   Resistance profiles of airborne *E. faecalis* in the enclosed chicken shed environment. Horizontal axis: antibiotics; vertical axis: resistance rates.

current study showed that more than 50% of airborne *E. faecalis* isolates from the chicken shed were resistant to penicillin, amoxicillin, erythromycin, gentamicin, streptomycin, and tetracycline. These results are consistent with previous studies conducted in chickens of Chinese farms, but higher than those from cattle, sheep, pigs, and other animals (Yang, et al., 2010; Liu et al., 2013). This may be related to the rearing practice and use of antibiotics on chicken farms. The airborne *E. faecalis* isolates had the lowest resistance rate to vancomycin, suggesting that vancomycin should still be the drug of choice for treatment of *Enterococcus* infection in chickens in Qingdao, China. However, continued surveillance of vancomycin resistance in *E. faecalis* from chickens should be conducted.

The current study showed that multi-drug resistance was widespread amongst airborne *E. faecalis* in the chicken shed environment. These multidrug-resistant strains not only lower the therapeutic efficacy of antibiotics and prolong the course of infection, but can also lead to complications that result in death of infected animals and subsequent economic losses (Radhouani, et al., 2010). Currently, the antibiotics used in the animal husbandry industry coincide with those used in treating human infection. Thus, antibiotic-resistant bacterial strains originating from animals may contaminate meat or meat products during slaughtering or processing, and be transmitted to humans through the food chain. Clinical management of human infection arising from these bacteria would be difficult owing to their multi-drug resistance. Another threat from these antibiotics-resistant strains is the spread of antibiotic-resistance genes between bacteria within animals, or between strains in animals and humans. Therefore, the control of emergence and transmission of zoonotic antibiotic-resistant bacteria is an important part of the greater problem of the control of general and worsening antibiotic-resistant bacterial infections of humans.

The current study showed that airborne *E. faecalis* had high rates of antibiotic resistance, and that their concentration was as high as 10^2 CFU/m^3. They were mainly captured on stage D of the Andersen-6 stage air sampler, and their aerodynamic radii were in the range of 1–2 μm. These particulates can thus reach the lower respiratory tract and even alveoli, and therefore pose a serious threat to the health of breeders and animals. Hence, we should focus on controlling airborne transmission of *E. faecalis*, through measures such as proper ventilation and regular sterilization, to control the risk of infection.

ACKNOWLEDGEMENTS

This study was supported by natural grants of Shandong province (ZR2013CM030 and ZR2011CL013), and the grant of Taishan Medical University (2013GCC07).

REFERENCES

Braga TM, Pomba C, Lopes MF. High-level vancomycin resistant *Enterococcus faecium* related to humans and pigs found in dust from pig breeding facilities. Vet Microbiol, 2012, 161: 344–349.

Clinical Laboratory Standards Institute. Performance Standards for Antimicrobial Susceptibility Testing: Twentieth Informational Supplement M100-S20. CLSI, Wayne, PA, USA, 2010.

Liu M, Dong YM, Xu AQ, et al. Clinical distribution, antimicrobial susceptibility and vancomycin genes of *Enterococcus*. Int J Lab Med, 2013, 34: 2392–2393.

Magiorakos AP, Srinivasan A, Carey RB, et al. Multidrug-resistant, extensively drug-resistant and pandrug-resistant bacteria: an international expert proposal for interim standard definitions for acquired resistance. Clin Microbiol Infect, 2012, 18: 268–281.

Radhouani H, Pinto L, Coelho C, et al. MLST and a genetic study of antibiotic resistance and virulence factors in vanA-containing *Enterococcus* from buzzards (Buteo buteo). Lett Appl Microbiol 2010;50:537–541.

Sapkota AR, Curriero FC, Gibson KE, et al. Antibiotic-resistant *enterococci* and fecal indicators in surface water and groundwater impacted by a concentrated swine feeding operation. Environ Health Perspect, 2007, 115: 1040–1045.

Yang Q, Yu YS, Ni YX, et al. CHINET 2009 surveillance of antibiotic resistance in *Enterococcus* in China. Chin J Infect Chemother, 2010, 10: 421–425.

Medicine Sciences and Bioengineering – Wang (Ed.)
© 2015 Taylor & Francis Group, London, ISBN: 978-1-138-02684-1

GC-MS fingerprint of *Acanthopanax brachypus* in China

Hao-bin Hu*, Xu-dong Zheng, Huai-sheng Hu & Yun Wu
College of Chemistry & Chemical Engineering, Longdong University, Qingyang, Gansu, China

ABSTRACT: The chromatographic fingerprint of *A. brachypus* was established by using GC-FID and GC-MS techniques, as well as computer-aided similarity evaluation system. Thirty-two different batches of samples collected from the different producing regions and the different parts of *A. brachypus* were studied. The results showed that the fingerprinting profiles were found to be consistent for the fresh stem bark acquired from various production areas, 48 common peaks were determined, but the relative abundance of peaks was varied. Except for the leaf, the chemical components among different parts of fresh plant were inconsistent with the stem bark. Besides, the varieties and relative levels of chemical components, in the fresh stem bark were more abundant than the dry counterpart.

1 INTRODUCTION

Acanthopanax brachypus belonging to the genus *Acanthopanax*, is a peculiar folk medicinal plant, narrowly distributed in the loess plateau of the northwest of China, mainly in Liupanshan, Ziwuling and Northern Shannxi. Studies showed that its rhizome extract had been used for the treatment of neurasthenic, male sexual dysfunction, secondary hypertension, hypotension and leucopenia disease, also had the function of preventing cancer and anti-cancer (Gansu Food and Drug Administration, 2009). Previous studies revealed that *A. brachypus* contained essential oil, flavonoids, triterpenoids, amino acids, and so on (Hu & Fan, 2012). However, to the best of our knowledge, there are no reports on the chemical fingerprint of *A. brachypus* up to now. In this regard, the present study seeks to establish the characteristic GC-MS fingerprint of *A. brachypus* for distinguishing the substitute or adulterant, and further assessing the differences of *A. brachypus* grown in various areas of China.

2 EXPERIMENT

2.1 Sample preparation

Representative samples were collected from three main distributions of *A. brachypus* (fresh stem bark ZWL1-10, fresh root ZWL11-14 and dry stem bark ZWL15-16 from Ziwuling, fresh stem bark LPS1-8 from Liupanshan, fresh stem bark NS1-8 from Northern Shannxi) in September of 2010, and authenticated by Prof. Xiaoqiang Guo. Fresh samples were lyophilized and analyzed according to the different parts, then ground to fine powder with a particle size of 40 mesh. The essential oils were extracted by hydrodistillation using a Clevenger-type apparatus.

---

*Correspondence to: H.B. Hu, College of Chemistry and Chemical Engineering, Longdong University, Lanzhou Road, Qingyang City 745000, Gansu Province, People's Republic of China. Phone: +86-934-8522487, Fax: +86-934-8651531, E-mail: hhb-88@ 126.com

Table 1. RPAs of characteristic peaks of samples of *A. brachypus* from various sources.

No	Chemical compound	Ziwuling Fresh stem bark (n = 10) RPA	Fresh leaf (n = 2) RPA	Fresh root (n = 2) RPA	Dry stem bark (n = 2) RPA	Liupanshan Fresh stem bark (n = 8) RPA	Northern Shaanxi Fresh stem bark (n = 8) RPA
1	*n*-Hexanal	0.10 ± 0.005	0.22 ± 0.012	0.13 ± 0.023		0.07 ± 0.015	0.09 ± 0.011
2	(*E*)-2-Hexenal	0.07 ± 0.012	0.14 ± 0.103			0.04 ± 0.084	0.06 ± 0.031
3	*α*-Thujene	0.22 ± 0.023	0.42 ± 0.069	0.32 ± 0.117	0.12 ± 0.078	0.24 ± 0.031	0.28 ± 0.028
4	Camphene	0.35 ± 0.005	0.65 ± 0.037	0.58 ± 0.089		0.40 ± 0.019	0.63 ± 0.219
5	Benzaldehyde	0.08 ± 0.037	0.20 ± 0.117		0.21 ± 0.015	0.12 ± 0.127	0.27 ± 0.024
6	*β*-Pinene	1	1	1	1	1	1
7	*β*-Myrcene	0.07 ± 0.011	0.16 ± 0.037			0.82 ± 0.030	0.20 ± 0.021
8	*n*-Octanal	0.06 ± 0.014	0.15 ± 0.061		0.36 ± 0.105	0.24 ± 0.126	0.12 ± 0.030
9	*p*-Cymene	0.74 ± 0.024	1.13 ± 0.091		0.59 ± 0.116	0.35 ± 0.016	0.15 ± 0.023
10	Limonene	0.10 ± 0.130	0.21 ± 0.061	1.02 ± 0.217	1.09 ± 0.093	0.95 ± 0.028	0.18 ± 0.042
11	*γ*-Terpinene	0.28 ± 0.034	0.71 ± 0.038	0.33 ± 0.118		0.24 ± 0.024	1.72 ± 0.013
12	Acetophenone	0.06 ± 0.119	0.15 ± 0.121		0.03 ± 0.063	0.16 ± 0.017	0.15 ± 0.117
13	Linalool	0.76 ± 0.116	0.89 ± 0.057	0.25 ± 0.041	0.15 ± 0.152	0.78 ± 0.216	0.12 ± 0.015
14	*β*-Thujone	0.24 ± 0.027				0.24 ± 0.021	0.13 ± 0.014
15	*trans*-Pinene hydrate	0.08 ± 0.033	0.28 ± 0.070			0.07 ± 0.032	0.48 ± 0.034
16	Camphor	0.25 ± 0.041	0.37 ± 0.068			0.06 ± 0.029	0.05 ± 0.065
17	*β*-Terpineol	0.12 ± 0.032	0.25 ± 0.107		0.45 ± 0.091	0.27 ± 0.067	0.22 ± 0.017
18	*trans*-Menthone	0.11 ± 0.229	0.27 ± 0.099	0.07 ± 0.069	0.24 ± 0.047	0.28 ± 0.041	0.41 ± 0.014
19	*endo*-Borneol	0.31 ± 0.075	0.86 ± 0.048		0.49 ± 0.029	0.80 ± 0.122	0.91 ± 0.009

No.	Compound						
20	Terpinen-4-ol	0.17 ± 0.247	0.29 ± 0.033	0.18 ± 0.083		0.30 ± 0.008	0.35 ± 0.211
21	p-Cymene-8-ol	0.21 ± 0.018	0.35 ± 0.027			0.31 ± 0.017	0.37 ± 0.024
22	trans-Piperitol	0.23 ± 0.021	0.25 ± 0.084			0.22 ± 0.015	0.29 ± 0.017
23	Verbenone	0.31 ± 0.022	0.53 ± 0.061	0.96 ± 0.097	0.28 ± 0.171	0.34 ± 0.234	0.49 ± 0.008
24	Citronellol	0.03 ± 0.314			0.07 ± 0.035	0.11 ± 0.009	0.26 ± 0.027
25	δ-Elemene	0.17 ± 0.023	0.23 ± 0.052		0.68 ± 0.062	0.53 ± 0.012	0.25 ± 0.057
26	α-Copaene	0.08 ± 0.032		0.28 ± 0.189	0.23 ± 0.134	0.97 ± 0.110	0.06 ± 0.023
27	β-Bourbonene	0.12 ± 0.097			0.03 ± 0.066	0.16 ± 0.033	0.09 ± 0.212
28	β-Elemene	0.13 ± 0.040	0.20 ± 0.084	0.07 ± 0.215		0.29 ± 0.026	0.23 ± 0.034
29	β-Caryophyllene	0.29 ± 0.034	0.09 ± 0.091	1.84 ± 0.167		0.26 ± 0.013	0.58 ± 0.051
30	α-Guaiene	0.18 ± 0.008	1.03 ± 0.062	0.49 ± 0.101		0.14 ± 0.011	0.09 ± 0.013
31	Alloaromadendrene	0.08 ± 0.016	0.24 ± 0.018			0.13 ± 0.027	0.10 ± 0.027
32	Germacrene-D	0.26 ± 0.024	0.54 ± 0.053	0.06 ± 0.047	0.27 ± 0.035	0.31 ± 0.135	0.29 ± 0.011
33	β-Selinene	0.09 ± 0.031	0.22 ± 0.324		0.41 ± 0.028	0.36 ± 0.026	0.09 ± 0.020
34	Valencene	0.06 ± 0.126	0.13 ± 0.094	0.39 ± 0.046		0.64 ± 0.024	0.08 ± 0.106
35	α-Muurolene	0.16 ± 0.037	0.21 ± 0.113		0.08 ± 0.065	0.15 ± 0.032	0.23 ± 0.024
36	(E)-α-Farnesene	0.09 ± 0.089				0.21 ± 0.075	0.12 ± 0.034
37	β-Cadinene	0.24 ± 0.021	0.53 ± 0.046		0.35 ± 0.072	0.25 ± 0.029	0.32 ± 0.085
38	Cadina-1,4-diene	0.13 ± 0.022	0.28 ± 0.215		0.20 ± 0.203	0.18 ± 0.030	0.18 ± 0.017
39	Spathulenol	0.35 ± 0.076	0.53 ± 0.037	0.52 ± 0.227	0.29 ± 0.086	0.34 ± 0.023	0.52 ± 0.012
40	Caryophyllene Oxide	0.17 ± 0.028	0.19 ± 0.034	0.74 ± 0.311	0.05 ± 0.139	0.17 ± 0.319	0.29 ± 0.009
41	Globulol	0.16 ± 0.034	0.22 ± 0.243	0.78 ± 0.036	0.03 ± 0.347	0.28 ± 0.312	0.26 ± 0.031

(Continued)

Table 1. (*Continued*) RPAs of characteristic peaks of samples of *A. brachypus* from various sources.

| | | Ziwuling | | | Liupanshan | | Northern Shaanxi |
| | | Fresh stem bark ($n = 10$) | Fresh leaf ($n = 2$) | Fresh root ($n = 2$) | Dry stem bark ($n = 2$) | Fresh stem bark ($n = 8$) | Fresh stem bark ($n = 8$) |
No	Chemical compound	RPA	RPA	RPA	RPA	RPA	RPA
42	α-Cadinol	0.10 ± 0.017		0.12 ± 0.072	0.45 ± 0.013	0.14 ± 0.039	0.65 ± 0.026
43	α-Bisabolol	0.06 ± 0.049			0.89 ± 0.218	0.20 ± 0.034	0.08 ± 0.021
44	β-Sinensal	0.07 ± 0.021	0.10 ± 0.087	0.18 ± 0.154	0.01 ± 0.056	0.16 ± 0.022	0.09 ± 0.037
45	(*E*,*E*)-Farnesol	0.16 ± 0.053	0.28 ± 0.158		0.68 ± 0.068	0.22 ± 0.056	0.21 ± 0.026
46	Palmitoleic acid	0.13 ± 0.214		1.14 ± 0.028	0.24 ± 0.049	0.14 ± 0.017	0.18 ± 0.139
47	Palmitic acid	0.05 ± 0.035	0.08 ± 0.067	0.20 ± 0.034	0.21 ± 0.009	0.12 ± 0.031	0.08 ± 0.026
48	Tetracosane	0.02 ± 0.029	0.06 ± 0.007	0.06 ± 0.105		0.05 ± 0.011	0.05 ± 0.031

2.2 Data analysis of chromatogram

By means of GC-FID and GC-MS techniques, the gas chromatogram and mass spectrogram of the essential oils were achieved. Components were analyzed and identified based on comparison of RT and RI and/or MS fragmentation pattern (Adams, 2007). A standard solution of n-alkanes (C_6-C_{30}) was used to obtain the retention indices. The correlation coefficients of entire chromatographic patterns among samples were calculated, and the simulative mean chromatogram was generated using the Computer-Aided Similarity Evaluation System. The fingerprint analysis was performed on the basis of RRT and RPA. β-Pinene was assigned as the reference peak.

3 RESULTS AND DISCUSSION

3.1 Chemical composition of the essential oils

Comparison of the composition of the essential oils from different parts of A. brachypus, showed that the dominant constituents were monoterpenes, sesquiterpenes, and their oxides, which were in accordance with most *Acanthopanax* plants. The fresh stem bark oil is rich in β-pinene, linalool, p-cymene, spathulenol, *endo*-borneol, camphene and verbenone. p-Cymene, α-guaiene, β-pinene, linalool, γ-terpinene, *endo*-borneol and camphene were the major constituents of the fresh leaf oil. β-Caryophyllene, palmitoleic acid, limonene, β-pinene, verbenone and globulol were the major constituents of the fresh root oil, whereas limonene, β-pinene, α-bisabolol, δ-elemene, (E,E)-farnesol and p-cymene were the major constituents of the dry stem bark oil. However, the constituents of the essential oils from the fresh root and dry stem bark were less than those from the fresh stem bark and leaf, only 13 of 48 constituents were in common, and their RPA values were also different. And can be seen from the above analysis, as the principal constituents of A. brachypus oil, linalool, β-pinene, limonene, verbenone, β-caryophy-llene, spathulenol and β-thujene have important pharmacological activities, which is in accordance with the medicinal effects of A. brachypus.

3.2 GC-MS fingerprint of fresh A. brachypus

Analyzed fresh stem bark acquired from different areas, the correlation coefficient between each chromatogram and respective simulative mean chromatogram were 0.971 ± 0.041 ($n = 10$, ZWL), 0.967 ± 0.008 ($n = 8$, LPS) and $0.9730.067$ ($n = 8$, NS), respectively. In general, the chromatographic fingerprinting profiles were highly similar to each other within the same source. However, the correlation coefficients among various sources were significantly different. The correlation coefficients with respect to the simulative mean chromatogram were evaluated as 0.712 (ZWL *vs.* LPS), 0.825 (ZWL *vs.* NS) and 0.693 (LPS *vs.* NS). Comparing the chemical components in various areas, the contents of compounds **9** and **16** were the highest in ZWL. The RPA of **16** in ZWL ($0.25 + 0.041$ for fresh stem bark, $0.37 + 0.068$ for fresh leaf) was four times higher than that of LPS ($0.06 + 0.029$), and about five times higher than that of NS ($0.05 + 0.029$). Furthermore, the contents of compounds **7**, **10**, **26**, **33** and **34** were the highest in LPS, the RPA values were $0.82 + 0.030$, $0.95 + 0.028$, $0.97 + 0.110$, $0.36 + 0.026$ and $0.64 + 0.024$, respectively. It was observed that the RPA of **26** in LPS ($0.97 + 0.110$) was 12 times higher than that in ZWL ($0.08 + 0.032$), and 16 times higher than that in NS ($0.06 + 0.023$). In contrast, the content of compound **11**, **15** and **42** was the highest in NS, with the RPA ($1.72 + 0.013$, $0.48 + 0.034$ and $0.65 + 0.026$) sextupled that in other sources. In this regard, fresh A. brachypus of different areas can be distinguished by comparing the relative contents of compounds **15**, **16** and **26**.

3.3 Comparison of chromatographic fingerprint among various medicinal parts

The correlation coefficients of the simulative mean chromatogram were $0.9420.023$ ($n = 2$, fresh leaf), $0.917 + 0.015$ ($n = 2$, fresh root), $0.936 + 0.011$ ($n = 2$, dry stem bark), 0.833 (fresh leaf *vs.* fresh stem bark), 0.421 (fresh leaf *vs.* fresh root), 0.479 (fresh stem bark *vs.* fresh root), 0.645 (fresh stem bark *vs.* dry stem bark), 0.281 (fresh leaf *vs.* dry stem bark), and 0.212 (fresh root *vs.* dry stem bark), respectively. Comparing the chemical compounds of various parts, the contents of compounds **11, 18, 19, 30, 31, 32** and **37** were the highest in the leaf, the RPA of **30** was almost 6 times more abundant than that in other parts. The level of compounds **10, 23, 29, 40, 41** and **46** were the highest in the root, the RPAs of **46** and **29** in the root were about 8 and 6 times higher than that in the stem bark, and RPA of **29** was about 20 times higher than that in the leaf. The results indicated that the fresh stem bark and leaf possessed high similarity in terms of overall chemical components, but the root possessed low similarity with the stem bark.

Comparing the fingerprinting profiles and chemical components between the fresh and dry stem bark, the contents of compounds **13, 41** and **44** were higher in the former, with the RPA generally five times higher than that of the latter. In contrast, the contents of compounds **8, 10, 33** and **43** were higher in the dry form with the RPA of **43** almost 15 times higher than in the fresh. It is worth noting that compounds **4, 11, 16, 20, 21, 22** and **30** were not observed in the dry stem bark, but were present in considerable abundance in the fresh counterpart. To sum up, the fresh and dry stem bark of *A. brachypus* from Ziwuling possessed similar fingerprinting profiles. However, there existed drastic differences in terms of chemical composition and quantities.

These differences can probably be attributed to the loss or decomposition of various components during the drying process.

4   CONCLUSION

By comparing the fingerprints, fresh samples acquired from different areas possessed drastic differences, which implies that the choice of production area should be carefully considered in order to maintain a consistent production of quality material. Besides, the fingerprinting profiles among different parts of the fresh samples possessed limited similarities to each other. It also revealed that the distribution of chemical compounds varied among those medicinal parts. Traditionally, the root was used as a medicinal part. However, the stem bark of *A. brachypus* was reported to have multifarious medicinal function (Hu *et al.*, 2009). Comparing the fingerprints of dry and fresh stem bark of *A. brachypus*, the number of chemical components for the latter was always more abundant than the former, as well as some bioactive components in particular compounds **13, 41** and **44** are always higher in content. Although, practically, it is difficult to use fresh *A. brachypus* in clinical application, preservation methods should nonetheless be developed with an aim to facilitate and popularize the use of these fresh medicinal materials.

ACKNOWLEDGEMENTS

This work was financially supported by the Natural Science Foundation of China (No. 2146202 6) and the Applied Chemistry Key Subject of Gansu Province (No. GSACKS201304).

REFERENCES

Adams, R.P. (2007) Identification of essential oil components by GC/MS (4 ed). Carol Stream, IL, USA., Allured Publishing Corporation. 56–119.
Gansu Food and Drug Administration (1st). (2009) Gansu Chinese Materia Medica Standards. Lanzhou, Gansu Culture Press. 59–61.
Hu, H.B., Fan, J. (2012) Chemical constituents from *Acanthopanax brachypus*, *Biochemical Systematics and Ecology*, 43, 67–72.
Hu, H.B., Zheng, X.D., Hu, H.S., Li, Y. (2009) Chemical compositions and anti-microbial activities of essential oils extracted from *Acanthopanax brachypus*, *Archives of Pharmacal Research*, 32, 699–710.

Medicine Sciences and Bioengineering – Wang (Ed.)
© *2015 Taylor & Francis Group, London, ISBN: 978-1-138-02684-1*

Research and practice of diversified pharmaceutical talent training model

Huan-qi Wang & Pei-ge Du*
College of Pharmacy, Beihua University, Jilin, China

ABSTRACT: In order to better adapt to the talent competition in the pharmaceutical market and the requirements for new pharmaceutical talents in the society, a diversified pharmaceutical talent training model was proposed. The model was aimed to cultivate the students to have an international vision, to be able to serve for the economic construction and social development. In this study, based on the characteristics of diversified training model, a training program with various contents and distinct characteristics was formulated, and the training methods and training approaches were designed and implemented according to the training program. The establishment of a pharmaceutical diversified talent training model and its teaching system can help to train the diversity of pharmaceutical talents, and should be in line with the requirements of social development for the talents. It is conducive to widening students' international horizon, and improving students' proficiency, innovation, market competitiveness and the quality of student training[1].

1   INTRODUCTION

In the 21st century, along with the rapid development of the life sciences, people had a deep understanding in the occurrence and mechanism of diseases, which has triggered a new revolution in drug research and development. Furthermore, the pharmaceutical education in China has entered a new era (D.H.Liu,2013). In order to better apt to the talent competition in the pharmaceutical market and the requirements for new pharmaceutical talents in the society, the teaching mode of higher pharmaceutical education must be constantly transformed and continuously reformed, its teaching philosophy must be innovated, and its development in various aspects must be further promoted. Aiming at a local pharmacy comprehensive university (D.H.Liu, 2013), the establishment of a training model of diversified pharmaceutical talent with an international vision, capable of serving for the economic construction and social development (C.P.Yang, 2013)was proposed, and studied and practiced by considering the reality of pharmacy and based on the previous experience on pharmaceutical teaching and teaching reform.

2   PREVIOUS WORK BASIS

In recent five years, in order to improve the quality of personnel training, we have increased our efforts to reform, launched two provincial items of the education reform, implemented an undergraduate tutorial system, attempted to carry out the bilingual teaching established a student research team relying on the undergraduate innovative experimental projects, and built open laboratories, which has helped establish a training model for the cultivation of applied pharmaceutical and innovative personnel. Several remarkable results in the research and practice in the exploration

---

First Author: Huanqi Wang. email: 1134442770@qq.com
*Corresponding author: Peige Du，email: 2207520094@qq.com

on the training model have been achieved. In our college, pharmacology and pharmaceutical analysis courses were named the excellent course of Jilin Province, and biotechnology pharmaceuticals was named the superior course of Jilin province. There is an excellent teacher team in our college, which has provided a good foundation for the teaching reform.

2.1 Establishment of diversified pharmaceutical personnel training model

To meet the needs of multi-level pharmacy personnel in society and to improve the quality of personnel training, based on the ranking of student test scores and the ranking of specific examination, the third-year students were divided into four parts who were trained in different directions from the first semester of the third year after they finished the general-knowledge and common basic courses according to the requirements of the training programs. The training directions included graduate training direction, to innovative talent training direction, applied talent raining direction and service talent training direction.

2.1.1 Graduate training direction

The students who had passed College English Test band 6 or 4 and whose scores of all courses were beyond 70 points were selected as the research objects. In the basis of the original curriculum stipulated by the undergraduate training program, they were asked to attend selected courses for preparing for the graduate entrance examination including English and pecialized courses. Teachers who had a higher English level and had received a good international education were invited to teach the professional intensified courses, to enhance their English language skills and professional competence.

2.1.2 Innovative talent training direction and applied talent training

Through an open selection way with an examination, the students with good skills were assigned to take part in scientific and technological innovation activities under the guidance of teachers with rich experiences on the practical teaching, and they were given more practical and related teaching in order to cultivate their innovative and applied capabilities. Moreover, as scientific research assistants, they could participate in some research projects for developing their scientific research capacity, and the outstanding could be selected to participate in the National Innovation Experiment Program, the National Pharmacy Practice Skills Competition and National Pharmacy Summit Forum.

2.1.3 Service talent training direction

The students who were willing to getting a job in the drug circulation, have a strong sense of service and dedication, and have a strong communication skill were selected to be trained toward this direction. In the selected courses, "Hundreds of Forums" were carried out, in which well-known entrepreneurs, as visiting professors, were invited to give the students lectures on marketing and to train them in vocational qualification, in order to develop their marketing capabilities.

2.2 Teaching system reform program for pharmacy diversified training model and its implementation

2.2.1 Establishment of innovative curriculum system

The curriculum system was established under the guidance of a diversified education thought, on the basis of update course content, centering on the building of core teaching materials and by integrating the multiple essential factors. The connotation construction and the reform of the curriculum were strengthened, and a new curriculum system in line with the requirements for the diversified talent training was established. An effort to build the national quality course of pharmacology and pharmaceutical analysis in our college, and the provincial quality course of pharmaceutical biotechnology was made. An innovative curriculum content was created, in which the teaching started from the source of drug development, the research principles and methods of new drug development, and the instances from well-known domestic and overseas pharmaceutical manufacturers and Institutes were added to the specialized courses to widen the students' horizons. In the teaching of pharmaceutics, pharmaceutical chemistry, pharmaceutical analysis and pharmacognosy courses, more attention was paid to combining the specialized pharmacy knowledge with the engineering technical knowledge, increasing the introduction of technical problems in the drug production of domestic and foreign pharmaceutical companies, focusing on the research and development of pharmaceutical preparation, to cultivate the students' innovative spirits. In undergraduates who were going to attend the graduate examination, the teaching of basic specialized knowledge was emphasized in the selected courses, realizing that the importance should be focused and the detail could be grasped. On the Pharmaceutical Marketing course, the analysis on the marketing cases was increased, and professionals from Bayer and Pfizer companies, the world's top 500 enterprises, were invited to teach how to develop new markets and increase the product market share.

2.2.2 *Establishment of an open practice teaching mode*

Practical teaching is one of important parts of high education, one of important steps comprehensively to examine students' theoretical knowledge, and can play a vital role in the cultivation of students' innovative spirit and scientific thinking. The implementation of an open practice teaching model can make the students transformed from a passive learning to an active learning, and their students' problem-analyzing and problem-solving skills will be further improved. The specific implementation steps included students' self-choice of projects within the curriculum program, self-design of experimental plan, analysis on the feasibility and self-performance after the improvement of the plan by teachers in the open laboratory, while the teachers only took responsibility for the instruction during the experiment. The assessment of open practice teaching model were based on a comprehensive evaluation of the students' design capabilities, operational skills, creative abilities, problem-analyzing, problem- solving skills, communication skills and self-learning capabilities. The core of open practice teaching model was to ask the students to get the best results with a scientific, simple and economical way. The results indicate that through the open practice teaching model, the students can gradually become knowledged, which should be beneficial to the improvement of quality of personnel training, and simultaneously help them have an ability to participate in reach college students participate in the National Innovation Experiment Program, the National Pharmacy Practice Skills Competition and National Pharmacy Summit Forum.

2.2.3 *Interactive research mode of undergraduates with graduates*

Currently interactive undergraduate and graduate research mode is a mode actively promoted in domestic and overseas universities, as well as the basic requirement for the construction of a teaching-research type of university. Our university is a teaching-research type of comprehensive university and there are a certain number of both undergraduates and graduates, which provides a condition for the implementation of interactive undergraduate and graduate research mode. In this study, a research team composed of tutors, graduates and undergraduates together was organized, in which the undergraduate were led by graduate students under the guidance of tutors. It is believed that in this mode, the undergraduates can learn more new research methods and techniques, especially the development of innovative thinking, which can lay a foundation for the future work. On the other hand, the implementation of this mode can also supplement the insufficiency in undergraduate teaching resources, and make undergraduates strengthen the theoretical knowledge and operational skills and improve their skills to solve practical problems.

2.2.4 *Introduction of innovative teaching methods and learning methods*

Combined with the actuality of college, PBL (Problem Based Learning) in theoretical teaching, RBL (Research Based Learning) in the practical teaching, and TBL (Team Based Learning) in class and after class have been implemented. The PBL teaching enables the students in advance to learn with questions proposed by the teachers, which can make their memories more deeply and improve their ability to accept new knowledge. The RBL teaching is a teaching method emphasizing that inquiry learning is taken as the purpose, which has been demonstrated effective in the students' comprehensive design experiment on mobilizing the students' learning initiative, enthusiasm and creativity, and enhancing the comprehensive practical ability. The TBL teaching is a learning mode focusing on problem-solving in team, and can be conducted both in class and after class. The goal is to solve the problem in team and to improve the students' unity cooperation ability (J.Hong, 2012).

3 SUMMARY

This study, based on the characteristics of diversified training model, a training program with various contents was formulated, and the training methods and training approaches were designed and implemented according to the training program. The establishment of a pharmaceutical diversified talent training model and its teaching system can help to train the diversity of pharmaceutical talents, be in line with the requirements of social development for the talents, especially the requirements of the National Twelfth Five-Year Development Strategy. It should be conducive to widening students' international horizon, and improving students' proficiency, innovation, market competitiveness and the quality of student training.

REFERENCES

Hong Jun. Analysis on personalized education oriented university diversified talent training [M] *Journal of Central South University Forestry & Technology* (Social Science), 2012.6(3):1–3.
Liu Dunhu. Research on diversified talent training model [M]. *Soft Science*, 2013. (9):23–31.
Yang Chuanping. Study and practice of the diversified forestry talent training model in Northeast Forestry University [M] *Forestry Education in China*, 2013, 31,(5):1–5.

Medicine Sciences and Bioengineering – Wang (Ed.)
© *2015 Taylor & Francis Group, London, ISBN: 978-1-138-02684-1*

Antioxidant study of the polysaccharides from *Cordyceps militaris*, natural quercetin and N-acetylneuraminic acid

Shou-dong Guo

Key Laboratory of Atherosclerosis in Universities of Shandong, Taishan Medical University, Taian, Shandong, China

ABSTRACT: From the year of 2000, lots of researches have focused on the antioxidant activity of polysaccharides of plant, algae or microbial origins, and it seems most of the polysaccharides bear good free radicals scavenging ability in vitro. In the past few years, we also screened the antioxidant ability on some of the polysaccharides of different sources, and the IC50 values were in the level of mg/mL, which were consistent with most of the other publications. In this paper, we investigated the in vitro antioxidant activity of the polysaccharides from Cordyceps militaris, the natural polyphenolic compound quercetin, and N-acetylneuraminic acid which distributed widely in cells or particles of mammalians. The results demonstrated that quercetin exhibit much stronger free radicals scavenging activity than the polysaccharides or N-acetylneuraminic acid. Additionally, quercetin could effectively protect HUVEC cells (EA.hy926) under oxidative stress condition. Therefore, our results indicated that polysaccharides may not be a kind of effective antioxidant with great potent application when compared with polyphenolic compound quercetin.

1 INTRODUCTION

Reactive Oxygen Species (ROS), e.g. superoxide anion radical, hydroxyl radical and hydrogen peroxide, can either be generated exogenously or produced intracellularly (Valko et al, 2007). The ROS produced is largely counteracted by an intricate antioxidant defence system that includes the enzymatic scavengers SOD, catalase (CAT) and glutathione peroxide, and a variety of non-enzymatic, low molecular mass molecules scanvengers, including ascorbate, flavonoids, pyruvate and so on (Finkel & Holbrook, 2000). However, the balance would often be broken due to the influences of inside and outside, and lead to the accumulation of ROS, the state of which is well known as "oxidative stress". The balance between ROS production and antioxidant defences determines the degree of oxidative stress. Increasing publications demonstrated that persistent oxidative stress is positively associated with various diseases (Valko *et al*, 2007; Blomhoff *et al.* 2008; Halvorsen *et al.* 2002; Hegde *et al.* 2005;), including cancer, cardiac and cerebro-vascular diseases, inflammation, aging (Wichens, 2001) and so on.

During the course of searching new natural antioxidant, polysaccharides have drawn much more attentions. In addition, polyphenols are mainly found in fruits and vegetables and are one of the most important sources of bioactive components of the human diet, and some of them such as flavonoids are important non-enzymatic compounds existing in human and other animals (Zhao *et al*, 1990; Finkel & Holbrook, 2000; Salim *et al*, 2004). In this study, the antioxidant activities of the polysaccharides from *Cordyceps militaris*, the natural quercetin and the widely distributed N-acetylneuraminic acid in cells or particles of mammalians were investigated at the same time via several commonly used investigation systems.

2 MATERIALS AND METHODS

2.1 *Materials*

1,1-diphenyl-2-picrylhydrazyl (DPPH), ascorbic acid, 1,2-phthalic dicarboxaldehyde and MTT were the products of Sigma–Aldrich (St. Louis, MO, USA). Standard quercetin, thiobarbituric acid (TBA), trichloroacetic acid (TCA) were from Beijing Prina Chemical Industry CO. LTD. N-acetylneuraminic acid (NANA) was provided by ACCOBIOTM (Jiangsu, China). All the other reagents used in this study were of the analysis grade.

2.2 *In vitro antioxidant assays*

Scavenging ability on DPPH, superoxide anion radicals and inhibition of lipid peroxidation was assessed according to the method reported by Shimada *et al.* (1992), and we previously published papers (Sun *et al*, 2009; Guo *et al*, 2010).

Human umbilical vein endothelial cell (HUVEC) cells (EA.hy926) were inoculated into 96 well plate, with 1×10^4 cells per well. After 4 hours preincubation in a humidified 5% CO_2 incubator at 37°C, samples were added, followed by adding 5 μL 1%H_2O_2, mixing and 12 hours' culture. Then, the culture medium was discarded and the cells were rinsed with PBS gently before the adding of 5 mg/mL MTT solution dissolved in PBS, 10 μL per well. The cells were cultured for another 4 hours and then the culture medium was discarded and the cells were rinsed with PBS gently. Finally, 100 μL DMSO was added to each well, mixed, and then measured at 570 nm.

2.3 *Statistical analysis*

All bioassay results were expressed as means ± standard deviation (SD). The experimental data were subjected to an analysis of variance (ANOVA) for a completely random design.

3 RESULTS

3.1 *In vitro antioxidant activity*

To make a comparative study between polysaccharides from *Cordyceps militaris* (CMPS) and polyphenolic compounds as well as an attempt to find the monosaccharide composition influence on the antioxidant activity of polysaccharides, the commonly reported antioxidant assays in vitro were used to evaluate the effect of quercetin, CMPS and the monosaccharide NANA.

Among the assays, all of the samples exhibited concentration dependent manner. As shown in Figure 1a, quercetin exhibited the strongest antioxidant activity. The DPPH radicals' scavenging effect was close to that of ascorbic acid, while CMPS and NANA exhibited significantly weaker DPPH scavenging effect than that of quercetin ($p \le 0.01$). At the highest concentration detected, the percentage scavenging effects of quercetin, CMPS and NANA were 85.77 ± 3.31, 57.23 ± 3.49 and 33.42 ± 2.31 μg/mL, respectively. Superoxide anion radicals scavenging assay was shown in Figure 1b. Although the effect of quercetin seemed near to ascorbic acid, from the concentration of 125 ug/mL to the maximum, the effect of quercetin was markedly lower than that of positive control ($p \le 0.05$). Both CMPS and NANA exhibited significantly weaker effect than that of quercetin. However, the effect of NANA on scavenging superoxide anion radicals was close to that of the polysaccharides CMPS ($p > 0.05$). The lipid peroxidation inhibition effect of quercetin was equal to that of ascorbic acid. At the concentration of 1 mg/mL, the percentage inhibitory effects of quercetin, CMPS and NANA were 83.69 ± 3.67, 52.13 ± 2.92 and 36.45 ± 2.81 μg/mL, respectively (Figure 2a).

Quercetin, CMPS and NANA were further studied on the scavenging activity of hydrogen peroxide and their antioxidant effect was evaluated by the survival rate of HUVEC cells under a

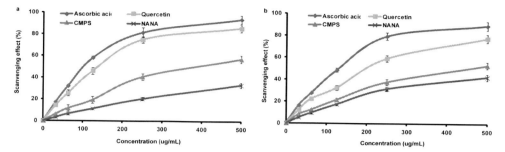

Figure 1. The percentage scavenging effect of quercetin, CMPS and NANA on DPPH (a) and superoxide anion (b) radicals.

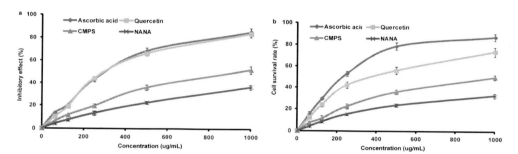

Figure 2. The percentage inhibitory effect of quercetin, CMPS and NANA on lipid peroxidation (a), and HUVEC cell survival rate (b) under different concentration of quercetin, CMPS and NANA.

oxidative stress condition. As shown in Figure 2b, at the dosage of 250 µg/mL, quercetin and the positive control ascorbic acid could protect half of the HUVEC cells from death, and quercetin showed a close protection effect compared to that of ascorbic acid. At the dosage of 1 mg/mL, about 50% HUVEC cells still alive under the protection of CMPS. In addition, NANA showed comparable protection effect at the highest dosage measured, compared with that of CMPS.

4 DISCUSSION

Our present results demonstrated that CMPS were weaker than that of quercetin in scavenging free radicals and lipid peroxidation inhibition effect. The in vitro antioxidant results of these measured polysaccharides were close to the extracellular polysaccharides PS1-1, PS1-2 and PS2-1 isolated from the marine fungus *Penicillium* sp. F23-2 (Sun *et al.* 2009), that previously reported protein-bound polysaccharide by Chen *et al.* (2008) and the extracellular polysaccharide isolated from *Pantoea agglomerans* strain KFS-9 (Wang *et al.* 2007).

Some researchers have indicated that the acidic monosaccharide may benefit the antioxidant activity of the polysaccharide, and our experiment demonstrated that NANA exhibited certain antioxidant activity. As has been reported the antioxidant mechanism of NANA is the same with that of pyruvate, both of which could counteract H_2O_2 through decarboxylation (Iijima et al, 2004). Additionally, protein may also benefit the antioxidant activity of the carbohydrates. For instance, Chen *et al.* (2008) found that the water soluble protein–bound polysaccharide from the fruiting bodies of *Ganoderma atrum* exhibited strong radical scavenging activities.

In order to detect the practical application of the samples, the adding of hydrogen peroxide (1%, 5 µL) was based on our previous experiment, which indicated without protection no more than 5% of the HUVEC cells could survive. Results demonstrated quercetin exhibited the best hydrogen peroxide scavenging activity, whose effect was near to that the positive control ascorbic acid. CMPS and NANA also showed certain protection effect under the extreme oxidative stress condition, at the concentration of 1 mg/mL.

5 SUMMARY

Although some polysaccharides could be good immune adjuvant and excellent industrial and pharmaceutical additive, however, our results indicated, at least in part, that polysaccharides may have less chances of being applied in clinic on account of their antioxidant activity.

ACKNOWLEDGEMENTS

This work was supported by Natural Science Foundation of China (31300639), Traditional Chinese Medicine of Shandong Province Science and Technology Research Project (2013-257), Natural Science Foundation of Shandong Province (ZR2013HQ014), and High Level Research Training Program of Taishan Medical University (330033).

REFERENCES

Blomhoff, R., Carlsen, M.H., Andersen, L.F., & Jacobs, D.R.J. (2008) Health benefits of nuts: Potential role of antioxidants. *British Journal of Nutrition*, 96, 52–60.

Chen, Y., Xie, M.Y., Nie, S.P., Li, C. & Wang, Y.X. (2008) Purification, composition analysisand antioxidant activity of a polysaccharide from the fruiting bodies of *Ganoderma atrum*. *Food Chemistry*, 107, 231–241.

Finkel, T. & Holbrook, N.J. (2000) Oxidants, oxidative stress and the biology of ageing. *Nature*, 408, 239–247.

Guo, S.D., Mao, W.J., Han, Y., Yang, C.L., Chen, Y., Chen, Y.L., Xu, J., Li, H.Y., Qi, X.H. & Xu, J.C. (2010) Structural characteristics and antioxidant activities of the extracellular polysaccharide produced by marine bacterium *Edwardsiella tarda*. *Bioresource Technology*, 101, 4729–4732.

Halvorsen, B.L., Holte, K., Myhrstad, M.C.W., Barikmo, I., Hvattum, E. & Remberg S.F. (2002) A systematic screening of total antioxidants in dietary plants. *Journal of Nutrition*,132, 461–471.

Hegde, P.S., Rajasekaran, N.S. & Chandra, T.S. (2005) Effect of the antioxidant properties of millet species on oxidative stress and glycemic status in alloxan-induced rats. *Nutrition Research*, 25, 1109–1120.

Iijima, R., Takahashi, H., Namme, R., Ikegami, S. & Yamazaki, M. (2004) Novel biological function of sialic acid (N-Acetylneuraminic acid) as a hydrogen peroxide scavenger. *FEBS Letters*, 561, 163–166.

Kweon, M.H., Hwang, H.J. & Sung, H.C. (2001) Identification and antioxidant activity of novel chlorogenic acid derivatives from bamboo (*phyllostachys edulis*). *Journal of Agricultural and Food Chemistry*, 49, 4646–4655.

Marklund, S. & Marklund, G. (1974) Involvement of superoxide anion radicals in the autoxidation of pyrogallol and a convenient assay for superoxide dismutase. *European Journal of Biochemistry*, 47, 469–474.

Salim, E.I., Kaneko, M., Wanibuchi, H., Morimura, K. & Fukushima, S. (2004) Lack of carcinogenicity of enzymatically modified isoquercitrin in F344/ DuCrj rats. *Food and Chemical Toxicology*, 42, 1949–69.

Shimada, K., Fujikawa, K., Yahara, K. & Nakamura, T. (1992) Antioxidative properties of xanthan on the autoxidation of soybean oil in cyclodextrin emulsion. *Journal of Agricultural and Food Chemistry*, 40, 945–948.

Sun, H.H., Mao, W.J., Chen, Y., Guo, S.D., Li, H.Y., Qi, X.H., Chen, Y.L. & Xu, J. (2009) Isolation, chemical characteristics and antioxidant properties of the polysaccharides from marine fungus *Penicillium* sp. F23-2. *Carbohydrate Polymers*, 78, 117–124.

Valko, M., Leibfritz, D., Moncol, J., Cronin, M.T.D., Mazur, M. & Telser, J. (2007) Free radicals and antioxidants in normal physiological functions and human disease. *The International Journal of Biochemistry & Cell Biology*, 39, 44–84.

Wang, H.Y., Jiang, X.L., Mu, H.J., Liang, X.T. & Guan, H.S. (2007) Structure and protective effect of exopolysaccharide from *P. agglomerans* strain KFS-9 against UV radiation. *Microbiology Research*, 162, 124–129.

Zhao, J., Zhang, C.Y., Xu, D.M., Huang, G.Q., Xu, Y.L. & Wang, Z.Y. (1990) The antiatherogenic effects of components isolated from pollen typhae. *Thrombosis research*, 57, 957–966.

Medicine Sciences and Bioengineering – Wang (Ed.)
© *2015 Taylor & Francis Group, London, ISBN: 978-1-138-02684-1*

Stability and antimicrobial activity of microencapsulated clove oil

Qing-lian Xu, Ya-ge Xing*, Dong Cao, Da-feng Zhang & Zhen-ming Che
Food Bio-technology Key Laboratory of Sichuan Province, College of Bioengineering, Xihua University, Chengdu, Sichuan, China

Wei-feng Han
School of Food Engineering, Luohe Vocational Technology College, Luohe, Henan, China

Ying Meng, Hong-bin Lin & Li Jiang
Food Bio-technology Key Laboratory of Sichuan Province, College of Bioengineering, Xihua University, Chengdu, Sichuan, China

ABSTRACT: In this investigation, characteristics of microencapsulated clove oil were investigated. The morphology of microencapsulated clove oil was also analyzed by SEM. The results indicated that the temperature and the relative humidity in the microenvironment around microencapsulation are two of the most important factors determined the release rate of clove oil. More important, the inhibitory zone was 20.67 mm, 23.48 mm and 22.61 mm for the microencapsulation against *E.coli*, *S. aureus* and *B. Subtilis*, respectively. The inhibitory zone was 43.25 mm, 39.50 mm and 57.15 mm for the microencapsulation against *A. flavus*, *R. nigricans* and *P. citrinum*, respectively. These results show that the microencapsulated clove oil exhibited high stability under different temperature and relative humidity and show good inhibited property against the growth of microorganism.

1 INTRODUCTION

Microbial contamination could increase the disease risk and further affect the quality of food products (Wanchaitanawong *et al.*, 2005). In recent years, some natural anti-microbial agents, such as essential oils, have been investigated by other researchers (Schelz *et al.*, 2006). Essential oils have been regarded as the potential alternatives for conventional antimicrobial agents due to their antimicrobial property (Singh *et al.*, 2002). Investigation on the antimicrobial activity of essential oils against food-related microorganisms has been reported recently (Deriu *et al.*, 2008).

Clove oil is not harmful to human health and the environment used as a natural preservative. Its antimicrobial activity has been reported to inhibit the growth of molds, yeasts and bacteria (Matan *et al.*, 2006). As reported by other researchers, the antimicrobial activity of clove oil should be due to its major competent of eugenol (Sukatta *et al.*, 2008). Eugenol has been reported to inhibit the growth of *E. coli* and *L. monocytogenes* (Blaszyk and Holley, 1998).

However, its application was restricted due to its quick release under the room temperature. Therefore, microencapsulation is a useful technology to improve its stability. Nevertheless, only a few investigations reported regarding the stability and antimicrobial activity of essential oils.

In this study, the stability of microencapsulated clove oil under different temperature and relative humidity was investigated. In addition, research on the *in vitro* antimicrobial activity of microencapsulatin containing clove oil was also conducted.

---

*Corresponding author. Fax: +86 2887720552; Email: xingyage1@aliyun.com

2 MATERIALS AND METHODS

2.1 *Preparation of microencapsulated clove oil*

Preparation of microencapsulation containing clove oil was prepared using a coprecipitation method (Bhandari *et al.*, 1998). β-cyclodextrin (β-CD) (6 g) was dissolved in 100 ml of distilled water at 75°C on a hot plate. After cooling to 42°C, clove oil in ethanol (1:1, v/v) was slowly added to the solution with continuous agitation, to give a molar ratio of clove oil/β-CD of 1:6. The vessel was stirred by a magnetic stirrer at room temperature for 4 h. Then the chitosan (1.0%), clove oil (0.3%), ethanol (15%) and Tween 80 (0.3%) were added. The obtained complex solution was stirred by the magnetic stirrer at room temperature for 1.5 h. The obtained solution was dried at 30°C for 50 h under vacuum condition.

2.2 *Morphological observation*

Morphological observation of microencapsulated clove oil was characterized by scanning electron microscopy (SEM). The powder was placed on the SEM stub using two-sided adhesive tapes and then SEM analyses after Pt sputtering.

2.3 *Stability of microencapsulated oil under different temperature*

Stability of microencapsulated clove oil at different temperature and relative humidity (5 or 25°C for 20 min) was investigated (Mandal *et al.*, 2006). Approximately 0.5 g of each dried powder was spread in thin layers in 15 mL glass bottles (20 mm I.D. × 48 mm), and placed in a desiccator with saturated salt solution in order to maintain a constant relative humidity at $43 \pm 5\%$, $75 \pm 5\%$, and $83 \pm 5\%$. The desiccators were held in an air bath at 20°C. The residual amount of clove oil in the power was measured.

2.4 *Determination of antimicrobial activity*

The agar diffusion method was used to determine the antimicrobial activity of microencapsulated clove oil (Pranoto *et al.*, 2005). For *E. coli*, *S. aureus* and *B. Subtilis*, microencapsulated clove oil (0.25 g) was placed on LB plate, which had been spread on 1.0 mL of inoculum containing approximately 10^6–10^7 CFU/mL of tested microorganism. The plates were incubated at 37°C for 24 h and then the diameters of the "inhibition zone" were measured. For antifungal activity inactivate *A. flavus*, *R. nigricans* and *P. citrinum*, microencapsulated clove oil (0.25 g) was placed on PDA plate, which had been spread on 1.0 mL of inoculum containing approximately 10^6–10^7 conidia/mL of tested fungi. The plates were incubated at 28°C for 72 h and then the diameters of "inhibition zone" were measured (Xing *et al.*, 2012).

2.5 *Statistical analysis*

The tests were carried out in triplicate and dates were analyzed by SPSS 13.0 software (SPSS Inc.). The one way analysis of variance procedure followed by least significant difference test was used to determine the significant difference ($p < 0.05$) between treatment means.

3 RESULTS AND DISCUSSION

3.1 *Morphology of microencapsulated clove oil*

Morphology of microencapsulated clove oil was characterized using SEM. As shown in Figure 1, morphological photos show that microencapsulation has an irregular shape with some forming agglomeration and show different particles size. During the preparation process, clove oil was enclosed in the β-cyclodextrin and chitosan coating. The water adsorption characteristics of chitosan may be one reason for the control release of clove oil in the microencapsulation, which

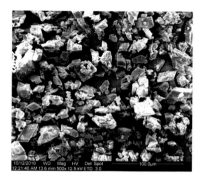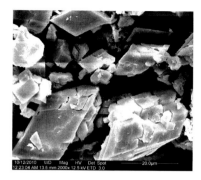

Figure 1.   Morphology of microencapsulation containing clove oil.

could impair the clove oil complexation and thereby the controlling effect of clove oil microcapsules on the release rate. Therefore, it is important to investigate the antimicrobial activity of microencapsulated clove oil.

3.2   *Stability of encapsulated oil under different temperature and relative humidity*

Effect of different temperature and relative humidity on the stability of microencapsulation containing clove oil was investigated and shown in Figure 2a and b. At RH 85%, the amount of oil released almost 60%, 67% and 90%, in 30 d when microencapsulated oil was stored at 25°C and 50°C, respectively. After storing at RH 75% for 30d and at RH 43% for 30d, the total amount of clove oil in the medium decreased drastically and was close to 50%, 56% and to 22%, 30%, when microencapsulated oil was stored at 25°C and 50°C, respectively. The results show that the release rate dramatically increased with increasing the temperature and the relative humidity of microenvironment. This indicated that the stability of microencapsulated clove oil may be closely related to the temperature and the relative humidity in the microenvironment around the powder. de Roos (2003) reported similar results for several esters. Such a change of temperature and relative humidity in the microenvironment had a great influence on the oil release (Soottitantawatet al., 2004). The RH-dependent and temperature-dependent characteristics of microencapsulated oil were evident in this investigation.

3.3   *In vitro antibacterial activity of microencapsulated clove oil*

The antibacterial properties of microencapsulated clove oil against *E. coli* and *S. aureus* can be seen from Figure 3. According to Figure 3, the antibacterial activity of microencapsulation

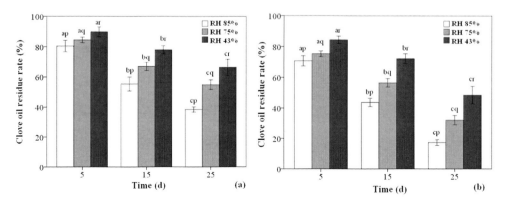

Figure 2.   Stability of microencapsulated clove oil during storage at 25°C (a) and 50°C (b).

673

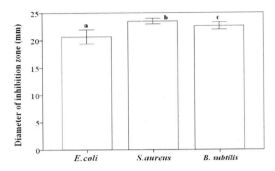

Figure 3. Antibacterial activity of encapsulated oil.

containing clove oil against *E. coli, S. aureus* and *B. Subtilis* was observed. The inhibitory zone was 20.67 mm, 23.48 mm and 22.61 mm for the microencapsulation against *E.coli, S. aureus* and *B. Subtilis*, respectively. The inhibitory effects of microencapsulated clove oil for *S. aureus* and *B. Subtilis* are stronger than that for *E. coli*. This result may be due to the difference structure and thickness of the membrane cell wall between *B. Subtilis, S. aureus* and *E. coli* (Li *et al.*, 2009). The antimicrobial activity of clove oil has been reported to inhibit the growth of molds, yeasts and bacteria (Matan et al. 2006). Eugenol, the main content in clove oil, is an antimicrobial compound having wide spectra of antimicrobial effects (Xing *et al.*, 2012).

3.4   *In vitro antifungal activity of microencapsulated clove oil*

The antifungal activity of microencapsulated clove oil against *A. flavus, R. nigricans* and *P. citrinum* can be seen from Figure 4. The inhibitory zone was 43.25 mm, 39.50 mm and 57.15 mm for the microencapsulation against *A. flavus, R. nigricans* and *P. citrinum*, respectively. The inhibitory effect of microencapsulated clove oil for *A. flavus* and *P. citrinum* is stronger than that for *R. nigricans*. Similar findings have been reported by other investigators (Farag *et al.* 1989). The antifungal activity of clove oil was evaluated in culture medium, and tomato paste was also investigated by Omidbeygi *et al.* (2007) and Xing *et al.*(2012).

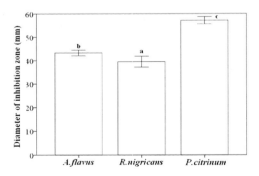

Figure 4. Antifungal activity of encapsulated oil.

4 SUMMARY

Microencapsulated clove oil was also analyzed by SEM. The results show that microencapsulated clove oil exhibited good antimicrobial activity. It was the temperature and the relative humidity in the microenvironment of microencapsulation that two of the most important factors determined the release rate of clove oil.

ACKNOWLEDGEMENTS

This study was supported by 2013 Industry cluster project of Chengdu (Integration and Industrialization of Key Technology for Mushroom Industry taking the intensive procedures as the core) and by Xihua University Young Scholars Training Program (01201413). This work was also financially supported by the Open Research Fund of Key Laboratory of Food Biotechnology, Xihua University (SZJJ2012-005, SZJJ2014-003 and SZJJ2014-002) the Key Research Foundation Program of Xihua University (Z1120539).

REFERENCES

Bhandari, B.R., D'arcy, B.R. &Bich, L. L. T. (1998) Lemon oil to beta-cyclodextrin ratio effect on the inclusion efficiency of beta-cyclodextrin and the retention of oil volatiles in the complex. J. Agricult. Food Chem. 46(4), 1494–1499.

Blaszyk, M. & Holley, R.A. (1998) Interaction of monolaurin, eugenol and sodium citrate on growth of common meat spoilage and pathogenic organisms. Int. J. Food Microbiol.,39, 175–183.

Deriu, A., Zanetti, S., Sechi, L.A., Marongiu, B., Piras, A., Procedda, S. &Tuveri, E. (2008) Antimicrobial activity of *Inula helenium* L. essential oil against gram-positive and gram-negative bacteria andCandidaspp. Int. J. Antimicrob. Agents,31, 588–590.

de Roos K. B. (2003). Effect of texture and microstructure on flavour retention and release. International Dairy Journal, 13(8), 593–605.

Matan, N., Rimkeeree, H., Mawson, A.J., Chompreeda, P., Haruthaithanasan, V. and Parker, M.(2006) Antimicrobial activity of cinnamon and clove oils under modified atmosphere conditions. Int. J. Food Microbiol.,107, 180–185.

Mandal , S., Puniya, A.K., Singh K. (2006) Effect of alginate concentrations on survival of microencapsulated Lactobacillus casei NCDC-298. International Dairy Journal, 16(10), 1190–1195.

Nanasombat, S.& Lohasupthawee, P. (2005) Antimicrobial activity of crude ethanolic extracts and essential oils of spices against salmonellae and other enterobacteria. KMITL Sci. Technol. J.,5, 527–538.

Pranoto, Y., Salokhe, V.M. &Rakshit, S.K. (2005)Enhancing antimicrobial activity of chitosan films by incorporating garlic oil, potassium sorbate and nisin. LWT-Food Sci. Technol.,38(8), 859–865.

Schelz, Z., Moinar, J. & Hohmann, J. (2006) Antimicrobial and antiplasmid activities of essential oils. Fitoterapia,77, 279–285.

Singh, G., Singh, O.P. & Maura, S. (2002) Chemical and biocidal investigations on essential oils of some Indian Curcuma species. Prog. Cryst. Growth Charact. Mater., 45, 75–81.

Soottitantawat, A.,Yoshii, H., Furuta, T., Ohgawara, M., Forssell, P., Partanen, R., et al. (2004). Effect of water activity on the release characteristics and oxidative stability of D-limonene encapsulated by spray drying. J. Agric.Food Chem., 52(5), 1269–1276.

Sukatta, U., Haruthaithanasan, V., Chantarapanont, W., Dilokkunanant, U. & Suppakul, P. (2008) Antifungal activity of clove and cinnamon oil and their synergistic against postharvest decay fungi of grapein vitro. Kasetsart J. (Nat. Sci.),42, 169–174.

Wanchaitanawong, P., Chaungwanit, P., Poovarodom, N.& Nitisinprasert,S. (2005) In vitro antifungal activity of Thai herb and spice extracts against food spoilage fungi. Kasetsart J. (Natural Sci.), 39, 400–405.

Xing, Y. Xu, Q. Li, X., Che Z. & J. Yun. (2012) Antifungal activities of clove oil against Rhizopus nigricans, Aspergilillus flavus and Penicillium citrinum in vitro and in wonded fruit test. Journal of Food Safety 32, 84–93.

Medicine Sciences and Bioengineering – Wang (Ed.)
© *2015 Taylor & Francis Group, London, ISBN: 978-1-138-02684-1*

Research on the test of gas emission control method of vehicular pyrolysis furnace for medical waste

Li-hua Wu, Jun-shu Han & Zheng Wang
Institute of Medical Equipment, Tianjin, China

ABSTRACT: The test of vehicular pyrolysis furnace for medical waste is introduced, and two kinds of gas emission control structures for pyrolysis furnace, including direct purification and purification by the coil, and the related tests are shown in detail. The method of purification by the coiled tube and the post-processing of underwater gently is proposed. If it can be done, the quality of vehicular pyrolysis furnace gas emissions can be effectively controlled and the synthetic impact on the environment from quadratic dioxins also can be significantly reduced. The test result has satisfied the national safety standards.

1 INTRODUCTION

Vehicular medical waste pyrolysis processing system has good mobility and can timely deal with medical waste, so it can be applied to medical garbage where output lessly, scatteredly rural towns and so on. It can also dispose many kinds of harmful waste caused by the natural disasters. But by the limitation of the vehicle chassis load size, width, length and so on, the gas emission system should not be too large or heavy, so it is a problem to solve the gas emission in a limited space. The research on gas emissions, especially dioxin and related tests were carried out in this article, and a feasible method of flue gas emission controlling was determined finally.

2 RESEARCH ON DIRECT PURIFICATION STRUCTURE AND EMISSION TEST

2.1 *Direct purification structure*

The principle of the direct purification method is to place a gas post-processing module directly after the pyrolysis furnace system, without changing the structure of the vehicular pyrolyzing furnace body. Spray alkaline solution neutralization, adsorption purification and some other methods are utilized in the processing module. This is the direct spray tower structure using in the test (Figure 1). The gas purification process is: gas emissions from the combustion chamber of the pyrolysis furnace gets into the spraying tower through the air inlet at the bottom of the tower, being cooled, sprayed, adsorb and then emitted into the atmosphere by the exhaust pipe.

2.2 *Emission test*

Test conditions and methods: **Pyrolytic sample:** medical waste from a military hospital, the ingredient proportion of the waste is 50% plastic products such as disposable infusion devices, 14% cotton fabric such as dressing, 2.5% operation waste, 3% test specimens, 0.5% disposable metal instruments and 30% glass bottles; **Neutralizing solution:** caustic soda; **Test equipment:** pyrolyzing furnace and direct purification spray tower; **The sample temperature:** 750°C in the furnace; **Sampling method:** higher 0.5 m than gas outlet, time interval is 1 H, each sample capacity is 0.5 m³; **Sample detection methods:** literature [Chinese Standard, HJ-77.2.2008].

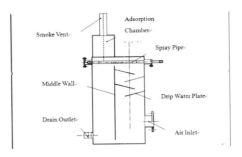

Figure 1. Direct purification spray tower structure chart.

Test result: The test results are shown in Table 1.

Test analysis: Relevant researches have shown that except the micro amount of dioxin-like materials contained in the waste, the dioxin-like materials in the smoke are mainly contributed through "creation within the furnace" and "low temperature resynthesis outside the furnace". According to the specific value of PCDFS and PCDDS, PCDFS/PCDDS, it can be deduced whether the creation pattern is "creation within the furnace" or "low temperature resynthesis outside the furnace": if the value of PCDFS/PCDDS is smaller than 1, "creation within the furnace" is much possible; if the value of PCDFS/PCDDS is larger than 1, "low temperature resynthesis outside the furnace". Calculated in accordance with the testing data in Table 1, the total volume of PCDFS in the smoke is 465.45 ng/m³, and the total volume of PCDDS is 112.09 ng/m³, making PCDFS/PCDDS = 4.15,

Table 1. Testing results of dioxin in gas at 750°C.

Test Items	Measured Concentration CS(ng/m³)	Equivalent Concentration C(ng/m³)	Conclusion I-TEQ (ng/m³)
2,3,7,8-TCDF	36.34563	24.41124	2.441124
1,2,3,7,8-PeCDF	35.10751	23.57967	1.178984
2,3,4,7,8-PeCDF	70.8377	47.57756	23.78878
1,2,3,4,7,8-HxCDF	48.12593	32.32339	3.232339
1,2,3,6,7,8-HxCDF	46.16159	31.00405	3.100405
2,3,4,6,7,8-HxCDF	55.99558	37.60897	3.760897
1,2,3,7,8,9-HxCDF	12.91317	8.673025	0.867302
1,2,3,4,6,7,8-HpCDF	118.9613	79.89937	0.798994
1,2,3,4,7,8,9-HpCDF	13.7708	9.249045	0.09249
OCDF	27.22102	18.28277	0.001828
2,3,7,8-TCDD	5.24619	3.52356	3.52356
1,2,3,7,8-PeCDD	12.0445	8.08959	8.08959
1,2,3,4,7,8-HxCDD	7.61122	5.112013	0.511201
1,2,3,6,7,8-HxCDD	9.71109	6.522374	0.652237
1,2,3,7,8,9-HxCDD	8.14783	5.472423	0.547242
1,2,3,4,6,7,8-HpCDD	39.81609	26.74215	0.267422
OCDD	29.55624	19.85121	0.001985
Total I-TEQ			52.85638

therefore, it can be deduced that the dioxin-like materials in the smoke tested in the test report are mainly contributed through "low temperature resynthesis outside the furnace". Analyzing with the 3T Theory for Control of Creation of Dioxin (Zhou Feng, Liu Yong & Guo Huaicheng, 2005), the reasons include: (1) pyrolyzing temperature is 750°C, which is slightly insufficient; (2) vehicular pyrolyzing furnace is small, the length of the pipe though which the smoke flow from incineration hearth is 5 m, with a flow rate 82 m³/h, passing time 1.19 s, which is comparatively short, and the smoke-flowing process is too smooth, making no eddy or turbulence; (3)the smoke passes through the spray tower with insufficient cooling rate, failing to keep away the 300~400°C low temperature resynthesis area of dioxin outside the furnace (Xu xu, 2002).

3 RESEARCH ON COILED PURIFICATION STRUCTURE AND EMISSION EFFECT TEST

3.1 *Coiled purification structure*

The design of the coil purification structure for smoke emission is as shown in Figure 2. This structure takes full advantage of the effective space within the incineration chamber, with the flue gas return coil purification structure designed to solve the problems of temperature, flue gas retaining time and formation of flue gas eddy, and the secondary underwater aeration quenching structure for flue gas spray purification. The gas purification process is as follows: the gas is emitted from the incineration chamber, enters into spray tank for dust and acid removal and cooling, then enters into the 24 m coiled pipe of the hearth for pyrolyzation again, where the temperature can reach over 900°C, after which the gas is introduced into the water tank for underwater aeration, making the temperature of the gas quenched down to less than 200°C, and then emitted into the atmosphere through the outlet.

3.2 *Emission test*

Test conditions and methods: **Pyrolytic sample:** medical waste from a military hospital, the ingredient proportion of the waste is 50% plastic products such as disposable infusion devices, 14% cotton fabric such as dressing, 2.5% operation waste, 3% test specimens, 0.5% disposable metal instruments and 30% glass bottles; **Neutralizing solution:** caustic soda; **Test equipment:** pyrolyzing furnace and coiled purification spray tower; **The sample temperature:** 750°C in the furnace; **Sampling method:** higher 0.5 m than gas outlet, time interval is 1H, each sample capacity is 0.5 m³; **Sample detection methods:** literature [1]

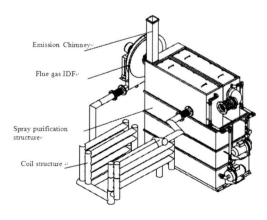

Figure 2.   Coil structure purification system.

Table 2. Testing results of dioxin in gas at 950°c.

Test Items	Measured Concentration CS (ng/m³)	Equivalent Concentration C (ng/m³)	Conclusion I-TEQ (ng/m³)
2,3,7,8-TCDF	0.19504	0.163899	0.0163899
1,2,3,7,8-PeCDF	0.13237	0.111235	0.0055618
2,3,4,7,8-PeCDF	0.23757	0.199639	0.0998193
1,2,3,4,7,8-HxCDF	0.13934	0.117092	0.0117092
1,2,3,6,7,8-HxCDF	0.14834	0.124655	0.0124655
2,3,4,6,7,8-HxCDF	0.21194	0.178101	0.0178101
1,2,3,7,8,9-HxCDF	0.0363	0.030504	0.0030504
1,2,3,4,6,7,8-HpCDF	0.47964	0.403059	0.0040306
1,2,3,4,7,8,9-HpCDF	0.04763	0.040025	0.0004003
OCDF	0.17205	0.14458	0.0001446
2,3,7,8-TCDD	0.01839	0.015454	0.0154538
1,2,3,7,8-PeCDD	0.03831	0.032193	0.0160966
1,2,3,4,7,8-HxCDD	0.02022	0.016992	0.0016992
1,2,3,6,7,8-HxCDD	0.03889	0.032681	0.0032681
1,2,3,7,8,9-HxCDD	0.04268	0.035866	0.0035866
1,2,3,4,6,7,8-HpCDD	0.21082	0.17716	0.0017716
OCDD	0.26356	0.221479	0.0002215
Total I-TEQ			0.213479

Test results: The test results are shown in Table 2.

Test analysis: Through Table 2, we can see that the toxic equivalent quantity of Dioxin is 0.21TEQ ng/m³, occupying only 42% of the national Dioxin standard for fixed waste treatment equipment, and is close to the American standard (Sheng Hongzhi, 2011).

4 TEST ANALYSIS

The analysis of results for two tests shows:

1. The total emission volume of dioxin-like materials is decreased from 577.54 ng/m³ to 2.43 ng/m³, the dioxin control effects of the new structure is remarkable.
2. For the emission of dioxin through coil purification structure, the total volume of PCDFS is 1.8 ng/m³, and the total volume of PCDDS is 0.63 ng/m³, making PCDFS/PCDDS = 2.85, and showing that the coiled pipe structure and spraying and underwater aeration structure effectively decreased the secondary synthesis of dioxin.
3. Spraying and underwater aeration structure can decrease the temperature rapidly and effectively avoid the 300–400°C temperature interval for the secondary synthesis of dioxin-like materials.
4. PCDFS/PCDDS = 2.85 shows that within the total emission volume of 2.43 ng/m³, secondary synthesis is still the main contributor; in other words, further improvement of the structure can further decrease the emission of dioxin.

5 SUMMARY

The control technology and flue gas aftertreatment quenching technology systematically used for vehicular pyrolysis furnance for medical waste, can effectively control the emission of dioxin and other gas quality, laying a good foundation for the further structural optimization and the research of dioxin emission control technology.

REFERENCES

Ambient air and waste gas Determination of polychlorinated dibenzo-dioxin(PCDDSs) and polychlorinated dibenzofurans(PCDFs). *Chinese Standard*, HJ-77.2.2008.(in Chinese).

Sheng Hongzhi. Measures and Plasma Technology for Reduction of Dioxin Emission during Waste Treatment. (2011).

Xu xu. Research on Creation and Emission Characteristics of Dioxin during Incineration. *Zhejiang University* (2002).

Zhou Feng, Liu Yong, Guo Huaicheng. Research on Key Parameters during Treatment of Medical Waste. *Journal of Environmental Science Research*, 2005, volume 18 (3); 24–28.

Medicine Sciences and Bioengineering – Wang (Ed.)
© 2015 Taylor & Francis Group, London, ISBN: 978-1-138-02684-1

Study for problems and solutions of the paperless electronic prescription

Ai-ning Li
Hebei Engineering and Technical College, Cangzhou, Hebei Province, China

Sheng-li Hu*
Central Hospital of Cangzhou, Cangzhou, Hebei Province, China

ABSTRACT: Purpose: Promote the development of paperless electronic prescription. Method: Studies on the advantages of paperless electronic prescription and a number of problems found in its legal status; electronic special prescription; the color of a special prescription; the protection of the right to know to patient; verification and safety of special project. Results: Put forward to the solutions, i.e., Improvement of laws and regulations; application of electronic signature; setting up a CA certification agency subject to hygienic industry; inputting the system of drug rational use; setting up a personalized prescription template; improvement of the management system, formulation of emergency plans; installation of self-service equipment. Conclusion: This paper plays a very important significance to set up a high-quality digital hospital.

1 INTRODUCTION

There are many discordant points existed in Prescription Administrative Policy (Hereinafter refers to Method), issued by Ministry of Health on May 1, 2007, which is different from that of an electronic prescription, in order to realize its paperless operation that there are many difficulties faced against electronic prescription. Electronic Signature Law of the People's Republic of China (Hereinafter refers to Electronic signature Law), launched on April 1, 2005, can effectively solve these difficulties on electronic prescription legalization, the others of which need us for further studies on paperless electronic prescription and its solutions (LI Chun-rong, 2012). The following discussions are its advantages, existing problems as well as its solutions of the paperless electronic prescription.

2 ADVANTAGES OF PAPERLESS ELECTRONIC PRESCRIPTION

2.1 *For the convenience of doctor and patient*

Doctor makes up a prescription while the patient can simultaneously scan the drug categories, description, quantity in stock, unit price, total price, etc., from the display, regulating the drugs and inspection items at any time according to their own economic status after communicating with the doctor. The price can only be known at the time when the prices are determined through learning from the prices and selection of drugs after a prescription is modified. No drug can be ordered as there is no drug in stock. Although there is a prescription, no drug can be ordered, to avoid the prescription which is repeatedly modified by the patient.

---

*Corresponding Author: Hu Shengli E-mail address: hushenglihsl@139.com

2.2 Avoid rechecking, improve the medical quality

Electronic prescription information can be kept in a database, the previous conditions for drug use and inspections of which can be provided for the patient, thus, to take a detailed guidance of drug use for the patient's subsequent visit in order to prevent repeated drug uses and inspections. The price of a prescription may also be controlled, with its statistics on categories, total quantity of drug use in the clinic controlled for its quality in order to provide technical support for Leadership Decision.

3 EXISTING PROBLEMS IN PAPERLESS ELECTRONIC PRESCRIPTION

3.1 The problem of electronizing special prescription

Electronic prescription also serves for a common prescription, but there has not been specified whether or not these prescriptions can be used in an emergency clinic, nerve anesthetization and pediatric prescription, we can conclude from Article 28 of the "Method".

3.2 Color problem of special prescription

Light yellow printed paper can be used in an emergency ward, light green in the pediatric ward and light red for the prescriptions of narcotics and the 1st category of psychotropic drugs. These all apparently aim at the stipulations for paper prescription, its purpose of which warns the pharmacist to be more careful about it. To realize paperless electronic prescription must solve the color problem of a special prescription, which is specified in Article 5 of the "Method".

3.3 Protection of right-to-know to patient

To realize a paperless electronic prescription, the right of choice and the right to know to patient will to some extent be damaged. In such case, if there has no prescription, patient cannot go out for purchase of drugs. A number of benefits owned by the patient should be protected upon use of electronic prescription.

3.4 Verification of special items

Applicability of prescription for drug use should be verified by a pharmacist, the verified content of which includes: For drugs stipulated for skin test, whether or not sensitivity test and results judgment are marked by prescription pharmacist. Most of present hospitals have no special template of skin test, as no skin test markings cannot be beneficial to verification of prescription, which is specified in Article 35 of the "Method".

4 SOLUTIONS ANALYSIS OF PAPERLESS ELECTRONIC PRESCRIPTION

4.1 Establishment and improvement of laws and regulations in the present medical & hygienic realm

Legal system of health &Medicine will be well improved, with hygienic laws and regulations improved. Aiming at the imperfection and the irrationality of the hygienic laws and regulations, the electronic special prescription and its color, present laws and regulations should be rechecked and modified. While, relevant stipulations of the printed paper prescription must be canceled. Relevant measures of electronic prescription normalization management should be supplemented in the system of prescription in order to realize a scientific, legalized electronic prescription. Aiming at the Electronic signature Law, the terms relevant to the medical realm should be added for the determination of the legal status of electronic signature in the application of the electronic prescription system, to solve contradictory problems of law lagging behind its application, pointed out in new medical policy.

4.2 *Applied electronic signature*

Technology of Applied Electronic Signature is used for signing and validating the prescription data, which adopts a certain degree of technical means to protect the safety of signature, and to protect prescription data which cannot be illegally falsified. Due to the data of electronic prescription characteristic of traceless falsification, in order to have electronic signature endowed with legal validity, Electronic signature must be reliable and safe for use. There are many technical means-technologies (Xu Huy, 2007) of PKI based, matured digital signature found its widely application, and stronger operability: Certification institution of digital certificate chosen by some hospitals has no approval and verification of MIIT, although authentication function of digital certificate is used in this system, it only adopts common signature, meaning that is only to prevent data falsification and to demonstrate transmitted main content, unable to protect electronic prescription data kept in a long-term effective status as an evidence for use. Therefore, at present, E-signature introduced by most of hospitals cannot truly resolve the problem of legal effect (Yan Yuqin, 2011).

4.3 *Input a monitoring system for rational drug use*

The monitoring system for rational drug use will be embedded in the electronic prescription system in order to automatically verify compatibility of medicine of prescription, dosage, drug side-effect, and can be used for the assessment of drug contraindication arising from patient disease according to drug allergy experiences, which relevant prompting is given out before doctor settles them down according to relevant prompting. After that, a prescription can be submitted. In such case, prescription errors may be eliminated on the generation phase, which irrational prescription is completely eradicated in order to promote rational drug use.

4.4 *Setup of the template for personalized prescription*

Prior to make up a prescription, common disease diagnostic and personalized prescription template libraries should be well maintained beforehand, which includes such templates as spirit, anesthesia, pediatrics and emergency prescriptions, with background color of prescription set as the ones to be stipulated in "Method", the personnel in Pharmacy Department will maintain well its name, specifications, unit, dosage, unit price of the drugs and etc, charges collection department well maintained for its name, number and remarks and other information of inspection items, as well as in practical applications with these to be continuously improved and supplemented. Only template can be tuned out when made up a prescription, with Pinyin Code input. Thus, well-maintained inspection items beforehand can be automatically tuned out, and in special circumstances may be automatically modified. In such case, the efficiency of making up prescription can be quickly enhanced.

In a prescription, a marking is set for a skin test in a special column and other special items in favor of pharmacist examination. With those medicines needed for skin test, dialog box can be automatically popped up, which indicates the required skin test.

4.5 *Improvement of a paperless electronic prescription management system*

Management of electronic prescription is largely different from that of hand-written prescription, with inventory information of electronic prescription shown as dynamic real-time display. In the general case, the drugs is not allowed to be borrowed, in case of an emergency rescue drugs needed for a patient, a drug-borrowing management procedure should be carried out. This drug inventory information will be temporarily prohibited for use.

A prescription includes Physician's Order Sheet for drug use in the wards of medical institution, operating it according to the module of clinic electronic prescription. Based on an original Physician's Order Sheet for drug use, with name, age, hospital admission number, clinical diagnosis, dosage and other contents of patient added in it, enabling Physician's Order Sheet in conformity with relevant stipulations of national prescription management system, which is stipulated in Article 2 of the "Method".

4.6 *All types of self-service equipments equipped in the apparent places of the hospital*

After a paperless electronic prescription is carried out in the hospital, in order to maximize the protection of patient's Right-to-Know, the doctor should enhance communicating with the patient when making up prescriptions, actively informing the patient of the category and price of drugs, and the prescription inquiry system will be equipped with an apparent place. Therefore, the drugs, prices and usage, and other contents can be inquired in the system, to meet maximum patient Right-to-Know. The prescription can be printed out after clinical patient inputs the number or swipes a card. Hence, freely purchase right of a patient can be effectively settled down.

5 CONCLUSION

Paperless electronic prescription is still developed in a starting phase with many imperfect aspects. This needs us to make a continuous effort for its further study in order to discover an effective solution. This plays an important significance for medical expenses saving and increasing of medical quality based on the patient.

REFERENCES

LI Chun-rong,XU Li,HUANG Zhi-yong. (2012) The application of electronic signature based on fingerprint recognition in the outpatient electronic prescribing system[J]. CHINESE JOURNAL OF DRUG APPLICATION AND MONITORING,09(4): 237–239.

Xu Huyi. (2007) First Exploration of Feasibility of Electronic Prescription[J], Chinese Pharmacy, 18(19):1454–1456.

Yan Yuqin, Zhang Bing, Li Xiuying.(2011) Application of Electronic Prescription System and Drugs Dispensing in the Ward of Our Hospital[J].China's Pharmaceuticals, 20(07):39–40.

Medicine Sciences and Bioengineering – Wang (Ed.)
© *2015 Taylor & Francis Group, London, ISBN: 978-1-138-02684-1*

Detection of genetically modified herbicide tolerant soybeans using multiplex-nested PCR

You-wen Qiu, Ming-hui Zhang, Ying Liu, Zhen Zhen, Ao-xue Wang,
Xue-jun Gao & Yan-bo Yu*
Key Laboratory of Agricultrual Biological Functional Genes, College of Life Science, Northeast Agricultural University, Harbin, China

ABSTRACT: A qualitative multiple nested PCR detection method for four kinds of genetically modified herbicide tolerant soybeans was established for commercialization. In addition, the sensitivity of the detection system was evaluated. The detection sensitivity of this method was 0.05% in the first round of PCR and 0.0005% in the second round of PCR. The results suggest that the genetically modified organization of genetically modified soybean products can be detected using the multiple nested PCR detection method established in the research. This detection method is effective, simple, quick and accurate, and it has an important practical significance.

1 INTRODUCTION

In recent years, due the development and application of genetically modified technology, a large number of new varieties of genetically modified plants have been emerging (James 2013). Herbicide-resistant genetically modified soybeans are the earlier commercialized genetically modified crops. The main varieties of genetically modified soybeans are GTS-40-3-2 and MON897 (EPSPS gene was transferred), and A2704-12 and A5547-127 (PAT gene was transferred).

Currently, there are two main methods in practice for the detection of the genetically modified plants. (1) Detection of the exogenous gene-specific DNA sequences and (2) detection of the proteins expressed by exogenous gene. In the methods of detecting the exogenous gene-specific DNA sequences, the PCR detection is the most widely used method, but the detection efficiency of the ordinary PCR method is low, and the cost of fluorescent PCR is high. The multiplex-nested PCR is a new method that has the advantage of high detection efficiency and low-cost spending. This technology is primarily used for the detection of animal viral diseases and human diseases (Gomez-Couso et al., 2004; Tafreshi et al., 2005; Formiga-Cruz et al., 2005), but rarely applied to the detection of genetically modified plants (Zhang Minghui et al., 2007; Ao Jinxia et al., 2011). In this test, a multiplex-nested PCR method was used to detect four kinds of commercialized genetically modified herbicide tolerant soybeans, and this test provides an experimental basis for the application of multiplex-nested PCR in the detection of genetically modified plants and its deep-processed products.

2 MATERIALS AND METHODS

2.1 *DNA extraction and purification*

Mix genetically modified soybean sample with non-genetically modified soybean sample to make the six genetically modified samples containing: 0.5%, 0.1%, 0.05%, 0.01%, 0.005% and 0.001%. DNA extraction of the test samples and the positive standard of genetically modified rice,

---

*E-mail: yw12_630@126.com

corn and canola were performed with plant genomic DNA Kit (Tiangen Biotech, Beijing Co., Ltd). The DNA concentrations were measured by absorbance at 260 nm and diluted to the same concentration.

2.2 Primers designing

Primers were designed based on NCBI Gene Bank sequence by Primer Premier V5.0 software. Lectin gene (Gene Bank No. K00821), genetically modified soybean A2704-12 (Gene Bank No.CS447634.1), genetically modified soybean A5547-127 (Gene Bank No. DM079061.1), genetically modified soybean MON89788 (Gene Bank No. x00806), genetically modified soybean GTS40-3-2 (Gene Bank No. AB209952.1). Primers (as shown in Table 1) were synthesized by Invitrogen (Shanghai, China).

2.3 Detection of genetically modified herbicide tolerant soybeans using multiplex nested PCR

2.3.1 Nested PCR system and conditions

In the first round PCR, the Reaction System was 20 μL and the composition is as follows: $1 \times$ PCR buffer, 0.25 mmol/L dNTP mix, 0.2 μmol/L upstream primer, 0.2 μmol/L downstream primer, 1U rTaq DNA polymerase and genomic DNA 50 ng. The PCR was performed using the following condition: one cycle of 95°C for 3 min; 32 cycles of 95°C for 30 sec, 56°C for 30 sec, and 72°C for 30 sec; and one cycle of 72°C for 3 min.

In the second round PCR, the Reaction System was the same as the first round PCR but the template was 1 μL of the PCR products (diluted100-fold) of the first round PCR. The PCR was performed using the following condition: one cycle of 95°C for 3 min; 26 cycles of 95°C for 30 sec, 56°C for 30 sec, and 72°C for 30 sec; and one cycle of 72°C for 3 min.

2.3.2 Verification of the validity of all templates

In order to verify the validity of all templates, all genetically modified soybeans and negative controls were detected with the corresponding reference gene by qualitative PCR amplification. The system and conditions of qualitative PCR were same as the first round PCR.

Table 1. The primers of multiple nested PCR.

Rounds	Primer name	sequences (5′→3′)	Gene	Size of amplified fragment(bp)
1	A27 KR A27 KF	TGAGGGGGTCAAAGACCAAG CCAGTCTTTACGGCGAGT	PAT	239
	A55 KR A55 KF	CGCCATTATCGCCATTCC GCGGTATTATCCCGTATTGA	PAT	317
	M89 KR M89 KF	TGTTGGTAACGGTGGACT CGACCTTCAAGACGGATG	CP4-EPSPS	450
	GTS KR GTS KF	CCTTCATGTTCGGCGGTCTCG GCGTCATGATCGGCTCGATG	CP4-EPSPS	498
2	A27 KR A27 KF	TATCAGCCAAGCATTCTAT CAGTCTTTACGGCGAGTT	PAT	206
	A55 KR A55 KF	CGCCATTATCGCCATTCC CGGTCGCCGCATACACTA	PAT	279
	M89 KR M89 KF	GTTGGTAACGGTGGACTC CAAGCAGAACAGCGGACT	CP4-EPSPS	304
	GTS KR GTS KF	GCGTCATGATCGGCTCGATG GGCGACGCCTCGCTCACAA	CP4-EPSPS	240

2.3.3 Detection of genetically modified herbicide tolerant soybeans using multiplex nested PCR and sensitivity analysis of multiplex nested PCR assay

Four kinds of genetically modified soybeans were detected with primers of multiple-nested PCR by multiplex-nested PCR. The system and conditions of multiple-nested PCR are shown in 2.3.1. Mix genetically modified soybean sample with non-genetically modified soybean sample to make the following genetically modified contains samples: 5%, 1%, $5 \times 10 - 1\%$, $5 \times 10 - 2\%$, $5 \times 10 - 3\%$, $1 \times 10 - 3\%$, $5 \times 10 - 4\%$ and $1 \times 10 - 4\%$. The sensitivity of the multiplex-nested PCR assay was detected and the system and conditions of multiple-nested PCR was the same as described previously.

3 RESULTS

3.1 Verification of the validity of all templates

In order to verify the validity of all templates, PCR amplification of soybean reference gene was completed. As expected, the PCR products appeared in all templates (Figure 1). This result suggested that all templates were normal and the PCR reaction system is not inhibited.

3.2 Detection of genetically modified herbicide tolerant soybeans using multiplex-nested PCR

In the PCR results, PCR products were not appeared in blank and negative controls, but appeared in all four kinds of genetically modified soybeans. It suggested that no pollution in the PCR reaction system and genetically modified soybeans could be detected by this way (Figure 2).

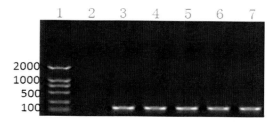

1:DL2000 DNA marker; 2: Blank; 3-7: PCR amplification of soybean reference gene (Lectin, 118 bp), the order of templates was non-genetically modified soybeans, genetically modified soybeans A2704-12, A5547-127, MON89788 and GTS40-3-2.

Figure 1. Verification of the validity of all templates.

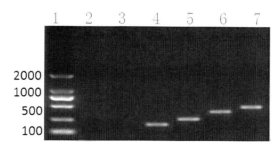

1:DL2000 DNA marker; 2: Blank; 3-7: non-genetically modified soybeans, genetically modified soybeans A2704-12, A5547-127, MON89788 and GTS40-3-2.

Figure 2. Detection of genetically modified herbicide tolerant soybeans using multiplex-nested PCR.

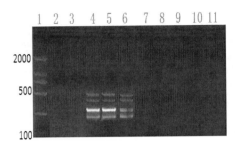 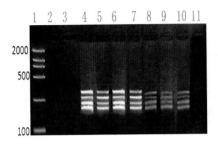

A, the frist round PCR amplification; B, the second round PCR amplification; M, DL-2000; 1, blank control; 2, negative control; 3, positive control; 4-11, the concentrations of transgenic are 5%, 1%, 5 × 10 − 1%, 5 × 10 − 2%, 5 × 10 − 3%, 1 × 10 − 3%, 5 × 10 − 4%, 1 × 10 − 4%.

Figure 3. Sensitivity analysis of the multiple PCR.

3.3 *Sesitivity analysis of multiplex-nested PCR assay*

In the first round PCR, the templates were 5 × 10 − 2% of positive mixed standard and four pairs of primers as previously mentioned. In the results, four PCR products appeared in all four pairs of primers suggested that the sensitivity of the first round PCR was 5 × 10 − 2% (Figure 3A). In the second round PCR, the templates were 5 × 10 − 4% of positive mixed standard and four pairs of primers as previously mentioned. In the results, four PCR products appeared in all four pairs of primers suggested that the sensitivity of the first round PCR was 5 × 10 − 4% (Figure 3B).

4 DISCUSSIONS

With the increase of genetically modified organization in the market, the challenge of detection of genetically modified crops was brought and an effective method of genetically modified detection is highly desirable (Van *et al.*, 2010). A key problem faced by current genetically modified organization detection industry is how to identify genetically modified samples quickly, accurately and scientifically (Zel *et al.*, 2006).

The nested PCR is one of the methods of detection of genetically modified crops. But the primer design and PCR cycles can affect the test results (Gonsalves , 1998). In this test, for the detection of genetically modified soybean with nested PCR, primer dimers and PCR cycles were considered and in order to analyse the sensitivity of the nested PCR, a multiplex-nested PCR was designed and applied. The test data show that the multiplex-nested PCR created by the test can detect the genetically modified organization and the detection sensitivity is 0.005%. The international standard of detection sensitivity of genetically modified organization is 0.1 % (Davison 2010).The detection sensitivity of the method in this test is better than the international standard and other multiplex PCR methods (Germini, et al., 2004; Forte et al., 2005). It suggests that this multiplex nested PCR fully can be used to detect the Herbicide-tolerant genetically modified soybeans and its deep-processed products.

5 SUMMARY

Based on the results of this research, the multiple-nested PCR detection method established in the research can detect the genetically modified soybeans and the genetically modified organization of genetically modified soybean-processing products. This detection method has the advantage of effectively, simple, quick and accurate, and it has an important practical significance.

ACKNOWLEDGMENTS

National Major Project of Breeding of Species of Transgenic genetically Modified Soybean (no. 2014ZX08004-002-002), Heilongjiang Postdoctoral Grant (no. LBH-Z13036), Foundation of Educational Committee of Heilongjiang Province of China (no. 12541047)

REFERENCES

Ao Jinxia, Li Qiangzhang, Gao Xuejun, Yu Yanbo, Li Lu, Zhang Minghui.(2011). A multiplex nested PCR assay for the simultaneous detection of genetically modified soybean, maize and rice in highly processed products. *Food control.* 2011, 22(10): 1617–1623.

Davison J. (2010).GM plants: Science, politics and EC regulations. *Plant Sci.* 178 (2): 94–98.

Formiga-Cruz M, Hundesa A, Clemente-Casares P. (2005). Nested multiplex PCR assay for detection of hu-man enteric viruses in shellfish and sewage. *J Virol Methods.*25 (2):111–118.

Forte V T, Di Pinto A, Martino C,. (2005). A general multiplex-PCR assay for the general detection of ge-netically modified soya and maize. *Food Control.* 16:535–539.

Germini A, Zanetti A, Salati C,. (2004).Development of a seven-target multiplex PCR for the simultaneous detection of transgenic soybean and maize in feeds and foods. *J Agric Food Chem.*52(11):3275–3280.

Gomez-Couso H,Freire-Santos F,Amar C F.(2004).De-tection of Cryptosporidium and Giardiain molluscan shellfish by multiplexed nested-PCR. *Int J Food Microbiol.* 91(3):279–288.

Gonsalves D. (1998).Control of papaya ringspot virus in pa-paya: a case study. *Annual Review of Phytopathology.* 36(1):415–437.

James C. (2013) Global status of commercialized biotech/GM crops: 2013. ISAAA brief no. 43. ISAAA, Ithaca.

Tafreshi N K, Sadeghizadeh M, Amini-Bavil-Olyaee S. (2005).Development of a multiplex nested consensus PCR for detection and identification of major human Herpesvirusesin CNS infections. *J Clin Virol.* 32(4):318–324.

Van B M, Lievens A, Barbau-piednoir E, Mbongolombella G, Roosens N, Sneyers M, Casi A. (2010).A theoretical introduction to "Combinatory SYBR Green qPCR Screening", a matrix-based approach for the detection of materials derived from genetically modified plants. *Anal Bioanal Chem.*396 (6): 2113–2123.

Zel J, Cankar K, Ravnikar M, Camloh M, Gruden K.(2006). Accreditation of GMO detection laboratories: Improving the reliability of GMO detection. *Accreditation and Quality Assurance: Journal for Quality, Comparability and Reliability in Chemical Measurement.* 10 (10): 531–536.

Zhang Minghui,Gao Xuejun,Yu Yanbo.(2007). Detec-tion of Roundup Ready Soy in highly processed products by triplex nested PCR. *Food Control.*18 (10):1277–1281.

Medicine Sciences and Bioengineering – Wang (Ed.)
© 2015 Taylor & Francis Group, London, ISBN: 978-1-138-02684-1

Research on the effect of attracting insects about the composite LED lamppost

Wang-biao Qiu* & Shu-yun Lin

College of Mechanical Engineering, Guizhou University, Guiyang, Guizhou Province, China

ABSTRACT: The composite LED lamppost mainly is used on the solar insecticidal streetlight. This experiment researches the effect of attracting insects through changing the proportion of the purple LED on the premise of the power of lamppost and the quantity of beads holding the line. It is obtained by comparing experiments that the lamppost of the purple LED accounted for 3/4 is the best; and the lamppost of the purple LED accounted for 1/2 followed, and all purple LED followed them.

1 INTRODUCTION

Agricultural production provides necessary materials for human life that are important for the society. The agricultural production mainly uses pesticide management control pests, and its effect is prominent, but the use of pesticides pollutes the environment, and the residual pesticide is an enormous threat for the human body health. As a new type of street lamp, if the LED solar insecticidal lamp can be widely installed to use in rural areas, it can kill the injurious insects so that reduce the use of pesticides, and improve agricultural production. It can greatly improve the lighting at night without extra power. While the LED lamp as a core component of the solar insecticidal streetlight, it must meet the requirements of the lighting and the requirements of trap. According to the study of Mikkola, about 18 kinds of Lepidoptera insects have UV tolerance capacity (Dong R&Wang J, Zhai Y Z. Study on Phototrop ic Law of Insects, *Journal of Anhui Agricultural*, 2010). In order to improve the trapping effect, the LED lamp post is mixed with purple LED and white LED. At the same time, the LED lamp can save energy. The following experiment provides important data for producing the LED lamppost and determines the ratio of purple and white LED .

2 MATERIALS AND METHODS

2.1 *Experimental lamppost*

The experimental lamppost is homemade. The length of lamppost is 70 mm and the diameter of lamppost is 46mm. The LED lamp with the white LED of 5 mm and the purple LED of 5 mm was chosen. The wavelength of white LED ranges from 460 to 465 nm, and the wavelength of purple LED ranges from 395 to 400 nm. Rated voltage of LED ranges from 3.2 to 3.4V, and rated current is 20 mA. The LED lamppost is supplied with 12V DC power as expressed in Fig.1. Three LED lights in series with a resistor and welding so that they do not burn because of the large current and voltage, and then each group of LED lights is connected in parallel.

---

*Wangbiao Qiu, the author for correspondence, Male, Professor, Tutor of master, Guizhou University, E-mial:qiuwangbiao@163.com.

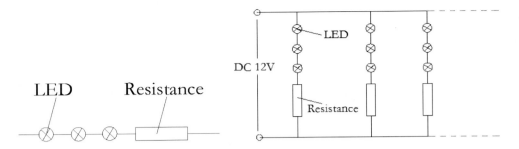

Figure 1 . The connected method of the LED lamppost.

The series-wound of LED Lamp resistance :

$$R_1 = \frac{12 - (3.2 \sim 3.4) \times 3}{20 \times 10^{-3}} = (90 \sim 120) \, \Omega \tag{1}$$

Resistance unified GB, in case of LED lights burn because of voltage and preventing excessive resistance and thus leaves the LED luminous intensity not to the higher level, so choose the resistance: R = 100Ω.

2.2 *Experimental apparatus and method*

The experiments was conducted in the field. In order to facilitate the experiment using the following experimental setup, the structure of this experimental device is simple. As shown in Fig. 2, 1 is bracket for fixing lamppost; 2 is lamppost; 3 is the basin, which is equipped with appropriate amount of water, and lampposts from the water about 10 cm. In the experiments, to ensure consistent power of lamppost and the consistent number of lamp beads, the trapping effects of different proportions of white and purple LED lamp were observed.

3 EXPERIMENTAL CONTENT AND ANALYSIS

Light attracts insects through phototaxis of insect, and the reason is that the retina of compound eyes has a kind of pigment, which absorbs specific wavelengths of light, stimulating the optic

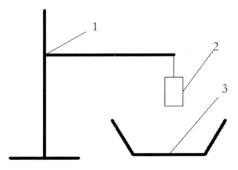

Figure 2. Schematic diagram of experimental device.

nerve so that the insect responds to a specific wavelength of light and tends to the light. According to the available experimental studies, the insects are more sensitive to short-wavelength visible light, therefore the light below 400 nm ha more obvious effect of attracting insects. The experimental time ranged from July to August in 2013 (Lin & Ao, Zhang, Re). The studies of solar LED lights for killing worms, Renewable Energy Resources, 2007).

3.1 *Trapping effect of different proportions of white-purple LED Lamp*

To ensure the overall power around 16w, the proportion of white and purple lamp post was changed and observed the change in the effect of attracting insects. From the foregoing that three LED lamps in a series, in order to facilitate mass production, choose the full-white, all purple , purple LED - white is 1 / 1, purple LED is 1/ 4, purple LED is 3 / 4. According to Table 1, 3 / 4 purple LED Lamp is best, and 1 / 2 followed .

3.2 *Comparison with black light about trapping effect*

To observe the difference between the trapping effect of the lamppost and conventional lamps luring effect, considering the lighting elements, the white-purple is 1/2 contrasting with black light and purple light. As shown in Table 2, the trapping effect of 1/2 purple LED closes to the black light, and the purple light is the worst one. Combing with the Table 1, the 3 / 4 purple LED lamppost is the best one , and better than conventional black light ,while the 1/ 2 purple closes to the black light.

4 CONCLUSION

Application of composite LED lamppost in insecticidal solar streetlight can reduce costs, save energy, and improve the efficiency of energy. According to the experiment, the ratio purple and white LED lamppost is 1/1 suitable for the insecticidal solar streetlight but the 3/4 one trapping effect is the best one which can be used in LED solar insecticidal lamp. Changing the ratio of purple and white of lamppost can improve the insecticidal efficiency and the utilization ratio of energy so that it has a very broad application prospects.

Table 1. The effect of attracting insects of different proportion.

	The proportion of purple					
Number	Time	All white	1/4	1/2	¾	All purple
Number	20:30–22:30	42	127	165	182	108

Table 2. The effect of attracting insects of different proportion light source.

	Kinds			
Number	Time	Purple	Black light	1/2 purple
	20:40–21:30	22	62	47
Number	21:30–22:15	63	45	65
	Total	85	107	112

ACKNOWLEDGEMENT

Contract of Branch building [2012102] 3-28 .

REFERENCES

Dong R&Wang J, Zhai Y Z. Study on Phototrop ic Law of Insects[J].Journal of Anhui Agricultural,2010,38(25):13563–13564.
Lin M,&ao B Y, Zhang Y H, Re Z W. The studies of solar LED lights for killing worms[J].Renewable Energy Resources,2007,25(3):79–80.
Wang B, Cheng X. Application of LED Lamp for Trapping Worms in Greenhouse[J].Journal of Anhui Agricultural,2010,38(15):8216–8217,8250.

Medicine Sciences and Bioengineering – Wang (Ed.)
© *2015 Taylor & Francis Group, London, ISBN: 978-1-138-02684-1*

Changes of functional connectivity patterns of V1 with eyes open and closed

Jiao-jian Wang

Key Laboratory for NeuroInformation of the Ministry of Education, School of Life Science and Technology, University of Electronic Science and Technology of China, Chengdu, China

Tian-zi Jiang*

Key Laboratory for NeuroInformation of the Ministry of Education, School of Life Science and Technology, University of Electronic Science and Technology of China, Chengdu, China
Brainnetome Center, National Laboratory of Pattern Recognition, Institute of Automation, Chinese Academy of Sciences, Beijing, China
The Queensland Brain Institute, University of Queensland, Brisbane, Australia

ABSTRACT: Recent studies have revealed that eyes open and eyes closed could reflect the interoceptive and exteroceptive state, respectively. The primary visual cortex (V1) which is one of the most important brain areas for perception receives visual input from the retina. Therefore, understanding the changes of functional activity of the primary visual cortex will provide fundamental insights into how the brain operates when eyes open and eyes closed. In this study, we used resting-state functional connectivity (RSFC) to evaluate the changes of functional connectivity of V1 under eyes open and eyes closed state. RSFC analyses revealed that compared to eyes closed state, the stronger functional connectivities were found in execution control network and attentional network. In addition, compared to eyes closed state, the decreased functional connectivities were also found in default model network and sensory-motor network. Our findings revealed that different functional connectivity patterns of V1 in eyes open and eyes closed condition, which indicated different "work" state under different resting-state. Thus, our finding might provide important reference for choosing the resting condition in MRI experiments.

1 INTRODUCTION

The primary visual cortex V1 which is located in the posterior pole of the occipital cortex is primarily responsible for processing visual stimuli. V1 is also related to the processing of externally and internally oriented stimuli. Recent studies on eyes open and eyes closed have suggested that eyes open and eyes closed could reflect the exteroceptive state and interoceptive state, respectively (Marx *et al.*, 2003; Marx *et al.*, 2004). However, the functional connectivity patterns of V1 under eyes open and eyes closed remain unclear.

Resting-state functional MRI can noninvasively assess brain function by measuring the temporal correlation of the spontaneous fluctuations of the blood oxygen level-dependent (BOLD) signal between regions (Biswal *et al.*, 1995; Zhang & Raichle, 2010). Therefore, resting-state functional connectivity (RSFC) is an effective way to detect the changes of functional activity of brain areas. In the current study, we also employed the RSFC to evaluate the changes of functional connectivity patterns of V1 when eyes open and eyes close to determine the influence of different resting conditions on the brain network of V1.

---

*The corresponding author of this article is Tianzi Jiang. jiangtz@nlpr.ia.ac.cn.

2   METHODS

2.1   *Participants*

Forty-six healthy, right-handed subjects (22 males and 24 females, mean age = 22.5 years, standard deviation = 2.17) were accessed from community-shared samples (Beijing: Eyes Open Eyes Closed Study, web link: http://fcon_1000.projects.nitrc.org/). This dataset includes 48 subjects' MRI images. During processing, two subjects were excluded because of unmatched time-points of resting-state functional images. From each subject, 240 volumes of echo planar images were acquired using a gradient-echo single-shot echo planar imaging sequence (TR = 2000 ms, echo time = 30 ms; 33 axial slices with slice thickness 3.5 mm). A structural scan was acquired for each participant in the same session, using a 3D T1 magnetization-prepared rapid acquisition gradient echo sequence (voxel size, 1.3×1×1.3 mm).

2.2   *Resting-state fMRI data preprocessing*

The preprocessing of the resting state fMRI data were carried out using SPM8 software. To allow for magnetization equilibrium, the first 10 volumes were discarded. The slice timing for the remaining images was corrected, and the images were realigned to the first volume for head motion correction. All the subjects with a maximum displacement of less than 1.5 mm and an angular motion of less than 1.5° were used in this study. All of the fMRI images were further normalized to the Montreal Neurological Institute (MNI) EPI template and resampled to a 3mm cubic voxel. Then, all the functional images were smoothed using a Gaussian kernel of 6mm full-width at half maximum (FWHM). Finally, six motion parameters, white matter and cerebrospinal fluid and global mean signals were regressed out and filtered with temporal band-path of 0.01~0.1Hz.

2.3   *Seed mask of V1 definition*

In this study, we aimed to explore the functional changes of V1 when eyes open and eyes closed. In order to map the functional connectivity of V1, we first defined the V1 mask on the basis of Brodmann atlas (Figure 1). And then the whole functional connectivity of V1 was calculated.

2.4   *Functional connectivity analyses*

The functional connectivity was defined by Pearson correlation coefficients between the time series. For each subject, the functional connectivity was calculated between each seed region and each voxel of the whole brain and then converted to z-values using Fisher's z transformation to

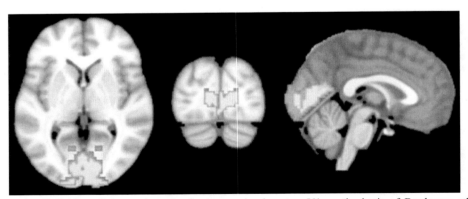

Figure 1.   Definition of the seed mask of primary visual cortex, V1 on the basis of Brodmann atlas. The extracted mask was overlaid on the MNI152 structural images.

improve normality. In order to establish the functional changes when eyes open and closed. Paired *t*-test was used to identify the exact regions that differed in their resting-state functional connectivity strengths under eyes open and eyes closed. For all the above voxel-wise comparisons, the false discovery rate (FDR) method was used for multiple comparison correction ($p < 0.001$), and only clusters that contained a minimum of 100 voxels were reported.

3 RESULTS

Functional difference analyses revealed that different functional connectivity when eyes open and eyes close. When eyes open, the stronger functional connectivities were found in bilateral anterior middle frontal gyrus, insula, superior occipital gyrus, fusiform gyrus, anterior and middle cingulate gyrus and right anterior supramarginal gyrus. In addition, the decreased functional connectivities were found in the bilateral posterior cingulate gyrus, angular gyrus, middle and superior temporal gyrus, dorsal primary motor cortex and secondary sensory cortex (Figure 2).

4 SUMMARY

In this study, we used resting-state functional connectivity to evaluate the changes of functional activity of primary visual cortex V1 when eyes open and eyes closed. The different functional connectivity patterns were found in the two different conditions. When eyes open, we found stronger functional connectivities with visual network and execution control network. Furthermore, the decreased functional connectivities with default model network and sensory-motor network were also found. These finding provide important references for the future acquisition of resting-state functional MRI data when choosing the type of a resting condition.

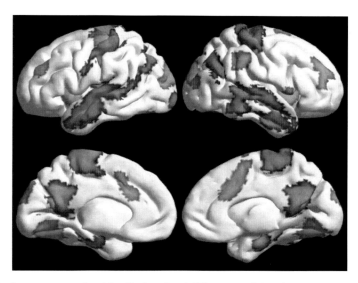

Figure 2. Paired t-test was used to identify functional differences of V1 when eyes open and eyes closed. False discovery rate (FDR) method was used for multiple comparison correction and only clusters that contained a minimum of 100 voxels were reported ((p < 0.001)).

ACKNOWLEDGEMENTS

This work was supported by the National Basic Research Program of China (973 program, 2011CB707801) and the Fundamental Research Funds for the Central Universities.

REFERENCES

Biswal, B., Yetkin, F.Z., Haughton, V.M., Hyde, J.S. (1995) Functional connectivity in the motor cortex of resting human brain using echo-planar MRI. Magnetic resonance in medicine, 34:537–41.

Marx, E., Deutschlander, A., Stephan, T., Dieterich, M., Wiesmann, M., Brandt, T. (2004) Eyes open and eyes closed as rest conditions: impact on brain activation patterns. NeuroImage, 21:1818–24.

Marx, E., Stephan, T., Nolte, A., Deutschlander, A., Seelos, K.C., Dieterich, M., Brandt, T. (2003) Eye closure in darkness animates sensory systems. NeuroImage, 19:924–34.

Zhang, D., Raichle, M.E. (2010) Disease and the brain's dark energy. Nature reviews. Neurology, 6:15–28.

Medicine Sciences and Bioengineering – Wang (Ed.)
© *2015 Taylor & Francis Group, London, ISBN: 978-1-138-02684-1*

Production of L-lactic acid by *Escherichia coli* JH12 using rice straw hydrolysate as carbon source

Ye Liu, Xiao Zhao, Jian-jian Gu & Jin-hua Wang
Key Laboratory of Fermentation Engineering (Ministry of Education), Hubei Provincial Cooperative Innovation Center of Industrial Fermentation, College of Bioengineering, Hubei University of Technology, Wuhan, China

Sheng-de Zhou
Key Laboratory of Fermentation Engineering (Ministry of Education), Hubei Provincial Cooperative Innovation Center of Industrial Fermentation, College of Bioengineering, Hubei University of Technology, Wuhan, China
Department of Biological Sciences, Northern Illinois University, DeKalb, USA

Wa Gao*
Key Laboratory of Fermentation Engineering (Ministry of Education), Hubei Provincial Cooperative Innovation Center of Industrial Fermentation, College of Bioengineering, Hubei University of Technology, Wuhan, China

ABSTRACT: This paper used brittle rice straw, a new kind of biomass resource, as the research object to ferment and produce L-lactic acid. The components of raw materials were compared between brittle rice straw and normal rice straw. Brittle rice straw and normal rice straw were pretreated by milling, 2% H_2SO_4 and enzymatic hydrolysis. The hydrolysate could be used for lipid fermentation by *Escherichia coli* JH12 without adding other carbon source. Shake-flask fermentation was carried out to produce L-lactic acid by *Escherichia coli* JH12 using the hydrolysate of normal and brittle rice straw as carbon source. Fermentation with brittle rice straw hydrolysate as carbon source achieved a L-lactic acid production of 22.6 ± 0.57 g/L, which was 26.3% higher than the L-lactic acid production (17.9 ± 0.62 g/L) with normal rice straw hydrolysate as carbon source.

1   INTRODUCTION

In recent years, lactic acid is an important product that has attracted a great deal of attention due to its wide-spread applications, mainly in cosmetic product, food, pharmaceutical and chemical industries (Mohamed Ali et al, 2013). Currently, it is regarded as an important material for biodegradable plastics such as polylactic acid (PLA; Tokiwa and Calabia, 2006). PLA has attracted a great deal of attention, because of the growing environmental concerns arisen from the excessive consumption of fossil fuels and the soaring of the price of oil (Wee et al., 2004). Rice straw is an abundant renewable resource that serves as a substrate in the production of alternative fuels, Rice straw – a potential source of ethanol has recently gained considerable interest in Asian countries (Karimi et al., 2006). Presently PLA production is considered a relatively mature technology at the industrial scale by fermentation. About 90 % of the worldwide lactic acid production comes from microbial fermentation because the biological production results in optical pure D or L-lactic acid and it is possible to use cheap renewable raw material as substrate (Hofvendhal and Hahn-Hagerdal, 2000).

---
*Corresponding author: Tel. + 86-27-59750481, email: wgao@mail.hbut.edu.cn

In the present study, rice straw subjected acidolysis followed by enzymolysis pretreatments. The hydrolysate as the inexpensive carbon source was applied to produce L-lactic acid. The production of L-lactic acid by *Escherichia coli* JH 12 was investigated using a 7 L fermenter.

2 MATERIALS AND METHODS

2.1 *Raw materials*

Rice straw was collected from experimental base of Hubei Agri-academy of Sciences. The rice straw was coarsely cut into < 3-mm-long pieces by cutter milling and air dried at 60°C. The contents of cellulose, hemicellulose and lignin in brittle rice straw and normal rice straw were determined using the method of Sluiter et al. (sluiter, 2012). The cutter-milled rice straw was subjected to two types of pretreatments, acidolysis followed by enzymolysis. In acidolysis, 2% sulfuric acid was used to liquefy and hydrolyze the fresh material to fermentative sugars. The effect of the enzyme mixture was investigated by supplementing cellulase (Sukehan cellulase, 30 FPU/g) at levels of 0–0.2% (v/w) at a ratio of 1:2 for fresh material and water.

2.2 *Microorganisms and production medium*

Escherichia coli JH 12 is an L-lactic acid producing strain, was provided by Key Laboratory of Fermentation Engineering of Hubei University of Technology, *E. coli* JH 12 was stored in 40% glycerol at -80°C. The strain was activated three times by streaking it out on Luria-Bertani (LB) agar plates and incubating at 37°C for 24 h. The strain was then transferred daily to glucose (20 g/L) mineral salts medium plates (Zhou et al. 2003) and incubated at 37°C to maintain active cells for fermentation.

2.3 *Batch fermentation process in a 7 L fermenter*

Starter cultures were prepared by transferring one colony from a slant to 50 mL of LB broth medium with an addition of 20 g/L xylose, followed by incubation at 37°C and 150 rpm until the OD reached 1.0-1.5. These starter cultures were used as inoculums for 4 L L-lactic acid production medium. The medium for L-lactic acid production consisted of the following ingredients (g/L): hydrolysate of rice straw, tryptone 10 g/L and yeast extract 5 g/L. The initial pH of all media was adjusted to 7.0 with NaOH. All culture media and the neutralizing agents were autoclaved at 121°C for 15 min. Working volumes of the 7 L bioreactors (Sartorius stedim Biotech, GmbH 37070) were 4 L and inoculum size of batch fermentations for production of L-lactic acid by *E. coli* JH 12 was 5 % (v/v). Agitation speed was set at 150 rpm. The fermentation was carried out under anaerobic condition at 37°C. Samples were withdrawn periodically from the culture broth to determine the production of L-lactic acid.

2.4 *Analysis*

Samples from fermentations were centrifuged to remove cells. After centrifugation, the supernatant was then filtered through a 0.22 μm membrane (Millipore, USA) and used for analysis. The concentrations of glucose, lactic acid and other organic acid byproducts were determined by high performance liquid chromatography (HPLC) equipped with a Bio-Rad HPX 87H column and a differential refracting index detector (RID-6A, Shimadzu). The analytical conditions were as follows: column temperature, 35 °C; mobile phase, 4 mM H_2SO_4; flow rate, 0.5 mL/ min.

3 RESULTS AND DISCUSSION

3.1 *The determianation of cellulose, hemicellulose and lignin contents in brittle rice straw and normal rice straw*

The contents of cellulose, hemicellulose and lignin in brittle rice straw and normal rice straw were determined using the method of Sluiter et. al (Sluiter, 2011). The results were shown in Table 1.

Table 1. Component differences between brittle rice straw and normal rice straw.

Component	Brittle straw (%)	Normal straw (%)
Cellulose*	31.2 ± 0.5	36.4 ± 0.5
Hemicellulose*	29.2 ± 0.6	24.9 ± 0.8
Lignin*	14.7 ± 0.3	13.9 ± 0.3

*indicates significant difference at $P < 0.05$ level.

Table 2. Comparison of productions by pretreated brittle rice straw and normal rice straw.

Material	Sugar compositions after enzymatic hydrolysis (g/L)			
	Glucose*	Xylose*	Arabinose	Total sugar*
Brittle straw	17.9 ± 0.4	12.4 ± 0.5	2.9 ± 0.6	35.1 ± 1.2
Normal straw	15.8 ± 0.3	9.6 ± 0.1	2.7 ± 0.5	29.4 ± 1.4

*indicates significant difference at $P < 0.05$ level.

The cellulose, hemicellulose and lignin in brittle rice straw were 31.22 ± 0.52%, 29.21 ± 0.61% and 14.73 ± 0.25%, whereas those in normal rice straw were 36.43 ± 0.53%, 24.93 ± 0.84% and 13.96 ± 0.32%. The cellulose content in brittle rice straw was relative lower than normal rice straw, while the hemicellulose and lignin contents were higher than the normal rice straw.

3.2 The sugar contents in hydrolysate

The sugar content in hydrolysate was analysed after acidolysis and enzymolysis, and the results were shown in Table 2. Total sugar content in brittle rice straw (35.1 ± 1.2 g/L) was higher than the normal rice straw (29.4 ± 1.4 g/L) obviously. The glucose and xylose contents in brittle rice straw were 17.9 ± 0.4 and 2.9 ± 0.6 g/L, which were higher than the contents in normal rice straw (15.8 ± 0.3 and 9.6 ± 0.1 g/L). There was no significant difference shown in arabinose between brittle rice straw and normal rice straw hydrolysate.

3.3 Batch fermentation process in a 7 L fermenter by E. coli JH 12

The hydrolysate of brittle rice straw and normal rice straw was applied as a carbon source in the following fermentation by *E. coli* JH 12. The time course for total sugar, glucose and xylose consumption, L-lactic acid production was shown in Figure 1. During the first 12 h, the time course for sugar, glucose and xylose consumption were similar. The values of sugar, glucose and xylose consumption increase significantly from 12 h to 60 h. The L-lactic acid content of brittle and normal rice straw increased significantly and reached the maximum value at 60 h, after which it decreased gradually up to 72 h. The maximum L-lactic acid content value of brittle rice straw and normal rice straw were 22.74 and 18.33 g/L.

During the fermentation the strain *E .coli* JH12 consumed glucose prior to xylose. In the first 24 h in the fermentation process, glucose was consumed completely both in brittle rice straw hydrolysate and normal rice straw hydrolysate. After 24 h, xylose was consumed and be used completely at 60 h both in two hydrolysate.

4 SUMMARY

After pretreated by sulfuric acid and cellulase, brittle rice straw hydrolysate contains relative higher total sugar, glucose and xylose. Brittle rice straw has more advantages than normal rice straw. Hemicellulose content in brittle rice straw is 17.2% higher than normal rice straw, while

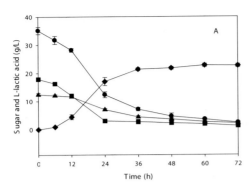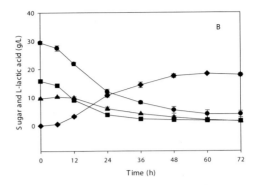

Figure 1. Time course of L-lactic acid production by *E. coli* JH12 with brittle and normal rice straw hydrolysate at pH7.0 and 37 °C. A: brittle rice straw; B: Normal straw. (●, total sugar; ■, glucose; ▲, xylose; ◆, L-lactic acid).

cellulose content is relative lower than the normal rice straw. Compare with cellulose, hemicellulose is easier to be hydrolysed by sulfuric acid. Brittle rice straw is easier to be pretreated by sulfuric acid. Both the brittle rice straw and normal rice straw hydrolysate could be used as carbon source to produced L-lactic acid by *E. coli* JH12. Our study provides a theoretical basis for application of rice straw and expands the usage of rice by-product biomass.

ACKNOWLEDGEMENTS

This research was supported by the National Science & Technology Pillar Program during the 12th Five-year Plan Period (Grant No. 2012BAD27B03), Nature Science Foundation of HuBei Province (Grant No.2011CDB076), Doctoral Scientific Research Foundation of HuBei University of Technology (Grant No. BSQD12047, No. BSQD12143 and No. BSQD13005).

REFERENCES

A. Sluiter B. H., R. Ruiz, C. Scarlata,J. Sluiter, D. Templeton, and D. Crocker. (2012) Determination of structural carbohydrates and lignin in biomass. National renewable energy laboratory.

Karimi K, Emtiazi G,Taherzadeh MJ. (2006) Ethanol production from dilute-acid pre-treated rice straw by simultaneous saccharification and fermentation with Mucor indicus, Rhizopus oryzae, and Saccharomyces cerevisiae. Enzyme Microb Technol, 40:138–44.

K.Hofvendhal, B. Hahn-Hagerdal. (2000) Factors affecting the fermentative lactic acid. Enzyme, Microb. Technol, 26: 87–107.

Mohamed Ali Abdel-Rahman, Yukihiro Tashiro, Kenji Sonomoto. (2013) Recent advances in lactic acid production by microbial fermentation processes. Biotechnology Advances, 31:877–902.

Tokiwa,Y., Calabia,B.P. (2006) Biodegrad ability and biodegradation of poly(lactide) , Appl. Microbiol. Biotechnol. 72: 244–251.

Tong-min W. C.-l. W. L.-q. M. (2012) Characterization and gene mapping of a brittle cuim mutant nbc(t)in rice. Journal of Huazhong Agricultural University, 31 (2): 159–164.

Wee YJ, Kim JN, Yun JS, Ryu HW. (2004) Utilization of sugar molasses for economical L(+)-lactic acid production by batch fermentation of *Enterococcus faecalis*. Enzyme Microb Technol, 35: 568–573.

Zhou, S., Causey, T.B., Hasona, A., Shanmugam, K.T., Ingram, L.O. (2003) Production of optically pure D-lactic acid in mineral salts medium by metabolically engineered *Escherichia coli* W3110. Appl. Environ. Microbiol. 69(1), 399–407.

Medicine Sciences and Bioengineering – Wang (Ed.)
© *2015 Taylor & Francis Group, London, ISBN: 978-1-138-02684-1*

Study on the multiple wavelength HPLC integration fingerprint of active fractions from a purified sample of Naodesheng

Bei Liu, Zhan-chao Li, Chao chen, Shu-mei Wang & Sheng-wang Liang*
School of Traditional Chinese Medicine, Guangdong Pharmaceutical University, Guangzhou, China

ABSTRACT: A five wavelength HPLC integration fingerprint for analyzing the purified sample of Naodesheng (pNDS) is described in the paper. On the basis of the results of the ultraviolet full wavelength scanning, data of five different wavelengths, i.e. 203nm, 250nm, 321nm, 350nm and 403nm, were exported in cdf format from Shimadzu LCsolution (Japan). HPLC fingerprint integration was set up by MATLAB software. The five-wavelength HPLC integration fingerprint of pNDS was established and 20 common characteristic peaks were acquired by taking the peak 5 of pueerarin as the reference peak (S). According to retention times and UV spectra of reference compounds, another four peaks were identified as HSYA, ferulic acid, vitexin-2"-O-rhamnoside and notoginsenoside R1, respectively. The integrated fingerprint gives the best abundance and the maximum number of compounds within one chromatographic window. It represents the characteristics of chemical constitutions of the complex medicine objectively, and is convenient for popularization and application. This method provides a theoretical basis for further research of Naodesheng as well as a reference for studies on the material foundation of Chinese medicine.

1   INTRODUCTION

With the deepening research in the field of food, life science, traditional Chinese medicine (TCM) and natural products, the increasing number of research projects possesses the characteristic of complexity and unknown. Seeking for ideas and methods for analysis of complex system has become one of the critical problems to solve. Compared with the simple system, the number of chemical components in a complex one is larger, and the contents of them vary from one to another. What's more, relationships of these chemicals are non-linear. To the Chinese herbal and preparations, research should be done following the principle of comprehensiveness and maximizing the feature information, thus giving a better understanding of the complex system (Luo *et al.*, 2009).

Fingerprint has gained more and more attention and been internationally accepted as a feasible means for the quality control of TCM. The chemical fingerprint obtained by HPLC-DAD has become the primary instrumentation among many other analytical tools. However, fingerprints were always compared under a single wavelength when evaluating the similarity. It is obvious that only one chromatogram under a wavelength can not fully express the quality characteristics, especially for complex systems such as TCM. Currently, the characteristic fingerprint of multi-dimensional and multi-data has been described for resolving problems in quality control of TCM (Luo & Wang, 2002). Luo Guo-an and his coworkers resorted to multi-wavelength fusion fingerprint for the analysis (Luo *et al.*, 2009).

With regard to fingerprint fusion, methods can generally be expressed in two aspects.*i*) Hyphenated techniques as to detectors, including HPLC/DAD-ELSD (Wang *et al.*, 2010; Li *et al.*, 2008), HPLC/DAD-MS (Li *et al.*, 2004; Feng *et al.*, 2007) and LC-MS-SPE-NMR (Hooft *et al.*,

---

*Corresponding author. Tel.: +86 20 39352172; fax: +86 20 39352174. E-mail address: swliang371@163.com

2011) are more commonly used by practitioners than combination one separation method with another. Recently, research on the coupled separation techniques has been a driving force in the development of instrumental analysis, a large number of methods has been developed and combined in various ways (Cao *et al.*, 2004).*ii*) Concerning data-level information fusion method, the software of "Digitized Evaluation System for Super-Information Characteristics of the Traditional Chinese Medicine Fingerprints 3.0" was described to establish and evaluate the fusion fingerprint, and then employed to Fuzilizhong pills (Sun & Wang, 2009; Ren *et al.*, 2009). The results showed that the information of fusion fingerprint was more abundant. The multi-wavelength fusion fingerprint analysis was highly reproducible and may serve for quality identification and comprehensive evaluation of Fuzilizhong pills. The computer-aided-similarity-evaluation (CASE) software, a pattern recognition program recommended by the Chinese Pharmacopoeial committee, was applied to set up the fusion fingerprints (Hua *et al.*, 2008). In addition to the software discussed above, it was reported that the all-time multi-wavelength fusion fingerprint was used to control the quality of Qizhiweitong granules, quantitative analysis of six components was done as well based on the fingerprint (Yao *et al.*, 2013). The method was simple, providing the basis for quality control of Qizhiweitong granules. The principal component analysis (PCA) was applied to data processing for HPLC fingerprint, taking *Gardenia jasminoides* Ellis as an example (Nie *et al.*, 2005). It was reported that the information of individual fingerprint was combined by using serial or parallel information fusion strategy at the raw data level; an algorithm based on information fusion was developed to evaluate the similarity of multiple chromatographic fingerprints of TCM (Fan *et al.*, 2006; Fan *et al.*, 2006).

Naodesheng, a TCM prescription, has functions of promoting blood flow to dissipate stasis, dredging channel meridians and waking up the brain. The present paper describes a five wavelength HPLC integration fingerprint for analyzing the purified sample of Naodesheng (pNDS). The integrated fingerprint gave the best abundance and the maximum number of compounds within one chromatographic window. It represented the characteristics of chemical constitutions of the complex medicine objectively, and was convenient for popularization and application. This method provides a theoretical basis for further research of Naodesheng as well as a reference for studies on the material foundation of Chinese medicine.

2 METHODOLOGY AND EXPERIMENTAL

2.1 *Methodology of multiple wavelength HPLC fingerprint integration*

On the basis of the results of the ultraviolet full wavelength scanning, data of five different wavelengths, i.e. 203nm, 250nm, 321nm, 350nm and 403nm, were exported in cdf format from Shimadzu LCsolution (Japan). HPLC fingerprint integration was set up by the MATLAB software according to the following principles:*i*) for eluting peaks of the same retention time from different chromatographic windows, compared the peak area and took the maximum one as the integrated peak;*ii*) for other eluting peaks, compared the peak intensity at each time point and took the maximum one as the intensity of an integrated peak. The integrated fingerprint gave the best abundance and the maximum number for characteristic compounds within one chromatographic window.

2.2 *Materials and reagents*

Samples of Sanchi (*Panax notoginseng*), Chuanxiong (*Ligusticum chuanxiong*), Safflower (*Carthamus tinctorius*), Kudzu Root (*Pueraria lobata*) and Hawkthorn (*Crataegus pinnatifida*) were purchased from the Guangzhou Zhixin Pharmaceutical Corporation Ltd. (Guangdong, China), and authenticated by Professor Shuyuan Li from Guangdong Pharmaceutical University.

Standards of notoginsenoside R_1, puerarin, ferulic acid and hydroxysafflor yellow A were purchased from the National Institutes for Food and Drug Control (Beijing, China). A pure compound of vitexin-2"-O-rhamnoside was purchased from the Chengdu Must Bio-technology Corporation Ltd (Sichuan, China).

HPLC-grade acetonitrile and acetic acid were from Honeywell (USA). Deionized water was obtained from a Milli-Q water system (Millipore, Bedford, MA, USA).

2.3 Apparatus and conditions

The HPLC system consisted of two delivery pumps (Shimadzu LC-20AD, Japan) and a PDA detector (Shimadzu, SPD-M20A, Japan). Chromatographic separation was carried out at 25°C using a Luna (2) C18 analytical column (250 mm×4.6 mm, 5 μm) supplied by Phenomenex (USA). The mobile phase consisted of water–acetic acid (A, 100:0.1, v/v) and acetonitrile–acetic acid (B, 100:0.1, v/v); A:B was as follows: 0-60 min, 5%→20% B; 60–80 min, 20%→40% B; 80-100 min, 40%→60% B; 100-101 min, 60%→80% B; 101-106 min, 80%→80% B. The flow rate was 1.0 ml/min.

2.4 Sample preparation

According to the formulation of Naodesheng, the medical materials of 7.8 g Sanchi, 7.8 g Chuanxiong, 9.1 g Safflower, 26.1 g Kudzu Root and 15.7 g Hawkthorn were smashed into crude powder and divided into two parts for further extraction. The powder of Safflower was denoted as Part II, and the others were denoted as Part I. Part I was extracted twice with 70% ethanol while Part II with distilled water. Both of them, then purified with different types of macroporous absorbent resins (MAR), respectively (Chen et al., 2011). Ethanol-H₂O extracts from each part was concentrated, dried under decompression at 40°C (vacuum pressure: 0.9 Mpa) and mixed with each other. Consequently pNDS was made. The whole fractionation process can be graphed in Figure 1.

0.1 g fine powder of the pNDS was accurately weighted, dissoluted with 50 ml of 30% methanol then filtered through a 0.22μm membrane filter. Ten microliters of the sample solution was injected to an HPLC column and separated under above chromatographic conditions.

2.5 Reference preparation

Dissolve 50.00 mg of notoginsenoside R_1, 50.00 mg of puerarin, 10.00 mg of ferulic acid, 40.00 mg of hydroxysafflor yellow A and 10.00 mg of vitexin-2"-O-rhamnoside in 50% methanol and dilute to 50.00 mL with the same solvent. Transfer 1.00 mL of this solution to a 10.00 mL volumetric flask and dilute to volume.

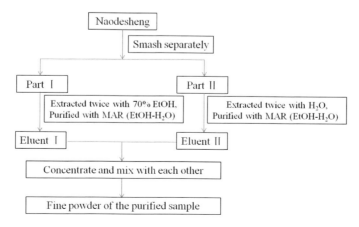

Figure 1. Flowchart of the fractionation process.

2.6 Method validation

The validation of the analytical method was carried out with reference solution and sample solution. Six injections of the reference solution to demonstrate system suitability were made before the sample injections. It is more reliable to ensure the general resolving power of the system that minimum 1.5 of resolution (R) from the sample solution between a peak identified as one of the five standards and a closely eluting compound. The instrument/injection precision (repeatability) was obtained by analyzing the variations of peak area of six injections. The stability of sample solution was evaluated in 48h while replicate samples from a single batch were prepared and analyzed in a single day, and the test was assessed by analyzing the variations of peak area of six determinations.

3 RESULTS AND DISCUSSION

3.1 Optimization of the chromatographic conditions

Generally, a well strategy of optimization parameters in HPLC was done on the basis of a sound theoretical foundation, predicting the retention time of solutes of complex sample. In the previous work, predictive model of the retention time and the grid search algorithm were employed to optimize the separation condition (Yin et al., 2007; Yin et al., 2010; Yin et al., 2007). The results could not meet the requirements of the separation as compared with that of articles reported. Finally, the optimization was done through investigating the influence regarding mobile phase, column temperature, flow-rate and sample amount.

3.1.1 Mobile phase

In this work, a mixture of acetonitrile and water was chosen as the mobile phase. Considering the presence of flavonoids and other polyphenols in the pNDS, a little amount of acetic acid was added to the mobile phase to reduce the ionization, thus lowering the polarity of these compounds. The optimum mobile phase was achieved with solvent A (H_2O + 0.1% acetic acid) and solvent B (acetonitrile + 0.1% acetic acid) in the gradient mode.

3.1.2 Column temperature and flow-rate

Column temperature is also specified as a key influence on the resolution of components, for it has a close relationship with retention behavior of solutes as well as the selectivity of the column. In the present study, 25°C was chosen as the optimum temperature. The retention time of eluting compounds became shorter with the rise of column temperature, while the results obtained at 20°C were not satisfied compared with that at 25°C in terms of peak intensity. The flow-rate was 1.0 mL/min, considering the majority of compounds were resolved well.

3.1.3 Sample amount

Sample concentration and injection volume should be appropriate in order to ensure the numbers of components are detected as many as possible. Without sacrificing the resolution and symmetry of chromatographic peaks, sample amount has several aspects:*i*) peak area of each common peak for the multiple wavelength HPLC integration fingerprint is at least three orders of magnitude;*ii*) flat peak is forbidden in the chromatogram. Consequently, the concentration of sample solution was 4 mg/mL and injection volume was 10 μL.

3.1.4 Detection wavelength for fingerprint integration

In order to obtain a large amount of detectable peaks in the HPLC chromatogram, the spectra of all peaks in the chromatogram of the sample were investigated with photodiode array detection. Given the relative homogeneity of wavelengths in the UV range, five wavelengths were chosen for further integration, i.e. 203nm, 250nm, 321nm, 350nm and 403nm, representing characteristic components of each raw medicinal material of NDS, namely notoginsenoside R_1, puerarin, ferulic acid, vitexin-2"-*O*-rhamnoside and HSYA, respectively.

Table 1. The results of the system suitability test (n = 6).

	HSYA	Puerarin	Ferulic acid	Vitexin-2"-O-rhamnoside	Notoginsenoside R_1
RSD (RT)	1.5	0.02	0.02	0.03	0.06
RSD (PA)	0.5	0.08	0.1	0.1	2.3
T	1.81	1.07	1.07	1.02	1.52
N	37169	92671	93409	45165	375349
R	2.44	7.66	1.87	3.33	1.98

RT: retention time; PA: peak area.

3.2 Validation of the analytical method

HPLC fingerprint method validations were carried out under the regulation of the Chinese Pharmacopoeia Commission (Chinese Pharmacopoeia Commission, 2002). Validation result was based on the five wavelength HPLC integration fingerprints. The result of the system suitability test was shown in Table 1. Method precision was based on replicated analysis of samples, with reported relative standard deviations (RSDs) less than 3.0% for relative peak area (RPA) of common peaks. The stability test was performed with a sample solution in 0, 4, 8, 16, 24 and 48 h. The RSDs of the RPA were found less than 3.0%. The method reproducibility was studied through six-replicated sample solutions. The corresponding RSDs of RPA were reported less than 3.0%. All of these results were in accordance with the requirement, indicating that the developed method was validated and applicable for sample analysis.

3.3 Five wavelength HPLC integration fingerprint of pNDS

The integration fingerprints were generated from five batches of pNDS [Figure 2 (a-e)]. Twenty peaks (which contributed >98% total peak area) were selected as the common characteristic peaks in the Table 2, generated by MATLB as well. Peak 5 of puerarin was selected as the reference peak (S). According to retention times and UV spectra of reference compounds, peak 4, 12,13

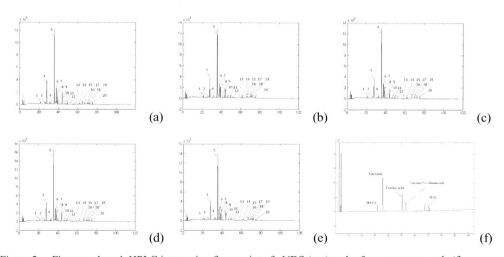

Figure 2. Five wavelength HPLC integration fingerprint of pNDS (a-e) and reference compounds (f).

Table 2. Five wavelength HPLC integration fingerprint of pNDS from five batches.

No.	S1 RPA	S2	S3	S4	S5
1	0.0411	0.0386	0.0394	0.0406	0.0413
2	0.0352	0.0370	0.0353	0.0356	0.0354
3	0.226	0.225	0.226	0.225	0.226
4	0.0228	0.0233	0.0228	0.0220	0.0230
5	1.00	1.00	1.00	1.00	1.00
6	0.182	0.180	0.181	0.181	0.177
7	0.175	0.175	0.176	0.177	0.175
8	0.0115	0.0113	0.0115	0.0113	0.0108
9	0.195	0.195	0.195	0.195	0.194
10	0.0243	0.0241	0.0241	0.0239	0.0237
11	0.0436	0.0438	0.0427	0.0434	0.0437
12	0.00424	0.00423	0.00421	0.00423	0.00434
13	0.0354	0.0343	0.0341	0.0357	0.0350
14	0.0438	0.0440	0.0418	0.0433	0.0429
15	0.00543	0.00561	0.00526	0.00560	0.00559
16	0.0251	0.0255	0.0248	0.0248	0.0238
17	0.00714	0.00707	0.00698	0.00729	0.00688
18	0.00613	0.00618	0.00610	0.00608	0.00601
19	0.0251	0.0251	0.0250	0.0248	0.0247
20	0.0355	0.0350	0.0352	0.0353	0.0358

and 18 were identified as HSYA, ferulic acid, vitexin-2"-O-rhamnoside and notoginsenoside R_1, respectively.

4 CONCLUSION

With the development of analytical methods and TCM theories, an increasing number of strategies for establishing a fingerprint and evaluating the conformability have been developed. Nowadays, mass spectrometry (MS) has the best sensitivity as well as the ability to identify unknown compounds on-line. Unfortunately, it is not very popular among practitioners because of the high-cost. In this study, a multiple wavelength HPLC integration fingerprint is proposed as a strategy for quality control of complex herbal medicines instead of reported single chromatographic fingerprinting. It objectively represents the whole characteristics of chemical constitutions of the analyte, and is convenient for popularization and application. As an example, five wavelength HPLC integration fingerprints of pNDS were developed for consistency assessment. The results indicate that multiple wavelength HPLC integration fingerprint could show the promising prospect for resolving problems in quality control of complex herbal medicines.

ACKNOWLEDGEMENT

We acknowledge the financial support by the National Natural Science Foundation of China (No. 81274059).

REFERENCES

Chinese Pharmacopoeia Commission (2002) *Guidance on chromatographic fingerprint experimental research of TCM injection* (in Chinese).

Cao, J., Xu, Y., Zhang, Y.Z., Wang, Y.M. & Luo, G.A. (2004) Integrated fingerprint chromatogram analysis for Gardenia.*Chinese Journal of Analytical Chemistry*, 32(7): 875–878.

Chen, C., Li, S.X., Wang, S.M. & Liang, S.W. (2011) A support vector machine based pharmacodynamic prediction model for searching active fraction and ingredients of herbal medicine: Naodesheng prescription as an example.*Journal of Pharmaceutical and Biomedical Analysis*, 56(2): 443–447.

Fan, X.H., Ye, Z.L. & Cheng, Y.Y. (2006) A computational method based on information fusion for evaluating the similarity of multiple chromatographic fingerprints of TCM.*Chemical Journal of Chinese Universities*, 27(1): 26–29.

Fan, X.H., Cheng, Y.Y., Ye, Z.L., Lin, R.C. & Qian, Z.Z. (2006) Multiple chromatographic fingerprinting and its application to the quality control of herbal medicines.*Analytica Chimica Acta*, 555(2): 217–224.

Feng, H.P., Yang, Z.L. & Hu, Y.Z. (2007) Chromatographic studies on fingerprints of Cortex *Magnoliae officinalis* and their processed products by HPLC-DAD-MS.*Chinese Traditional Patent Medicine*, 29(1): 84–88.

Hua, R.F., Huang, K.E., Ke, X.H. & Chen, J.F. (2008) Analysis of dual-wavelength fingerprint chromatogram of Buzhong Yiqi decoction.Traditional Chinese Drug Research & Clinical Pharmacology, 19(1): 42–47.

Hooft, J.J.J., Mihaleva, V., Vos, R.C.H., Bino, R.J. & Vervoort, J. (2011) A strategy for fast structural elucidation of metabolites in small volume plant extracts using automated MS-guided LC-MS-SPE-NMR. *Magnetic Resonance in Chemistry*, 49(S1): S55–S60.

Luo, G.A. & Wang, Y.M. (2002) Classification and Development of TCM Fingerprint.*Chinese Journal of New Drugs*, 11(1): 46–51.

Li, S.L., Lin, G., Chung, H. & Tam, Y. (2004) Study on fingerprint of rhizoma Chuanxiong by HPLC-DAD-MS.*Acta Pharmaceutica Sinica*, 39(8):621–626.

Li, W.L., Yu, Y.Y., Zhao, J., Wang, X.D., Hu, Z.T. & Xu, D. (2008) Fingerprinting analysis of glycosides in JinKui Shenqi pill by HPLC-DAD-ELSD.*Chin Pharm J*, 43(13): 968–970, 1032.

Luo, G.A., Liang, Q.L. & Wang, Y.M. (2009) *TCM Fingerprint: Evaluation, Quality Control, New Drug Research and Development.*Beijing, Chemical Industry Press.

Nie, L., Hu, Z., Luo, G.A., Wang, Y.M. & Cao, J. (2005) Fusion technology of TCM fingerprints.*Chinese Journal of Analytical Chemistry*, 32(6):898.

Ren, P.P., Sun, G.X. & Sun, L.N. (2009) Study on multi-wavelength fusion HPLC fingerprint of Fuzilizhong pills. *Chinese Journal of Pharmaceutical Analysis*, 29(3): 411–415.

Sun, G.X. & Wang, J.Q. (2009) Quality of Radix et rhizoma glycyrrhizae by systematic quantified fingerprint based on dual wavelength fingerprints and their fusion fingerprints.Central South Pharmacy, 7(5): 378–383.

Wang, H.L., Yao, W.F., Zhu, D.N. & Hu, Y.Z. (2010) Chemical Fingerprinting by HPLC-DAD-ELSD and Principal Component Analysis of *Polygala japonica* from Different Locations in China.*Chinese Journal of Natural Medicines*, 8(5): 343−348.

Yin, X.Y., Yao, W.F. & Hu, Y.Z. (2007) Predictive model of the retention time for solutes based on multiple regression under linear gradient condition.*Journal of China Pharmaceutical University*, 38(3):236–242.

Yin, X.Y., Yao, W.F. & Hu, Y.Z. (2007) Fast optimization method of linear gradient elution condition for herbal medicine's chromatographic fingerprint separation.*Chinese Journal of Analytical Chemistry*, 35(6): 839–844.

Yin, X.Y., Luo, Y.M. & Hu, Y.Z. (2010) Optimization of separation condition for TCM *Pueraria thomsoniics* chromatographic fingerprint from different gradient profile.*Chinese Journal of Pharmaceutical Analysis*, 30(7): 1218–1221.

Yao, D., Meng, X.S., Wang, S., Bao, Y.R., Pan, Y. & Han, L. (2013) Study on all-time multi-wavelength fusion fingerprint of Qizhiweitong granules and multi-component quantitative analysis. *China Journal of Chinese Materia Medica*, 38(10): 1513–1517.

Medicine Sciences and Bioengineering – Wang (Ed.)
© *2015 Taylor & Francis Group, London, ISBN: 978-1-138-02684-1*

Kinetics study of glutathione peroxidase 4 mutant using H_2O_2 as oxidizing substrate

Xiao Guo, Zhen-lin Fan, Yang Yu, Yin-long Zhang, Shuan Wang, Chuang Ma & Jing-yan Wei*
College of Pharmaceutical Science and Institute of Theoretical Chemistry, Jilin University, Changchun, Jilin, China

Jian Song, Rui-qing Xing, Da-li Liu & Hong-wei Song*
College of Electronic Science and Engineering, Jilin University, Changchun, Jilin, China

ABSTRACT: Glutathione peroxidase 4 (GPx4) is a critical selenoenzyme which could reduce hydrogen peroxide, membrane-bound phospholipid and cholesterol hydroperoxides. However, it has been difficult to produce recombinant human GPx4 (hGPx4) in *E. coli* for a long time due to the complicated expression mechanism of selenocysteine (Sec)-containing protein. In this study, seleno-hGPx4 mutant was expressed in an *E. coli* BL21(DE3)*cys* auxotrophic strain and the kinetics of recombinant hGPx4 mutant based on H_2O_2 was studied. The results shows that the mutant exhibited a typical "ping-pong" mechanism, which is similar to native GPx4. It provides an important theoretical foundation to study the recombinant GPx produced in *E.coli*.

1   INTRODUCTION

Phospholipid hydroperoxide glutathione peroxidase (GPx4, EC 1.11.1.12) is a selenium-dependent GPx. As a radical scavenger, GPx4 protects cells and tissues from oxidative damage like other glutathione peroxidases (GPxs) and plays an essential role in cellular differentiation during embryonic development (Imai *et al.*, 2003). GPx4 is a monomeric enzyme in contrast to other members of the GPx family (Ran *et al.*, 2004). In addition, an oligomerization loop exposed on the surface is present in the other selenium-dependent tetrameric GPxs, but absent in GPx4. The oligomerization loop is considered to participate in the tetramer assembly and limit the accessibility of the active site to the large substrates (Scheerer *et al.*, 2007). Because of its unique structure, GPx4 exhibits much broader substrate specificity than the other members of the GPx family.

Selenocystein (Sec) in the N-terminal region of GPx4 is encoded by UGA, usually regarded as a stop codon. And the fact that the mechanism of seleno-protein expression differs from prokaryotes to eukaryotes makes it difficult to heterologously express hGPx4 in *E. coli*. In this study, a hGPx4 mutant with all Cyestine (Cys) residues changed to Serine (Ser) residues was prepared by *E. coli* BL21(DE3)*cys* auxotrophic strain (Strub *et al.*, 2003). And kinetics of the mutant based on H_2O_2 was studied.

2   MATERIALS AND METHODS

2.1   *Materials*

BL21(DE3)*cys* auxotrophic strain was a generous gift from professor Marie-Paule Strub and August Bock. Plasmid pMazF and MiniBEST Plasmid Purification Kit were purchased from

---

*The corresponding authors: Jingyan Wei and Hongwei Song. Tel.:186–431-85619716. E-mail: jingyanweijluedu@163.com and songhw@jlu.edu.cn.

Takara. Plasmid pCGPx4 encoding hGPx4 with all Cys residues changed to Ser has been constructed. Reduced nicotinamide adenine dinucleotide phosphate (NADPH), ethylenediaminetetraacetic acid (EDTA), glutathione reductase, Sec and antibodies were purchased from Sigma. Other chemicals were obtained from the Beijing Chemical Factory, China.

2.2 Overexpression and purification of seleno-hGPx4 mutant

E. coli BL21(DE3)cys auxotrophic strain was used to produce selenoenzyme via tRNA^{Cys} mis-loading. The auxotrophic strain was cotransformed with plasmid pCGPx4 and pMazF containing mazF gene. The production of selenoprotein was carried out according to the method described previously (Guo et al., 2014). Purification of recombinant proteins from E.coli was carried out by immobilized metal affinity chromatography.

2.3 Steady-state kinetics of seleno-hgpx4 mutant

Steady-state parameters were determined using the same assay with the concentration of one substrate varied while the other was kept fixed. The k_{cat} and K_m values were calculated from Lineweaver-Burk plots. GPx activities were measured using the method as described above.

2.4 Molecular modeling

molecular modelings were performed with Insight II package, version 2000 (Accelrys, San Diego, CA). Crystal structure of GPx4 (PDB: 2OBI) was used for calculations. Resulting models were refined by MD simulations and analyzed with Profile-3D and Procheck (Guo et al., 2013).

3 RESULTS

3.1 Overexpression and purification of seleno-hGPx4 mutant

The purified selenoprotein showed a single band of molecular mass ~20 kDa on SDS-PAGE and Western blotting (Figure 1), indicating that seleno-hGPx4 mutant was successfully expressed and purified from E.coli BL21(DE3)cys.

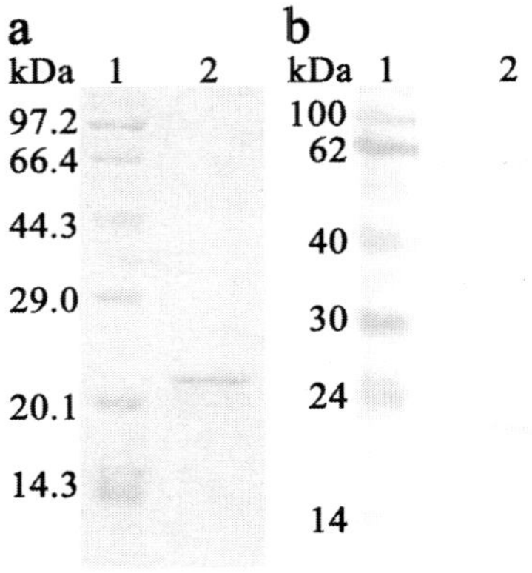

Figure 1.   SDS-PAGE (a) and Western blotting (b) analysis of various purified seleno-hGPx4 mutant.

3.2 Assay of enzyme activity

The GPx activity of seleno-hGPx4 mutant was about 646 ± 48 U/μmol. Non-seleno-hGPx4 exhibited no GPx activity. It was shown that the catalytic activity was attributed to Sec in the catalytic center. This mutant was 653-fold more efficient than Ebselen (0.99 U/μmol) (Mugesh and Singh, 2000), but showed lower activity than native GPx4 (3100 U/μmol) (Ursini et al., 1985).

3.3 Steady-state kinetics of seleno-hGPx4 mutant

Double-reciprocal plots of $[E_0]/v_0$ versus the reciprocal concentration of one substrate at various fixed concentrations of the second substrate give a set of parallel lines (Figure 2). This result indicated that seleno-hGPx4 mutant followed a "ping-pong" mechanism. Steady-state kinetic parameters were determined by fitting the experimental data to Equation 1 and the values of the kinetic parameters are summarized in Table 1. The $k_{cat}/K_m^{H_2O_2}$ value of the mutant is two orders of magnitude lower than that of native GPx4 (1.8×10^8) (Takebe et al., 2002), indicating the rate of reaction between the mutant and H_2O_2 is slower than between native GPx4 and H_2O_2.

$$\frac{v_0}{[E]_0} = \frac{k_{cat}[GSH][ROOH]}{K_m^{GSH}[ROOH] + K_m^{H_2O_2}[GSH] + [ROOH][GSH]} \tag{1}$$

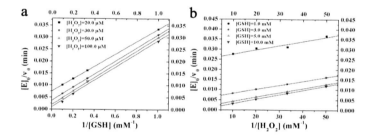

Figure 2. Double-reciprocal plots for the reduction of H_2O_2 by GSH catalyzed by seleno-hGPx4 mutant. (a) $[E]_0/v_0$ versus $1/[GSH]$(mM^{-1}) at $[H_2O_2] = 20.0$ μM (■), 30.0 μM (●), 50.0 μM (▲), and 100 μM (▼). (b) $[E]_0/v_0$ versus $1/[H_2O_2]$ (mM^{-1}) at $[GSH] = 1$ mM (■), 3 mM (●), 5 mM (▲), and 10 mM (▼).

Table 1. Steady-state kinetic parameters for glutathione peroxidase 4 mutant.

[GSH] (mM)	k_{cat} (min^{-1})	$K_m^{H_2O_2}$ (M)	$k_{cat}/K_m^{H_2O_2}$ (M^{-1}min^{-1})
1	39 ± 6	$(5.7 \pm 0.13) \times 10^{-6}$	$(6.8 \pm 0.21) \times 10^6$
3	149 ± 3	$(2.9 \pm 0.20) \times 10^{-5}$	$(5.1 \pm 0.13) \times 10^6$
5	480 ± 10	$(1.0 \pm 0.06) \times 10^{-4}$	$(4.8 \pm 0.06) \times 10^6$
10	1094 ± 35	$(2.0 \pm 0.33) \times 10^{-4}$	$(5.7 \pm 0.25) \times 10^6$

[H$_2$O$_2$] (mM)	k_{cat} (min^{-1})	K_m^{GSH} (M)	k_{cat}/K_m^{GSH} (M^{-1}min^{-1})
0.02	139 ± 11	$(3.9 \pm 0.12) \times 10^{-3}$	$(3.6 \pm 0.20) \times 10^4$
0.03	274 ± 15	$(7.5 \pm 0.32) \times 10^{-3}$	$(3.7 \pm 0.03) \times 10^4$
0.05	980 ± 36	$(2.8 \pm 0.28) \times 10^{-2}$	$(3.5 \pm 0.34) \times 10^4$
0.1	2001 ± 10	$(5.9 \pm 0.19) \times 10^{-2}$	$(3.4 \pm 0.15) \times 10^4$

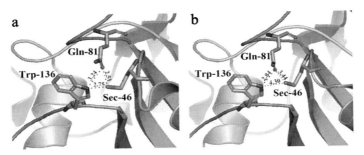

Figure 3. Stereo view of the active site of putative native GPx4 (a) and seleno-hGPx4 mutant (b) The cartoon representations were generated in PyMol.

3.4 Molecular modeling

The Profile-3D scores of putative native GPx4 and seleno-hGPx4 mutant are 74.06 and 72.7, respectively, compared with the expected high score of 74.72 and the expected low score of 33.63. Ramachandran plot analysis showed more than 80% of residues in each model in the core region. These results suggested that the conformations of putative native GPx4 and seleno-hGPx4 are reliable. The catalytic triad consisting of Sec-46, Gln-81 and Trp-136 was detected in the two models. But it was obviously that the distances between each of these atoms in seleno-hGPx4 mutant were longer than them in the putative hGPx4 (Figure 3).

4 DISSCUSSION

GPx4 catalyses the reduction of hydroperoxides with GSH and protects organism from oxidative damage (Ran et al., 2004). Owing to the fact that the incorporation of Sec into protein requires a special mechanism, the heterologous expression of seleno-GPx with high activity from E. coli has not been reported for a long time. The mischarging of tRNA^{Cys} with Sec in the E. coli BL21(DE3) cys auxotrophic strain makes it possible to achieve this goal. And c-GPx4 is a single poly-peptide chain protein and does not undergo any major post-translational modification, thus it is suitable for its production in E. coli. Considering the fact that Ser has similar properties to Cys, so Cys residues in native human GPx4 were changed to Ser residues to minimize the negative effects caused by the replacement of Cys with Sec residues.

In the catalytic reaction of GPx4, the rapid reaction of the E-SeOH with GSH appears to be very important, because this reaction ensure the regeneration of E-SeH and thereby maintain the catalytic efficiency of the selenoenzyme. Although the structure of E-SeSG has not been solved to date, we envision that the orientation of selenenic group of E-SeOH might be one of the essential factors for the reduction of selenenic acid. As shown in Fig. 3, the orientation of the selenenic group in seleno-hGPx4 was similar to that in putative native GPx4. The results led us to propose a hypothesis that the structure of Sec-46 in putative native GPx4 and seleno-hGPx4 may facilitate the interaction between the selenenic group and GSH.

Although the activity of the enzyme was higher than some of GPx mimics, it was still lower than native GPx4. The apparent second-order rate constant k_{cat}/K_m^{GSH} was lower than that of native one, indicating the enzyme had a lower catalytic efficiency. The reduction in catalytic efficiency observed for this mutant might be attributed to the conformational changes in the active site. And that might be the main reason for the loss of the activity of seleno-hGPx4 compared with native GPx4. In this study, a seleno-hGPx4 mutant with high activity was successfully prepared by using the Cys auxotrophic strain. Kinetics study of the mutant using H_2O_2 as oxidizing substrate showed that catalytic mechanism was similar with native GPx and explained the reason why the activity of this mutant was lower than the natural one.

ACKNOWLEDGEMENTS

The authors thank Prof Marie-Paule Strub and August Böck for providing the *E. coli* cysteine ausotrophic strain, BL21(DE3)*cys*. This work is supported by the National Natural Science Foundation of China (No.30970633 and 31270851), Doctoral Funding Grants, Norman Bethune Health Science Center of Jilin University (No.470110000006) and Graduate Innovation Fund of Jilin University (No.2014067 and No.2014060).

REFERENCES

Guo, X., Song, J., Yu, Y. & Wei, J. (2013) Can recombinant human glutathione peroxidase 1 with high activity be efficiently produced in Escherichia coli? *Antioxid Redox Signal.*

Guo, X., Yu, Y., Liu, X., Zhang, Y., Guan, T., Xie, G. & Wei, J. (2014) Heterologous expression and characterization of human cellular glutathione peroxidase mutants. *Iubmb Life,* 66, 212–219.

Imai, H., Hirao, F., Sakamoto, T., Sekine, K., Mizukura, Y., Saito, M., Kitamoto, T., Hayasaka, M., Hanaka, K. & Nakagawa, Y. (2003) Early embryonic lethality caused by targeted disruption of the mouse PHGPx gene. *Biochem Biophys Res Commun,* 305, 278–286.

Maiorine, M., Roveri, A., Ursini, F. & Gregolin, C. (1985) Enzymatic determination of membrane lipid peroxidation. *J Free Radic Biol Med,* 1, 203–207.

Mugesh, G. & Singh, H. B. (2000) Synthetic organoselenium compounds as antioxidants: glutathione peroxidase activity. *Chemical Society Reviews,* 29, 347–357.

Ran, Q., Liang, H., Gu, M., Qi, W., Walter, C. A., Roberts, L. J., Herman, B., Richardson, A. & Van Remmen, H. (2004) Transgenic mice overexpressing glutathione peroxidase 4 are protected against oxidative stress-induced apoptosis. *Journal of Biological Chemistry,* 279, 55137–55146.

Scheerer, P., Borchert, A., Krauss, N., Wessner, H., Gerth, C., Hhne, W. & Kuhn, H. (2007) Structural Basis for Catalytic Activity and Enzyme Polymerization of Phospholipid Hydroperoxide Glutathione Peroxidase-4 (GPx4), §. *Biochemistry,* 46, 9041–9049.

Strub, M. P., Hoh, F., Sanchez, J. F., Strub, J. M., Bock, A., Aumelas, A. & Dumas, C. (2003) Selenomethionine and selenocysteine double labeling strategy for crystallographic phasing. *Structure,* 11, 1359–67.

Takebe, G., Yarimizu, J., Saito, Y., Hayashi, T., Nakamura, H., Yodoi, J., Nagasawa, S. & Takahashi, K. (2002) A comparative study on the hydroperoxide and thiol specificity of the glutathione peroxidase family and selenoprotein P. *Journal of Biological Chemistry,* 277, 41254–41258.

Medicine Sciences and Bioengineering – Wang (Ed.)
© *2015 Taylor & Francis Group, London, ISBN: 978-1-138-02684-1*

Study on the job satisfaction of public health staff

Wen-juan Zhong[a] & Wei-di Yang
Wuhan Polytechnic University, Wuhan, China

Bin Li[*]
Tongji Medical College of Huazhong University of Science and Technology, Wuhan, China

ABSTRACT: The objective of this study is to survey the job satisfaction of public health staff in HanChuan to provide a basis for its decision-making. **Methods** Using the self-made questionnaire for the cluster sampling method, questionnaire survey and the statistical methods for result analysis. **Results** The main factors affecting the satisfaction of public health staff included the performance appraisal system, working emphasis, income satisfaction, lack of experimental material, no cooperation teamwork, earned income. **Conclusion** It is very important to establish an effective performance evaluation system and protection mechanism of a public health personnel talent, improve salary and welfare and people's thinking and understanding of public health issues, increase government attention and investment efforts so as to enhance the overall job satisfaction of public health staff.

1   INTRODUCTION

Public health is a basic guarantee for citizens in a whole country or in a whole region, which is correlated to every citizen's physical and psychological health. Our country's construction of public health aims at improving rural primary health care service and urban basic medical service, satisfying the need of rural and urban citizens for basic health services. Job satisfaction means after one evaluates his job or his work experience, he feels happy and vibrant. Public health personnel is the main force who provide public health service. Therefore, paying due attention to their job satisfaction is the way to bring into full play their enthusiasm to do well their own work, which will improve the present level of our country's public health. We surveyed the public health personnel in HanChuan city of Hubei province and made an investigation of their job satisfaction.

2   OBJECTIVES AND METHODS

2.1   *The survey and its content*

We selected Hanchuan public health personnel for the research object, adopted the self-designed questionnaire survey which included personal basic condition, basic working condition and job satisfaction including ten aspects. Measurement scales of the questionnaire for public health staff's job satisfaction is used from very dissatisfied to very satisfied with the Likert five-point scale, where 5 means very satisfied, gradually decreasing, each person's overall job satisfaction at 0–50 points, with higher scores on behalf of higher satisfaction.

By testing the reliability and validity of the job satisfaction questionnaire, it showed that the questionnaire cronbach α coefficient is 0.920, and its reliability is fair; by using factor analysis to analyze the validity of the questionnaire results, the exploratory factor analysis showed the cumulative variance contribution rate of job satisfaction including 10 common factors is more

[a]E-mail:wjzhong8616@126.com

than 40%, in which each measurement item on a common higher load factor is greater than 0.4. It indicates that the construct validity of this questionnaire is sound.

300 survey questionnaires were distributed in total, and 286 valid questionnaires were returned. The effective rate was 95.33%.

2.2 Data processing

SPSS13.0 statistical software is used to establish a database and do the statistical analysis.

3 RESULTS

3.1 The basic information of the respondents

As to the 286 investigated public health workers, in terms of gender 149 were male, accounting for 52.1%, while female were 137, accounting for 47.9%. In terms of their educational background, 124 people got secondary technical school degree or lower, accounting for 43.4%, 127 people got college degree, accounting for 44.4%, 34 people got master degree, accounting for 11.9%, and the other 1, accounting for 0.3%. From the perspective of the title structure, 84 people have no title, accounting for 29.4%, 135 people have got the junior technical title, accounting for 47.2%, 59 people got the intermediate technical title, accounting for 20.6%, and six people got the vice senior technical title, accounting for 2.1%. But two people omitted this item, accounting for 0.7%. From the perspective of the local income level, only one person's income is above the average, accounting for 0.3%, 22 people's reaches the middle level, accounting for 7.7%, and 89 people's is below the average, accounting for 31.1%, 174 people's reaches the low level, accounting for 60.8%. From the perspective of their age, the oldest one is 62 years old, the youngest is 19 years old, and their average age is 35.21 years old. The longest working years is 45 years, the shortest is 6 months, and the average is 12.95 years .

3.2 Analysis of job satisfaction of public health staff

3.2.1 Relationship Between The Factors of Public health staff and Their Job Satisfaction

To analyze the relationship between the job satisfaction of public health staff and their factors such as gender, age, education background, job title, income level and working years, we used variance analysis and found out the influence of these factors on job satisfaction was no statistically significant ($P > 0.05$).

3.2.2 Analysis of multiple factors of public health staff

The job satisfaction level of public health staff was treated as the dependent variable, and the general characteristic variables (age, gender, education background, job title, income level, working years) and survey items of the basic working conditions were treated as independent variables. The multiple stepwise regression analysis is used. The results are shown in Table 1.

From Table 1, according to the standard regression coefficient, it shows that the reasons that impact on job satisfaction from most important to less important are: performance appraisal system, unappreciated work, income satisfaction, inadequate experimental material, non-cooperative teamwork, extra income.

4 SUMMARY

From the survey results, we draw a conclusion that the performance appraisal system is the main factor influencing the job satisfaction of public health stuff. Therefore, the establishment of an effective performance appraisal system has a positive effect on gaining the job satisfaction of public health stuff .

Table 1. The Analysis of The Multiple Factors of Public Health Staff.

	Unstandardized Coefficient		Standardized Coefficient		
	Coefficient b	Standard Error	Coefficient β	t	p
Constant Term	48.663	4.404		11.050	0.000
Performance Appraisal System	−3.286	0.611	−0.330	−5.731	0.000
Unappreciated Work	−3.273	0.859	−0.216	−3.811	0.000
Income Satisfaction	−2.727	0.748	−0.234	−3.648	0.000
Inadequate Experimental Material	−3.074	0.981	−0.169	−3.134	0.002
Non-cooperative teamwork	−2.326	0.820	−0.139	−2.835	0.005
Extra Income	−2.064	0.844	−0.121	−2.444	0.015

From the present situation, the clinical worker's income and status are significantly better than those of prevention staff, which is attributed to China's basic national conditions. Consequently, many public health workers think their work is unappreciated and feel unsatisfied with their income, longing to increase their extra income.

The construction of a stable funding mechanism is the way to ensure that public health staff get well paid, to increase public health workers' job satisfaction, so that they will be motivated to provide better public health services for the society. Besides inadequate experimental material and non-cooperative teamwork are another two problems they meet in their work. Therefore, to solve those problems the government should put emphasis on the investment of public health.

Public health has a close relationship to the healthy body of the people of a country or a region. It is an important symbol of social progress and human comprehensive development. To equally provide the basic public health services for the public is an important foundation for social harmony and stability and the prerequisite to improve the healthy conditions of the public .

To deal with a variety of serious public health emergencies, some developed countries have incorporated the public health system into the construction of national security and economic security concerned with large modern safety issues. However, most people of China don't acquire an understanding of public health, and even some leaders don't fully understand it and fail to recognize the importance of public health. Therefore, there's a great need to deepen people's understanding of public health issues, and give much publicity with them (such as publicizing scientific knowledge about health issues etc.).

Governments should also remedy the shortcomings of health care, such as the irrational health worker staffing and the limitations in the investment of public health. By establishing personnel security mechanisms in public health, increasing public health professionals, providing the further education opportunities for the professionals who can meet the needs of the society, enhancing the basic skills of the public health workers on the job, the overall quality of public health personnel will be improved, so that our public health will be further developed .

REFERENCES

Liang ,J.F. & Liu, Y.Z.(2010)Satisfaction of Community Health Care Service in Taiyuan. *Journal of China Modern Doctor*.48(9).70–71.

Liu,Z.J. (1997)The Assessment of the Reliability and Validity of Questionnaire . *Chinese Journal of Prevention and Control*. 5:174–177.

Liu ,L. (2007)Analysis and Strategy on Satisfaction Degree of Nurse to Personal Occupation. *Journal of Chinese Modern Nursing* .4 (17).1557–58.

Liu, F. Luo, L. Shu ,D.etal.(2011)*Investigation and Comparative Study on Job Satisfaction of Health Care Staff* . Journal of Chinese Hospital Management. 31 (7).20–22.

Howard, M.Weiss. (2002)Deconstructing job satisfaction: separating evaluations, belief and affective experiences. *Journal of Human Resource Management Review.* 12:174.

Zhang, X.D. Xu ,Y. Liu Y. (2008)Sampling Survey on The Job Satisfaction of Workers in TB Prevention and Control Institution in China . *Journal of Modern Preventive Medicine.* (8).1453–1455.

Medicine Sciences and Bioengineering – Wang (Ed.)
© 2015 Taylor & Francis Group, London, ISBN: 978-1-138-02684-1

Study on extracts constituents of *nux prinsepiae uniflorae*

Yun Wu, Xu-dong Zheng, Hao-bin Hu & Jun-ying Zhao
College of Chemistry and Chemical Engineering, Longdong University, Qingyang, Gansu, China

ABSTRACT: The extracts of *nux prinsepiae uniflorae* growing in the Qingyang region, Gansu province of China, were isolated by the solvent-extraction method and analyzed by gas chromatography and gas chromatography-mass spectrometry. A total of 60 components were identified in the extracts, representing 91.92 % of the total integrated chromatographic peaks. The major compounds were found to be β-Bourbonene (13.24 %), β-Caryophyllene (11.94 %), τ-Muurolol (9.66 %), α-Copaene (8.87 %), Palmitic acid (4.25 %), Margaric acid (3.59 %). The results indicated that the levels of total sesquiterpene fraction (61.24 %) were more than 6.9 times higher than those of monoterpene components (8.87 %).

1 INTRODUCTION

Prinsepia uniflora is a kind of deciduous shrub from the Rosaceae family. The nucleolus of this plant named *nux prinsepiae uniflora* has been used in traditional Chinese medicine. Therapeutic activities of dispelling wind, therming dissipine, nourishing the liver and improving visual acuity have been reported for the applications of the *nux prinsepiae uniflora* in Chinese medicine (Yang *et al.*, 2008; Li *et al.*, 2012).

As far as our literature survey could ascertain, the constituents of extracts or essential oil of *nux prinsepiae uniflora* have not been published previously, although there is only one report on essential oil constituents of dry stems and leaves of *prinsepia uniflora* (Li *et al.*, 2012), and some other reports on the biological characteristic observation, the cultivation technology, green environmental protection, application in food and medicine (Wang *et al.*, 2012).

In the present work, we investigated the chemical composition of the extracts isolated from *nux prinsepiae uniflora* for the first time by the solvent-extraction method with ethyl ether as the solvent.

2 EXPERIMENT

2.1 *Plant materials and chemicals*

The *nux prinsepiaes uniflora* were collected during the fruiting stage in August 2013 in the Qingyang region (Gansu province,China).

The anhydrous ethyl ether (analytical grade) was purchased from Xian Chemical Reagent Co. (Xian, China).

2.2 *Isolation procedure*

20 grams of shelled and powdered plant materials were immersed with 200 mL anhydrous ethyl ether at room temperature for 24 h. After evaporation of the solvent under reduced pressure, the remaining material was dried over anhydrous sodium sulfate and stored at 4°C in the dark. The extracts yielded 52.4% of a yellow pale oil based on the dried weight.

2.3 GC-FID analysis

Analytical gas chromatography was carried out in a Hewlett Packard 6890 (Agilent Technologies, Palo Alto, CA, USA) equipped with a FID detector. A HP-Innowax capillary column (30 m × 0.25 mmi.d., 0.25 μm film thickness) was used for the separation. Nitrogen was used as carrier gas with a flow rate of 1.6 mL/min at 50°C and constant pressure 12 psi. injection was performed at 250°C in split mode (1: 60), and flame ionization detection (FID) was set at 300°C. The temperature was programmed from 40°C(10 min) to 205°C(10 min) at a rate of 3°C/min. The injection volume for the sample was 0.1 μm.

2.4 GC-MS analysis

Analyses were carried out in a Hewlett-Packard 6890 gas chromatograph coupled with a Hewlett Packard model 5973 mass detector. A HP-5MS capillary column (60 m × 0.25 mm i.d., 0.25 μm film thickness) was used for the separation. The column temperature was programmed from 50°C(3 min) to 150°C(1 min) at a rate of 5°C/min, and from 150°C to 280°C(20 min) at a rate of 3°C/min. The injector was performed at 250°C and the detector was set at 300°C. Helium was used as carrier gas with a flow rate of 1.2 mL/min at 60°C, split ratio was 60:1. Mass spectra were recorded in full-scan mode at 70 eV with a mass range of 35–450 m/z.

3 RESULTS AND DISCUSSION

A total ion chromatogram obtained from the GC-MS analysis is presented in Figure1, and the chemical composition of the extracts of nux prinsepiaes uniflora was summarized in Table 1, where all compounds are listed in the order of their elution on HP-5MS capillary column, most oil components were identified by comparing the obtained mass spectra of the analytes with those of authentic standards from the NIST (National Institute of Standards and Technology), and with the mass spectra published previously (Adams,1995; Zhao & Chen et al., 1999). The relative level of each component was calculated by comparing its GC peak area to the total area that were summed from all detected peaks, the results of peak area percentage were also listed in Table 1.

Sixty components representing 91.92 % of the oil were identified. This oil was characterized by the presence of a high content of sesquiterpenes (61.24 %) while monoterpenes represented 8.87% of the total amount, the levels of total sesquiterpene fraction were more than 6.9 times higher than those of monoterpene components. Among all components, monoterpenes hydrocarbon (5.77 %), oxygenated monoterpennes (3.1%), sesquiterpenes hydrocarbon (44.98 %), oxygenated sesquiterpenes (16.26 %), acids (10.45 %), esters (2.6 %), alcohols (4.33 %), aldehydes (1.25%), ketones (1.23 %), phenols (0.34 %) and heterocyclic compounds (1.61 %). The main constituents were

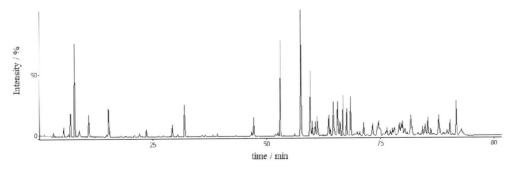

Figure 1.   GC-MS total ion chromatogram of *nux prinsepiaes uniflora*.

Table 1. Percentage composition of extract components identified in *nux prinsepiaes uniflora*.

No.	RI (HP-5MS)	RI (HP Innowax)	Compound	MF	Contents/%
1	854	1231	(E)-2-Hexenal	$C_6H_{10}O$	0.02
2	902	1195	Heptanal	$C_7H_{14}O$	0.03
3	906	1395	(E,E)-2,4-Hexadienal	C_6H_8O	0.45
4	936	1038	α-Pinene	$C_{10}H_{16}$	1.35
5	951	1076	Camphene	$C_{10}H_{16}$	3.36
6	959	1541	Benzaldehyde	C_7H_6O	0.04
7	978	1118	β-Pinene	$C_{10}H_{16}$	1.06
8	990	1243	2-n-Pentylfuran	$C_9H_{14}O$	1.27
9	996	1233	Ethyl hexanoate	$C_8H_{16}O_2$	0.01
10	1009	1506	(E,E)-2,4-Heptadienal	$C_7H_{10}O$	0.02
11	1045	1662	Phenylacetaldehyde	C_8H_8O	0.12
12	1094	1513	Linalool	$C_{10}H_{18}O$	0.02
13	1103	1390	n-Nonanal	$C_9H_{18}O$	0.38
14	1145	1550	Camphor	$C_{10}H_{16}O$	1.43
15	1167	1719	Borneol	$C_{10}H_{18}O$	0.02
16	1186	1489	cis-3-Hexenylbutyrate	$C_{10}H_{16}O_2$	0.03
17	1189	1798	Methyl salicylate	$C_8H_8O_3$	0.01
18	1231	1663	Pulegone	$C_{10}H_{16}O$	0.03
19	1256	1857	Geraniol	$C_{10}H_{18}O$	1.56
20	1263	1639	2-Decenal	$C_{10}H_{18}O$	0.01
21	1271	1288	Perillaldehyde	$C_{10}H_{14}O$	0.04
22	1286	1571	Borneyl acetate	$C_{12}H_{20}O_2$	0.24
23	1291	2472	Indole	C_8H_7N	0.34
24	1307	1827	(E,E)-2,4-Decadienal	$C_{10}H_{16}O$	0.18
25	1341	1479	δ-Elemene	$C_{15}H_{24}$	1.46
26	1352	1456	α-Cubebene	$C_{15}H_{24}$	1.23
27	1356	2186	Eugenol	$C_{10}H_{12}O_2$	0.34
28	1375	1451	α-Copaene	$C_{15}H_{24}$	8.87
29	1383	1509	β-Bourbonene	$C_{15}H_{24}$	13.24
30	1391	1594	β-Elemene	$C_{15}H_{24}$	1.68
31	1394	2050	Methyl cinnamate	$C_{10}H_{10}O_2$	0.51
32	1412	1571	α-Cedrene	$C_{15}H_{24}$	0.32
33	1418	1612	β-Caryophyllene	$C_{15}H_{24}$	11.94
34	1453	1663	α-Humulene	$C_{15}H_{24}$	0.98
35	1472	1709	Dodecanol	$C_{12}H_{26}O$	1.53
36	1476	1726	Germacrene D	$C_{15}H_{24}$	1.59
37	1481	1958	(E)-β-Ionone	$C_{13}H_{20}O$	1.23
38	1485	1718	β-Selinene	$C_{15}H_{24}$	1.31
39	1498	1715	Ledene	$C_{15}H_{24}$	1.04
40	1510	1729	β-Bisabolene	$C_{15}H_{24}$	0.78
41	1529	1758	δ-Cadinene	$C_{15}H_{24}$	0.54
42	1561	2050	trans-Nerolidol	$C_{15}H_{26}O$	0.74
43	1566	2505	Lauric acid	$C_{12}H_{24}O_2$	0.31
44	1574	2128	Spathulenol	$C_{15}H_{24}O$	0.77
45	1581	2003	Caryophyllene oxide	$C_{15}H_{24}O$	1.08
46	1598	2121	α-Cedrol	$C_{15}H_{26}O$	1.48
47	1603	1998	β-Oplopenone	$C_{15}H_{24}O$	1.10
48	1606	2134	Cedrenol	$C_{15}H_{24}O$	1.34
49	1642	2217	τ-Muurolol	$C_{15}H_{26}O$	9.66
50	1685	2221	α-Bisabolol	$C_{15}H_{26}O$	0.09

(*Continued*)

Table 1. Percentage composition of extract components identified in *nux prinsepiaes uniflora*. (*Continued*)

No.	RI (HP-5MS)	RI (HP Innowax)	Compound	MF	Contents/%
51	1762	2655	Benzyl benzoate	$C_{14}H_{12}O_2$	0.47
52	1769	2713	Myristic acid	$C_{14}H_{28}O_2$	0.37
53	1870	2822	Pentadecylic acid	$C_{15}H_{30}O_2$	0.17
54	1925	2208	Methylhexadecanoate	$C_{17}H_{34}O_2$	1.33
55	1949	2622	Phytol	$C_{20}H_{40}O$	2.80
56	2012	2931	Palmitic acid	$C_{16}H_{32}O_2$	4.25
57	2074	2975	Margaric acid	$C_{17}H_{34}O_2$	3.59
58	2122	3157	Linoleic acid	$C_{18}H_{32}O_2$	1.06
59	2140	3193	Linolenic acid	$C_{18}H_{30}O_2$	0.20
60	2185	3402	Stearic acid	$C_{18}H_{36}O_2$	0.50

β-Bourbonene (13.24 %), β-Caryophyllene (11.94 %), τ-Muurolol (9.66 %), α-Copaene (8.87 %) Palmitic acid (4.25 %) and Margaric acid (3.59 %).

Comparison of the results from this study with those reported previously (Li *et al.*, 2012; Wang, *et al.*, 2012; Li, *et al.*, 2009) indicated that 53 components were identified for the first time in this plant except eugenol, β-Caryophyllene, spathulenol, palmitic acid, linoleic acid, linolenic acid and stearic acid.

β-Bourbonene was the highest amount component in the oil, which had a significant inhibitory effect on *Staphylococcus aureus*, *Escherichia coli*, *Pneumonia bacilli*, *Pseudomcnas aeruginosa*, *Candidaal bicans* and pathomycete (Mirjana *et al.*, 2006). β-Caryophyllene was another main component, and it was mainly used for topical anesthesia and the treatment of colitis and cough. In addition, some studies show that β-Caryophyllene have biological activities to plants, microorganisms and insects in different degree (Chen, *et al.*, 2010).

ACKNOWLEDGEMENT

This study was supported by the Applied Chemistry Key Subject of Gansu Province (No. GSACK20130113).

REFERENCES

Chen, X.B., Tong, C. & Chen, G.Y. (2010) Advances in the research of β-Caryophyllene. *Shandong Chemical Industry*.40(37):34.

Li, N., Li, H.X., Meng, D.L. & Li, X.(2009) Chemical constituents of Nux Prinsepiae(II). *Journal of Shenyang Pharmaceutical University*.26(11),871–873.

Li, Y., Zheng, X.D., Hu, H.B.& Zhu, J.H.(2012)Analysis on Essential oil Constituents of Prinsepia uniflora Batal. *Chinese Journal of Spectroscopy Laboratory*.29(3):1823–1825.

Mirjana S, Nada B, & Valerija D.(2006)Phytochemical composition and antimicrobial activities of the essentialoils from Satureja subspicata Vis growing in Croatia. *Food Chemistry*,96(1), 20–28.

R.P.Adams,(1995)Identification of Essential Oil Components by Gas Chromatography-Mass Spectris- copy, Illinois, Allured Publishing.

Wang, Y.M., Tai, Y.L., Zhang, Q.& Zhu, G.L., Wei, X.Z. (2012) Research on Chemical Constituent in Leaves of Prinsepia uniflora Batal. *Wild plant resources in China*.31(5):44–47.

Yang, F.H., Zhao, X.M., Zhao, H.Y.& Yong,Y.X.(2008) Research Progress in Prinse p ia Uniflora Batal. *Journal of Shan xi Agricultural Sciences*.36(9),94–96.

Zhao, S.N., Chen, Y.S., Xie, J.S.& Gong, Y.H.(1999)Handbook of Terpenoid, vol.I, Kunming, Yunnan Science and Technology Press.

Medicine Sciences and Bioengineering – Wang (Ed.)
© 2015 Taylor & Francis Group, London, ISBN: 978-1-138-02684-1

Optimization of fermentation conditions for bacteriocin production by *Lactobacillus plantarum* 153

Lin-xia Jie, Hui Liu, Tao Han, Hong-xing Zhang & Yuan-hong Xie*

Beijing Key Laboratory of Agricultural Product Detection and Control of Spoilage Organisms and Pesticide Residue, Beijing Laboratory of Food Quality and Safety, Faculty of Food Science and Engineering , Beijing University of Agriculture, Beijing, China

ABSTRACT: In this paper, based on MRS medium, the medium and culture conditions for bacteriocin production of *Lactobacillus plantarum* 153 were optimized, including the temperature, the pH value of the medium, the carbon source and the nitrogen source. The results indicated that when the culture temperature was 30°C, pH 7.0, the antibacterial activity of bacteriocin produced by *Lactobacillus plantarum* 153 reached the maximum. Then an orthogonal experiment was used to optimize the concentrations of carbon source and nitrogen source on bacteriocin production of *Lactobacillus plantarum* 153. Orthogonal experiments indicated that cultured in the medium containing 1% casein peptone, 0.5% beef extract and 3% fructose, the bacteriocin titer produced by *Lactobacillus plantarum* 153 reached 282.12, which increased 36.5% compared with the control.

1   INTRODUCTION

Lactic acid bacteria are a genus term for a group of bacteria which are capable of fermenting sugars to produce generic lactic acid (Kjos *et al.*, 2011). It is an antiseptic protein or polypeptide bactericidal substances secreting into the environment in the metabolic process which inhibits a class of the same species or closely related to the species (Klaenhammer, 1933). Lactic acid and other acidic materials produced by fermentation have the function of preventing product corruption, and some strains of lactic acid bacteria can also produce bacteriocins with bacteriostasis and germicidal action (Stiles, 1996). The bacteriocin has received considerable attention with its high efficiency, no toxic, no residue, no drug resistance and its safe use in food. With its variety and ubiquitous in nature, bacteriocin is widely used in food additives and feed additives (Cotter *et al.*, 2005). Bacteriocins as a feed additive prevent contamination of feed by pathogenic bacteria. With the increasing problem of antibiotic resistance, bacteriocin will play an important role in terms of prevention and treatment of human diseases, animal health and food antisepsis and freshness and so on (Picot, & Lacroix, 2014).

More than 40 bacteriocins have been described (De Vuyst, & Leroy, 2007), which are produced by strains of the bacteria, such as *Pediococcus*, *Bifidobacterium*, *Enterococcus*, *Leuconostoc*, *Streptococcus*, *Lactococcus* and *Bacillus* (Mathara *et al.*, 2008; Marugg *et al.*, 1992). In this research, we focused on the optimal conditions of *Lactobacillus plantarum* 153 on the bacteriocin activity, the optimum temperature, pH and medium carbon, nitrogen, volume fraction of stimulating factor Tween 80.

---

*Correspondence: xieyuanh@163.com

2   MATERIALS AND METHODS

2.1   *Strains*

Listeria monocytogenes ATCC54003 was used as the indicator strain. *Lactobacillus plantarum* 153 is a bacteriocin-produced strain selected from Fujian homemade meatballs stuffed. *Lactobacillus plantarum* 153 was cultured in improved MRS medium, *Listeria monocytogenes* was cultured in TSBYE medium.

2.2   *Bacteriocin assay*

Lactobacillus plantarum 153 was picked into MRS medium formulation, vertical shake, cultured 24 hours in a constant temperature incubator at 30°C. The culture was centrifuged at 10000r/min, and the supernatant was obtained. The bacteriocin activities were assayed using the agar diffusion method (Marugg *et al.*, 1992), 100 microliters fermentation broth were added into Oxford cup, *Listeria monocytogenes* ATCC54003 was used as indicator strain.

2.3   *Optimization of culture conditions and medium component for the bacteriocin activity*

The culture temperatures were selected as 30°C, 37°C and 42°C, respectively. And the initial pH values were 4.0, 5.0, 6.0, 7.0, 8.0, and 9.0, respectively. The bacteriocin activities of the fermentation were investigated by the agar diffusion method (Marugg *et al.*, 1992). Carbon sucrose: maltose, glucose and fructose in place of glucose in MRS medium respectively. Nitrogen sucrose: peptone, casein, peptone, soy peptone instead of tryptone in MRS medium, respectively. Then the optical density (OD600) of *Lactobacillus plantarum* 153 and the antibacterial activity of bacteriocins were examined according to the method (Marugg *et al.*, 1992).

2.4   *Orthogonal experiments*

There levels of fructose (1%, 2% and 3%), casein peptone (0.5%, 1% and 1.5%) and beef extract (0.5%, 1% and 1.5%) concentrations were set up to optimize the production of *Lactobacillus plantarum* 153 and bacteriocin production. Then the optical density (OD600) of *Lactobacillus plantarum* 153 and the antibacterial activity of bacteriocins were examined according to the method (Marugg *et al.*, 1992).

3   RESULTS AND DISCUSSION

3.1   *Optimization of culture conditions*

As shown in Figure 1, cultured at 37°C for 24h, the OD value of *Lactobacillus plantarum* 153 was obviously higher than that at 30°C and 42°C. When cultured at 30°C, the antibacterial activity produced by *Lactobacillus plantarum* 153 reached maximum, which suggests that the optimum temperature of bacterial growth and bacteriocins production is different. It also shows that the bacteriocin is a stress regulation. When faced with a discomfort growth environment, bacteriocins produce positive physiological and biochemical reactions (Klaenhammer, 1933).

3.2   *Optimization of medium pH*

As shown in Figure 2, the bacteriocin activity also increased when the medium pH increased from 4.0 to 7.0. While the range of medium pH is 7–9, with the increase of pH value, antibacterial activity reduced. So, we concluded that when the medium pH is 7.0, the bacteriocin activity and OD value of *Lactobacillus plantarum* 153 reached the highest. Many bacteriocins have strong

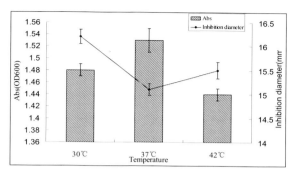

Figure 1.   Temperature effects on the bacteriocin production of *Lactobacillus plantarum* 153.

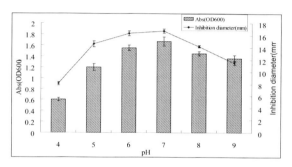

Figure 2.   pH effects on the bacteriocin production of Lactobacillus plantarum 153.

antibacterial activity at low pH environment, which may be due to different pH environment causing bacteriocins conformational changes in the protein structure, thus, change the antimicrobial activity (Mathara *et al.*, 2008).

3.3   *Optimization of Carbon and Nitrogen of Medium*

As shown in Figure 3, when fructose was used as carbon source, the bacteriocin activity produced by *Lactobacillus plantarum* 153 was obviously higher than other carbon sources. Sucrose has strongest inhibitory effect in disaccharide. Therefore, fructose can be used as the carbon source.

Tryptone in MRS medium was replaced with tryptone, peptone, casein, peptone, soy peptone to culture *Lactobacillus plantarum* 153. As shown in Figure 4, *Lactobacillus plantarum* 153 can use peptone, tryptone, peptone, casein peptone as a nitrogen source to produce bacteriocin, and when using casein peptone as nitrogen, fermentation broth has strongest inhibitory effect.

3.4   *Orthogonal experiments*

Three factors and three level orthogonal experiments were set up to determine the components of the medium for bacteriocin production, fructose and casein peptone were used as carbon source and nitrogen source, beef extract was used as growth factors, with the volume fraction of 0.3% Tween 80 in medium. As shown in Table 2, the three factors order to the bacteriocin yield is A > B > C, in other words fructose > beef extract > casein peptone. The optimized medium is 1% casein peptone, 0.5% beef extract, 3% fructose.

In this work, using MRS medium, when cultured at 30°C and pH 7.0, the bacteriocin activity produced by *Lactobacillus plantarum* 153 was highest. Moreover, the best carbon source and nitrogen source were fructose and casein peptone in optimization culture medium for bacteriocin

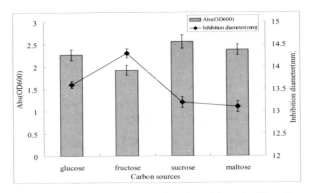

Figure 3.   Effect of carbon sources on bacteriocin productuion of Lactobacillus plantarum 153.

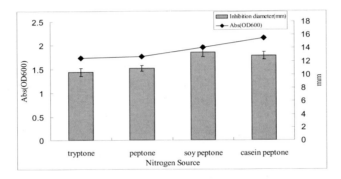

Figure 4.   Effect of nitrogen sources on bacteriocin production of *Lactobacillus plantarum* 153.

Table 1.   Orthogonal experimental results of medium optimization.

Grade	Fructose%	Casein peptone%	Beef extract%	Inhibition zone diameter/mm
1	1	0.5	0.5	20.1
2	1	1.0	1.0	19.3
3	1	1.5	1.5	17.9
4	2	0.5	1.0	19.0
5	2	1.0	1.5	19.2
6	2	1.5	0.5	20.1
7	3	0.5	1.5	21.2
8	3	1.0	0.5	21.6
9	3	1.5	1.0	20.0
R1	57.3	60.3	61.8	
R2	58.3	60.1	58.3	
R3	62.8	58	59.7	
R	5.5	2.3	2.1	

production of *Lactobacillus plantarum* 153. Orthogonal experiments indicated that cultured in the medium containing 1% casein peptone, 0.5% beef extract and 3% fructose, the bacteriocin titer produced by *Lactobacillus plantarum* 153 reached 282.12, which increased 36.5% compared with the control.

ACKNOWLEDGEMENTS

The research was financially supported by National High-tech R&D Program (863 Program) (No. 2012AA101606-05), Importation and Development of High-Caliber talents project of Beijing Municipal Institutions (CIT&TCD20140315) and Key Construction Discipline Program of Beijing Municipal Commission of Education (PXM2014-014207-0000029).

REFERENCES

Cotter, P.D., Hill, C., Ross, R.P. (2005) Bacteriocins: developing innate immunity for food. *Nat Rev Microbiol*, 3: 777–788.

De Vuyst, L., Leroy, F. (2007) Bacteriocins from lactic acid bacteria: production, purification, and food applications. *J Mol Microbiol Biotechnol*, 13:194–199.

Kjos, M., Borrero, J., Opsata, M., Birri, D.J., Holo, H., Cintas, L.M., Snipen, L., Hernández, P.E., Nes, I.F., Diep, D.B. (2011) Target recognition, resistance, immunity and genome mining of class II bacteriocins from Gram-positive bacteria. *Microbiology*, 157:3256–3267.

Klaenhammer, T.R. (1993) Genetics of bacteriocins produced by lactic acid bacteria. *FEMS Microbiol Rev*, 12:39–85.

Mathara, J.M., Schillinger, U., Kutima, P.M., Mbugua, S.K., Guigas, C., Franz, C., Holzapfel, W.H. (2008) Functional properties of *Lactobacillus plantarum* strains isolated from Maasai traditional fermented milk products in Kenya. *Curr Microbiol*, 56: 315–321.

Marugg, J.D., Gonzalez, C.F., Kunka, B.S., Ledeboer, A.M., Pucci, M.J., Toonen, M.Y., Walker, S.A., Zoetmulder, L.C., Vandenbergh, P.A.(1992) Cloning, expression, and nucleotide sequence of genes involved in production of pediocin PA-1, and bacteriocin from *Pediococcus acidilactici* PAC1.0. *Appl Environ Microbiol*, 58: 2360–2367.

Picot, A., Lacroix, C. (2014) Encapsulation of *bifidobacteria* in whey protein-based microcapsules and survival in simulated gastrointestinal conditions and in yoghurt. *International Dairy Journal*, 14: 505–515.

Stiles, M.E. (1996) Biopreservation by lactic acid bacteria. *Antonie Van Leeuwenhoek*, 70: 331–345.

Medicine Sciences and Bioengineering – Wang (Ed.)
© 2015 Taylor & Francis Group, London, ISBN: 978-1-138-02684-1

Study on characteristic of apple pectins of pH-modification and heat-modification

Jiao Dou, Yu-rong Guo* & Jie Li

College of Food Engineering and Nutritional Science, Shaanxi Normal University, Xi'an, China

Lei Liu

College of Veterinary Medicine, Gansu Agricultural University, Lanzhou, China

Hong Deng

College of Food Engineering and Nutritional Science, Shaanxi Normal University, Xi'an, China

ABSTRACT: Apple pectins of pH-modification and heat-modification, which were extracted from Cold-Extracting Apple Flesh Pomace (CEAFP) and were evaluated in the study. The solubility, galacturonic acid content, Degree of Esterification (DE), intrinsic viscosity and molecular weight of apple pectins (NAP, PMAP and HMAP) were determined, respectively. The results indicated that modifications could increase the solubility and the galacturonic acid content of pectins, but decrease the degree of esterification, intrinsic viscosity and molecular weight significantly ($P < 0.05$). Moreover, the color values of NAP were better than PMAP and HMAP. It could be concluded that pH-modification and heat-modification had a significant influence on the quality of apple pectin.

1 INTRODUCTION

Pectin is a kind of polysaccharide polymer which commonly exists in vegetables and fruits with a relative molecular mass between 10,000–400,000. It has been reported that pectin can inhibit the proliferation and metastasis of cancer cells and promote the apoptosis of cancer cells. However, it may hinder or limit its role in anticancer because of its large molecular weight and the poorly solubility. As we all know, pectin modification can generate shorter and less branched sugar chain so as to lower its molecular weight and esterification degree and to increase the content of galacturonic acid and solubility (Wai *et al*, 2010). Yan et al discovered that the pH-modified citrus pectin can inhibit the proliferation of human and rat prostate cancer cells, and induce the apoptosis cancer cells (Yan & Katz, 2010). Jackson *et al*. reported that heat-modified citrus pectin can strongly promote apoptosis of prostate cancer cells (Jackson *et al*., 2007). The objectives of this study are to investigate the quality differences of apple pectins (NAP, PMAP and HMAP) and provide a theoretical basis for the further study of functional activities of modified apple pectin.

2 MATERIALS AND METHODS

2.1 *Materials and instruments*

CEAFP is provided by the Shaanxi normal university, which is the by-product of juice production line; Galacturonic acid, Ethanol, Phenolphthalein, Carbazole and other reagents were obtained from Sinopharm Chemical Reagent Co., Ltd. (Shanghai, China).

2.2 Methods

2.2.1 Preparation of apple pectin

CEAFP was dried at 60°C and crushed into power (60 mesh) by a disintegrator. The conventional acid method was adopted to extract natural apple pectin (NAP) from the powder and the extraction parameter was as follows: ratio of solid to liquid 1:10, pH 2.0, temperature 90°C and time 90 min.

2.2.2 Preparation of pH-modified apple pectin and heat-modified apple pectin

The pH-modification of NAP was performed according to the method reported by Wai et al. and Nangia et al. to obtain the pH-modified apple pectin (PMAP) (Wai et al., 2010; Nangia et al., 2002). The heat-modification of NAP was performed according to Jackson et al. to generate the heat-modified apple pectin (HMAP) (Jackson et al., 2007).

2.2.3 Physical and chemical properities of NAP, PMAP and HMAP

Degree of esterification (DE) was determined by a direct titrimetric method (Jiang et al., 2012). The content of galacturonic acid was measured by carbazole-sulfuric acid method with D-galacturonic acid as the standard. The water solubility of pectin was determined gravimetrically. The color value of pectins was measured by hunter L*a*b* color-expressing system under reflection mode. Intrinsic viscosity and viscosity-average molecular were determined according to Kar et al. (Kar & Arslan, 2007).

3 RESULTS AND ANALYSIS

3.1 Identification of pectin products

According to the methods of GB 25533-2010, the samples obtained by different methods were pectin products after identification. The yield of NAP was 12.49% based on the mass of apple flesh pomace. After modification, the yields of PMAP and HMAP were 90.71% and 92.99% based on the mass of NAP, respectively.

3.2 Effect of modification on the quality of apple pectins

The quality differences of NAP, PMAP and HMAP were shown in Table. 1. The results indicated that the solubility of pectin increased significantly after modification as the solubility of NAP was only 78.28% and the solubilities of PMAP and HMAP were 94.29% and 92.59%, respectively. The galacturonic acid contents of NAP, PMAP and HMAP were 72.67%, 82.26% and 84.61%, respectively. Moreover, the esterification degree of NAP, PMAP and HMAP were 78.71%, 56.44% and 53.50%, respectively. Depending on the degree of esterification, NAP belonged to high ester super fast setting pectin and PMAP and HMAP were high ester super slow setting pectin.

Table 1. Effect of pH-modification and heat-modification on the quality of apple pectin.

Material	NAP	PMAP	HTAP
Solubility (%)	78.28 ± 0.736a	94.29 ± 0.858b	92.59 ± 1.242b
Purity (%)	72.67 ± 1.250a	86.62 ± 2.253b	84.61 ± 1.507b
Esterification degree (%)	78.71 ± 0.803a	56.44 ± 0.928b	58.50 ± 1.159c

Note: Values are means ± standard deviations (SD) of triplicates, and means in every column with different letters are significantly different ($P < 0.05$).

3.3 *Effect of modification on the color values*

Effect of modification on apple pectin color values is shown in Table 2. The results indicated that L*, b*, C and h values of PMAP and HMAP were significantly lower than that of NAP, but a* value of PMAP and HMAP were higher than NAP. It could be due to the browning of pectin, which made the color value of PMAP and HMAP darker than NAP during the pH-modification and heat-modification.

3.4 *Effect of modification on intrinsic viscosity and viscosity-average molecular weight*

Intrinsic viscosity was determined on the basis of Huggins and Kramer equation. The viscosity-average molecular weight was calculated by empirical equation $[\eta]=kM_\eta^\alpha$. It could be observed apparently in Table 3 that NAP exhibited the highest intrinsic viscosity, followed by HMAP and PMAP and the corresponding viscosity-average molecular weight were 71264Da, 531200Da and 395664Da, respectively. Additionally, the reduced viscosity of pectin solutions increased in a concentration-dependant manner as shown in Figure 1. This could be due to different degree of degradations during modifications, and then led to the decrease of viscosity-average molecular weight. It was reported that the decrease of viscosity-average molecular weight contributed to the increase of pectin functional abilities as low molecular weight pectin may easier access to the body cells (Zhang *et al.*, 2012).

Table. 2.   Effect of pH-modification and heat-modification on color values of apple pectin.

Meterial	L*	a*	b*	C	h
NAP	78.02±1.15a	-8.04±0.27a	25.22±0.77a	20.25±0.81a	80.90±2.51a
PMAP	69.35±0.90b	3.29 ±0.05b	14.82±0.28b	15.18±0.28b	77.50±0.08b
HMAP	70.42±0.07b	3.92±0.10c	14.12±0.14c	14.66±0.13c	74.49±1.51b

Table. 3.   Effect of pH-modification and heat-modification on the intrinsic viscosity and molecular weight of apple pectins.

Material	[η](mPa.s)			M_η^α		
	Huggins	Kramer	Average	Huggins	Kramer	Average
NAP	1.40	1.71	1.56	630957	794328	712642
PMAP	0.87	1.02	0.94	354813	436515	395664
HMAP	1.17	1.23	1.20	512861	549540	531200

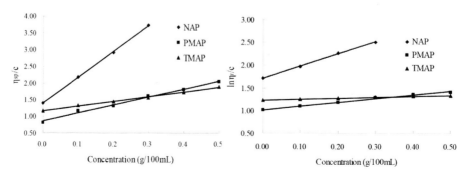

Figure 1.   Intrinsic viscosity of NAP, PMAP and HMAP with Huggins and Kramer equations.

4 CONCLUSION AND DISCUSSION

In the present study, pH-modification and heat-modification were adopted to modify apple pectins and the quality differences were evaluated after modifications. The results indicated that the content of galacturonic acid and solubility increased after modification, while the esterification degree and viscosity-average molecular weight of pectins decreased. Moreover, the microstructures of PMAP and HMAP were obviously different from that of NAP. To our knowledge, pectin is mainly composed of the negatively charged of galacturonic acid (Zhang et al., 2010). Anticancer activities of high galacturonic acid content of pectin are ascribed to the interaction between the negative charges of pectin and some cytokines in the body (Sathisha et al., 2007). In addition, esterification degree can affect the hydrophobicity of pectin and the decrease of esterification degree can improve the solubility of pectin (Bergman et al., 2009). Compared to NAP, pH-modification and heat-modification could decrease the molecular weight of pectin and further increase its solubility. Thus, modified pectins were easier access to cancer cells and interacted with drug targets, thereby to inhibit the proliferation, metastasis of cancer cells and to promote the apoptosis. In this regard, modified pectins play similar roles with antineoplastic drugs. Therefore, it is necessary to decrease the molecular weight and esterification degree and to select the high galacturonic acid content of pectin so as to improve the anticancer activities. All data presented above indicate that pH-modification and heat-modification could be used as a means to improve the antitumor activity of pectin.

ACKNOWLEDGEMENTS

This research was supported by an earmarked fund for China Agriculture Research System (CARS-28) and fundamental research funds for the Central Universities (GK261001330).

REFERENCES

Bergman M., Djaldetti M. & Salman H. (2009) Effect of citrus pectin on malignant cell proliferation. *Biomedicine & Pharmacotherapy*, 2824, 4.

Jackson C. L., Dreaden T. M. & Theobald L. K. (2007) Pectin induces apoptosis in human prostate cancer cells: correlation of apoptotic function with pectin structure. *Glycobiology*, 17(8), 805–819.

Jiang Y., Du Y. X. & Zhu X. M. (2012) Physicochemical and comparative properties of pectins extracted from Akebia trifoliata var. australis peel. *Carbohydrate Polymers*, 87, 1663–1669.

Kar F. & Arslan N. (2007) Characterization of orange peel pectin and effect of sugars, L-ascorbic acid, ammonium persulfate, salts on viscosity of orange peel pectin solutions. *Carbohydrate Polymers*, 40, 285–291.

Nangia M. P., Hogan V. & Honjo Y. (2002) Inhibition of human cancer cell growth and metastasis in nude mice by oral intake of modified citrus pectin. *Journal of the National Cancer Institute*, 94, 1854–1862.

Sathisha U. V., Jayaram S. & Nayaka M. A. H. (2007) Inhibition of galectin-3 mediated cellular interactions by pectic polysaccharides from dietary sources. *Glycoconjugate*, 24(8), 497–507.

Wai W. W., Abbas F. M. & Azhar M. E. (2010) Comparing biosorbent ability of modified citrus and durian rind pectin. *Carbohydrate Polymers*, 79, 584–589.

Yan J. & Katz A. (2010) Pectasol-C modified citrus pectin induces apoptosis and inhibition of proliferation in human and mouse androgen-dependent and –independent prostate cancer cells. *Integrative Cancer Therapies*, 9(2), 197–203.

Zhang Y. Y., Mu T. H. & Zhang M. (2012) Effects of modified sweet potato pectins on the proliferation of cancer cells. *Scientia Agricultura Sinica*, 45(9), 1798–1806.

Zhang W. B., Liu C. Z. & Gao L. (2010) Modified citrus pectin: preparation, characterization and anti-cancer activities. *Chemical Journal of Chinese Universities*, 31(5), 964–969.

Medicine Sciences and Bioengineering – Wang (Ed.)
© 2015 Taylor & Francis Group, London, ISBN: 978-1-138-02684-1

Study on kinetics of sludge reduction in domestic wastewater with nitrogen removal filler

Ling-hui Gao
School of Environmental Science and Engineering, Suzhou University of Science and Technology, Suzhou, China
Suzhou Purification and Environmental Research Institute, Suzhou, China

Jing-ming Liu*
Suzhou SuJing Environmental Protection New Material Co., Ltd, Suzhou, China
Suzhou Purification and Environmental Research Institute, Suzhou, China

Hong-zhuan Wang, Jia-jun Wang & Le Shi
Suzhou SuJing Environmental Protection New Material Co., Ltd, Suzhou, China

Yao-liang Shen*
School of Environmental Science and Engineering, Suzhou University of Science and Technology, Suzhou, China

ABSTRACT: This is a small pilot study about sewage treatment plant in Shaanxi Fengxiang A^2O sewage treatment process. The raw water COD was up to 608.00 mg / l, TN 110.75 mg / l, total phosphorus 3.59 mg / l, SS was 302.60 mg / l. By adding Sujing efficient denitrification filler in oxic tank, COD of effluent water quality packing down 80 mg / l or less, ammonia down to 5 mg / l or less, which can efficiently remove nitrogen and packing of organic pollutants in sewage. With ammonia as a standard method, we get the apparent growth rate is 0.079, and calculating the apparent growth factor activated sludge micro-organisms Yobss and the apparent growth factor biofilm microorganisms Yobsb, respectively, were 0.023 and 0.093. COD as a standard the apparent growth rate was 0.073, Yobss and Yobsb were 0.022, 0.223.

1 INTRODUCTION

With the improvement of living standards, rapid economic development and enhanced awareness of environmental protection, so as to increase domestic sewage and industrial wastewater emissions, the government sewage treatment plants have a more stringent emissions standards, but most of the municipal wastewater treatment plants are mainly using activated sludge at this stage, in which sewage purification will also generate a lot of primary sedimentation and sludge. It is estimated that China's urban sewage treatment plant sludge emissions is about 1.3 million tons per year (dry weight), and the annual growth rate was approximately 10%, accounting for 3.2% of the total amount of solid waste, the dealing with remaining sludge is a major problem being faced by China's sewage treatment plant.

2 MATERIALS AND METHODS

Laboratory water was taken from the Fengxiang treatment plant's anaerobic tank effluent wastewater, and the water quality is shown in Table 1.

---

*Corresponding Author:
Jing-ming Liu: Professor, Doctor, liujingmingnail@aliyun.com
Yao-liang ShenZ: Professor, ylshen@mail.usts.edu.cn

Table 1. Compositions of the waste water.

COD (mg/L)	TN (mg/L)	NH$_3$–N(mg/L)	methyl orange alkalinity (mg/L)	SS (mg/L)	TP (mg/L)	pH
608.00	110.75	92.40	900.90	302.60	3.59	8.00

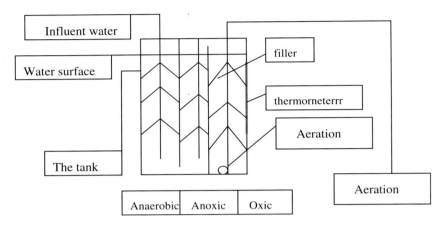

Figure 1. The sketch map of the experimental equipment.

Experiments using aerobic reactor is cylindrical as shown in Figure 1, analog ordinary aerobic reaction vessel, the total volume is 1.5L, the effective volume is 1L, the temperature controller with a temperature of about 35 °C , using it as aeration device. Test equipment and process shown in Figure 1.

3 MEASURING METHOD

CODcr used potassium dichromate, TB used the titration method, NH$_3$ -N was used in Nessler reagent, TP was used with ammonium molybdate spectrophotometry, SS was used in gravimetric method.

4 RESULTS AND DISCUSSIONS

4.1 *Data analysis*

Reflux ratio of the influent water is 1, in the first place of the small-scale aerobic process is domestication of microbial strains, microbial acclimation and its adaptation of the water took about four days time. Changed the water three times during this period, the best results is ammonia from 47 mg / l down to 1mg / l or less within 7 hours, ammonia, COD, SS treatment effect is as follows during official operation.

4.1.1 *Ammonia COD treatment effect during test run*
As can be seen from Figure 2, aerobic was running good, influent ammonia was 45.3 mg / L, effluent ammonia decreased to 1.35mg / L in treatment for 8h, packing system using nitrogen removal rate reached to 97%. Sujing net developed water denitrification filler with great ammonia removal ability and impact resistance ability, furthermore nitrifying bacteria during domestication has fully adapted to the water, and quickly absorb ammonia treatment reactor, the ammonia is converted to nitrate anaerobic zone thus formed inside the filler discharged outside the reactor by the denitrifying bacteria treated as nitrogen.

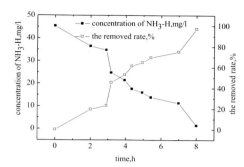

Figure 2.   Ammonia removal.

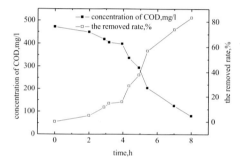

Figure 3.   COD removal.

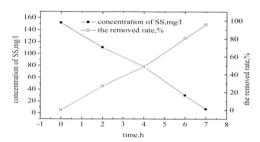

Figure 4.   SS removal.

Figure 3 shows that the aerobic reactor influent COD was 472mg / L, within 7h it can be reduced to 100mg / L or less, mainly because Sujing developed nitrogen filler biofilm filling, forming a dissolved oxygen gradient outside the biofilm layer of aerobic bacteria, in the middle of anoxic bacteria. The inner layer of anaerobic bacteria and is formed much of microscopic A² / O process, simultaneous nitrification and denitrification, while beneficial to a large number of microbial growth, forming a longer microorganisms chain, these heterotrophic microorganisms multiply growth requires a lot of carbon, thereby resulting COD rapid decline in consumption, 7 hours COD removal efficiency that reaches 83%.

4.1.2   *Suspended solids treatment effect during the trial*

As can be seen from Figure 4, after 7 hours of aerobic aeration treatment system SS concentration from 150 mg / L reduced to 5 mg / L or less, the removal rate is 95%, can effectively reduce the sludge aerobic segment growth.

4.2 *The apparent growth factor model*

In the complex biofilm treatment COD, ammonia and nitrate were processed, under steady-state conditions, the amount of activated sludge process of COD and ammonia can be expressed by the formula (1) (Liu Jingming, 2010). Formula (1) can be re-expressed as Equation (2). Through the test, formula (1) and formula (2) can be obtained.

$$VXqNmaxN/(Ks+N)=Q(No-N)-aVJ \tag{1}$$

$$aVJ=Q(1-F_s)(N_o-N) \tag{2}$$

4.2.1 *With ammonia as the standard*

By the $1 / q_N = Ks / q_{Nmax}N_{NH3-N} +1 / q_{Nmax}$ relationship, based on data derived from Figure 5, the linear regression equation can be expressed as 1: $1 / q_N = 1.1764/ N_{NH3-N} +0.3164$, where $Ks / q_{Nmax} = 1.1764, 1 / q_{Nmax} = 0.3164$, obtained: $q_{Nmax} = 3.161$, $Ks = 3.712$.

Q is 125 ml / h, V is 1L, X is 30gVSS / m³, a is 3500 m²/m³, substitute them into the formula (1), J may be obtained 0.00127g / (m²h). Substituting (2) can be obtained Fs = 0.192.

Eqs. (3) and (4) denote the apparent growth factor Fs and activated sludge and biofilm Yobs, thereby obtaining a composite biological activated sludge Yobss and and biofilm Yobsb (Wang, 2011).

$$Fs=(Ms/Yobss)/[(Ms/Yobss)+(Mb/Yobsb)] \tag{3}$$

$$Yobs=FsYobss+(1-Fs)Yobsb \tag{4}$$

The relationship of Y and Kd:

From $1/\theta c = Y(SO-Se)/tX\theta-kd$ and Linear equation 2 in Figure 6, we can get Linear equations: $Y = 0.0807X-0.0037$, so $Y = 0.0807$ $Kd = 0.0037$, then get Yobs = 0.079, M_s is 0.005kg, M_b is 0.017kg, so substitute them into (3)and (4), to obtain $Y_{obss} = 0.023$ $Y_{obsb} = 0.093$.

4.2.2 *With COD as the standard*

By the $1 / q_N = Ks / q_{Nmax} N_{COD} +1 / q_{Nmax}$ relationship, based on data derived from Figure 7, the linear regression equation 3: $1 / q_N = 1.2479/ N_{COD} +0.0187$, where $Ks / q_{Nmax} = 1.2479, 1 / q_{Nmax} = 0.0187$, obtained: $q_{Nmax} = 53.48$, $Ks = 66.74$.

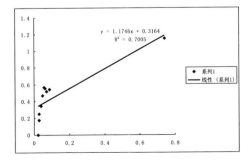

Figure 5.   Linear equations 1.

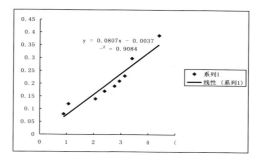

Figure 6.　Linear equations 2.

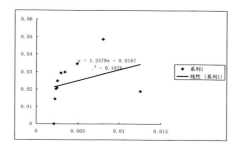

Figure 7.　Linear equations 3.

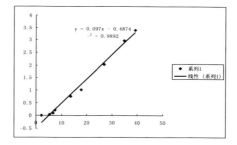

Figure 8.　Linear equations 4.

Q is 125ml / h, V is 1L, X is 30gVSS / m^3, a is 3500m^2/m^3, take them into the formula (1), J may be obtained 0.0036g / (m^2h). Substituting (2) to obtain Fs = 0.747.

The relationship of Y and Kd:

From $1/\theta c = Y(SO-Se)/tX\theta - kd$ and Figure 8, we can get Linear equations: Y = 0.097X−0.4874, so Y = 0.097 Kd = 0.4874. then get Yobs = 0.073 M_s is 0.005kg, M_b is 0.017kg, so get them into(3) and(4), obtained Y_{obss} = 0.022 Y_{obsb} = 0.223.

5 SUMMARY

1. The use of Sujing nitrogen filler developed for the processing of sewage can well meet the national standard A, and can effectively reduce emissions of sludge.
2. Within 7 hours, COD removal efficiency can reach 83%, ammonia can remove 95%, SS can remove 95%. The effluent COD, ammonia, SS were, respectively, 80 mg / L,1.35 mg / L, 6.5 mg / L.

3. With ammonia as the standard method, we get the apparent growth rate 0.079, and calculating biologically activated sludge Yobss and biofilm Yobsb were 0.023,0.093. COD as a standard the apparent growth rate is 0.073, Yobss and Yobsb were 0.022,0.223.

ACKNOWLEDGEMENTS

Authors gratefully acknowledge Financial supports from science and Technology Depatment of Jiangsu Province (BK20131197) and Foundation of Technological Bureau of Suzhou City, Jiangsu Province (No.SS-201235).

REFERENCES

Liu Jingming, Sun Dongdong, Liu Hui. (2010)Biodegradation Kinetics for Pre-treatment of Klebsiella pneumoniae Waste with Autothermal Thermophilic Aerobic Digestion.Chinese *Journal of Chemical Engineering,* 18(6), 905–909.
Wang H, Liu J, Yu S, Lin J, Shi L, Chen Y. (2011)Study on Biodegradation Characteristics of Simulated in-suit Remediation in Taihu Lake by Four Fillers. *Procedia Environ. Sci,* 10, 89.

Medicine Sciences and Bioengineering – Wang (Ed.)
© 2015 Taylor & Francis Group, London, ISBN: 978-1-138-02684-1

Effect of steam blanching on drying characteristics of Jin Yin Hua, the flower bud of *Lonicera japonica* Thunb.

Zhi-hua Liu & Xue-sen Wen*
School of Pharmaceutical Sciences, Shandong University, Jinan, Shandong, China

Guo-dong Wei
Shandong College of Traditional Chinese Medicine, Yantai, Shandong, China

Yong-qing Zhang
School of Chinese Materia Medica, Shandong University of Traditional Chinese Medicine, Jinan, Shandong, China

ABSTRACT: Jin Yin Hua is a commonly used health food and herbal medicine in Asian countries. To reveal its drying characteristics and improve its quality, thin-layer drying experiments of both steam blanched and untreated samples were conducted at 50, 60, 70 and 80°C, with an air velocity of 0.5 m/s in a laboratory dryer. It was found that all dryings belonged to falling rate drying, and the Midilli model could well describe the drying behaviour of Jin Yin Hua. By plotting the natural logarithm of moisture ratio versus drying time, the drying curves were divided into two stages. Based on the drying data of stage 1, activation energy was calculated; it was 59.28 kJ/mol for steam blanched sample, and 80.04 kJ/mol for control. The content of chlorogenic acid, the quality marker of Jin Yin Hua, was found much higher in steam blanched samples than in untreated controls. Therefore, this pretreatment was strongly advised for industrial drying of Jin Yin Hua.

1 INTRODUCTION

Lonicera japonica Thunb. (family Caprifoliaceae) is native to East Asia including China, Japan and Korea. Its flower bud, Jin Yin Hua in Chinese, is traditionally used as a health food and a crude drug (Shang *et al.*, 2011). Traditionally, it was dried in the open air, which is a time-consuming process. Sulphur fumigation could successfully accelerate its drying and overcome the browning phenomenon, however it was forbidden in China for the residue of sulphur and unpleasant odour.

In recent years, several drying methods have been recommended, including hot air drying, vacuum drying and freeze drying, or hot-air drying combined with microwave, steam or baking pretreatment (Chen, 2006; Hou & Luo, 2010; Ji & Zhu, 2008; Li & Yang, 2011; Liu *et al.*, 2010; Qi *et al.*, 2010). Among them, hot air drying is cost-effective and time-saving, and it has become the primary method for industrial drying of Jin Yin Hua. However, hot-air drying characteristics of Jin Yin Hua remain largely unknown up to now.

Fresh Jin Yin Hua has a high level of polyphenol oxidase (PPO) (Liu *et al.*, 2013). Steam blanching is a common pre-treating method to inactivate the enzyme with several advantages, such as feasible and convenient to be applied, accelerating drying rate, and reducing bacteria (Kozempel *et al.*, 2002; Qin *et al.*, 2011). Therefore, hot-air drying characteristics of steam-blanched Jin Yin Hua were compared with the untreated controls in this paper, and chlorogenic acid content was also determined in the resulting products.

2   MATERIALS AND METHODS

2.1   *Materials and chemicals*

Fresh flower bud of *L. japonica* was collected in medicinal plant garden of Shandong University according to the traditional practice (Li, 2010). The dry matter content was 15.0 ± 1.0%. Chlorogenic acid was obtained from Sichuan Weikeqi Biological Technology Co., Ltd. (Chengdu, China). The other chemicals were obtained from local commercial source.

2.2   *Experimental procedure*

A drying apparatus was designed to conduct thin layer drying experiment as described in our previous work (Zhu *et al.*, 2014). The dryer was set at 50°C, 60°C, 70°C or 80°C with the air velocity of 0.5 m/s. Aliquots (ca. 40g) of the flower bud were spread on a stainless steel mesh (15 cm in diameter) and steamed for 60 s in a steamer, and then cooled to room temperature. The drying was not stopped until sample weight (automatically recorded with a 10-min interval) became about 15–18% of the initial weight. Each drying was repeated twice.

2.3   *Determination of chlorogenic acid*

The content of chlorogenic acid was determined according to the method of Chinese Pharmacopoeia with slight modification (Chinese Pharmacopoeia Committee, 2010). Chromatographic separation was achieved using an ODS C18 column (250 × 4.6 mm, 5 μm, Phenomenex, USA) on a Simadzu LC-10ATvp chromatographic system, Data were acquired and processed using N2000 chromatography software (Zhejiang University, China).

2.4   *Data analysis*

2.4.1   *Moisture content, drying rate and mathematical modelling*
Moisture content of the material was expressed in moisture ratio (*MR*). The drying data were fitted to ten drying models commonly used in literatures, and the criteria of the fitness, R^2, *P*, χ^2 and RMSE, were calculated as our previous works (Qin *et al.*, 2011; Zhu *et al.*, 2013; Zhu *et al.*, 2014).

2.4.2   *Calculation of activation energy*
Generally, biomaterial drying obeys first order kinetics. Drying rate constant (*k*) in Lewis model has been found well fitted to the Arrhenius equation (Kholmanskiy *et al.*, 2013; Sawhney *et al.*, 1999; Zhu *et al.*, 2013), therefore, the activation energy of Jin Yin Hua was estimated according to the relationship.

3   RESULTS AND DISCUSSION

3.1   *Drying curves of Jin Yin Hua and mathematical modelling*

There is a close dependence of *MR* on air temperature for both steam blanched samples and corresponding untreated controls (Figure 1). It is clearly shown that the dryings all belong to falling rate drying, although there is an initial increasing rate drying period for control dryings at lower temperatures. The drying curves of the steam blanched sample and the control nearly overlap at 80°C, however, the discrepancies between them increase rapidly as hot air temperature decreases from 80°C to 50°C. That may be due to the destruction of cuticular layer induced by steam blanching, which facilitates moisture diffusion across the cuticular layer. In view of the fact that the drying kinetics of the plant food products depend primarily on hot air temperature, but is hardly sensitive to the air flow velocity and humidity (Krokida *et al.*, 2003), their effects were not examined in this work.

The drying data were fitted to ten mathematical models. The four assessment criteria, R^2, P, χ^2 and RMSE, ranged from 0.9573 – 0.9999, 0.92% – 64.03%, 0.058 × 10⁻⁴ – 29.2 × 10⁻⁴, and 0.23 × 10⁻⁴–13.96 × 10⁻⁴, respectively. Among them, Midilli model was considered to be the best one to describe the drying processes of both steam blanched and control samples with the R^2, P, χ^2 and RMSE values of 0.9994 – 0.9999, 1.16% – 5.36%, 0.1 × 10⁻⁴ – 0.5 × 10⁻⁴, and 0.349 × 10⁻⁴ – 0.659 × 10⁻⁴, respectively. Previously, Page model have been selected to describe the vacuum far-infrared radiation drying of Jin Yin Hua (Liu *et al.*, 2010). However, it is inferior to Midilli model for hot air drying of both control and steam blanched samples. The fitness of Midilli model was shown as Figure 2.

3.2 *Calculation of activation energy*

The fitness of Lewis model is not the best one comparing with the other models. By plotting Ln*MR* versus drying time, the curves are not straight lines for most of the dryings as shown in Figure 2. The deviation mainly occurred at the later stage (when Ln*MR* was < –2.8), thus, the drying can be divided into two stages (Figure 2). The majority of the moisture (93.8%) was removed in stage 1; the activation energy was therefore calculated mainly based on the k values in stage 1. It was 59.28 kJ/mol for

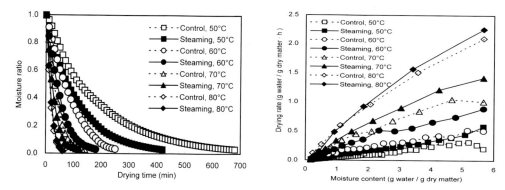

Figure 1. Drying curves (left) and drying rates (right) of thin-layer hot air drying of control and steam blanched Jin Yin Hua at different temperatures.

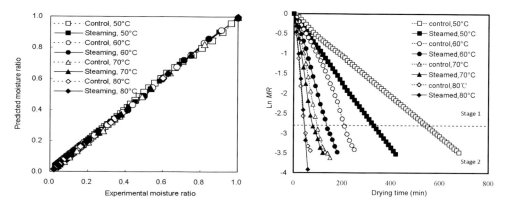

Figure 2. Fitness (left) of the experimental and Midilli model predicted moisture ratios and the relationship between LnMR and drying time (right) of control and steam blanched Jin Yin Hua.

steam blanched sample, and 80.04 kJ/mol for control. The result indicates that moisture movement becomes much easier upon the pretreatment.

3.3 Chlorogenic acid determination

The level of chlorogenic acid in steamed samples, regardless of drying temperature, is about 50 mg/g dry mass, much higher than the minimum content required in Chinese Pharmacopoeia (15 mg/g dry mass) (Chinese Pharmacopoeia Committee, 2010), which indicates that chlorogenic acid is insensitive to drying temperature at the condition of this study. However, the remained chlorogenic acid in control samples dried at 50, 60, 70 and 80°C is 61.23%, 2.69%, 5.73% and 51.96% of that in the corresponding steamed samples. The result suggests that inactivation of PPO is vital for postharvest drying of Jin Yin Hua, which agree with the results of Hou & Luo (2010) and Peng *et al.* (2006).

4 SUMMARY

The result of this study indicates that steam blanching can distinctly speed up the drying process, reduce the activation energy of hot air drying, and improve the product quality. Midilli model could well predict the drying behaviour of both control and steam blanched sample. Accordingly, steam blanching is strongly advised for the industrial drying of Jin Yin Hua.

ACKNOWLEDGEMENT

This research was funded by National Key Technology Research and Development Program from the Ministry of Science and Technology of China (2011BAI06B01).

REFERENCES

Chen, D. J. (2006) A study on the effect of drying methods on the quality of honeysuckle. *Food Science*, 27 (11): 277–279.

Chinese Pharmacopoeia Committee (2010) *Pharmacopoeia of the People's Republic of China.* Beijing: China Medical Science Press.

Hou, S. & Luo, L. (2010). The mechanism of honeysuckle color degeneration in hot air drying. *Acad Period Farm Prod. Process*, 10, 63–66.

Ji, Y. Q. & Zhu, W. X. (2008). Experimental study on the drying technique of Flos Lonicerae. *Food Science and Technology*, 6, 79–82.

Kholmanskiy, A., Tilov, A., and Sorokina, E. Y. (2013). Drying kinetics of plant products: Dependence on chemical composition. *Journal of Food Engineering*, 117 (3), 378–382.

Kozempel, M., Radewonuk, E. R., Scullen, O., and Goldberg, N. (2002). Application of the vacuum/steam/vacuum surface intervention process to reduce bacteria on the surface of fruits and vegetables. *Innovative Food Science & Emerging Technologies*, 3 (1), 63–72.

Krokida, M. K., Karathanos, V., Maroulis, Z., and Marinos-Kouris, D. (2003). Drying kinetics of some vegetables. *Journal of Food Engineering*, 59 (4), 391–403.

Li, J. & Yang, J. J. (2011). Determination of processing methods of Lonicerae Japonicae Flos in production place. *Journal of Xinyang Agricultural College*, 21 (3), 114–115.

Li, X. (2010). Effects of different collecting time, flowering phase and drying method on the content of chlorogenic acid in Xiushan honeysuckle. *Journal of Anhui Agricultural Sciences*, 38 (6), 2938–2939.

Liu, N. N., Liu, W., Wang, D. J., Zhou, Y. B., Lin, X. J., Wang, X., and Li, S. B. (2013). Purification and partial characterization of polyphenol oxidase from the flower buds of Lonicera japonica Thunb. *Food Chemistry*, 138 (1), 478–483.

Liu, Y. L., Zhu, W. X., and Ma, H. L. (2010). Kinetics modelling of vacuum far-infrared radiation drying on honeysuckle. *Transactions of the Chinese Society for Agricultural Machinery*, 41 (5), 105–109.

Peng, J. Y., Gong, Y. H., Wang, J. R., Liu, Y., and Liang, Z. S. (2006). Effects of different drying methods on officinal qualities of (Flos lonicerace). *Acta Botanica Boreali-Occidentalia Sinica*, 26 (10), 2044–2050.

Qi, H., Sheng, H., and Zhang, C. (2010). Effects of different drying methods on quality of Flos Lonicerace. *China Pharmaceuticals*, 19 (14), 36–37.

Qin, S., Wen, X., Shen, T., and Xiang, L. (2011). Thin layer drying characteristics and quality evaluation of steam blanched chrysanthemum. *Transactions of the Chinese Society of Agricultural Engineering*, 27 (6), 357–364.

Sawhney, R., Sarsavadia, P., Pangavhane, D., and Singh, S. (1999). Determination of drying constants and their dependence on drying air parameters for thin layer onion drying. *Drying Technology*, 17 (1), 299–315.

Shang, X., Pan, H., Li, M., Miao, X., and Ding, H. (2011). *Lonicera japonica* Thunb.: Ethnopharmacology, phytochemistry and pharmacology of an important traditional Chinese medicine. *Journal of Ethnopharmacology*, 138 (1), 1–21.

Zhu, B. M., Wen, X. S., and Wei, G. (2014). Effect of pre-treatments on drying characteristics of Chinese jujube (*Zizyphus jujuba* Miller). *Journal of Agricultural and Biological Engineering*, 7 (1), 94–102.

Zhu, B. M., Wen, X. S., and Wei, G. D. (2013). Hot-air drying of rehmannia root: Its kinetic parameter, shrinkage and mathematical modelling. *International Journal of Engineering Research and Technology*, 2 (11), 1172–1178.

Medicine Sciences and Bioengineering – Wang (Ed.)
© *2015 Taylor & Francis Group, London, ISBN: 978-1-138-02684-1*

Optimization of oligonucleotide pools amplification for SELEX

Cong-xiao Zhang, Xue-fei Lv, Xiang-han Wang, Hong Qing* & Yu-lin Deng*
School of Life Science, Beijing Institute of Technology, Beijing, China

ABSTRACT: In order to realize the amplification of oligonucleotide pools for aptamer selection, this investigation studied the Optimization of oligonucleotide amplification pools for SELEX. The PCR conditions were optimized including cycles, annealing temperature, primer concentrations and template concentrations. The study will be helpful with the aptamer selection for aptamer candidate amplification.

1 INTRODUCTION

Aptamers are the ligands which are screened via target specific interaction of the target oligonucleotide from a specific oligonucleotide library (DNA or RNA) by exponential enrichment evolutionary technology (systematic evolution of ligands by exponential enrichment, SELEX) (Bock *et al.*, 1992; Ellington & Szostak, 1990). Aptamers are able to bind the target molecule with high affinity and specifity via specific base pair formed by three-dimensional structure, such stem loops, ahairpins, pockets or the G-tetrad(Keniry & Owen, 2013; Hermann & Patel, 2000). In the process of aptamer screening, it's needed to amplify the oligonucleotides library which was chemically synthesized in order to meet the requirements of ssDNA in the selection process (Marimuthu *et al.*, 2012). Since oligonucleotide library includes many types and huge quantity of oligonucleotide chain, it is essential to optimize the condition of oligonucleotide amplification pools for SELEX.

2 MATERIALS AND METHODS

2.1 *Oligonucleotide library and primers*

The oligonucleotide ssDNA library contained a randomized sequence of 40 nucleotides in the center flanked by two 20-nt primer hybridization sites (5'-CCC AAG CTT GGG TAT GAG AG-40-nt-GAA GTT ATC GCG GAT CCG CG-3'). The capacity of ssDNA pool with 40nt oligo nucleotide random sequence is 10^{24}.

2.2 *Amplification conditions*

The basic condition of PCR was that pre-denaturation at 94°C for 4 min; several cycles of denaturation at 94°C for 55 s, annealing for 50 s and elongation at 72°C for 40 s; followed by final extension for 72°C for 10 min. The PCR conditions were optimized including cycles, primer concentrations, template concentrations and annealing temperatures.

---

*Corressponding author: Yulin Deng, deng@bit.edu.cn; Hong Qing, hqing@bit.edu.cn.

2.3 *Characterization of amplification products*

The PCR products were analyzed by electrophoresis in a 3% agarose gel at 110 V for 1hour. The products were stained with the fluorescence dye Genecolour (Beijing Genebio Biotech Co. Ltd). The DNA band were observed under UV light and taken the image in the gel.

3 RESULTS AND DISCUSSIONS

3.1 *Cycles number of amplification*

Increasing the cycle numbers could enhance the amplification reaction, but the increasing cycles may also lead to generate spurious bands and to smears composed of the other unexpected products. Representative s cycles including 8, 15, 25cycles of amplification were carried out to estimate the proper cycles for oligonucleotide amplification. As is shown in Figure 1, 25 cycles is appropriate for oligonucleotide pools amplification.

3.2 *Annealing temperature*

Annealing temperature is an important factor to influence the success of amplification, so that it is critical to optimize the annealing temperature in PCR. We initiated the experiment for a given set of reaction conditions approximately from 50 to 65 degree centigrade. The results in Figure 2 showed that there was no apparent difference for the annealing temperature in the range of 50 to 65 degree centigrade in the oligonucleotide pools amplification. We choose 55 degree centigrade for the amplification.

3.3 *Primer concentrations*

The high concentration of primer will make an increase in dimers and multimers of products while low concentration of primer will yield little target product. Thus, suitable concentration of primer is critical to produce the required amount and quantity of target DNA. As is shown in Figure 3, there is an increasing amount in 80nt band with the increasing concentration from 0 to 4 µM of primer while other by-products increase simultaneously. According to the results, the concentration 3 µM were adopted to the amplification reaction of oligonucleotides.

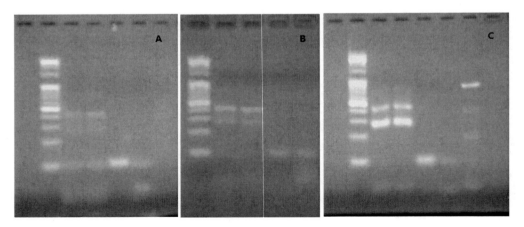

Figure 1. Various cycles of DNA pools amplification. A: 8 cycles; B: 15 cycles; C: 25 cycles. The main 20 bp ladder: 20 40 60 80 100 200 500.

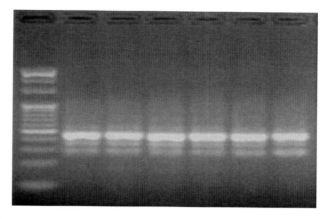

Figure 2.　Annealing temperature gradient: 50.5, 53.1, 56.5, 60.0, 63.3, 65.6°C. The main bands of Taraka 20 bp ladder: 20, 40, 60, 80, 100, 200, 500.

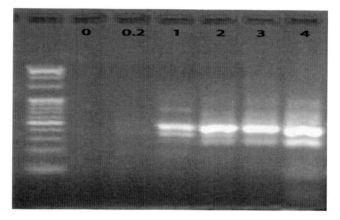

Figure 3.　Various concentration (0-4 μM) of primer in DNA amplification. The main bands of Taraka 20 bp ladder: 20, 40, 60, 80, 100, 200, 500.

3.4　*Template concentrations*

The template concentration is also a key factor to influence the processing of amplification reaction. The low template concentration will reduce the productivity of target DNA; the high template concentration will increase the producing of multiple products or a high-molecular-weight smear. The results shown in Figure 4 indicated that the template concentration variety had little effect on the productivity of amplification, but the by-products including dimers and multimers increased with the increasing concentration of template. According to the results , the concentration 0.5 ng/μL were adopted to the amplification reaction of oligonucleotides.

4　SUMMARY

In order to realize the amplification of oligonucleotide pools for aptamer selection, this investigation studied the Optimization of oligonucleotide amplification pools for SELEX. The PCR conditions were optimized including cycles, annealing temperature, primer concentrations

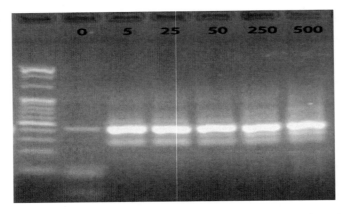

Figure 4. Various amounts (0–500 ng) in 50 μL of primer in DNA amplification. The main bands of Taraka 20bp ladder: 20, 40, 60, 80, 100, 200, 500.

and template concentrations. The study will be helpful with the aptamer selection for aptamer candidate amplification.

ACKNOWLEDGEMENTS

This work was financially supported by the National Natural Science Foundation of China (21275019) and the National Special R&D Programme for Key Scientific Instruments and Equipment (2012YQ04014005).

REFERENCES

Bock, L.C., Griffin, L.C., Latham, J.A., Vermaas &E.H., Toole, J.J. (1992) Selection of single-stranded DNA molecules that bind and inhibit human thrombin. Nature 355, 564–566.

Ellington, A.D. &Szostak, J.W. (1990) In vitro selection of RNA molecules that bind specific ligands. Nature 346, 818–822.

Hermann, T. &Patel, D.J. (2000) Adaptive recognition by nucleic acid aptamers. Science 287, 820–825.

Keniry, M.A.&Owen, E.A.(2013) Insight into the molecular recognition of spermine by DNA quadruplexes from an NMR study of the association of spermine with the thrombin-binding aptamer. Journal Of Molecular Recognition 26, 308–317.

Marimuthu, C., Tang, T.H., Tominaga, J., Tan, S.C.&Gopinath, S.(2012) Single-stranded DNA (ssDNA) production in DNA aptamer generation. Analyst 137, 1307–1315.

Medicine Sciences and Bioengineering – Wang (Ed.)
© *2015 Taylor & Francis Group, London, ISBN: 978-1-138-02684-1*

Antioxidant responses of two *in vitro* shoots of snow lotus (*Saussurea involucrata* Kar.et Kir.) to salt stress

Yuan Ou
School of Life Science, Beijing Institute of Technology, Beijing, China
Institue of Forensic Science, Ministry of Public Security, Beijing, China

Lei Zhao, Jing Sun, Xing-chun Zhao & Jian Ye[*]
Institue of Forensic Science, Ministry of Public Security, Beijing, China

ABSTRACT: The effects of salt stress on the growth and antioxidant system of two *in vitro* shoots of snow lotus (*Saussurea involucrata* Kar.et Kir.) were investigated. Salinity significantly declined the Relative Growth Rate (RGR) of the two shoots and Relative Water Content (RWC). Salt-tolerant shoot H had higher RGR and RWC than salt-sensitive shoot B. Soluble protein content was negative correlation to the NaCl concentrations. However, the contents of proline, lipid peroxidation and hydrogen peroxide were positive correlation to NaCl concentrations. Compared with salt-sensitive shoot B, salt-tolerant H had higher soluble protein and proline contents, lower lipid peroxidation and hydrogen peroxide content. Salt treatments resulted in chlorophyll a, chlorophyll b, total chlorophyll and carotenoid contents loss in both shoots. It was observed that salt-tolerant shoot H had higher photosynthetic pigments than salt-sensitive shoot B. Salt stress elevated antioxidant enzyme activities, regardless of SOD, APOX, CAT and GR. The antioxidant enzyme activities of salt-tolerant shoot H were significantly higher than those of salt-sensitive shoot B.

1 INTRODUCTION

Salinity is considered a major factor in limiting plant growth and production. Being the major common abiotic stress, high exogenous salt concentrations cause an imbalance of the cellular ions resulting in a sort of physiological and biochemical changes such as ion toxicity, osmotic stress and production of activated oxygen species, and disrupt the integrity of cellular membranes, the activities of the various enzymes, function of photosynthetic apparatus and many other processes. Plant cells have developed an array of enzymatic and non-enzymatic mechanism for scavenging these toxic components to protect cellular and subcellular systems from the cytotoxic effects of these oxygen species (AOS), including superoxide dismutase (SOD), catalase (CAT), ascorbate peroxidase (APOX), glutathione reductase (GR), polyphenol oxidase (PPO) and non-enzymatic ascorbate and glutathione. SOD removes superoxide anion free radicals accompanying with formation of hydrogen peroxide (H_2O_2), which is then detoxified by CAT and POD. In the ascorbate-glutathione cycle, APOX reduces H_2O_2 using ascorbate as an electron donor. Oxidized ascorbate is then reduced by GSH generated from GSSG catalyzed by GR at the expense of NADPH. There are many reports about effects of salt stress on plant growth and antioxidant system. The plants involved include lentil (Ebru Bandeoğlu and Füsun Eyidogan, 2004), wheat (R.K. Sairam et al., 2005), olive, Cassia angustifolia (S. Agarwal and V. Pandey, 2004) and so on. However, no information is available on the effects of salt stress on the AOS metabolism and antioxidant system in different shoots of snow lotus (Saussurea involucrata Kar.et Kir.). Snow lotus is an endangered medicinal plant distributed in the Tianshan and Kunlun mountain ranges of China, and is very sensitive to salinity. Studies of antioxidant mechanism on snow lotus seedlings under

---

[*] Corresponding author :Ye Jian, Tel:+86-10-66269548, E-mail:yejian77@126.com.

salt stress would be beneficial in large scale cultivation this medicinal plant in saline areas. This present work studied the antioxidant responses of two shoots of snow lotus to salt stress.

2 MATERIALS AND METHOD

2.1 *Plant materials, growth conditions and treatments*

Two cultivar seeds of snow lotus (*Saussurea involucrata* Kar.et Kir.) were collected from Hejing County (H) and Balikun County (B) of Xinjiang Uigur Autonomous Region of China, respectively. The seeds were soaked in 70% (v/v) ethanol for 1 min and washed three times with sterile distilled water, and then, the seed surface was sterilized in 2% NaClO for 10 min then rinsed with sterilized water 5 times. Surface-sterilized seeds were aseptically planted into vermiculite. The shoots were induced from the leaf explant of *S. involucrata* Kar.et.Kir. in our laboratory. The shoots were treated with the MS medium containing 0, 50, 100, 200 mM NaCl, respectively. The plants were cultured under natural light at 25°C. One week after NaCl treatment, the shoots were harvested and correlative parameters were measured.

2.2 *Estimation of soluble protein and proline contents*

Soluble protein contents were estimated by the method of Bradford using bovine serum albumin as standard. Proline determination was carried out according to the method of Bates et al.. The absorbance of fraction with toluene aspired from liquid phase was read at 520 nm. Proline concentration was calculated by standard curve.

2.3 *Estimation of lipid peroxidation and hydrogen peroxide*

Seedlings were homogenized under 0.1% (v/v) chilled TCA. The extract was centrifuged at $10000 \times g$ for 10min. Two milliliter of the reactant mixture consisted of 0.5ml supernatant, 0.5 ml 10 mM potassium phosphate buffer (pH 7.0), and1ml 1M KI, and the absorbance was read at 390 nm. Hydrogen peroxide content was calculated by standard curve.

2.4 *Estimation of photosynthetic pigments*

The fresh leaves were homogenized with 80% chilled acetone as the solvent. The extract was centrifuged at $10000 \times g$ for 10 min and the absorbance of the supernatant was read at 645 nm, 663 nm and 470 nm using a spectrophotometer.

2.5 *Enzyme activity assays*

Enzyme extract for SOD, APOX, and CAT was prepared from shoots samples (0.2g), and homogenized under 10ml chilled extraction buffer consisting of 0.1M phosphate buffer, pH 7.5, 0.5 mM EDTA for SOD and CAT, or 0.1 M phosphate buffer, pH 7.5, 0.5mM EDTA, 1mM ascorbic acid in the case of APOX.

2.6 *Statistical analysis*

The experiment within the greenhouse was setup in a completely randomized design. All the experiments were repeated three times. In each treatment, at least five replicates were used. Prior to statistical analyses, the percentage data were transformed into arc sine square roots. One-way analyses of variance were calculated using the PROC ANOVA of SAS version 6.12 at 95% confidence interval. The means were separated by Duncan's Multiple Range Test (DMRT), and the term significant has been used to denote the differences for which $p \leq 0.05$.

3 RESULTS

3.1 *Effects of salt treatments on growth and water status of two snow lotus shoots*

Salt treatments led to a significant decline in the growth and relative water content of two snow lotus shoots. The RGR of the shoots remarkably decreased under different salt concentrations of two snow lotus shoots. The RGR was reduced from 0.139 gg^{-1} d^{-1}(shoots H) and 0.138 $gg^{-1}d^{-1}$ (shoots B) to 0.072 gg^{-1} d^{-1} (shoots H) and 0.068 $gg^{-1}d^{-1}$ (shoots B) in the range from 0 to 200 mM NaCl respectively. Compared to shoots H, the salt treatments had larger effect on B growth (Fig.1a). The RWC reduced significantly with the increase of salt concentration. The RWC was 94.3%, 91.9%, 90.2% (H) and 91.5%, 88.6%, 86.3 (B) of non-NaCl treatment respectively. There were significant differences in RWC between two shoots. The RWC decrease degree of B was larger than that of H (Fig.1b).

3.2 *Effects of salt treatments on soluble protein and proline contents of two snow lotus shoots*

Salt stress induced a significant decrease in soluble protein content of two snow lotus shoots. The soluble protein contents of H reduced 13.3%, 29.7% and 43.0% under different salt treatment respectively. Compared with H, those of B reduced 15.5%, 27.0% and 43.9% respectively. There were no significant differences in soluble protein content between two shoots (Fig.1c). The proline contents of two shoots increased with increasing salt concentration. The proline content increased 0.17 fold, 0.81 fold, 1.32 fold (H) and 0.18 fold, 0.69 fold, 1.14 fold (B) under different salt concentrations. The results showed that proline accumulation of H shoot was larger than that of B shoot (Fig.1d).

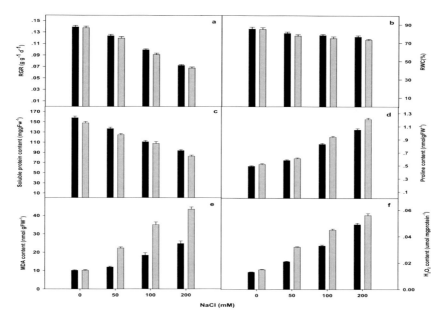

Figure 1.   Responses of two *in vitro* shoots of snow lotus (*Saussurea involucrata* Kar.et Kir.) to salt stress. (H)-seeds collected from Heijing County. (B)-seeds collected from Balikun County. (a) RGR, (b) RWC, (c) soluble protein content, (d) proline content, (e) MDA content, (f) H_2O_2 content. Vertical bars show mean ± SE of three independent experiments with five replicates.

3.3 Effects of salt treatments on lipid peroxidation and hydrogen peroxide contents of two snow lotus shoots

Lipid peroxidation was determined by measuring malondialdehyde (MDA) formation. MDA contents of both shoots significantly increased with increasing salinity. MDA accumulation was much higher in B compared to H at all salt concentrations. Moreover MDA contents of B were 1.15, 1.52, 1.36 and 1.14 times as those of H at corresponding concentration respectively (Fig.1e). Hydrogen peroxide content of both shoots increased under salt stress. Moreover, B maintained higher hydrogen peroxide content under all treatments than H (Fig.1f).

3.4 Effects of salt treatments on photosynthetic pigment contents of two snow lotus shoots

Compared with non-NaCl treatment, the contents of photosynthetic pigments under salt stress were markedly decreased. For chlorophyll a content, there were significant differences under different concentration NaCl treatment in H shoot. Moreover, chlorophyll a contents were significant differences under 0 mM, 50 mM and 100 mM salt concentrations in B shoot, but no significant difference between 100 mM and 200 mM. For chlorophyll b content, there were significant differences at all salt concentrations in both shoots. For total chlorophyll content, the change trend was the same as chlorophyll a in two shoots. There were obviously decreased in carotenoid content under salt treatments in two shoots. Compared with the contents of photosynthetic pigments of B shoot, those of H shoot maintained much higher magnitude at all salt treatments except for the carotenoid contents at 100 mM and 200 mM NaCl treatments (Table 1).

4 SUMMARY

Salt stress could increase the lipid peroxidation level, which induce the formation of AOS. AOS could destroy the integrality of cellular membrane. So, lipid peroxidation often acted as an indicator of oxidative damage under salt stress (Filiz et al., 2004). Measurement of H_2O_2 in plant tissues under salt stress conditions is important because it can be a precursor of highly AOS. Compared with the salt-sensitive shoot B, MDA and H_2O_2 contents of salt-tolerant shoot H were lower in all salt concentration treatments.

It is widely believed that the assembly of the reaction centers of photosystem (PS) I and PS II are dependent on chlorophyll a. Chlorophyll b is required for formation of the light harvesting complexes. There is a correlation between the processes of biosynthesis of protein and biosynthesis of chlorophylls. The light harvesting complexes also contain certain carotenoids, which fulfill light-harvesting and photo-protective functions in photosynthetic membranes. Because carotenoids are readily oxidized, under stress conditions they protect the photosynthetic

Table 1. Effect of NaCl treatments on photosynthetic pigments of two snow lotus *in vitro* shoots.

NaCl (mM)	Chl a content (ug/cm²)		Chl b content (ug/cm²)		Total Chl content (ug/cm²)		Carotenoid content (ug/cm²)	
	H	B	H	B	H	B	H	B
0	12.45 ± 1.02a	10.03 ± 0.98a	3.73 ± 0.69a	3.54 ± 0.71a	16.18 ± 0.31a	15.23 ± 0.25a	2.32 ± 0.31a	2.16 ± 0.25a
50	9.36 ± 0.83b	8.19 ± 0.74b	3.07 ± 0.56b	2.87 ± 0.49b	12.43 ± 0.24b	11.06 ± 0.19b	1.79 ± 0.28b	1.75 ± 0.31b
100	7.45 ± 0.76c	6.47 ± 0.69c	2.83 ± 0.67c	2.64 ± 0.62c	10.28 ± 0.24c	9.11 ± 0.21bc	1.68 ± 0.29c	1.70 ± 0.32bc
200	6.09 ± 0.97d	5.62 ± 0.83c	2.45 ±0.54d	2.46 ± 0.53d	8.54 ± 0.20d	8.08 ± 0.18c	1.53 ± 0.21c	1.57 ± 0.23c

Note:Data are presented as mean ±SE of three independent experiments with five replicates. Chl is abbreviation of chlorophyll. (H)-seeds collected from Heijing County. (B)-seeds collected from Balikun County. Data followed by different low case letters are significant difference at P < 0.05 level according to Duncan's multiple range test.

apparatus from the damaging effect of oxidative radicals and singlet oxygen, which is produced as a result of interaction of molecular oxygen with excited triplet states of chlorophyll (I. S. Vasil'eva et al., 2003). Our results concluded that salt stress significantly reduces photosynthetic pigment content, the reduced degree of salt-tolerant shoot H was lower than that of salt-sensitive shoot B (Table 1).

In conclusion, the results in this study indicated that salt stress inhibited the growth of two snow lotus shoots, reduced soluble protein content and photosynthetic pigment contents, increased proline content, elevated lipid peroxidation and H_2O_2 levels and induced antioxidant enzyme activities. Two snow lotus shoots had different response to salt stress. H shoot had better tolerant response to salt stress than B shoot.figures and tables

REFERENCES

Ebru Bandeoğlu & Füsun Eyidogan. (2004) Anti oxidant responses of shoots and roots of lentil to NaCl-salinity stress. Plant Growth Regul. 42: 69–77.

Filiz Özdemir, Melikebor, Tijen Demiral & İsmail Türkan. (2004) Effects of 24-epibrassinolide on seed germination, seedling growth, lipid peroxidation, proline content and antioxidative system of rice (*Oryza sativa* L.) under salinity stress. Plant Growth Regul. 42: 203–211.

I. S. Vasil'eva, S. A. Vanyushkin, S. V. Zinov'eva, Zh. V. Udalova, Yu. V. Bolychevtseva & V. A. Paseshnichenko. (2003) Photosynthetic pigments of tomato plants under conditions of biotic stress and effects of furostanol glycosides. Appl Biochem and Micro. 39:606–612.

R.K. Sairam, G.C. Srivastava, S. Agarwal & R.C. Meena. (2005) Differences in antioxidant activity in response to salinity stress in tolerant and susceptible wheat genotypes. Biol. Plantarum 49 (1): 85–91.

S. Agarwal and V. Pandey. (2004) Antioxidant enzyme responses to NaCl stress in *Cassia angustifolia.* Biol. Plantarum 48 (4): 555–560.

Medicine Sciences and Bioengineering – Wang (Ed.)
© 2015 Taylor & Francis Group, London, ISBN: 978-1-138-02684-1

Research progress on chemical compositions of *Hymenocallis littoralis*

Yu-bin Ji, Yu-bo Liang*, Ning Chen, Dan Zhao, Dong-xue Song,
Chang-ru Xu & Xiu-ming Cao
*Engineering Research Center of Natural Anticancer Drugs, Ministry of Education, Harbin University of
Commerce, Harbin, China*

ABSTRACT: *Hymenocallis littoralis* is a member of the *Hymenocallis* genus of the *Amaryllidaceae* family, which is native to the tropical American region and the West Indies. In recent years, it has been cultivated in Fujian, Guangdong, Guangxi, Yunnan provinces in China. Its leaves and bulbs have the effect of relaxing tendons, and they relieve swelling and pain. Research shows that the pancratistatine of *Hymenocallis* has a distinct anti-tumor effect. This paper mostly reviews the current achievements on chemical composition and pharmacological effects of *H. littoralis*.

1 INTRODUCTION

Hymenocallis littoralis is a member of *Hymenocallis* genus of *Amaryllidaceae* family. Also called *Hymenocallis americana Roem, Hymenocallis speciosa, Spider Lily* etc. Amaryllidaceae plants belong to the monocotyledon, and there is a wide variety of that.

H. littoralis Scapes is hard and flat, The flowers are green and white, with aroma, and flower in the summer and autumn. Capsule presents as ovoid or circular, succulent-like, opens at maturity, its seeds are green spongy. *H. littoralis* suitable for growing in warm and humid climate, also can grow in humus and clayey soil (As shown in Figure 1).

2 CHEMICAL COMPOSITION

Amaryllidaceae is a widely reputable family for its high alkaloidal content. The alkaloids from the extracts of Amaryllidaceae plants have been the object of chemical investigations for nearly 200 years (Lin Lz et al., 1995). The Hymenocallis Salisb. genus was first phytochemically studied in 1920, which resulted in the isolation of lycorine. Despite a variety of biological activities reported for Hymenocallis alkaloids, these compounds received little scientific interest until 1993, from which the antineoplastic alkaloid pancratistatin had been isolated, was reclassified as *H. littoralis* Salisb.

Pettit extracted and isolated a variety of Lycoris type alkaloids from *H. littoralis* (Pettit G R, 1995). Xuan separated and identified five alkaloids from the bulb of *H. littoralis* which was planted in Nanning. They were *crinine acetate, O-acetyldihydrocrinine, diacetyl lycorine, bowdensine,* and *norpluviine diacetate.* Amina and Abou-Doniaa (Amina & Abou-Donia, 2008) separated four alkaloids and two flavonoids from the bulb of *H. littoralis* which was cultivated in Egypt. They were *lycorine, hippeastrine, 11-hydroxyvittatine, (+)-8-O-demethylmaritidine, quercetin 3'-O-glucoside, rutin.* The specific name, chemical formula and relative molecular mass of the chemical composition are shown in Table 1, the structural formula are shown in Figure 2.

*liangyubo1987@126.com

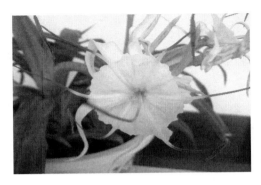 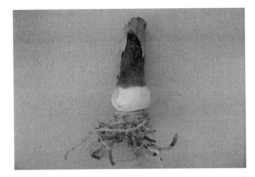

Figure 1.   The flower and bulb of *Hymenocallis littoralis*.

Table 1.   The chemical components and molecular weight of alkaloids in bulbs.

No	Name of compound	Molecular formula	Molecular weight
1	pancratistatin	$C_{14}H_{15}NO_8$	325.2708
2	narciclasine	$C_{14}H_{13}NO_7$	307.2555
3	7-deoxy-narciclasine	$C_{14}H_{13}NO_6$	291.2561
4	7-deoxy-trans-dihydronarciclasine	$C_{14}H_{15}NO_6$	293.2724
5	littoraline	$C_{18}H_{21}NO_5$	331.3630
6	haemanthamine	$C_{17}H_{19}NO_5$	317.3365
7	hippeastrine	$C_{17}H_{17}NO_5$	315.3206
8	6-O-methyllycorenine	$C_{19}H_{25}NO_4$	331.4061
9	lycorine	$C_{16}H_{17}NO_4$	287.3105
10	homolycorine	$C_{18}H_{21}NO_4$	315.3636
11	lycorenine	$C_{18}H_{23}NO_4$	317.3795
12	lycoramine	$C_{17}H_{23}NO3$	289.3694
13	vittatine	$C_{16}H_{17}NO_3$	271.3111
14	demethylmaritidine	$C_{16}H_{19}NO_3$	273.3270
15	pretazettine	$C_{18}H_{21}NO_5$	331.3630
16	tazettine	$C_{18}H_{21}NO_5$	331.3630
17	5,6-dihydrobicolorine	$C_{15}H_{13}NO_2$	239.2692
18	macronine	$C_{18}H_{19}NO_5$	329.3472
19	crinine acetate	$C_{18}H_{19}NO_4$	313.3478
20	O-Acetyldihydrocrinine	$C_{18}H_{21}NO_4$	315.3636
21	diacetyl lycorine	$C_{20}H_{21}NO_6$	371.3838
22	bowdensine	$C_{21}H_{25}NO_7$	403.4257
23	norpluviine diacetate	$C_{20}H_{23}NO_5$	357.4003

The volatile constituents of the plant flowers were analyzed by GC/MS, which led to the identification of a number of known compounds. They were *citronellal, hydroxycitronellal, farnesene, cyclohexanone, geranyl acetone, methyl 4-methoxycinnamate, germacrene A, farnesyl acetone C* and so on.

3 PHARMACOLOGICAL EFFECTS

- An anti-tumor effect: Pettit found that pancratistatin for a variety of other tumor cell melanoma, renal cancer cells, colon cancer cells, lung cancer cells, brain tumor cells have certain effects. McLachlan, who found that pancratistatin for SHSY-5Y cells significantly inhibited the proliferation. Patrick Dumont (Dumont *et al.*, 2007), who conducted experiments on Narciclasine doxycycline has found significant inhibition of tumor cell growth and promote tumor cell apoptosis.
- Anti-RNA viral effect: Gabrielsen found that pancratistatin improved 100% of mice infected with Japanese encephalitis survival with anti-RNA viral effect.
- Antimalarial: Liang Zhengfen (Liang Zhengfen, 2009) found that Lycorine and Tazettine type alkaloids have good antimalarial.

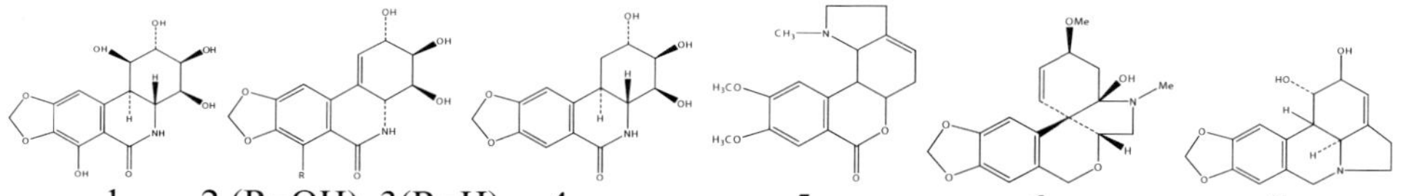

1 2 (R=OH) 3(R=H) 4 5 6 7

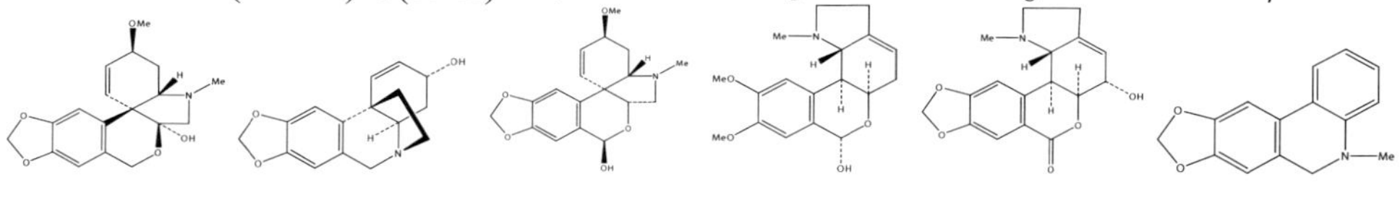

8 9 10 11 12 13

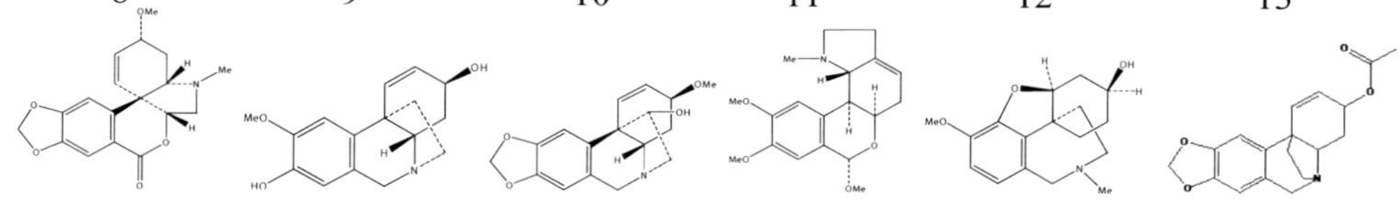

14 15 16 17 18 19

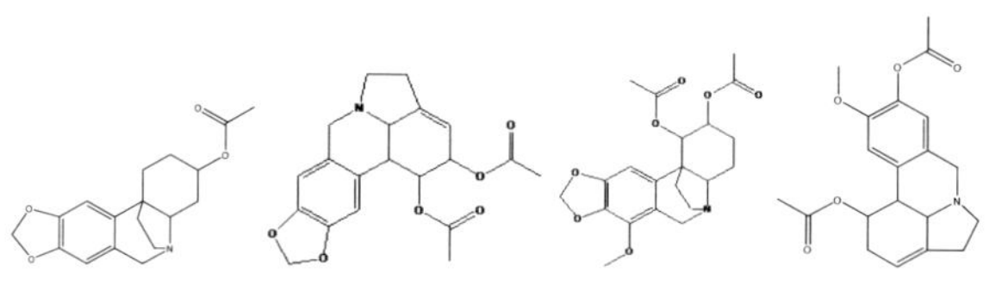

20 21 22 23

1:pancratistatin;2(R=OH)narciclasine;3:(R=H)7-deoxynarciclasine;4:7-deoxy-trans-dihydronarciclasine; 5:homolycorine; 6: littoraline; 7: lycorine; 8: tazettine; 9: haemanthamine; 10: pretazettine; 11: lycorenine; 12: hippeas-trine; 13: 5,6-dihydrobicolorine; 14: macronine; 15: demethylmaritidine; 16: vittatine; 17: 6-O-methyllycorenine; 18: lycoramine; 19: crinine acetate; 20: O-Acetyldihydrocrinine; 21: diacetyl lycorine; 22: bowdensine; 23: norpluviine diacetate

Figure 2. Structural formula of alkaloids.

- Anti-leukemia effect: Carly Griffin (Carly Griffin, 2010) for pancratistatin studied, experimental results show that pancratistatin can obviously cause apoptosis in peripheral blood mononuclear cells of patients with leukemia and normal cells on small.
- Other effects: Qin Kunming (Qin Kunming, 2009) reported that Lycorine in *H. littoralis* have anti-inflammatory effects. Jin proved Lycorine have a significant sedative effect to rabbits and mice in animal experiments. Foreign scholars also studied the inhibitory effect of acetylcholine enzyme for 23 kinds of Amaryllidaceae alkaloids, they found that lycoremine and Lycorine have fine inhibitory effect of acetylcholine enzyme. Carly Griffin (Griffin C, 2007) found that *H. littoralis* through the mitochondrial pathway of apoptosis induced by tumor without affecting normal cells.

4 CONCLUSION

H. littoralis contains high levels of alkaloids having anti-tumor properties. So far, there was not integrated research in the chemical constituents of *H. littoralis*. This paper summarized the chemical composition and pharmacological activity of each position of *H. littoralis*. It will lay the foundation for the extraction and separation of chemical and pharmacological studies of *H. littoralis*.

ACKNOWLEDGEMENTS

Natural Science Foundation of Heilongjiang Province (C201123) and Heilongjiang Provincial Department of Education key technology projects (12541210) .

REFERENCES

Amina H & Abou-Donia. (2008) Phytochemical and Biological Investigation of Hymenocallis littoralis Salisb. *Chemistry & Biodiversity*, 5:332–339.
Carly Griffin. (2010) Primary research Pancratistatin induces apoptosis in clinical leukemia samples with minimal effect on non-cancerous peripheral blood mononuclear cells. *Cancer Cell International*, 10(6), 1–7.
Dumont P, Ingrassia L & Ribaucour S. (2007) The Amaryllidaceae isocarbostyril narciclasine induces apoptosis by activation of the death receptor and/or mitochondrial pathways in cancer cells but not in normal fibroblasts. *Neoplasia*, 9, 766–776.
Griffin C. (2007) Selective cytotoxicity of Pancratistatin-related natural Amaryllidaceae alkaloids: evaluation of the activity of two new compounds. *Cancer Cell International*, 7, 1–7.
Lin Lz, Hu SH F & Chai H B. (1995) Lyeorine alkaloids from Hymenocallis littoralis. *Phytochernisty*, 40(4), 1295–1298.
Liang Zhengfen. (2009) Research advances plant used in antimalarials. *China Agricultural Bulletin*, 25(08), 256–261.
Pettit G R. (1995) Antineoplastic agents, 301. an investigation of the amaryllidaceae genus Hymenocallzs . *Journal of Natural Products*, 58(5), 756–759.
Qin Kunming. (2009) Pharmacological effects and its derivatives Lycoris Research Survey. *Journal in Beijing Union University*, 23(1):6–10.

Medicine Sciences and Bioengineering – Wang (Ed.)
© 2015 Taylor & Francis Group, London, ISBN: 978-1-138-02684-1

A study on the influence of living habits on indoor air quality

Wei-he Wang
Institute of Applied Remote Sensing & Information Technology, Zhejiang University, Hangzhou, Zhejiang, China

Jin Xu
Soil and Fertilizer Station of Zhejiang Province, Hangzhou, Zhejiang, China

Jian-she Liang[*]
Institute of Applied Remote Sensing & Information Technology, Zhejiang University, Hangzhou, Zhejiang, China

ABSTRACT: A pilot investigation has been conducted on the influence of several typical daily lifestyles on indoor air quality in terms of environmental PM concentration. The results show that hourly levels of PM 2.5 of different sites in the living room revealed obvious differences due to human activities. However, a good linear regression relationship exists between the indoor and outdoor PM 2.5 values. Besides, smoking in an airtight room rapidly worsened the air quality, making the values of PM greatly exceed the national limit specified by the Air Pollution Index (API). While food was fried or stir-fried in the kitchen, the values of PM 2.5 significantly increased, which may cause a lot of kitchen pollution. Moreover, by the installation of air purifiers, the indoor air quality can be significantly improved.

1 INTRODUCTION

It has been reported that as high as 80%–90% of human cancers are related to environment, while carcinogens in the environment can cause mutations and deletions in human tumor-associated genes, eventually making cells carcinogenesis an indisputable fact (Xu, 2006). The data released by the Chinese Ministry of Health indicated that about 260 million people have been diagnosed with chronic diseases, with the death rate up to 85%, higher than the world average. Some people think that an increase in chronic diseases is related not only to diet and lifestyle, but also to environmental pollution (Zhou *et al.*, 2003).

PM2.5 represents fine particles per cubic meter of the air, and the higher the value is, the more serious air pollution will be. Epidemiological researches indicate that aerosols less than 2.5μm in diameter can get into the lungs and deposit in the alveoli. As for aerosols, the smaller particles are, the more easily they will be absorbed by human beings, such some harmful matters as heavy metals, organic matter, bacteria and viruses. Actually, PM2.5 is most harmful to human health. (Choudhury *et al.*, 1997, Carlton *et al.*, 1999)

As people spend more and more time in indoor activities, there's a high possibility of fine particles in the air constituting great harm to the human body by damaging respiratory and cardiovascular systems, transforming lung function and its structure, altering immune function, increasing the incidence of cancers, such as lung cancer (Wu *et al.*, 1999). Pope *et al.* (2002) have carried out a long-term follow-up survey on tens of thousands of Americans and found that with the increase of PM2.5 in every 10μg/m³, the mortality of cardiopulmonary and lung cancer increased respectively by 6% and 8% with an increase of 4% in total mortality. PM2.5 derives not only from air pollutants entering the room, but also from fuel combustion, especially indoor smoking (Zhao *et al.*, 1997). Qian *et al.* (2005; Meta-Analysis of Association Between Air Fine Particulate Matter and Daily Mortality) have

---

[*]Corresponding author: Jianshe Liang, E-mail: jianshel@126.com

established an exposure-response relationship about the residents of short-term exposure to atmospheric PM pollution, and concluded that once PM2.5 concentration in the atmosphere increased by 100 μg/m³, the death incidence of residents would increase by 12.07%. In this paper, a research on the influence of common living habits on indoor air quality was carried out to explore the possibility that different living habits may lead to the change of air quality and damage to human health.

2 RESEARCH METHODS AND INSTRUMENTS

The location of this study was chosen in a flat of the residential compound in the Chunjiang Huayue Community on the north side of the Qiantang River in Hangzhou. A few investigators worked from 7 am to 10 pm every day for 4 consecutive weeks to measure PM2.5 and PM10 in eight different spots, analyzing air pollution levels, spatial distribution and inner variation characteristics of different sites in the flat. Specifically, what may result in changes of indoor PM2.5 and PM10 concentration was analyzed based on different living habits of family members.

2.1 Methods

A flat on the eighth floor of a residential compound in Chunjiang Huayue Community was selected for a test site. The investigators monitored indoor PM2.5 and PM10 in the air every hour in eight functional spots from 7 am to 10 pm between October 1st and 28th, 2013. During the investigation, the temperature was maintained between 15 and 26°C, with the predominant weather of being clear to overcast and cloudy and wind speed being less than Level 3. The eight testing functional spots were respectively in the front balcony, sitting room, study, master bedroom, guest room, and secondary bathroom, kitchen and back balcony. For SPSS software analysis, the eight functional spots above were given the values of 1 to 8 accordingly. The causes of the change in PM values were explored by means of the functional relation between different PM values in different spots at different times.

Meanwhile, the main smoking area (secondary bathroom) of the host and the cooking area (kitchen) of the hostess were selected respectively for monitoring PM2.5 and PM10. The main purpose of this paper is to study the influence of human living habits on indoor air quality and assess the possible danger of PM to human health.

2.2 Instruments

In this research, a laser diode and chips (Thomas Company, USA) as the main accessory of the CW-HAT200 high-precision handheld PM2.5 automatic analyzer was adopted. The detection range of particles is between 0 and 10 μm. The monitor directly displays the record of PM2.5 and PM10 mass concentration in the air. Connected with the sensor equipment of relative humidity and outside temperature, the machine can simultaneously read data on temperature and humidity. The machine was sent to the factory for calibration a week before it was used and it had to be reset just after each measurement.

3 FIGURES AND TABLES

We have used the automatic analyzer to detect PM2.5 values at 16 timing nodes every day and at eight spots. The PM2.5 and PM10 data were gathered during 4 weeks in October 2013.

3.1 Figures

Figure 1 is the variation of indoor PM2.5 values. As can be seen, it clearly showed that from the morning to noon, PM2.5 value was on the rise, while between the noon and night, PM2.5 value was on the decline, reaching highest between 12 pm and 14 pm.

Figure 2 revealed that all PM curves at the horizontal axis 6 (i.e., the secondary bathroom), were up to highest values, forming a triangular peak, which means that PM2.5 values are greater than those in the rest spots of the flat. The fact is that the secondary bathroom is the daily fixed smoking place of the host on most of the weekdays at home.

By expressing indoor PM2.5 change in a linear diagram (Figure 3), as can be seen from below, PM2.5 values outdoors are always higher than those indoors. In this regression analysis, we took outdoor PM2.5 as a dependent variable and indoor PM2.5 as an independent variable. The results turn out $F = 18.094$, $P = 0.002 < 0.01$ and $t = 4.254$, which indicate that an extremely significant linear regression relationship exists between outdoor and indoor PM2.5. The regression can be formulated by $Y = 0.418 + 1.255 x$.

Figure 4 shows that PM concentration was on the decrease inside the bedroom after the air purifier was turned on. As you can see, 30 minutes after the air purifier was turned on, PM2.5 value

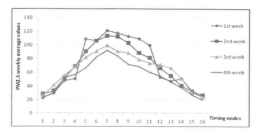

Figure 1.   Weekly PM2.5 average values at 16 point in 4 weeks.

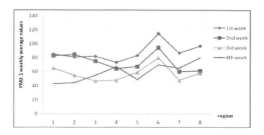

Figure 2.   Weekly PM2.5 average values in 8 spots in four weeks.

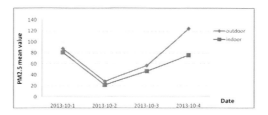

Figure 3.   Liner diagram of indoor and outdoor PM2.5 mean value variance.

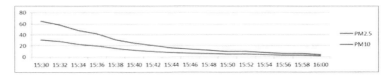

Figure 4.   PM concentration variation after the air purifier was placed in the bedroom.

Table 1. PM values obtained before and after smoking in the secondary bathroom.

PM type	Four means before smoking	Four means after smoking
PM2.5	50, 51, 52,51	447, 487, 524, 487
PM10	105, 107, 110, 106	938, 1098, 1100, 1095

Table 2. PM values obtained in the kitchen while food was stir-fried.

Time	16:18	16:19	16:20	16:21	16:22	16:23	16:24	16:25
PM2.5	43	49	45	302	341	213	106	316
PM10	90	102	95	621	716	447	222	663

Table 3. PM values obtained in the kitchen while food was fried.

Time	16:44	16:45	16:46	16:47	16:48	16:49	16:50	16:51
PM2.5	45	42	44	196	336	509	1007	1238
PM10	94	88	92	402	705	1068	2190	2599

Table 4. PM values obtained in the kitchen while food was steamed.

Time	17:11	17:12	17:13	17:14	17:15	17:16	17:17	17:25
PM2.5	49	44	44	47	39	45	47	47
PM10	102	92	92	94	81	98	93	94

declined from 33 to 2 before it remained stable, which indicates that air purifiers have a significant effect on the reduction of indoor PM.

3.2 Tables

The monitoring results shown in Table 1 indicate average PM2.5 and PM10 values before smoking, respectively, 51 and 107 in the secondary bathroom, air quality on good level.

In order to study the influence of different cooking ways on indoor PM, we measured the variable data of PM2.5 and PM10 in the kitchen in the process of cooking in terms of per minute frequency on September 12 (Table 2, Table 3, and Table 4).

4 SUMMARY

Human living habits have an obvious influence on the fluctuation of PM levels. In different spots of the room, PM value will change with human activities. Indoors or outdoors, the fluctuation of PM2.5 follows a good linear regression relationship. Besides, smoking in an airtight room can quickly worsen indoor air quality, making indoor PM value far higher than the upper limit specified by Air Pollution Index in China. This study also found that serious air pollution formed in the kitchen while food was fried or stir-fried due to a sharp increase in PM2.5 value, which may constitute severe health risks. As a countermeasure, air purifiers are recommended as they have a significant effect of improving air quality by reducing PM value.

ACKNOWLEDGEMENT

Supported by Science and Technology Department of Zhejiang Province (2010C32018).

REFERENCES

Carlton, A.G., Turpin B.J., Johnson W., Buckley B.T., Simcik M., Eisenreich S.J. and Porcja R.J. (1999) *Microanalysis methods for characterization of personal aerosol exposures.* Aerosol Science and Technology 31(1): 66–80.

Choudhury, A.H., Gordian M.E. and Morris S.S. (1997) *Associations between respiratory illness and PM 10 air pollution.* Archives of Environmental Health: An International Journal 52(2): 113–117.

Pope III, C.A., Burnett R.T., Thun M.J., Calle E.E., Krewski D., Ito K. and Thurston G.D. (2002) *Lung cancer, cardiopulmonary mortality, and long-term exposure to fine particulate air pollution.* JAMA: the journal of the American Medical Association 287(9): 1132–1141.

Qian, X.L., Kan H.D. and Song W.M. (2005) *Meta-Analysis of Association Between Air Fine Particulate Matter and Daily Mortality.* Journal of Environment and Health 22(4): 246–248.

Wu G.P., Hu W., Teng E.J., Wei F.S. (1999) *PM2.5 and PM10 pollution level in the four cities in China.* China Environmental Science 19(2):133–137.

Xu, L.Z. (2006) *Life habits and the prevention of cancer.* Anticancer (3): 42–43.

Zhao, L. (1997) *Research progress of atmospheric particulate matter on human health effects.* Shandong Environment 1: 40–41.

Zhou, J., Cai G.Y. and Chen Y. (2003) *Significance and approach of PM2.5 in city air pollution control.* Gansu Environmental Study and Monitoring 16(1): 29–31.

Medicine Sciences and Bioengineering – Wang (Ed.)
© *2015 Taylor & Francis Group, London, ISBN: 978-1-138-02684-1*

Separation of polysaccharide from wolfberry fruit and determination by infrared spectroscopy based on nonlinear modeling

Heng Zhang
School of Life Science and Chemical Engineering, Huaiyin Institute of Technology, Huaian, Jiangsu, China

Zhao-tang Xu
School of Traffic Engineering, Huaiyin Institute of Technology, Huaian, Jiangsu, China

Hai-shan Zhao
School of Life Science and Chemical Engineering, Huaiyin Institute of Technology, Huaian, Jiangsu, China

ABSTRACT: The aim was to develop a nonlinearity model of quantitative analysis of polysaccharide content by infrared spectroscopy and to provide a theoretical basis for nondestructive testing of polysaccharide content in wolfberry fruit. An absorption peak of about $1600 cm^{-1}$ was selected as characteristic absorption peak to set up a linearity or nonlinearity model. The result shows that the nonlinearity model, with a correlation coefficient of 0.9952, had more nicety than that of the linearity model. It was feasible and effective to determine the polysaccharide content of wolfberry fruit by infrared spectroscopy based on nonlinear modeling.

1   INTRODUCTION

Lycium Barbarum plays an important role in traditional Chinese medicine, which the mature fruit is known as wolfberry fruit. *Lycium barbarum* polysaccharide (LBP) belongs to proteoglycan, is mainly composed of arabinose, glucose, galactose, mannose, xylose, rhamnose and amino acid (Sun & Zuo, 2010). LBP has important application value due to having biological function such as adjusting immunity, scavenging free radicals, anti-aging, fatiguing, and so on (Miao, Xiao & Jiang, 2010). The method of hot solvent extraction was usually adopted to separate polysaccharide from wolfberry fruit. This method declines polysaccharide activity because of operating in high temperature. In addition, there are some defects containing residual solvent and long extraction time. Ultrasonic-assisted method can enhance yield, which has short extraction time, low energy consumption, and high efficiency (Gou, Gou & Zhang, 2012). Usually, the polysaccharide was determined with linear model, based on the nonlinear model that can make more accurate quantitative results, this method was rarely reported.

2   MATERIALS AND METHODS

2.1   *Sample*

Wolfberry fruits (WF) were obtained from sold.

2.2   *Infrared spectrometer parameters*

The scanning was repeated by 32 times with a resolution of $4 cm^{-1}$; data interval was $1.926 cm^{-1}$; IR light source; scanning spectral ranged from 4 000 to $400 cm^{-1}$; pyroelectric detector DTGS; KBr tabletting; the spectral data of analyte are the average of 8 times of scanning.

2.3 Extraction of polysaccharide from wolfberry fruit

The process of water-extraction and alcohol-precipitation method (WEAP) is as follows: wolfberry fruit → drying → degreasing → extraction with water → precipitation with alcohol → washing → freeze drying → crude polysaccharide.

The process of ultrasonic-assisted enzymolysis method (UAE) is as follows: wolfberry fruit → drying → degreasing → ultrasonic-assisted extraction with water → enzymolysis → deproteinization → precipitation with alcohol → washing → freeze drying → crude polysaccharide. The protein in wolfberry fruit was removed by papain enzymolysis joint Sevage method.

2.4 Orthogonal design

The extraction temperature, solid-liquid ratio and extraction time were considered as treatment factors as shown in Table 1. These three factors and three levels of orthogonal test were designed to examine the polysaccharide yield.

2.5 Polysaccharide assay

The polysaccharide was measured according to infrared spectroscopy based on nonlinear modeling UV spectrophotometry (Zhang, Xu & Chen, 2009).

2.6 The determination of crude polysaccharide yield

The yield was determined by the gravimetric method (Wei, Shang, Zhang & Zheng, 2009).

3 RESULTS AND DISCUSSIONS

3.1 Comparison of two extraction methods

The polysaccharide was separated from wolfberry fruit according to the process of WEAP and UAE, respectively. The results are shown in Table 2.

As shown in Table 2, the crude polysaccharide yield with UAE is significantly higher than that of WEAP. The WEAP method can accelerate the release of polysaccharide from cell, shorten extraction time, increase extraction yield, deproteinize favorbale effect.

3.2 The operating condition optimizing of UAE

As shown in the combination of the factors in Table 1, the crude polysaccharide was obtained from *Fructus lycii*. Using the orthogonal design, nine experiments were carried out. Table 3 shows the detailed assignment and the results.

According to Table 3, the tendency chart of indicator of each factor was drawn as shown in Figure 1.

From Table 3 and Figure 1, we can see that the extraction temperature and time played important roles and the influence of temperature was more remarkable than that of time. The effect of factor on the yield in a descending order was temperature > time > solid-liquid ratio. Optimal operating condition was $A_2B_2C_2$, namely extraction temperature 60°C, solid-liquid ratio1:15, and extraction time 50 min. The test result for verification shows that reproducibility is good (see Table 4).

3.3 Feature of infrared spectrum of polysaccharide from wolfberry fruit

The infrared spectrum of polysaccharide of wolfberry fruit was obtained (see Figure 2). In Figure 2, ① for standard substance, ② for extract.

Table 1. $L_9(3^4)$ orthogonal design.

Levels	Factors		
	A, Temperature/°C	B, Solid-liquid ratio	C, Time/min
1	50	1:10	40
2	60	1:15	50
3	70	1:20	60

Table 2. Comparison with the crude polysaccharide yield.

Process	Yield /g / 100g WF			Average / %	RSD / %
WEAP	3.12	3.09	3.23	3.15	2.34
UAE	5.52	5.43	5.63	5.53	1.81

Table 3. Results of $L_9(3^4)$ orthogonal experiment.

Test No.	A, Temperature/°C	B, Solid-liquid ratio	C, Time/min	D	Yield//g/100g WF
1	1 (50)	1 (1:10)	1 (40)	1	4.37
2	1 (50)	2 (1:15)	2 (50)	2	5.09
3	1 (50)	3 (1:20)	3 (60)	3	4.89
4	2 (60)	1 (1:10)	2 (50)	3	5.77
5	2 (60)	2 (1:15)	3 (60)	1	5.87
6	2 (60)	3 (1:20)	1 (40)	2	4.92
7	3 (70)	1 (1:10)	3 (60)	2	5.10
8	3 (70)	2 (1:15)	1 (40)	3	5.06
9	3 (70)	3 (1:20)	2 (50)	1	5.34
K_1	14.35	15.24	14.35	15.58	
K_2	16.56	16.02	16.20	15.11	
K_3	15.50	15.15	15.86	15.72	
k_1	4.78	5.08	4.78	5.19	
k_2	5.52	5.34	5.40	5.04	
k_3	5.17	5.05	5.29	5.24	
R	2.21	0.87	1.85	0.61	

Source of variance	A	B	C	D	
SS	0.81	0.15	0.65	0.068	
df	2	2	2	2	
MS	0.41	0.076	0.32	0.034	
F	11.97	2.24	9.5	F0.10(2,2) = 9.00	

There is no different spectrum standard substance and extract as shown in Figure 2. According to Meng *et al.* (2006), 2900 cm[-1] frequency zone is commonly vibration frequency intervals of aldehyde group. There are typical absorption peaks of hydroxyl group near the range of 1000–1200 cm[-1] and 3000–3700 cm[-1], acetamido group near the range of 1600 cm[-1]. The acetamido

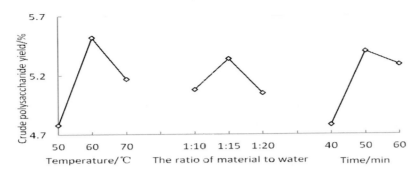

Figure 1. The change tendency of factors and index.

Table 4. The result of verification test.

Optimal process	Yield/g /100g WF	Average	RSD / %
$A_2B_2C_2$	5.97 6.03 5.89	5.96	1.18

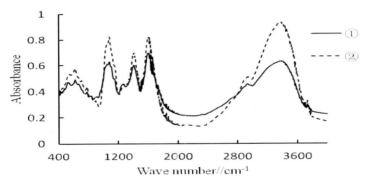

Figure 2. The infrared spectrum of polysaccharide of wolfberry fruit.

group is a basic structure of active polysaccharide intracellular, thus, this zone was chosen to analyse wolfberry fruit polysaccharide as basis (see Figure 2).

3.4 *Establishment and verification for quantitative model of polysaccharide analysis*

The preparation of polysaccharide concentration gradient was according to the KBr tablet weight and the different ratios of polysaccharide samples and KBr. The infra-red spectra of different levels of polysaccharide content showed that the spectra of different sample contents was very similar, with the polysaccharide content decreasing, the absorbance of corresponding wave also decreased, and the spectral removed downward.

Near the 1600 cm⁻¹, with the different content of polysaccharide, the intensity of peaks changed significantly. The concentration of polysaccharide in slice was taken as the X-axis, while the absorbance value near the 1600 cm⁻¹ was taken as the Y-axis to establish the linear and nonlinear models (Figure 3).

Meanwhile, the polysaccharide content (W/W) was considered as the independent variable (x), while the corresponding absorbance was taken as the dependent variable (y) to establish a linear model (Eq. 1) and non-linear model (Eq. 2), based on MATLAB and Statistica software (Ma & Yin, 2002).

$$y = 0.2548x - 0.1965 \qquad r = 0.9784 \tag{1}$$

$$y = 0.0011x^5 - 0.031x^4 + 0.296x^3 - 1.249x^2 + 2.404x - 1.303 \qquad r = 0.9952 \tag{2}$$

Linear model is a kind of traditional quantitative model, widely used in the quantitative analysis because its modeling is relatively simple; whereas the nonlinear model needs more mathematics basis with a certain degree of difficulty, thus is not widely used at present.

Figure 3 and Table 5 show that with the polysaccharide content changing, the absorbance at 1600 cm^{-1} changed significantly with specific vibration wave characteristics of molecular vibration, that was, the changing trend was non-linear. Therefore, the traditional linear model could not express this changing trend with the vibration characteristics. The fitting degree of the model suggested that the correlation degree of nonlinear model was significantly greater than that of the linear model, indicating the larger error of the linear model, whereas the accuracy of nonlinear model was much greater than that of linear model.

4 CONCLUSIONS

The extraction temperature and time play important roles and the influence of temperature is more remarkable than that of time. The effect of factor on the yield in a descending order was temperature > time > solid-liquid ratio. This operating condition was optimal at extraction temperature 60°C, solid-liquid ratio1:15, and extraction time 50 min.

Two kinds of quantitative models were established and compared in this study. It could be concluded that linear model has a narrow applicability, which is only applicable within the linear intervals of model; while the nonlinear model has a more extensive adaptability and thus

Table 5. The calculation results of two models

Type	Content /%			Average/%	RSD/%
Nonlinearity	4.4337	4.4387	4.4322	4.4349	0.076
Linearity	4.0479	4.7236	4.7822	4.5179	9.034

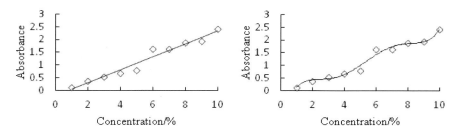

Figure 3. Two quantitative models of standard polysaccharide of wolfberry fruit.

could be used for quantitative prediction of the samples. The correlation coefficient of linear model was 0.9784, and nonlinear model 0.9952. This shows that the determination of polysaccharide of wolfberry fruit by infrared spectroscopy based on nonlinear modeling is a feasible and reliable.

REFERENCES

Gou C. L., Gou J. P. & Zhang Y. (2012) Study on composition and separation of lycium barbarum polysaccharide. *Ningxia Journal of Agri. And Fores. Sci & Tech*, 53(5), 89–90.

Ma Z. F. and Yin X. (2002) *Engineering Application of Mathematics Calculation Methods and Software.* Chemical industry press, Beijing, pp.225–266, 2002. (in Chinese)

Meng Q. Z., Li C. R., Dong Y. H. & Zhou C.S. (2006) *Chinese Journal of Spectroscopy Labortory*, 23, 911–912.

Miao Y, Xiao B X, Jiang Z, et al. (2010) Growth inhibition and cell-cycle arrest of human gastric cancer cells by Lycium barbarum polysaccharide. *Medical Oncology*, 3(27), 785–790.

Sun G. J. & Zuo P. G. (2010) Functions of lycium barbarum polysaccharide and itsapplicational status. *Journal of Southeast Univ. (Medical Science)*, 29(2), 209–215.

Wei Y. X., Shang X. L., Zhang J. & Zheng X. D. (2009) Progress on the extraction of natural active substances from lycium barbarum. *Shandong Chemical Industry*, 38(7), 18–20. (in Chinese)

Zhang H., Xu Z. T. & Chen Y. (2009) Determination of moisture content in druggery by infrared spectroscopy based on wavelet theory. *Journal of Instrumental Analysis*, 28(8), 905–908.

Medicine Sciences and Bioengineering – Wang (Ed.)
© *2015 Taylor & Francis Group, London, ISBN: 978-1-138-02684-1*

Transformation of trichothecene acetyldeoxynivalenol to deoxynivalenol by bacterial acetyltransferase

Wence Wang
College of Animal Science, South China Agricultural University, Guangzhou, China
Guelph Food Research Center, Agriculture and Agri-Food Canada, Guelph, ON, Canada

Sameh S. M. Soliman
Guelph Food Research Center, Agriculture and Agri-Food Canada, Guelph, ON, Canada
Department of Pharmacognosy, Faculty of Pharmacy, Zagazig University, Zagazig, Egypt

Xiu-Zhen Li & Hong-hui Zhu
Guelph Food Research Center, Agriculture and Agri-Food Canada, Guelph, ON, Canada

Lin Yang
College of Animal Science, South China Agricultural University, Guangzhou, China

Yu-long Yin
College of Animal Science, South China Agricultural University, Guangzhou, China
Research Center of Healthy Breeding of Livestock and Poultry, Hunan Engineering and Research Center of Animal and Poultry Science, Hunan, China
Key Laboratory of Agro-ecological Processes in Subtropical Region, Institute of Subtropical Agriculture, Chinese Academy of Sciences, Changsha, Hunan, China

Ting Zhou*
Guelph Food Research Center, Agriculture and Agri-Food Canada, Guelph, ON, Canada

ABSTRACT: Trichothecene-detoxifying enzyme, trichothecene-3-O-acetyltransferase (Tri101), and its reversible acetylation of DON suggested that Tri101 is a Fusarium self-defensive enzyme, and hence used to generate DON-resistant crops following Tri101-transformation. Bacterial isolates and their protein extracts showed deacetylation activity of 3-acetyldeoxynivalenol (3ADON), an intermediate in DON biosynthesis, similar to certain Fusarium species. Dot blot and Southern blot assays using Tri101 probe showed positive signals with 8 out of 16 tested bacterial isolates. Polymerase chain reaction (PCR) using normal and degenerate primers created from conserved Tri101 sequences showed amplified bands, none of them were Tri101 but some possessed transferase domain. The phylogenetic relationship indicated clustering of Fusarium Tri101 with somewhat closer relation to one of the bacterial isolates, Barpee. These results revealed a Tri101-like function from certain bacterial strains and a possible bacterial acetyltransferase targeting trichothecenes as its substrate.

1 INTRODUCTION

Trichothecenes are sesquiterpene biosynthesized through mevalonate pathway. Production of isotrichodermin under the effect of trichothecene-3-O-acetyltransferase (*Tri101*) is considered as the rate-limiting step in the biosynthesis of the well-known trichothecenes, including DON and T-2 toxin (Fig. 1), with different activities depending on their oxygenation levels (Zamir *et al.*, 1996; Ueno *et al.*, 1973). Bacterial O-acetyltransferases involved in several metabolic process including peptidoglycan O-acetylation and cell wall biosynthesis (Moynihan and Clarke,

---

*Corresponding authors: Yulong Yin email: Yinyulong@isa.ac.cn and Ting Zhou email: Ting@agr.gc.ca.

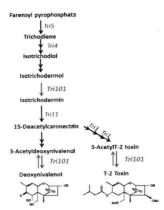

Figure 1. Biosynthetic pathway for trichothecenes and the suggested reversible and irreversible reactions of Tri101.

2010), bacterial survival (Yang *et al.*, 2007), bacterial virulence (Lewis *et al.*, 2006) and antibiotic resistance (Leslie, 1990). Recently, a proposed bacterial *O*-acetylesterase was assigned an *O*-acetyltransferase function instead (Moynihan and Clarke, 2010), indicating that the activity of both acetylestearase and acetyltransferase cannot be distinguished. In this research, several bacterial isolates were studied for the existence of an acetyltransferase with *Tri101*-like function, targeting trichothecenes substrates.

2 MATERIALS AND METHODS

2.1 *Chemicals and culture media*

Deoxynivalenol and 3-acetyldeoxynivalenol (3ADON) were purchased from Sigma-Aldrich (Oakville, Canada). Medium L10 broth and corn meal broth (CMB) were followed the method by Guan *et al.* (2009).

2.2 *Microbial detoxification activity, Protein extraction and acetyltransferase assay*

Sixteen bacterial isolates are listed in Table 1. The process of mycotoxin analysis was followed the method described by Young *et al.* (2007). Acetyltransferase assay was processed and evaluated according the method described by Kimura *et al.* (1998).

2.3 *PCR identification of Tri101 in bacteria and fungi and phylogenetic tree*

Bacterial and fungal DNA was extracted respectively. The Tri101 normal and degenerate primer sequences were designed from conserved *Fusarium* Tri101 sequences as shown in Table 1. *O*-acetyltraferase protein sequences from 29 different taxa including *Tri101* from several *Fusarium* spp. were downloaded from Genebank and used to construct phylogenetic tree.

2.4 *Dot blot hybridization and southern blot*

DNA probes were amplified from *Fusarium* Tri101 gene using 5′ -GGCATCAGCGAAGG-AAACA -3′ and 5′ -CCCAGTCCAAACCCAAAGTC -3′ primers to amplify 339bp sequences (Fig. 2A). *E. coli* used as the negative control, and *Fusarium* as positive control. Southern blot was carried out using the DIG High Prime DNA Labeling and Detection Starter Kit (Roche, Germany).

Table 1. List of primers used in this study.

Primer name		Primer sequence	Amplicon (bp)
Tri101	Forward	5'- GGCATCAGCGAAGGAAACA -3'	659bp
	Reverse	5'- CCCAGTCCAAACCCAAAGTC -3'	
Primer1	Forward	5'- GGCATCAGCGAAGGAAACA-3'	993bp
	Reverse	5' CCCAGTCCAAACCCAAAGTC - -3'	
Primer2	Forward	5'- ACCGCCTCTTCTTTCAATCTA -3'	712bp
	Reverse	5' AGTCTTTGTGGCTGCGTCTT - -3'	
Primer3	Forward	5'-GAAAGACGCAGCCACAAAGA-3'	1510bp
	Reverse	5'- GAAATGGACGCCGTAAACTC-3'	
Primer1*	Forward	5'- CAAGCGTCATCTTTCTCAGCGC-3'	
	Reverse	5' GGATGGAACGCTTCGACCAC - -3'	
Primer2*	Forward	5'- ATGGCTTTCAAGATACAGCTCG -3'	
	Reverse	5' CTAACCAACGTACTGCGCATACT -3'	
Primer3*	Forward	5'-CACATCATCCATATGGTCGCAACG-3'	
	Reverse	5'- CTCTGATCAATGGCTACTAGCTTC-3'	
Acety 1Nest	Forward	5'-ATGACATTAGGATTAAGAGGATTAACA-3'	235bp
	Reverse	5'-TTGCAGAACAAGACATACCAGTTAAAC-3'	
Acety 2 Nest	Forward	5'-AATGGAATTGGAGGAAGAGGAGAT-3'	252bp
	Reverse	5'-AAGATTTTAAACGCCACAAACTGGTGG-3'	
Acety 2 degenerate	Forward	5'-AAYGGNATHGGNGGNWSNGGIGAY-3'	300bp
	Reverse	5'-RAGNTYHTAYACNCCNCARACNGGNGG-3'	
Acety 2Nest degenerate	Forward	5'-AATGGAATTGGAGGAAGAGGAGAT-3'	327bp
	Reverse	5'-NTGYAGYACRAGNCAYACYAGHTAYAC-3'	

* Published primer sequences

3 RESULTS

3.1 *Ability of bacterial isolates and their protein extracts to deacetylate ADON to DON*

Activities of 16 bacteria isolated were tested against DON and their biosynthetic intermediate 3ADON in comparison to *E. coli* as a negative control, and several Fusarium spp. as positive controls. Eight bacterial isolates (50%) showed the ability to deacetylate 3ADON to DON with different rates ranging from only a portion ($\leq$ 10%) to complete deacetylation (Table 2).

3.2 *A potential Tri101-like gene in bacterial isolates with a close distance relation to Fusarium Tri101*

A Dot Blot assay to screen the possible presence of bacterial Tri101-like gene was performed using a Tri101 probe (sequence in Fig. 2A) isolated from *F. graminearum*. *E. coli* was used as the negative control and *F. graminearum* was the positive control. In comparison to the positive signal, high positive signals were detected in Fish2, ADS47, SS3, LS107, LS100 and Barpee, and low positive signals were detected in Fish1, Fish3, and LS94. Other bacterial isolates including *E. coli* (the negative control) showed negative results (Fig. 2B). A confirmation was performed using

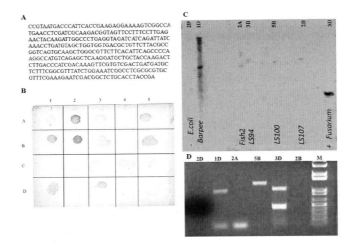

Figure 2. Searching of Fusarium Tri101 in bacterial isolates. (A) Fusarium Tri101 probe sequence. (B) Dot Blot assay. Samples were spotted onto nylon membranes and hybridized with biotin-labelled Fusarium Tri101 probe. Positive samples were as follows; 1A (Fish1), 2A (Fish2), 3A (Fish3), 5A (ADS47), 1B (SS3), 2B (LS107), 3B (LS94), 5B (LS100), 3C (LS117), 4C (LS121), 5C (LS129), and 1D (Barpee). 2D (*E.coli*) and 3D (Fusarium) as negative and positive controls, respectively. (C) Southern blot assay. Samples were spotted onto nylon membranes and hybridized with biotin-labelled Fusarium Tri101 probe. Positive samples were as follows; LS107, LS100, LS94, Fish 2 and Barpee. Fusarium and E.coli as positive and negative controls, respectively. (D) PCR. Samples were as follows; LS107, LS100, Fish2, barpee. Fusarium and E.coli as positive and negative controls, respectively. M is molecular size marker.

Table 2. Bacteria and their detoxification function.

Microbe	Source	Culture medium	Modification effect	
			3ADON to DON	DON to other forms
SS-3	Chicken gut	L10	0%	No change
LS-61	Chicken gut	L10	0%	No change
LS-72	Chicken gut	L10	0%	No change
LS-83	Chicken gut	L10	100%	No change
LS-94	Chicken gut	L10	100%	No change
LS-100	Chicken gut	L10	100%	dE-DON**
LS-107	Chicken gut	L10	0%	No change
LS-117	Chicken gut	L10	0%	No change
LS-121	Chicken gut	L10	0%	No change
LS-129	Chicken gut	L10	0%	No change
Fish1	Fish gut	FM	P*	No change
Fish2	Fish gut	FM	P	No change
Fish3	Fish gut	FM	P	No change
Fish4	Fish gut	FM	P	No change
Barpee (E17-8)	Soil	CMB	100%	epiDON***
ADS47	Soil	NB	P	dE-DON**
F. avenaceum	Lab	YPD	P	No change
F. lateritium	Lab	YPD	P	No change
F. sporotrichioides	Lab	YPD	P	No change
F. graminearum	Lab	YPD	100%	No change
E. coli	Lab	LB	0%	No change

* Partial conversion ≤ 10%
** DeepoxyDON
*** 3-Epi-DON

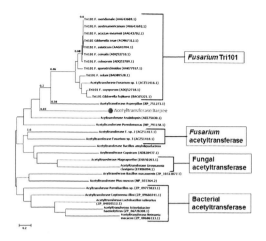

Figure 3. Evolutionary relationships of Tri101 protein and other taxa acetyltransferases. The optimal tree with the sum of branch length = 21.39292003 is shown. The tree is drawn to scale, with branch lengths in the same units as those of the evolutionary distances used to infer the phylogenetic tree.

southern blot assay with the same probe. While LS107, LS100, LS94, Fish 2 and Barpee showed potential positives, but with different band size (Fig. 2C). PCR using normal and degenerate primers created from conserved sequences of Fusarium. Tri101 showed amplified products from LS100 and Barpee, none of the PCR products were Tri101, but some of them have transferase domain including chloramphenicol acetyltransferase, glycosyltransferase and lipoyltransferase (Fig. 2D).

A phylogeny analysis of Tri101 and acetyltransferases from fungi, bacteria, plants and animals was conducted using the transferase domain. Tri101 showed a unique position in this phylogenetic tree (Fig. 3). All Fusarium Tri101 sequences were clustered together with far distance relation to Fusarium acetyltransferases, other fungal acetyltransferases or bacterial acetyltransferases. Aspergillus acetyltransferase and Barpee acetyltransferase showed somewhat closer relation (Fig. 3).

4   DISCUSSION

In this study, our results has revealed that a Tri101-like function from certain bacterial strains or a possible bacterial acetyltransferase targets trichothecenes as its substrate. In the first part of the results, although all the bacterial isolates tested have been reported possessing certain functions in DON detoxifications (Islam et al., 2012; He and Zhou, 2012; Karlovsky, 2011; Yu *et al.*, 2010), only three bacterial isolates with higher 3ADON deacetylation activity showed same DON-detoxification activities (Table 2), that is, LS-100 (100%), Barpee (or E17-8, 100%) and ADS47 (partial deacetylation, $\leq$ 10%). Total protein extracts from bacterial isolates Barpee, LS100 and ADS47 were used for further confirmation of the Tri101-like function of the bacterial isolates (Table 3). Second part of our results indicates that the aforementioned bacterial isolates possessed 3ADON deacetylation function similar to that of certain Fusarium species. Both bacterial isolates and the Fusarium species favored deacetylation of ADON rather than DON acetylation under the tested conditions. This indicated that Barpee might have an acetyltransferase with potential Tri101-like activity and a domain similarity. Because both Fusarium spp. and bacterial isolates favored the irreversible deacetylation activity without reverse under lab condition, one can suggest that there might be specific conditions requested for the bidirectional activity.

Table 3. Acetyltransferase assay of total protein extract.

Microbe	Modification effect	
	3ADON to DON	DON to other forms
Barpee	100%	EpiDON
ADS47	No change	dE-DON
LS100	100 %	dE-DON
E. coli	No change	No change
F. graminearum	100%	No change

Tri101 is required for the biosynthesis of trichothecenes including DON via the deacetylation step. The reverse reaction, i.e., acetylation, by Fusarium has never been reported. The activity of Tri101 might depend on the host metabolism partially or other regulatory changes within the host. That might explain why the Fusarium species and the bacterial isolates merely showed the deacetylation reaction under the conditions tested. On the other hand, because the deacetylation process is the confirmed mechanism in this work and the known mechanism by Fusarium to biosynthesis trichothecenes, it endangers the possibility of using Tri101-transformed crops as Fusarium-resistant crops. Enzymes or micro-flora of certain animals might have deacetylation function, which may change the less toxic acetylated trichothecenes to more toxic trichothecenes. Bacterial deacetylation of ADON might have another potential detoxification activity such as DON acetylation but still need to be investigated under various conditions or epimerization as reported earlier by Karlovsky. In particular that epimerization was processed on the same hydroxyl group at 3C position. Barpee genome sequencing will be a promising strategy in future to identify genes related to the deacetylation/detoxification process.

REFERENCES

Guan S, He JW, Young JC, Zhu HH, Li XZ, Ji C, Zhou T (2009) Transformation of trichothecene mycotoxins by microorganisms from fish digesta. Aquaculture 290: 290–295.

He J, Zhou T (2012) Bacterial isolate, methods of isolating bacterial isolates and methods for detoxification of trichothecene mycotoxins. Patent. In: Application USP, ed. *Patent*. US: Agri-FoodHer Majesty The Queen In Right Of Canada, As Represented By The Minister Of Agriculture, 1–17.

Islam R, Zhou T, Young JC, Goodwin PH, Pauls KP (2012) Aerobic and anaerobic de-epoxydation of mycotoxin deoxynivalenol by bacteria originating from agricultural soil. World J Microb Biot 28: 7–13.

Karlovsky P (2011) Biological detoxification of the mycotoxin deoxynivalenol and its use in genetically engineered crops and feed additives. Appl Microbiol Biotechnol 91: 491–504.

Kimura M, Kaneko I, Komiyama M, Takatsuki A, Koshino H, Yoneyama K, Yamaguchi I (1998) Trichothecene 3-O-acetyltransferase protects both the producing organism and transformed yeast from related mycotoxins: Cloning and chracterization of Tri101. J Biol Chem 273: 1654–1661.

Leslie AG (1990) Refined crystal structure of type III chloramphenicol acetyltransferase at 1·75 Å resolution. J Mol Biol 213: 167–186.

Lewis AL, Hensler ME, Varki A, Nizet V (2006) The group B Streptococcal sialic acid O-acetyltransferase is encoded by neuD, a conserved component of bacterial sialic acid biosynthetic gene clusters. J Biol Chem 281: 11186–11192.

Moynihan PJ, Clarke AJ (2010) O-acetylation of peptidoglycan in gram-negative bacteria: Identification and chracterization of peptidoglycan O-acetyltransferase in *Neisseria gonorrhoeae*. J Biol Chem 285: 13264–13273.

Saitou N, Nei M (1987) The neighbor-joining method: a new method for reconstructing phylogenetic trees. Mol Biol Evol 4: 406–425.

Ueno Y, Nakajima M, Sakai K, Ishii K, Sato N, Shimada N (1973) Comparative toxicology of trichothec mycotoxins: Inhibition of protein synthesis in animal cells. J Biochem 74: 285–296.

Yang Y, Qin S, Zhao F, Chi X, Zhang X (2007) Comparison of envelope-related genes in unicellular and filamentous cyanobacteria. Compar funct genom: 25751–25761.

Young JC, Zhou T, Yu H, Zhu H, Gong J (2007) Degradation of trichothecene mycotoxins by chicken intestinal microbes. Food Chem Toxicol 45: 136–143.

Yu H, Zhou T, Gong J, Young C, Su X, Li XZ, Zhu H, Tsao R, Yang R (2010) Isolation of deoxynivalenol-transforming bacteria from the chicken intestines using the approach of PCR-DGGE guided microbial selection. BMC Microbiol 10: 182–191.

Zamir LO, Nikolakakis A, Devor KA, Sauriol F (1996) Biosynthesis of the trichothecene 3-acetyldeoxynivalenol: Is isotrichodermin A biosynthetic precursor? J Biol Chem 271: 27353–27359.

Medicine Sciences and Bioengineering – Wang (Ed.)
© 2015 Taylor & Francis Group, London, ISBN: 978-1-138-02684-1

Binuclear lanthanide complexes derived from aroylhydrazines with 8-hydroxyquinoline-2-carboxyaldehyde and a series of DNA intercalators

Rui-xia Lei*, Dong-ping Ma, Xiao-wei Zhang, Yong-chun Liu,
Xu-dong Zheng & Jian-ning Liu
*Cooperative Innovation Center of Industrial Surfactant, College of Chemistry and Chemical Engineering,
Longdong University, Qingyang, Gansu, China*

Zheng-yin Yang
*State Key Laboratory of Applied Organic Chemistry, College of Chemistry and Chemical Engineering,
Lanzhou University, Lanzhou, China*

ABSTRACT: La^{III} and 8-hydroxyquinoline-2-carboxyaldehyde-(benzoyl)hydrazone can form a binuclear and 1:1 metal-to-ligand stoichiometry complex by nine-coordination at La^{III} center with the structure of $[LaL(NO_3)(DMF)_2]_2$ indicated by X-ray crystal structural analyses. The ligand acts as a dibasic tetradentate ligand, binding to La^{III} through the phenolate oxygen atom, nitrogen atom of quinolinato unit, the C=N group of methylene and $^-$O–C=N– group of the benzoyldrazone side chain. Dimerization of the monomeric unit occurs through the phenolate oxygen atoms leading to a central planar four-membered $(LaO)_2$ ring. In fact, lanthanide metal ions and structurally similar 8-hydroxyquinoline-2-carboxyaldehyde-aroylhydrazones can form a series of structurally similar binuclear and 1:1 metal-to-ligand stoichiometry complexes by nine-coordination at Ln^{III} center with geometry of distorted edge-sharing mono-capped square-antiprism of $[LnL(NO_3)(DMF)_2]_2$ ($Ln = La^{3+}, Nd^{3+}, Sm^{3+}, Eu^{3+}, Gd^{3+}, Tb^{3+}, Dy^{3+}, Ho^{3+}, Er^{3+}$) except for Yb^{III} complex by eight-coordination at Yb^{III} center with geometry of distorted edge-sharing dodecahedron of $[YbL(NO_3)(DMF)]_2$. All these complexes, strongly binding to calf thymus DNA by intercalation with binding constants at $0.1422{\sim}28.53 \times 10^6$ L·mol^{-1}, may be used as potential anticancer drugs.

1 INTRODUCTION

The bioactivities of lanthanides such as antimicrobial, antitumor, antivirus, anticoagulant action, enhancing NK and Macrophage cell activities, prevention from arteriosclerosis, etc., have been explored in recent decades (Parker *et al.*, 2002; Albrecht *et al.*, 2005). The chemistry of quinoline and its derivatives have also attracted special interest due to their therapeutic properties. Quinoline sulphonamides have been used in the treatment of cancer, tuberculosis, diabetes, malaria, and convulsion (Schmidt, 1969; El-Asmy *et al.*, 1990). DNA is an important cellular receptor, many chemicals exert their antitumor effects through binding to DNA thereby changing the replication of DNA and inhibiting the growth of the tumor cells, which is the basis of designing new and more efficient antitumor drugs and their effectiveness depends on the mode and affinity of the binding (Zeng *et al.*, 2003; Pyle *et al.*, 1990; Barton *et al.*, 1986). A number of metal chelates, as agents for mediation of strand scission of duplex DNA and as chemotherapeutic agents, have been used as probes of DNA structure in solution (Mahadevan & Palaniandavar, 1997; Lippard, 1978; Hecht, 1986). Additionally, Schiff-bases are able to inhibit the growth of several animal tumors, and some metal chelates have shown good antitumor activities against animal tumors

---

*Corresponding author. E-mail: rxlei1972@163.com

(Hodnett & Mooney, 1970; Hodnett & Dunn, 1972). So, well designed organic ligands enable a fine tuning of special properties of the metal ions. Previously, parts of lanthanide complexes were prepared from lanthanide metal ions and 8-hydroxyquinoline-2-carboxyaldehyde with aroylhydrazines (Liu et al., 2013; Liu & Yang, 2009; Liu & Yang, 2010; Liu et al., 2010; Liu et al., 2011). It is found that these lanthanide complexes have similarly structures and present stronger affinities of binding to calf thymus DNA through intercalation. This study will present the crystal structures of La^{III} complex prepared from 8-hydroxyquinoline-2-carboxyaldehyde and benzoylhydrazine. Moreover, the DNA binding properties of these lanthanide metal complexes will be summarized.

2 EXPERIMENTAL

2.1 *Materials*

Calf thymus DNA (CT-DNA) and Ethidium bromide (EB) were obtained from Sigma–Aldrich Biotech. Co., Ltd. 8-Hydroxyquinoline-2-carboxadehyde was obtained form J&K Chemical Co., Ltd. All the stock solutions (1.0 mmol·L^{-1}) of the investigated compounds were prepared by dissolving the powder materials into appropriate amounts of DMF solutions, respectively. CT-DNA stock solution was prepared by dissolving the solid material in 5 mmol·L^{-1} Tris–HCl buffer (pH 7.20) containing 50 mmol·L^{-1} NaCl. Then, the solution was kept at 2~8 °C. The CT-DNA concentration in terms of base pair L^{-1} or nucleotide^{-1} was determined spectrophotometrically as the literature (Zsila et al., 2004). EB was dissolved in 5 mmol·L^{-1} Tris–HCl buffer (pH 7.20) and its concentration was determined assuming a molar extinction coefficient of 5600 L mol^{-1} cm^{-1} at 480 nm (Suh & Chaires, 1995).

2.2 *Methods*

The melting points of the compounds were determined on an XT4–100X microscopic melting point apparatus (Beijing, China). Elemental analyses of C, N and H were carried out on an Elemental Vario EL analyzer. The metal ion content was determined by complexo-metric titration with EDTA after destruction of the complex in the conventional manner. The IR spectra were recorded on a Nicolet Nexus 670 FT-IR spectrometer using KBr disc in the 4000–400 cm^{-1} region. ESI-MS (ESI-Trap/Mass) spectra were recorded on a Bruker Esquire6000 Mass spectrophotometer.

Viscosity titration experiments were carried on an Ubbelohde viscometer in a thermostated water-bath maintained at 25.00 ± 0.01 °C. Relative viscosities for DNA either in the presence or absence of compound were calculated from the following relation (Suh & Chaires, 1995; Satyanarayana et al., 1992):

$$\eta = (t - t_\circ) / t_\circ \tag{1}$$

Fluorescence spectra were recorded using RF–5301PC spectrofluorophotometer (Shimadzu, Japan) with a 1 cm quartz cell. Both of the excitation and emission band widths were 10 nm. The binding constants were obtained by McGhee & von Hippel model (Chaires et al., 1982; McGhee & von Hippel, 1974):

$$\frac{r}{C_f} = K_b (1 - nr) \left[\frac{1 - nr}{1 - (n-1)r} \right]^{n-1} \tag{2}$$

EB-DNA quenching assay was performed as literatures (Krishna et al., 1998). Stern–Volmer equation was used to determine the fluorescent quenching mechanisms (Suh & Chaires, 1995):

$$F_\circ / F = 1 + K_q \tau_\circ [Q] = 1 + K_{SV} [Q] \tag{3}$$

2.3 Preperation of La^{III} complexes

Four Schiff-base ligands, 8-hydroxyquinoline-2-carboxyaldehyde-(benzoyl)hydrazone (**1a**), 8-hydroxyquinoline-2-carboxyaldehyde-(2′-hydroxybenzoyl)hydrazone (**1b**), 8-hydroxyquinoline-2-carboxyaldehyde-(4′-hydroxybenzoyl)hydrazone (**1c**) and 8-hydroxyquinoline-2-carboxyalde-hyde-(isonicotinyl)hydrazone (**1d**), were prepared as literatures (Liu & Yang, 2009; Liu *et al.*, 2013). Complex **2a** was prepared by refluxing and stirring equimolar amounts of a 40 mL methanol solution of ligand **1a** (0.058g, 0.2 mmol) and La(NO$_3$)·6H$_2$O on a water-bath. After refluxed for 30 min, tri-ethylamine (0.020 g, 0.2 mmol) was added into the reaction mixtures dropwise. Then, the mixtures were refluxed and stirred continuously for 8 h. After cooling to room temperature, the precipitate was centrifugalized, washed with methanol and dried in vacuum over 48 h. Yield: 84.6% (0.089 g), color: orange, m.p.: > 300 °C. Elemental analyses, found (calcd. %) for C$_{34}$H$_{30}$N$_8$O$_{14}$La$_2$: C, 38.69 (38.77); H, 2.85 (2.85); N, 10.68 (10.64); La, 26.47 (26.40). ESI-MS (DMF): *m/z* 1272.6 [M]$^+$, *m/z* 636.4 [M/2]$^+$, *m/z* 637.2 [M/2+H]$^+$, *m/z* 292.1 [M+H]$^+$ (ligand **1a**). IR (ν_{max}/cm^{-1}): 3423, 1628, 1548, 1104, 1501, 1310, 1040, 839, 733, 953, 687, 553, 481. Λ(DMF): 40.4 cm^2 Ω^{-1} mol^{-1}. Complex **2b**, **2c** and **2d** were prepared from equimolar amounts of La(NO$_3$)·6H$_2$O and **1b**, **1c** and **1d** as the way of **2a**, respectively.

2b: Yield: 86.7% (0.094 g), color: orange, m.p.: > 300 °C. Elemental analyses, found (calcd. %) for C$_{34}$H$_{30}$N$_8$O$_{16}$La$_2$: C, 37.69 (37.62); H, 2.78 (2.77); N, 10.34 (10.33); La, 25.57 (25.62). ESI-MS (DMF): *m/z* 1304.9 [M]$^+$, *m/z* 1305.8 [M+H]$^+$, *m/z* 652.4 [M/2]$^+$, *m/z* 653.3 [M/2+H]$^+$, *m/z* 308.2 [M+H]$^+$ (ligand **1b**). IR (ν_{max}/cm^{-1}): 3558, 3383, 1602, 1542, 1274, 1101, 1493, 1307, 1037, 841, 732, 935, 666, 561, 478. Λ(DMF): 33.1 cm^2 Ω^{-1} mol^{-1}.

2c: Yield: 90.4% (0.098 g), color: orange, m.p.: > 300 °C. Elemental analyses, found (calcd. %) for C$_{34}$H$_{30}$N$_8$O$_{16}$La$_2$: C, 37.66 (37.62); H, 2.78 (2.77); N, 10.37 (10.33); La, 25.66 (25.62). ESI-MS (DMF): *m/z* 1305.2 [M]$^+$, *m/z* 653.0 [M/2+H]$^+$, *m/z* 308.2 [M+H]$^+$ (ligand **1c**). IR (ν_{max}/cm^{-1}): 3425, 3233, 1584, 1546, 1294, 1106, 1499, 1332, 1035, 847, 733, 936, 651, 553, 483. Λ(DMF): 30.8 cm^2 Ω^{-1} mol^{-1}.

2d: Yield: 86.3% (0.091 g), color: orange, m.p.: > 300 °C. Elemental analyses, found (calcd. %) for C$_{32}$H$_{28}$N$_{10}$O$_{14}$La$_2$: C, 36.36 (36.42); H, 2.65 (2.66); N, 13.24 (13.28); La, 26.40 (26.35). ESI-MS (DMF): *m/z* 1274.7 [M]$^+$, *m/z* 1275.8 [M+H]$^+$, *m/z* 638.7 [M/2+H]$^+$, *m/z* 293.2 [M+H]$^+$ (ligand **1d**). IR (ν_{max}/cm^{-1}): 3425, 1636, 1590,1544, 1102, 1499, 1311, 1060, 839, 733, 940, 699, 558, 480. Λ(DMF): 37.6 cm^2 Ω^{-1} mol^{-1}.

2.4 Determination of crystal structure

The orange transparent, X-ray quality crystals of **1a** complex was obtained by vapor diffusion of diethyl ether into DMF solution of the metal complex (recrystallization in DMF suitable for X-ray measurements) at room temperature for 2 weeks. X-ray diffraction data for a crystal were performed with graphite-monochromated Mo *Kα* radiation (0.71073 Å) on a Bruker APEX area-detector diffractometer and collected by the ω–2θ scan technique at 298(2) K. The crystal structure was solved by direct methods. All non-hydrogen atoms were refined anisotropically by full-matrix least-squares methods on F^2. A partial structure was obtained by direct methods and the remaining non-hydrogen atoms were located from difference maps. Hydrogen atoms were located in geometrically defined positions and not refined. All calculations were performed using the programs SHELXS-97 and SHELXL-97 (Sheldrick, 1990).

3 RESULTS AND DISCUSSION

3.1 Structure analyses of La^{III} complexes

All these La^{III} complexes are stable in air, and soluble in DMF and DMSO, but slightly solu-ble in methanol, ethanol, acetonitrile, ethyl acetate and acetone, THF and CHCl$_3$. The data of

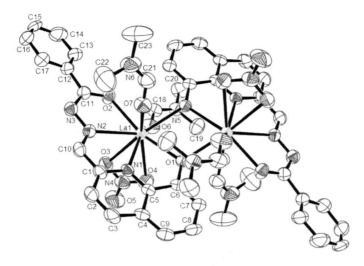

Figure 1. The Ortep structure of [LaL(NO$_3$)(DMF)$_2$]$_2$ complex.

molar conductance of the La^{III} complexes in DMF solution indicate that all of them act as non-electrolytes (Geary, 1971). Fig. 1 shows that the composition of La^{III} complex is of [LaL(NO$_3$)(DMF)$_2$]$_2$. Crystal and experimental data of La^{III} complex (CCDC No. 993158) were collected in Table 1.

Ligand **1a** acts as a dibasic tetradentate ligand, binding to La^{III} through the phenolate oxygen atom, nitrogen atom of quinolinato unit and the C=N group, ‾O–C=N– group enolized and deprotonated from O=C–NH– of the benzoylhydrazone side chain, where the C–O‾ bond length is 1.279(6) Å and the N=C double bond length is 1.321(6) Å. In addition, one DMF molecule is binding orthogonally to the ligand-plane from one side to the metal ion, while another DMF and a bidentate nitrate anion are simultaneously binding from the other. Dimerization of the monomeric unit occurs through the phenolate oxygen atoms leading to a central planar four-membered (LaO)$_2$ ring with a La···La separation of 4.0911(6) Å. At the dimerization site, a "set off" of the two parallel "LaL-planes" by an approximately 2 Å takes place. The center of symmetry according to the coordinates is located in the middle of the four-membered (LaO)$_2$ ring formed by two La atoms and the phenolic oxygen atoms. The deprotonization and enolization result the complex acting as non-electrolytes, may well be due to the addition of triethylamine

Factually, lanthanide metal ions and structurally similar Schiff bases **1a**, **1b**, **1c** and **1d** can form a series of structurally similar binuclear and 1:1 metal-to-ligand stoichiometry complexes by nine-coordination at Ln^{III} center with geometry of distorted edge-sharing mono-capped square-antiprism of [LnL(NO$_3$)(DMF)$_2$]$_2$ (Ln = La^{3+}, Nd^{3+}, Sm^{3+}, Eu^{3+}, Tb^{3+}, Dy^{3+}, Ho^{3+}, Er^{3+}) except for Yb^{III} by eight-coordination at Yb^{III} center with geometry of distorted edge-sharing dodecahedron of [YbL(NO$_3$)(DMF)]$_2$ (Liu *et al.*, 2013; Liu & Yang, 2009; Liu & Yang, 2010; Liu *et al.*, 2010; Liu *et al.*, 2011). This difference may be due to the small size of Yb^{III}. Comparison of the structural parameters of this ligand binding to different metal centers is shown in Table 2. It is obvious that from La^{III} to Yb^{III}, the bond lengths of metal ions linked with oxygen and nitrogen atoms gradually decrease; the distance of M···M separation gradually decrease too, whereas the angles of metal ions linked with oxygen and nitrogen atoms gradually increase.

Table 1. Crystal and experimental data of La^{III} complex (CCDC No. 993158).

Complex	[LaL(NO$_3$)(DMF)$_2$]$_2$
Chemical formula	C$_{46}$H$_{50}$N$_{12}$O$_{14}$La$_2$
Formula weight	1272.80
T (K)	298(2)
Wavelength (Å)	0.71073
Radiation	Mo Kα
Crystal system	Monoclinic
Space group	$P2_1/n$
a (Å)	10.4009(9)
b (Å)	21.2288(18)
c (Å)	12.0955(11)
α (°)	90.000
β (°)	98.8510(10)
γ (°)	90.00
V (Å^3)	2638.9(4)
Z	2
D_c (g cm^{-3})	1.602
μ (mm^{-1})	1.671
$F(000)$	1272
Crystal size (mm)	0.27 × 0.18 × 0.13
$\theta_{\text{min/max}}$ (°)	2.59–25.02
Index ranges	$-8 \leq h \leq 12, -25 \leq k \leq 21, -14 \leq l \leq 14$
Reflections collected	13171
Independent reflections	4660 ($R_{\text{int}} = 0.0433$)
Absorption correction	Semi-empirical from equivalents
Max. and min. transmission	0.8120 and 0.6611
Refinement method	Full-matrix least-squares on F^2
Data / restraints / parameters	4660 / 0 / 338
Goodness-of-fit on F^2	1.044
Final R indices [$I > 2\sigma (I)$]	$R_1 = 0.0373, wR_2 = 0.0761$
R indices (all data)	$R_1 = 0.0619, wR_2 = 0.0905$
$\rho_{\text{min/max}}$ (e Å^{-3})	0.786 / −0.587

3.2   DNA binding properties

Viscosity measurements are very sensitive to changes in the length of DNA, as viscosity is proportional to L^3 for rod-like DNA of length L. With the ratios of the investigated compounds to DNA increasing, the relative viscosities of DNA increase steadily (data not shown), indicating that there exist intercalations between all these lanthanide complexes with DNA helix (Suh & Chaires 1995; Palchaudhuri & Hergenrother 2007). Compared with the value of constant ($K_b = 3.166 \times 10^6$ L·mol^{-1}) of DNA binding to ethidium bromide (EB, a classic DNA intercalator), all these complexes can strongly binding to calf thymus DNA by intercalation with the binding constants K_b at $0.1422{\sim}28.53 \times 10^6$ L·mol^{-1} studied by fluorescent quenching and McGhee & von Hippel model. Moreover, at CF_{50}, the molar concentration of the tested compound that causes a 50% loss in the fluorescence intensity of EB-DNA system, all the molar concentration ratios of the investigated complexes to DNA are largely under 100:1, indicating that all these lanthanide complexes, as a series of DNA intercalators, may be used as potential anticancer drugs (Li et al., 1991).

Fig. 2 shows the binding constants of these complexes binding to DNA with the changes of 4f electronic numbers of metal ions. Obviously, the complexes derived from ligand **1b** and **1c**

Table 2. Comparison of the crystal structural parameters of ligand 8-hydroxyquinoline-2-carboxyaldehyde-(benzoyl))hydrazone binding to a series of lanthanide metal ion centers.

M^{III}	La	Nd	Sm	Eu	Tb	Dy	Ho	Er[1]	Yb[2]
M–O1	2.527(3)	2.4840(13)	2.462(7)	2.443(3)	2.428(2)	2.429(2)	2.4072(18)	2.385(11)	2.341(7)
M–N1	2.643(4)	2.5538(16)	2.545(8)	2.510(4)	2.484(3)	2.492(2)	2.464(2)	2.460(14)	2.401(7)
M–N2	2.666(4)	2.6087(15)	2.591(9)	2.566(3)	2.546(3)	2.551(3)	2.526(2)	2.552(13)	2.435(8)
M–O2	2.468(4)	2.4165(13)	2.374(8)	2.349(3)	2.330(2)	2.335(2)	2.312(2)	2.331(12)	2.254(7)
M′–O1	2.497(3)	2.4269(13)	2.420(7)	2.407(3)	2.388(2)	2.3981(19)	2.3729(17)	2.392(10)	2.309(7)
O1–M–N1	62.28(11)	64.06(4)	65.0(3)	64.99(11)	65.57(9)	65.94(8)	66.07(7)	66.3(4)	67.7(3)
N1–M–N2	59.67(13)	61.66(5)	61.6(3)	62.01(13)	62.29(11)	62.45(9)	62.64(8)	62.6(5)	64.3(3)
N2–M–O2	59.94(12)	60.67(5)	61.5(3)	61.74(13)	62.20(10)	62.38(8)	62.52(8)	62.8(5)	64.4(3)
M···M′	4.0911(6)	4.0356(7)	4.0713(12)	4.0349(4)	4.0090(4)	4.027	3.990	4.003	3.7553(9)

[1] The ligand is 8-hydroxyquinoline-2-carboxyaldehyde-(2′-hydroxybenzoyl)hydrazone.
[2] The ligand is 8-hydroxyquinoline-2-carboxyaldehyde-(isonicotinyl)hydrazone.

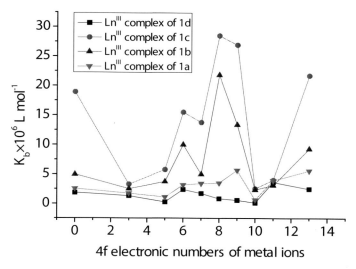

Figure 2. The plot of binding constants of lanthanide complexes binding to CT-DNA with the changes of 4f electronic numbers of metal ions.

consisting of hydroxyl substitutes present stronger binding to DNA than those derived from ligand **1a** and **1d** in that hydroxyl substitutes can bond well with base pairs of DNA through hydrogen bond besides the strong stacking interaction between the aromatic chromophore of the complexes and base pairs of DNA. Furthermore, the complexes derived from electron-deficient center ions and electron-affluent ions, such as La^{3+}, Eu^{3+}, Gd^{3+}, Tb^{3+}, Dy^{3+} and Yb^{3+}), present stronger binding to DNA, which may be due to a fine tuning of special properties of the metal ions. Additionally, Gd^{3+} complex present a slight hump, which may be related to the $4f^7$ electron effect. However, their pharmacodynamical, pharmacological and toxicological properties should be further studied *in vivo*.

4 SUMMARY

La^{III} and 8-hydroxyquinoline-2-carboxyaldehyde-(benzoyl)hydrazone can form a binuclear and 1:1 metal-to-ligand stoichiometry complex by nine-coordination at La^{III} center with the structure of $[LaL(NO_3)(DMF)_2]_2$ indicated by X-ray crystal structural analyses. In fact, lanthanide metal ions and structurally similar 8-hydroxyquinoline-2-carboxyaldehyde-aroylhydrazones can form a series of structurally similar binuclear and 1:1 metal-to-ligand stoichiometry complexes by nine-coordination at Ln^{III} center with geometry of distorted edge-sharing mono-capped square-antiprism of $[LnL(NO_3)(DMF)_2]_2$ (Ln = La^{3+}, Nd^{3+}, Sm^{3+}, Eu^{3+}, Gd^{3+}, Tb^{3+}, Dy^{3+}, Ho^{3+}, Er^{3+}) except for Yb^{III} complex by eight-coordination at Yb^{III} center with geometry of distorted edge-sharing dodecahedron of $[YbL(NO_3)(DMF)]_2$. All these complexes, strongly binding to calf thymus DNA by intercalation with the binding constants at $0.1422{\sim}28.53 \times 10^6$ L·mol⁻¹, may be used as potential anticancer drugs. However, their pharmacodynamical, pharmacological and toxicological properties should be further studied *in vivo*.

5 APPENDIX

CIF files for the X-ray crystal structures have been deposited with the Cambridge Crystallographic Data Center (CCDC No. 993158). Copies of this information may be obtained free of charge from the Director, CCDC, 12 Union Road, Cambridge, CB2 1EZ, UK (fax: +44 1223 336033; e-mail: deposit@ccdc.cam.ac.uk or http://www.ccdc.cam.ac.uk).

ACKNOWLEDGEMENTS

This study was supported by Gansu Applied Chemistry Key Subject Fund (No. GSACKS20130113) and Longdong University Doctor Fund.

REFERENCES

Albrecht, M., Osetska, O. & Fröhliich, R. (2005) 2-[(8-Hydroxyquinolinyl)methylene]hydrazinecarboxamide: expanding the coordination sphere of 8-hydroxyquinoline for coordination of rare-earth metal (III) ions. *Dalton Trans*, 23: 3757–3762.

Barton, J.K., Goldberg, J.M., Kumar, C.V. & Turro, N.J. (1986) Binding modes and base specificity of tris(phenanthroline)ruthenium(II) enantiomers with nucleic acids: tuning the stereoselectivity. *J Am Chem Soc*, 108, 2081–2088.

Chaires, J.B., Dattagupta, N. & Crothers, D.M. (1982) Studies on interaction of anthracycline antibiotics and deoxyribonucleic acid: equilibrium binding studies on the interaction of daunomycin with deoxyribonucleic acid. *Biochemistry*, 21, 3933–3940.

El-Asmy, A.A., El-Sonbati, A.Z., Ba-Issa, A.A. & Mounir, M. (1990) Synthesis and properties of 7-formyl-8-hydroxyquinoline and its transition metal complexes. *Transit Metal Chem*, 5, 222–225.

Geary, W.J. (1971) The use of conductivity measurements in organic solvents for the charaterisation of coordination compounds. *Coord Chem Rev*, 7, 81–122.

Hecht, S.M. (1986) The chemistry of activated bleomycin. *Accounts Chem Res*, 19, 383–391.

Hodnett, E.M. & Dunn, W.J. (1972) Cobalt derivatives of Schiff bases of aliphatic amines as antitumor agents. *J Med Chem*, 15, 339–339.

Hodnett, E.M. & Mooney, P.D. (1970) Antitumor activities of some Schiff bases. *J Med Chem*, 13, 786–786.

Krishna, A.G., Kumar, D.V., Khan, B.M., Rawal, S.K. & Ganesh, K.N. (1998) Taxol–DNA interactions: fluorescence and CD studies of DNA groove binding properties of taxol. *Biochimica et Biophysica Acta*, 1381, 104–112.

Lippard, S.J. (1978) Platinum complexes: probes of polynucleotide structure and antitumor drugs. *Accounts Chem Res*, 11, 211–217.

Liu, Y.C., Jiang, X.H., Yang, Z.Y., Zheng, X.D., Liu, J.N. & Zhou, T.L. (2010) Fluorescent and Ultraviolet–Visible Spectroscopy Studies on the Antioxidation and DNA Binding Properties of Binuclear Tb(III) Complexes. *Appl Spectrosc*, 64, 980–985.

Liu, Y.C., Xu, X.Y., Lei, R.X., Zhang, X.W., Wu, Y. & Yang, Z.Y. (2013) Anti-oxidation and DNA binding properties of La(III) complexes. *Chemical Research and Application*, 25 (11), 1475–1483.

Liu, Y.C. & Yang, Z.Y. (2009) Synthesis, crystal structure, anti-oxidation and DNA binding properties of binuclear Ho(III) complexes of Schiff-base ligands derived from 8-hydroxyquinoline-2-carboxyaldehyde and four aroylhydrazines. *J Organomet Chem*, 694, 3091–3101.

Liu, Y.C. & Yang, Z.Y. (2009) Crystal structures, anti-oxidation and DNA binding properties of Eu(III) complexes with Schiff-base ligands derived from 8-hydroxyquinoline-2-carboxyaldehyde and three aroylhydrazines. *J Inorg Biochem*, 103, 1014–1022.

Liu, Y.C. & Yang, Z.Y. (2009) Anti-oxidation and DNA binding properties of binuclear Nd(III) complexes with Schiff-base ligands derived from 8-hydroxyquinoline-2-carboxyaldehyde and four aroylhydrazides. *Inorg Chem Commun*, 12, 704–706.

Liu, Y.C. & Yang, Z.Y. (2009) Crystal structures, antioxidation and DNA binding properties of Dy(III) complexes with Schiff-base ligands derived from 8-hydroxyquinoline-2-carboxyaldehyde and four aroylhydrazines. *Eur J Med Chem*, 44, 5080–5089.

Liu, Y.C. & Yang, Z.Y. (2009) Crystal structures, anti-oxidation and DNA binding properties of Yb(III) complexes with Schiff-base ligands derived from 8-hydroxyquinoline-2-carbaldehyde and four aroylhydrazines. *Biometals*, 22, 733–751.

Liu, Y.C. & Yang, Z.Y. (2010) Antioxidation and DNA-binding properties of binuclear Er(III) complexes with Schiff-base ligands derived from 8-hydroxyquinoline-2-carboxaldehyde and four aroylhydrazines. *J Biochem*, 147, 381–391.

Liu, Y.C., Yang, Z.Y., Zhang, K.J., Wu, Y., Zhu, J.H. & Zhou, T.L. (2011) Crystal Structures, Antioxidation, and DNA Binding Properties of Sm^{III} Complexes. *Aust J Chem*, 64, 345–354.

Li, Z.L., Chen, J.H., Zhang, K.C., Li, M.L. & Yu, R.Q. (1991) Fluorescent study on the primary screening for nonplatinum type of Schiff-base antitumor complexes. *Science in China Series B: Chemistry*, 11, 1193–1200.

Mahadevan, S. & Palaniandavar, M. (1997) Spectroscopic and voltammetric studies of copper(II) complexes of bis(pyrid-2-yl)-di/trithia ligands bound to calf thymus DNA. *Inorg Chim Acta*, 254, 291–302.

McGhee, J.D. & von Hippel, P.H. (1974) Theoretical aspects of DNA-protein interactions: Co-operative and non-co-operative binding of large ligands to a one-dimensional homogeneous lattice. *J Mol Biol*, 86, 469–489.

Palchaudhuri, R. & Hergenrother, P.J. (2007) DNA as a target for anticancer compounds: methods to determine the mode of binding and the mechanism of action. *Curr Opin Biotechnol*, 18, 497–503.

Parker, D., Dickins, R.S., Puschmann, H., Crossland, C. & Howard, J.A.K. (2002) Being Excited by Lanthanide Coordination Complexes: Aqua Species, Chirality, Excited-State Chemistry, and Exchange Dynamics. *Chem Rev*, 102, 1977–2010.

Pyle, A.M., Morii, T. & Barton, J.K. (1990) Probing microstructures in double-helical DNA with chiral metal complexes: recognition of changes in base-pair propeller twisting in solution. *J Am Chem Soc*, 112, 9432–9434.

Satyanarayana, S., Dabrowiak, J.C. & Chaires, J.B. (1992) Neither Δ-nor Λ-Tris(phenanthroline)ruthenium(II) Binds to DNA by Classical Intercalation. *Biochemistry*, 31, 9319–9324.

Schmidt, L.H. (1969) Chemotherapy of the Drug-Resistant Malarias. *Ann Rev Microbiol*, 23, 427–454.

Sheldrick, G.M. (1990) Phase annealing in SHELX-90: direct methods for larger structures. *Acta Crystallogr A*, 46, 467–473.

Suh, D. & Chaires, J.B. (1995) Criteria for the mode of binding of DNA binding agents. *Bioorg Med Chem*, 3, 723–728.

Zeng, Y.B., Yang, N., Liu, W.S. & Tang, N. (2003) Synthesis, characterization and DNA-binding properties of La(III) complex of chrysin. *J Inorg Biochem*, 97, 258–264.

Zsila, F., Bikádi, Z. & Simonyi, M. (2004) Circular dichroism spectroscopic studies reveal pH dependent binding of curcumin in the minor groove of natural and synthetic nucleic acids. *Org biomol Chem*, 2, 2902–2910.

Medicine Sciences and Bioengineering – Wang (Ed.)
© *2015 Taylor & Francis Group, London, ISBN: 978-1-138-02684-1*

Analysis of two pairs of grape early-ripening bud sports varieties based on iPBS markers

Da-long Guo & Xiao-yu Zhang
College of Forestry, Henan University of Science & Technology, Luoyang, China

ABSTRACT: Two grape varieties 'Jingya', and 'Kyoho' and their corresponding early-ripening bud sports 'Luopuzaosheng', 'Fengzao' were analyzed using inter-primer binding site (iPBS) markers in order to explore their genomic differences between early-ripening bud sports and their parents. With primer 2395 of iPBS, a differential fragment about 500 bp was amplified and further cloned to be sequenced. The percentage of sequences homology between 'Jingya', 'Kyoho' and their early-ripening bud sports 'Luopuzaosheng', 'Fengzao' ranged from 29.8% to 99.9% and the cluster analysis divided the sequences into seven groups. Group I and Group II covered 26.7% of the total. In addition, their amino acid sequences showed many termination codon mutations and frameshift mutations. The results provide a direction on the genomic difference of early-ripening varieties.

1 INTRODUCTION

Grape (*Vitis vinifera* L.) is an important economic fruit around the world, and has been grown in China for more than 2000 years. The appropriate berry ripening time influenced a lot on the commodity value of grapes berry and wine. A selection of early-ripening grape varieties is one of the main breeding aims. In China, due to the influence of historical and traditional planting patterns, the availability of suitable early-maturing grape variety for cultivation is not enough. The present early-ripening grape varieties have many problems such as small berries, low yield, poor stress-resistance, easy cracking or low fresh-eating quality.

Bud sport is a kind of somatic mutation. As a way of grape breeding, selection of bud sport has unique advantages than other breeding methods (Seedling selection, cross breeding, induced mutation breeding, biotechnology breeding, etc.), and it is easy to be observed in the field and can be kept through grafting without the juvenility.

Retrotransposons are abundant mobile genetic elements in most species. They can mobilize by a replicative mechanism by which many copies are generated and inserted into the genome, therby increasing the genome size (D'Onofrio *et al.* 2010; Kalendar *et al.* 2010b).

iPBS is a new DNA fingerprinting technology, whose primers were based on the conserved parts of primer binding site (PBS) sequences. Because the method could be applicable not only to endogenous retroviruses, but also to *Gypsy* and *Copia* LTR retrotransposons, and without the need for prior sequence knowledge (Kalendar *et al.* 2010b), it is more comparable or even more efficient than other retrotransposons-based markers.

The aims of the present work were intended to discover the differences of grape early-ripening bud sports based on the iPBS markers.

2 MATERIALS AND METHODS

2.1 *Plant materials and DNA extraction*

Two grape varieties 'Jingya', 'Kyoho' and their corresponding early-ripening bud sports' Luopuzaosheng', 'Fengzao' were used. DNA was extracted from fresh, young leaf tissue according to the method as reported (Marsal et al. 2011). All four varieties were collected from the national grape germplasm repository of the Zhengzhou Fruit Research Institute at Chinese Academy of Agricultural Sciences.

2.2 *iPBS-PCR amplification*

Original forty-one 18-mer iPBS primers designed by published literature (Kalendar et al. 2010a) were synthesized and screened. Primer 2395 was used in this study for all the four samples; sequence of the primer is TCCCCAGCGGAGTCGCCA. iPBS-PCR amplification conditions was performed as reported previously (Kalendar et al. 2010a) with slight modifications. The PCR reaction was carried out in 20μL, comprised of 30 ng of template DNA, 0.6 μmol•L^{-1} primer, 1.5 mmol•L^{-1} Mg^{2}+, 0.4 mmol•L^{-1} dNTPs, and 1.0 U of Taq polymerase. PCR program consisted of: 1 cycle at 95°C for 3 min; 30 cycles of 95°C for 15 s, 55°C for 60 s, and 68°C for 60 s; a final extension step of 72°C for 5 min. The resulting PCR products were separated on 1.0% agarose gel in 1 × TBE buffer at 5 V/cm, stained with UltraPowerTM dye and visualized and photographed under White/Ultraviolet Transilluminator (UVP; Spring Scientific, New York, USA).

2.3 *PCR products purifying and cloning*

The amplification products were analyzed by agarose gel electrophoresis and the differential DNA fragments around 500 bp between 'Kyoho' and 'Fengzao', 'Jingya' and 'Luopuzaosheng' were excised. The size of gel slice was minimized by removing extra agarose. Purify the PCR product by Agarose gel DNA recovery kit (Beijing Bioteke Biotechnology Company). Vector pMD18-T (Takara Biotechnology Co., Ltd.) was used on the vector ligation. Follow the steps by the manual of pMD™18-T Vector Cloning Kit. Transform the productions of linkage into competent cells, coated plates, select monoclonal colony amplified in LB culture solution for 12 hours.

2.4 *Sequencing and analysis*

A total of 23 clones were sequenced at Beijing Sunbiotech Co. Ltd. The homology of the sequences were compared based on BLAST and DNAman, DNAstar software was employed to analyze the sequences (Kalendar et al. 2010a)

3 RESULTS

3.1 *Sequence analysis of differential fragments*

The profile of the agarose gel electrophoresis and the gel extraction were shown in Figure 1. A total of 15 of 23 sequences were successfully sequenced, numbered from 9 to 23. Number 9 to 13 from 'Jingya', 14 to 16 from 'Luopuzaosheng', 17, 18 from 'Kyoho' and 19 to 23 from 'Fengzao'. All the 15 sequences were compared with known sequences listed in the GenBank database, and the max identity of these sequences ranged from 89% to 99%, which means the results can be used for further analysis. Big differences of homology can be found after comparing the 15 sequences using MegAlign software of DNAstar. The sequences homology of the 10th from 'Jingya' and the 23th from 'Fengzao'up to 99.9%, and the 10th from 'Jingya' with the 17th from 'Kyoho' also reach to 99.7%, while the 21st and 22nd from 'Fengzao'can be as low as 29.8%. It indicates that common origin exist in the high homology sequences while mutation may occur for some reasons during transposition in the low homology sequences which means the retrotransposons in some sequences are transcription activity.

3.2 *Cluster analysis of sequences*

Cluster analysis of 15 fragments obtained by PCR was performed by using MegAlign software of DNAstar, phylogenetic tree was shown in Figure 2 in order to explore the correlation between the

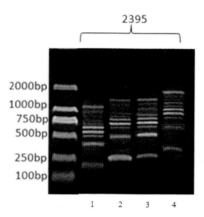

Figure 1.   Electrophoretogram of PCR product from iPBS marker 2395. Lane 1-4 are 'Kyoho', 'Fengzao', 'Jingya' and 'Luopuzaosheng', respectively.

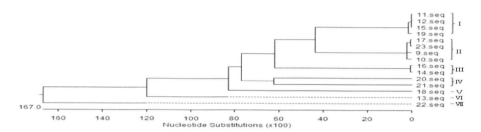

Figure 2.   Polygenetic tree of base sequences of the 15 grape gene segments.

gene segments. According to the phylogenetic tree analysis, seven groups exist. The uniformity of Group I is 93.7%, Group II is 89.43% and 99.13% in Group III, there is base substitution in these nucleotide sequences. The uniformity of Group IV is 40.90%. Group V, VI and VII all have one sequence, which length is 700 bp, 660 bp and 720 bp, respectively, the deletion mutant of nucleotide sequences may cause the greater genetic distances between them and the other groups.

3.3   *Sequence alignment of amino acid*

Translated the base sequences into an amino acid, then the sequence alignment by DNAman software ins shown in Figure 3. The presence of terminator codon may cause the functional loss of retrotransposon of reverse transcriptase, and silence the gene during evolutionary time. Different quantities of terminator codon and point mutation in the 15 amino acid sequences may be the reason generates the heterogeneity of the grape DNA fragments. In addition, all 15 sequenes showed non-conservative and a quantity of frameshift mutation which might be another important reason of heterogeneity.

4   DISSCUSSION

On the basis of the earlier works of primer screening, 'Jingya', 'Kyoho' and their early-ripening bud sports 'Luopuzaosheng', 'Fengzao' were analyzed by using inter-primer binding site (iPBS) markers in this study. The differential fragments were cloned and sequenced to compare the differences between the wild type and their early-ripening bud sports. Most of the sequences are around

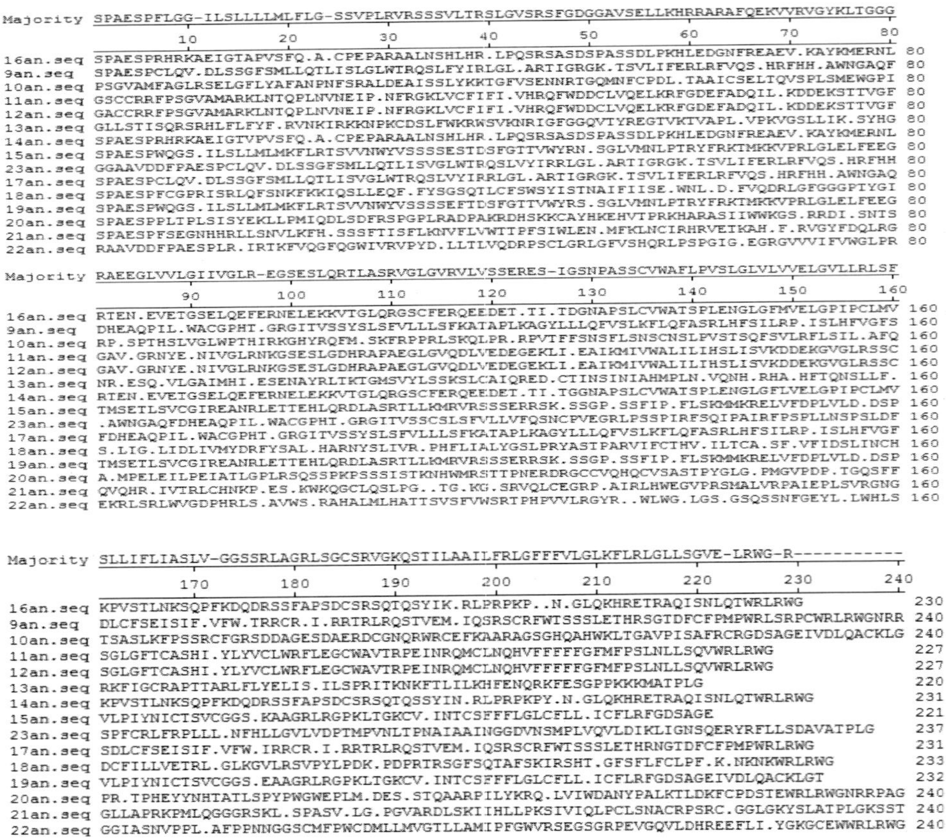

```
Majority   SPAESPFLGG-ILSLLLLMLFLG-SSVPLRVRSSSVLTRSLGVSRSFGDGGAVSELLKHRRARAFQEKVVRVGYKLTGGG
                  10        20        30        40        50        60        70        80
           |........|.........|.........|.........|.........|.........|.........|.........|
16an.seq   SPAESPRHRKAEIGTAPVSFQ.A.CPEPARAALNSHLHR.LPQSRSASDSPASSDLPKHLEDGNFREAEV.KAYKMERNL   80
9an.seq    SPAESPCLQV.DLSSGFSMLLQTLISLGLWTRQSLFYIRLGL.ARTIGRGK.TSVLIFERLRFVQS.HRFHH.AWNGAQF   80
10an.seq   PSGVAMFAGLRSELGFLYAFANPNFSRALDEAISSLYKKTGFVSENNRTGQMNFCPDL.TAAICSELTQVSPLSMEWGPI   80
11an.seq   GSCCRRFPSGVAMARKLNTQPLNVNEIP.NFRGKLVCFIFI.VHRQFWDDCLVQELKRFGDEFADQIL.KDDEKSTTVGF   80
12an.seq   GACCRRFPSGVAMARKLNTQPLNVNEIP.NFRGKLVCFIFI.VHRQFWDDCLVQELKRFGDEFADQIL.KDDEKSTTVGF   80
13an.seq   GLLSTISQRSRHLFLFYF.RVNKIRKKNPKCDSLFWKRWSVKNRIGFGGQVTYREGTVKTVAPL.VPKVGSLLIK.SYHG   80
14an.seq   SPAESPRHRKAEIGTAPVSFQ.A.CPEPARAALNSHLHR.LPQSRSASDSPASSDLPKHLEDGNFREAEV.KAYKMERNL   80
15an.seq   SPAESPWQGS.ILSLLMLMKFLRTSVVNWYVSSSSESTDSFGTTVWYRN.SGLVMNLPTRYFRKTMKKVPRLGLELFEEG   80
23an.seq   GGAAVDDFPAESPCLQV.DLSSGFSMLLQTLISVGLWTRQSLVYIRRLGL.ARTIGRGK.TSVLIFERLRFVQS.HRFHH   80
17an.seq   SPAESPCLQV.DLSSGFSMLLQTLISVGLWTRQSLVYIRRLGL.ARTIGRGK.TSVLIFERLRFVQS.HRFHH.AWNGAQ   80
18an.seq   SPAESPFCGPRISRLQFSNKFKKIQSLLEQF.FYSGSQTLCFSWSYISTNAIFIISE.WNL.D.FVQDRLGFGGGPTYGI   80
19an.seq   SPAESPWQGS.ILSLLMLMKFLRTSVVNWYVSSSEFTDSFGTTVWYRS.SGLVMNLPTRYFRKTMKKVPRLGLELFEEG   80
20an.seq   SPAESPPLTIPLSISYEKLLPMIQDLSDFRSPGPLRADPAKRDHSKKCAYHKEHVTPRKHARASIIWWKGS.RRDI.SNTS   80
21an.seq   SPAESPFSEGNHHHRLLSNVLKFH.SSSFTISFLKNVFLVWTIPFSIWLEN.MFKLNCIRHRVETKAH.F.RVGYFDQLRG   80
22an.seq   RAAVDDFPAESPLR.IRTKFVQGFQGWIVRVPYD.LLTLVQDRPSCLGRLGFVSHQRLPSPGIG.EGRGVVVIFVWGLPR   80

Majority   RAEEGLVVLGIIVGLR-EGSESLQRTLASRVGLGVRVLVSSERES-IGSNPASSCVWAFLPVSLGLVLVVELGVLLRLSF
                  90       100       110       120       130       140       150       160
           |........|.........|.........|.........|.........|.........|.........|.........|
16an.seq   RTEN.EVETGSELQEFERNELEKKVTGLQRGSCFERQEEDET.TI.TDGNAPSLCVWATSPLENGLGFMVLGIPICLMV   160
9an.seq    DHEAQPIL.WACGPHT.GRGIITVSSYSLSFVLLLSFKATAPLKAGYLLLQFVSLKFLQFASRLHFSILRP.ISLHFVGFS   160
10an.seq   RP.SPTHSLVGLWPTHIRKGHYRQFM.SKFRPPRLSKQLPR.RPVTFFSNSFLSNSCNSLPVSTSQFSVLRFLSIL.AFQ   160
11an.seq   GAV.GRNYE.NIVGLRNKGSESLGDHRAPAEGLGVQDLVEDEGEKLI.EAIKMIVWALILIHSLISVKDDEKGVGLRSSC   160
12an.seq   GAV.GRNYE.NIVGLRNKGSESLGDHRAPAEGLGVQDLVEDEGEKLI.EAIKMIVWALILIHSLISVKDDEKGVGLRSSC   160
13an.seq   NR.ESQ.VLGAIMHI.ESENAYRLTKTGMSVYLSSKSLCAIQRED.CTINSINIAHMPLN.VQNH.RHA.HFTQNSLLF.   160
14an.seq   RTEN.EVETGSELQEFERNELEKKVTGLQRGSCFERQEEDET.TI.TDGNAPSLCVWATSPLENGLGFMVLGIPICLMV   160
15an.seq   TMSETLSVCGIREANRLETTEHLQRDLASRTLLKMRVRSSSERRSK.SSGP.SSFIP.FLSKMMKRELVFDPLVLD.DSP   160
23an.seq   .AWNGAQFDHEAQPIL.WACGPHT.GRGITVSSCSLSFVLLVFQSNCPVEGRLPSSPIRFSQIPAIRFPSPLLNSPSLDF   160
17an.seq   FDHEAQPIL.WACGPHT.GRGIITVSSYSLSFVLLLSFKATAPLKAGYLLLQFVSLKFLQFASRLHFSILRP.ISLHFVGF   160
18an.seq   S.LIG.LIDLIVMYDRFYSAL.HARNYSLIVR.PHFLIALYGSLPRYASTPARVIFCTHV.ILTCA.SF.VFIDSLINCH   160
19an.seq   TMSETLSVCGIREANRLETTEHLQRDLASRTLLKMRVRSSSERRSK.SSGP.SSFIP.FLSKMMKRELVFDPLVLD.DSP   160
20an.seq   A.MPELEILPEIATLGPLRSQSSPKPSSSISTKNHWMRSTTPNERDRGCCVQHQCVSASTPYGLG.PMGVPDP.TGQSFF   160
21an.seq   QVQHR.IVTRLCHNKP.ES.KWKQGCLQSLPG..TG.KG.SRVQLCEGRP.AIRLHWEGVPRSMALVRPAIEPLSVRGNG   160
22an.seq   EKRLSRLWVGDPHRLS.AVWS.RAHALMLHATTSVSFVWSRTPHPVVLRGYR..WLWG.LGS.GSQSSNFGEYL.LWHLS   160

Majority   SLLIFLIASLV-GGSSRLAGRLSGCSRVGKQSTILAAILFRLGFFFVLGLKFLRLGLLSGVE-LRWG-R----------
                 170       180       190       200       210       220       230       240
           |........|.........|.........|.........|.........|.........|.........|.........|
16an.seq   KPVSTLNKSQPFKDQDRSSFAPSDCSRSQTQSYIK.RLPRPKP..N.GLQKHRETRAQISNLQTWRLRWG            230
9an.seq    DLCFSEISIF.VFW.TRRCR.I.RRTRLRQSTVEM.IQSRSCRFWTSSSLETHRSGTDFCFPMPWRLSRPCWRLRWGNRR   240
10an.seq   TSASLKFPSSRCFGRSDDAGESDAERDCGNQRWREECFKAARAGSPDHAWKLTGAVPISAFRCRGDSAGEIVDLQACKLG   240
11an.seq   SGLGFTCASHI.YLYVCLWRFLEGCWAVTRPEINRQMCLNQHVFFFFFGFMFPSLNLLSQVWRLRWG              227
12an.seq   SGLGFTCASHI.YLYVCLWRFLEGCWAVTRPEINRQMCLNQHVFFFFFGFMFPSLNLLSQVWRLRWG              227
13an.seq   RKFIGCRAPTTARLFLYELIS.ILSPRITKNKFTLILLKHFENQRKFESGPPKKKMATPLG                   220
14an.seq   KPVSTLNKSQPFKDQDRSSFAPSDCSRSQTQSSYIN.RLPRPKPY.N.GLQKHREATRAQISNLQTWRLRWG         231
15an.seq   VLPIYNICTSVCGGS.KAAGRLRGPKLTGKCV.INTCSFFFLGLCFLL.ICFLRFGDSAGE                   221
23an.seq   SPFCRLFRPLLL.NFHLLGVLVDPTMPVNLTPNAIAAINGGDVNSMPLVQVLDIKLIGNSQERYRFLLSDAVATPLG    237
17an.seq   SDLCFSEISIF.VFW.IRRCR.I.RRTRLRQSTVEM.IQSRSCRFWTSSSLETHRNGTDFCFPMPWRLRWG          231
18an.seq   DCFILLVETRL.GLKGVLRSVPYLPDK.PDPRTRSGFSQTAFSKIRSHT.GFSFLFCLPF.K.NKNKWRLRWG        233
19an.seq   VLPIYNICTSVCGGS.EAAGRLRGPKLTGKCV.INTCSFFFLGLCFLL.ICFLRFGDSAGEIVDLQACKLGT         232
20an.seq   PR.TPHEYYNHIATLSPYPWGWEPLM.DES.STQAARPILYKRQ.LVIWDANYPALKTLDKFCPDSTEWRLRWGNRRPAG   240
21an.seq   GLLAPRKPMLQGGGRSKL.SPASV.LG.PGVARDLSKIIHLLPKSIVIQLPCLSNACRPSRC.GGLGKYSLATPLGKSST   240
22an.seq   GGIASNVPPL.AFPPNNGGSCMFPWCDMLLMVGTLLAMIPFGWVRSEGSGRPEVGQVLDHREEFLI.YGKGCEWWRLRWG   240
```

Figure 3. Sequence alignment of amino acid sequences of the 15 grape gene segments.

670 bp in length. Compared the sequences with known sequences listed in the GenBank database showed that the max identity of these sequences ranged from 89% to 99%, which means the result can be used for analysis. Homogeneous analysis demonstrates a large difference between all these 15 sequences. The homology of the 10th sequence from 'Jingya' and the 23rd from 'Fengzao' up to 99.9%, the 10th from 'Jingya' and 22th from 'Fengzao' can be as low as 29.8%.

The cluster analysis showed that different genomic sequence may categorized into one group. The 11th and 12th from 'Kyoho', the 15th from 'Luopuzaosheng' and the 19th from 'Fengzao' may categorize into one group for instance. Translate these 15 base sequences into amino acid sequences and compared by DNAman software. The amino acid sequence similarity of 'Jingya' and 'Luopuzaosheng' is 84.44%, the similarity of 'Kyoho' and 'Fengzao' is 83.85%.

In grape, molecular markers have been applied to the assessment of seedless (Gustafson et al. 2006), skin color (Giannetto et al. 2008), berry color (Lijavetzky et al. 2006) and disease resistance (Riaz et al. 2008), and so on. But there are few reports on the early identification of grape early-ripening bud sports, much less on using iPBS-PCR to study the grape early-ripening bud sports has described at present. In this study, the sequences of genes of 'Jingya', 'Kyoho' and their early-ripening bud sports were cloned and sequenced to ascertain the differences.

However, only 500 bp in length of the PCR product has been studied is the main limitation of this study. The sequencing result showed a big difference between the sequences isolated from the same variety. This may correlate with the base insertions, deletions and substitutions during the transcription of the retrotransposon.

Further investigation focuses on comparing the gene expression profiling of bud sports and wild type to screen the specific related genes which control the grape early-ripening characteristics. Thus constitute the theoretical basis and practical significances for identifying the grape early-ripening bud sports and genetically modified the grape.

ACKNOWLEDGEMENTS

This work was partly supported by Natural Science Foundation of China (NSFC: 31372026), Program for Science & Technology Innovation Talents in Universities of Henan Province (13HASTIT004) and key Technologies R & D Program of He'nan Scientific Committee (132102110029).

REFERENCES

D'Onofrio, C., De Lorenzis, G., Giordani, T., Natali, L., Cavallini, A. & Scalabrelli, G. (2010). Retrotransposon-based molecular markers for grapevine species and cultivars identification. *Tree Genetics & Genomes*, 6: 451–466.

Giannetto, S., Velasco, R., Troggio, M., Malacarne, G., Storchi, P., Cancellier, S., De Nardi, B. & Crespan, M. (2008). A PCR-based diagnostic tool for distinguishing grape skin color mutants. *Plant Science*, 175: 402–409.

Gustafson, J., Cabezas, J., Cervera, M., Ruiz-García, L., Carreño, J. & Martínez-Zapater, J. (2006). A genetic analysis of seed and berry weight in grapevine. *Genome*, 49: 1572–1585.

Kalendar, R., Antonius, K., Smýkal, P. & Schulman, A. H. (2010a). iPBS: a universal method for DNA fingerprinting and retrotransposon isolation. *Theoretical and Applied Genetics*, 121: 1419–1430.

Kalendar, R., Flavell, A., Ellis, T., Sjakste, T., Moisy, C. & Schulman, A. H. (2010b). Analysis of plant diversity with retrotransposon-based molecular markers. *Heredity*, 106: 520–530.

Lijavetzky, D., Ruiz-García, L., Cabezas, J. A., De Andrés, M. T., Bravo, G., Ibáñez, A., Carreño, J., Cabello, F., Ibáñez, J. & Martínez-Zapater, J. M. (2006). Molecular genetics of berry colour variation in table grape. *Molecular Genetics and Genomics*, 276: 427–435.

Marsal, G., Baiges, I., Canals, J. M., Zamora, F. & Fort, F. (2011). A Fast, Efficient Method for Extracting DNA from Leaves, Stems, and Seeds of Vitis vinifera L. *American Journal of Enology and Viticulture*: ajev. 2011.10082.

Riaz, S., Tenscher, A., Rubin, J., Graziani, R., Pao, S. & Walker, M. (2008). Fine-scale genetic mapping of two Pierce's disease resistance loci and a major segregation distortion region on chromosome 14 of grape. *Theoretical and Applied Genetics*, 117: 671–681.

Medicine Sciences and Bioengineering – Wang (Ed.)
© 2015 Taylor & Francis Group, London, ISBN: 978-1-138-02684-1

Antimicrobial characters of bacteriocin produced by *Streptococcus lactis* S5-3

Jun-chao Zhang, Hui Liu, Yuan-hong Xie & Hong-xing Zhang[1]
Beijing Key Laboratory of Agricultural Product Detection and Control of Spoilage Organisms and Pesticide Residue, Beijing Laboratory of Food Quality and Safety, Faculty of Food Science and Engineering , Beijing University of Agriculture, Beijing, China

ABSTRACT: In this paper, functional characterization of the bacteriocin produced by *Streptococcus lactis* S5-3 selected from ham products of Zhejiang province was examined to lay the theoretical foundation for the development of natural and safe food preservative. Studying on the thermal stability and pH stability, our results indicate that the bacteriocin S5-3 still has antibacterial activity at 100°C for 30 min, and has strong antibacterial activity in the range of pH 2.0–6.0, but has no antibacterial activity after trypsin, proteinase K and pronase E treatment. The antibacterial spectrum of bacteriocin S5-3 suggested its good inhibitory effect on proliferation of *Listeria monocytogenes*, and had a certain inhibitory effect on other Gram-positive bacteria and other Gram-negative bacteria determined by the Oxford cup method. Above all show that bacteriocin S5-3 has the characteristics of good thermal and pH stability, broad antimicrobial spectrum.

1 INTRODUCTION

Lactobacillin are a class of extracellular proteins or peptides with antibacterial activity produced by ribosome biogenesis mechanism of lactic acid bacteria's metabolic processes (Jack *et al.*, 1995). Nisin is a kind of bacteriocins produced by *Lactococcus lactis subsp. Lactis* and is a safe biological preservative (Gálvez *et al.*, 2007). The bacteriocins inhibit their relative strains, and have antibacterial activity for most Gram-positive bacteria including *Listeria, Enterococcus, Staphylococcus, Streptococcus, Micrococcus, Mycobacterium, Corynebacterium and Lactobacillus,* etc. In recent years, its antibacterial mechanism is not entirely clear (Hasper *et al.*, 2004). We screened *Streptococcus lactis* S5-3, having obvious inhibitory effect on proliferation of *Listeria monocytogenes*, from traditional fermented foods, studied the antibacterial activity of the bacteriocin, analyzed its antibacterial spectrum, and studied the characteristics of thermal stability of bacteriocins, pH stability, enzyme stability. This provides a reference for further research and application of lactobacillin.

2 MATERIALS AND METHODS

2.1 *Determination of antibacterial activity*

The antibacterial activity was tested using the Oxford cup method (O' Shea *et al.*, 2012): *Listeria monocytogenes* strain ATCC54003 was used as indicator strain, and indicator bacteria was diluted to 10^7CFU/mL and mixed with solid medium and melted. About 15 mL of melted medium

---

[1] Correspondence: hxzhang51@163.com

was poured into the petri dish, until solidified. Then, 100 µL lactic acid was added into Oxford Cup on the petri dish for fermentation. Finally, after the petri dish stayed in 4°C refrigerator to diffuse for 4h, cultured at 37°C for 12 h. The appearance of the zone of inhibition was observed (De Kwaadsteniet et al., 2006).

2.2 Determination of bacteriocin titer

The bacteriocin activity was measured using the Oxford cup method and twice echelon dilution of the fermentation supernatant as samples (Tahiri et al., 2004). The bacteriocin titer was expressed in arbitrary units per ml (AU/mL). One AU was defined as the reciprocal of the highest serial twofold dilution with MRS (pH 6.0) broth that shows a clear zone.

2.3 Thermal, pH and enzyme stability assay

The fermentation supernatant of Streptococcus lactis S5-3 was made the following treatment: no treatment; at 60°C for 10 min; at 60°C for 30 min; at 60°C for 90 min; 100°C for 10 min; 100°C for 30 min; 100°C for 90 min; 121°C for 15 min. These fermentation supernatant were cooled to room temperature, the antibacterial activity was determined by the Oxford cup method (O' Shea et al., 2012). Experiments were carried out in triplicate.

The fermentation supernatant of Streptococcus lactis S5-3 was respectively adjusted to pH 2.0, 4.0, 6.0, 8.0, 10.0, 12.0, in 37°C for 2h, the supernatant was adjusted to pH 6.0. The Oxford cup method was used to determine antimicrobial activity of fermentation supernatant (O' Shea et al., 2012). Experiments were carried out in triplicate.

The fermentation supernatant respectively treated with catalase, α-amylase, pronase E, trypsin and proteinase K under the respective optimum pH. The final concentration of the enzymes were 1 mg/mL, in 37°C for 2h, the supernatant was transferred to pH 6.0. The Oxford cup method was used to determine antimicrobial activity of fermentation supernatant. The control was the fermentation supernatant without treatment at pH 6.0. Experiments were carried out in triplicate.

2.4 Streptococcus lactis S5-3 growth curve

Growth curve was made by turbidimetric method. The two-fold dilution method and the Oxford cup method were used to measure the antimicrobial activity of fermentation supernatant (8). Changes in optical density (600 nm) were recorded every four hours for 24h.

2.5 Antibacterial spectrum

The fermentation supernatant of Streptococcus lactis S5-3 adjusted to pH 6.0 was determined its inhibitory spectrum. These indicator bacterias and their culture conditions are listed in Table 1. The antibacterial activity was determined by the Oxford cup method (O' Shea et al., 2012).

3 RESULTS AND DISCUSSION

3.1 Growth curve and bacteriocin production of Streptococcus lactis S5-3

As shown in Figure 1, cell concentration of Streptococcus lactis S5-3 increased rapidly from 4 hours to 16 hours which reached the logarithmic phase. After 16 hours of fermentation, optical density of cells eventually reached 1.87 (OD600). Meanwhile, as the fermentation progresses, antibacterial activity of the bacteriocin also increased, and reached 640AU after the 16 hours of fermentation.

3.2 Thermal, pH and enzyme stability of bacteriocin S5-3

As shown in Figure 2A, with the increase of temperature and time, antibacterial of bacteriocin gradually decreased. When bacteriocin was treated at 100°C, inhibitory effect declined, and at 121°C for 15min, there was a certain inhibitory effect. The results show that bacteriocin is relatively stable at 121°C. Similar characteristics have been reported for several bacteriocins (De Kwaadsteniet *et al.*, 2006).

As shown in Figure 2B, at pH 2.0–12.0, with the increased pH, antibacterial activity of bacteriocin gradually decreased. And at pH 2.0–10.0, the inhibitory effect was of stability. The result indicates that the bacteriocin S5-3 has good pH stability.

Our results show that bacteriocin antibacterial activity completely inactivated after treating with trypsin and proteinase K, indicates trypsin and proteinase K decompose bacteriocin (Figure 2C). The bacteriocin antibacterial activities were basically the same after treating with catalase and nothing. This indicates that the antibacterial substance is bacteriocin, and not hydrogen peroxide. After treatment with α-amylase inhibitory activity has been reduced, indicating that this bacteriocin antibacterial activity is dependent on glycosylation.

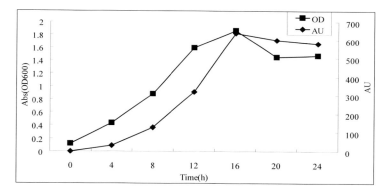

Figure 1. Bacteriocin production during growth of *Streptococcus lactis* S5-3 in MRS broth.

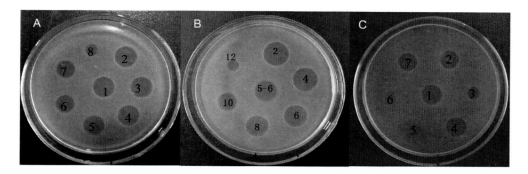

A: Effect of temperature on bacteriocin activity. 1, Cell-free supernatant (pH 6.0); 2, 60°C, 10 min; 3, 60°C, 30 min; 4, 60°C, 90 min; 5, 100°C, 10 min; 6, 100°C, 30 min; 7, 100°C, 90 min; 8, 121°C, 15 min. B: Effect of pH on bacteriocin activity. C: Effect of enzyme on bacteriocin activity. 1, Cell-free supernatant (pH 6.0); 2, treated with catalase; 3, treated with a-amylase; 4, treated with pronase E; 5, treated with trypsin; 6, treated with proteinase K; 7, treated with pepsin.

Figure 2. Effect of temperature, pH and enzyme on bacteriocin activity.

Table 1. The antimicrobial spectrum of bacteriocin S5-3.

Indicator organism	Strain[a]	Medium, incubation temperature (°C)	Sensitivity[b]
Escherichia coli	CDC85933	LB, 37	−
Enterococcus facealis	AS1.2984	MRS, 37	+++
Listeria monocytogenes	ATCC54003	TSBYE, 37	+++
Lactobacillus delbrueckii	AS1.2625[T]	MRS, 37	++
Lactobacillus acidophilus	Our strain collection	MRS, 37	+
Lactobacillus johnsonii	Our strain collection	MRS, 37	−
Lactobacillus delbrueckii	Our strain collection	MRS, 37	+
Lactobacillus casei	ATCC334	MRS, 37	+
Lactobacillus pentosus	ATCC8041	MRS, 37	++
Lactobacillus curvatus	Our strain collection	MRS, 37	+
Salmonella	ATCC50041	BPY, 37	+
Staphylococcus aureus	ATCC6535	LB, 37	+
Shigella	ATCC51253	GN, 37	+

NOTE: "−" Indicates no inhibition, "+" represents inhibition zone diameter (d) is 1 ~ 8 mm, "+ +" means 9–14 mm, "+ + +" indicates 15 ~ 21 mm.

3.3 Antimicrobial spectrum of bacteriocin S5-3

As shown in Table 1, bacteriocin S5-3 has a strong inhibitory effect on Gram-positive, such as *Listeria monocytogenes* ATCC54003 and *Enterococcus faecalis* AS1.2984. For Gram-negative bacteria, such as *Salmonella, Staphylococcus aureus,* also have a weak inhibitory effect, but does not inhibit the growth of *E. coli, Lactobacillus, Lactobacillus bulgaricus.* The results indicate that bacteriocin S5-3 can act against some Gram-positive and Gram-negative bacteria. Similar findings have been reported by Tahiri *et al.* (Tahiri *et al.*, 2004) and Yang *et al.* (Yang *et al.*, 1992).

In conclusion, an anti-*Listeria* bacteriocin produced by *Streptococcus lactis* S5-3 was isolated from a traditional Chinese meat product. This bacteriocin showed a broad inhibition spectrum, which includes some food-spoiling and pathogenic organisms in food, such as *L. monocytogenes, S. aureus* and *Salmonella*. Bacteriocin S5-3 is heat-resistant and stable over a pH range of 2.0–10.0, our findings will lay a theoretical foundation for the application of this bacteriocin as a natural biopreservative in the food industry.

ACKNOWLEDGEMENTS

The research was financially supported by National High-tech R&D Program (863 Program) (No. 2012AA101606-05), Importation and Development of High-Caliber talents project of Beijing Municipal Institutions (CIT&TCD20140315) and Key Construction Discipline Program of Beijing Municipal Commission of Education (PXM2014-014207-0000029).

REFERENCES

De Kwaadsteniet, M., Fraser, T., Van Reenen, C.A., Dicks, L.M. (2006) Bacteriocin T8, a novel class IIa sec-dependent bacteriocin produced by *Enterococcus faecium* T8, isolated from vaginal secretions of children infected with human immunodeficiency virus. *Appl Environ Microbiol*, 72:4761–4766.
Gálvez, A., Abriouel, H., López, R.L., Ben Omar, N. (2007) Bacteriocin-based strategies for food biopreservation. *Int J Food Microbiol*, 120:51–70.
Hasper, H.E., de Kruijff, B., Breukink, E. (2004) Assembly and stability of nisin-lipid II pores. *Biochemistry*, 43:11567–11575.

Jack, R.W. Tagg, J.R. Ray, B. (1995) Bacteriocins of gram-positive bacteria. *Microbiol Rev*, 59: 171–200.

O' Shea, E.F., O' Connor, P.M., Raftis, E.J., O' Toole, P.W., Stanton, C., Cotter, P.D., Ross, R.P., Hill, C. (2012) Subspecies diversity in bacteriocin production by intestinal *Lactobacillus salivarius* strains. *Gut Microbes*, 3:468–473.

Tahiri, I., Desbiens, M., Benech, R., Kheadr, E., Lacroix, C., Thibault, S., Ouellet, D., Fliss, I. (2004) Purification, characterization and amino acid sequencing of divergicin M35: a novel class IIa bacteriocin produced by *Carnobacterium divergens* M35. *Int J Food Microbiol*, 97:123–136.

Yang, R., Johnson, M.C., Ray, B. (1992) Novel method to extract large amounts of bacteriocins from lactic acid bacteria. *Appl Environ Microbiol*, 58:3355–3359.

Medicine Sciences and Bioengineering – Wang (Ed.)

Quality characteristics of WCA and PCA during cold storage

Yang-ya ng Li, Yu-rong Guo*, Ge Bai, Jiao Dou & Hong Deng
Shaanxi Normal University, College of Food Engineering and Nutritional Science, Xi'an, China

ABSTRACT: Taking Well-Color Apple (WCA) and Poor-Color Apple (PCA) (red area > 80% WCA, red area < 20% PCA) as materials, the variations of color value and texture were investigated during cold storage. The result showed that their color values changed during the cold storage and pH values rose gradually. Firmness of PCA declined faster than that of WCA. Protopectin content of the two treatments decreased significantly while water-soluble content pectin increased obviously, meanwhile MDA content of both kept increasing. Correlation analysis indicated that their b* value correlated with the pH value but a* value had no significant correlation (p < 0.05), and the firmness had extremely significant correlation (P < 0.01) both pectin and MDA.

1 INTRODUCTION

China is the largest country in acreage and yield of apples in the world. As China mainly cultivates various varieties of apple, Fuji apple's taste and flavor are popular to the consumers. However, the improvement of living standards and the rising requirements of exterior quality and texture lead to the difficulty of storage (Bai Shasha *et al.*, 2011). In this regard, studying of changes in various factors and exploring rules to provide theoretical basis for apple storage are necessary. Color is one of the important factors which significantly influence exterior quality. While firmness is one of the important factors that have influence on texture, so judging the correlation between firmness and other factors has important significance.

Some researches have reported that fruit softening attributed to the function and structure of cell wall and cytomembrane. With apple maturing, the organizations gradually soften and polysaccharides of the cell wall become soluble. There are a lot of pectins deposited in fruit born cell wall and mesogloea. In the unripe fruit, pectin exists in the form of protopectin, which makes the fruit solid and hard (Sun lijun *et al.*, 2012). However, during fruit maturing, pectin turns into water-soluble substance and makes the fruit tissue flabby, softening which lead to the decrease of firmness. MDA is one of membrane lipid peroxidation productions which leads to the peroxidation of membrane lipid. For these reasons, MDA has bad effect on physiological and biochemical reaction and apple quality in the storage finally.

2 MATERIALS AND METHODS

2.1 *Materials*

Luochuan Fuji apples (WCA and PCA) with no hurt and consistent size were collected from shaanxi Huasheng Fruit Co., Ltd.

2.2 *Methods*

2.2.1 *Color value*
L*, a*, b* were measured by CR-400 Colorimeter directly.

2.2.2 *Firmness*

FT-327Durometer 11mm bulk detector was used to measure the firmness.

2.2.3 *pH value*

Use PHS-3C pH Meter to measure each pH value.

2.2.4 *Pectin extraction and determination*

Water-soluble pectin was extracted by hot water and protopectin was extracted by conventional acid method. The purity of pectin was detected according to the method of carbazole-sulfuric acid colorimetry (Wang dongmei, 2009).

2.2.5 *MDA extraction and determination*

MDA was extracted by TCA and then reacted with TBA. The reaction solution absorbance was measured at a wavelength of 450 nm, 532 nm and 600 nm, respectively. Then the contents of MDA were calculated.

2.3 *Analysis and Statistics*

All processes were repeated three times, and the data were analyzed by SPSS16.0 software.

3 RESULTS AND ANALYSIS

3.1 *The change of color value during storage*

During the storage, their pH values rose gradually. Meanwhile a* value of WCA was first down and then up gradually while the PCA kept lowing all the time, b* value of WCA first rose and then declined but the PCA continued rising (Tables 1, 2). As shown in Table 3, pH value had significant correlation with b* value while had no significant correlation with a* value.

Table 1. pH and Color value of WCA during storage.

Item	pH value	a*	b*
0d	3.68 ± 0.03^a	34.89 ± 3.07^a	13.63 ± 2.13^a
50d	3.67 ± 0.02^a	33.49 ± 2.32^a	14.61 ± 1.93^{ab}
100d	3.78 ± 0.02^a	31.17 ± 5.87^a	19.16 ± 4.70^{bc}
150d	4.04 ± 0.06^b	31.82 ± 3.77^a	15.01 ± 1.95^c
200d	4.07 ± 0.13^b	34.96 ± 2.40^a	17.05 ± 2.36^c

Note: The different letters on the same list mean significant difference ($p < 0.05$).

Table 2. pH and Color value of PCA during storage.

Item	pH value	a*	b*
0d	3.70 ± 0.04^a	25.60 ± 4.89^a	19.79 ± 5.25^a
50d	3.58 ± 0.02^{ab}	18.63 ± 5.00^b	20.35 ± 3.75^a
100d	3.76 ± 0.06^b	18.68 ± 6.98^{bc}	21.86 ± 4.43^a
150d	4.03 ± 0.12^c	23.37 ± 4.15^{bc}	22.67 ± 2.89^a
200d	4.06 ± 0.06^c	14.57 ± 3.58^d	27.71 ± 2.24^b

Note: The different letters on the same list mean significant difference ($p < 0.05$).

3.2 The firmness of apple during storage

From Figure 1, we can conclude that with the extension of storage, firmness of PCA declined more obviously than WCA (0.21%, 0.13%).

3.3 Changes of water-soluble pectin and protopectin content during storage

The content of water-soluble pectin increased while protopectin decreased during the storage. Water-soluble pectin of WCA was a little higher than PCA, peotopectin of WCA was higher than PCA (Figure 2).

3.4 Change of MDA content during storage

Figure 3 indicated that the content of MDA kept increasing and WCA was always higher than PCA.

3.5 Correlation analysis of pectin, MDA and firmness

Water-soluble pectin and MDA exhibited a significant negative correlation with firmness while there was a significant positive correlation between protopectin and firmness (Table 4).

Table 3. Correlation analysis of color value and pH value during storage.

Item	a*	b*
pH (WCA)	−0.39	0.90**
pH (PCA)	−0.2	0.65**

*: $p < 0.05$, **: $p < 0.01$, n = 15.

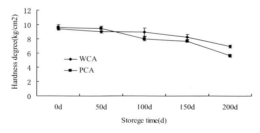

Figure 1. Firmness during storage.

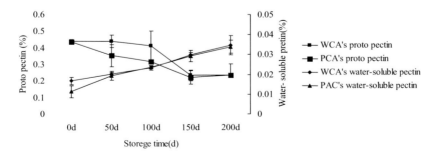

Figure 2. Change of Pectin content during storage.

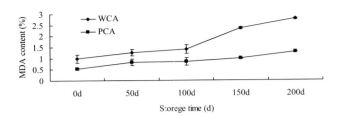

Figure 3.   Change of MDA during storage.

Table 4.   Correlation Analysis of Pectin, MDA and Firmness.

Item	WCA	PCA
Water-soluble pectin	−0.90**	−0.89**
Protopectin	0.72**	0.80**
MDA	−0.80**	−0.78**

4   DISCUSSION

We studied on the change of apple quality characteristics of WCA and PCA in cold storage and focused on color value and firmness. The result showed that WCA and PCA exhibited different color value trends and that pH value also had different correlation with their color value. Wang et al. (2006) analyzed the correlation between Litchi chinensis peel color and pH value during its maturing and indicated that pH value had significant correlation with fruit color index and that the increasing of pH value contributed to fruit color. Hence, we can conclude that pH value had significant correlation with b* color value whereas had negative correlation with a* value.

Pectin is one of the main factors affecting fruit firmness and in the normal maturation process, the dissociation of galactan and arabinose branch led to the decrease of protopectin and the increase of water-soluble pectin. Wei (Wei baodong et al., 2005) had studied that tomato firmness had a significant positive correlation with water-insoluble pectin and had a significant negative correlation with water-soluble pectin. This study suggested that firmness of the two treatments had a significant negative correlation with water-soluble pectin. However, the firmness had a significant positive correlation with protopectin.

Fruit softening was closely related to peroxidation of mermbane lipids, which directly led to the damage of membrane structure and the increase of permeability and thus caused the softening of fruit. Liu jianfeng et al. (2003) studied on "Texture of Postharvest Pear in Relation to Ca²⁺, Pectin, MDA and Ethylene" showed that MDA content had a significant negative correlation with fruit hardness. The present study also indicated that MDA content had extremely significant correlation with the firmness.

ACKNOWLEDGEMENT

This research was supported by an adrmarked fund for China Agriculture Research System (CARS-28).

REFERENCES

Bai Shasha, Bi Jinfeng, Fangfang et al. (2011) Current research progress and prospect of the technologies of apple quality evaluation. *Food Science*, 32 (3), 286–290.
Liu jianfeng, Zhang hongyan, peng shuang. (Cacas, 2003) Texture of postharvest pear in relation to Ca²⁺, pectin, MDA and ethylene. *Journal of Huazhong Agricultura University*, 22 (3), 270–273.

Sun lijun, Guo yurong, Tisn lanlan. (2012) Research progress of apple pectin. *Science and Technology of Food Industry*, 33 (4), 445–449.

Wang dongmei. (2009) *Biochemistry experiment instruction*. Beijing, Science Press.

Wang jiabao, Liu zhiyuan, Du zhongjun et al. (Cacas, 2006) Analysis of the factors related to pericarp color formation during fruit development of Litchi. *Chinese Journal of Tropical Crops*, 27 (2),11–17.

Wei baodong, Jiang bingyi, Feng hui. (Cacas, 2005) Studies on changes of firmness of tomato fruit affected shelf-life. *Food Science*, 26 (3), 249–252.

Medicine Sciences and Bioengineering – Wang (Ed.)
© *2015 Taylor & Francis Group, London, ISBN: 978-1-138-02684-1*

Ionic liquids improve the biotransformation of isoeugenol to vanillin by *Bacillus fusiformis* CGMCC1347

Li-qing Zhao
School of Bioscience and Bioengineering, South China University of Technology, Guangzhou, China
College of Chemistry and Chemical Engineering, Shenzhen University, Shenzhen, Guangdong, China
Guangdong Huanxi Biological Technology CO., LTD, Puning, Guangdong, China

Rou-xuan Chen & Yu-lin Chen
College of Chemistry and Chemical Engineering, Shenzhen University, Shenzhen, Guangdong, China

Jia-Mao Fang & Wei-bin Chen
Guangdong Huanxi Biological Technology CO., LTD, Puning, Guangdong, China

Ju-fang Wang*
School of Bioscience and Bioengineering, South China University of Technology, Guangzhou, China

ABSTRACT: An Ionic Liquid (IL)-containing buffer system was first applied in the conversion of isoeugenol to vanillin by *Bacillus fusiformis* CGMCC1347. High substrate solubility was achieved to enhance the efficiency of the reaction. Nine ILs were selected as co-solvents to assist catalytic reactions in this biotransformation process. 1-ethyl-3-methylimidazolium methylsulfate [C_2mim][MetSO_4] was the suitable ionic liquid to be tested for this biotransformation. The optimal biotransformation conditions were as follows: Ionic liquid 40 µL, isoeugenol 400 µL for 10 mL reaction liquid in 50-mL flask, phosphate buffer (pH 7.0) 50 mM, 37°C, 180 r/min for 60 h. The Maximum vanillin concentration reached 1.38 g/L.

1 INTRODUCTION

As one of the most important components of natural flavors, vanillin (4-hydroxy-3- methoxybenzaldehyde) is widely used in foods, beverages, perfumes, pharmaceuticals, medical industries and so on. In the medical industry, vanillin is an important raw material in many pharmaceutical and synthetic intermediates, and it has become the most promising areas of vanillin application. It is the important intermediate for L-dopa, which for Parkinson's disease and other drugs for hypertension, respiratory tract infections and heart disease. Natural vanillin extracted from vanilla pods features both an expensive price up to $3,000/Kg and a limited supply of about 20–50 tons per year due to the availability restriction of vanilli pods plant (Priefert *et al.*, 2002). More and more researches on the alternative or equivalent product of natural vanillin were conducted. According to EEC legislation, natural products are those obtained from plant materials or animal organisms through physical, enzymatic or microbiological processes (Druaux *et al.*, 1997).

Natural eugenol and isoeugenol from essential oil are more available and economical for the production of vanillin by bioconversion other than the substrates as ferulic acid, phenolicstilbenes and lignin. Therefore, the bioconversion of isoeugenol to vanillin becomes more and more attractive (Ashengroph *et al.* 2011, Su *et al.* 2011, Ashengroph *et al.* 2012, Ashengroph *et al.*, 2013, Ryu *et al.*, 2013).

The yield of vanillin production is generally low not only for the product inhibition, but also for the poor solubility of the substrate. In previous studies, the reaction and separation systems combining the addition of resin HD-8 and the isoeugenol/aquoeus biphasic system were established for the biotransformation of isoeugenol to vanillin by *Bacillus fusiformis* CGMCC1347 and successfully solve the problem of product inhibition (Zhao *et al.*, 2005; Zhao *et al.*, 2006).

Ionic liquids (ILs), having no measurable vapor pressure, are an interesting class of tunable and designer solvents, and they have been used extensively in a wide range of applications including enzymatic biotransformation. As compared to those observed in conventional organic solvents, the use of enzymes in ionic liquids has presented many advantages such as high conversion rates, high enantioselectivity, better enzyme stability, as well as better recoverability and recyclability (Moniruzzaman, 2010). The aim of this study was to investigate the effects of ionic liquids as the co-solvents on biotransformation of isoeugenol to vanillin by *Bacillus fusiformis* CGMCC1347 cells.

2 MATERIALS AND METHODS

2.1 *Materials and microorganisms*

Vanillin (99%) and isoeugenol (98%, *cis/trans* mixture) were obtained from Sigma Co. (St Louis, MO, USA). Methanol was of HPLC grade and other chemicals were of analytical grade.

2.2 *Microorganism*

Bacillus fusiformis CGMCC1347 was isolated from soil and kept at China General Microbiological Culture Collection Center (CGMCC).

2.3 *Cultivation and conversion*

Cultures were grown in 250-mL flasks containing 50 mL medium comprising corn steep 55 g/L, urea 1 g/L, $K_2HPO_4 \times 3H_2O$ 2 g/L and $MgSO_4 \times 7H_2O$ 1 g/L, at pH 7.5, 37°C and 180 rpm for 16 h. 0.36 g wet cells (obtained at $3\,000 \times g$, 10 min, 4°C, and equivalent to 0.05 g dry weight cells), 4% (v/v) isoeugenol and 40 µL ionic liquid were added into the 10 mL phosphate buffer pH7.0, 50 mM reaction solution (in 50-mL flask) and were shaken at 180 rpm and 37°C for 72 h (Zhao *et al.*, 2006).

2.4 *Vanillin and isoeugenol analysis*

Samples were diluted by ethanol to certain range (vanillin concentration 0.01 g/L to 0.1 g/L) and analyzed by HPLC (Li *et al.*, 2004).

3 RESULTS AND DISCUSSION

3.1 *Effects of different kinds of ionic liquids*

Ionic liquids (ILs) represent a class of promising and 'green' non-molecular solvents that have increasingly attracted attention as the green, high-tech reaction media of the future (Yang *et al.*, 2012). In this reaction, isoeugenol as the substrate was difficult to be solved in water. As shown in Fig.1, ILs as co-solvents were found a significantly increase in vanillin production such as 1-ethyl-3-methylimidazolium methylsulfate [C_2mim][MetSO_4] and 1,3-dimethylimidazolium methylsulfate. [C_2mim][MetSO_4] was the most effective ionic liquid for this biotransformation. As a result, it was selected for further research in this paper.

The amount of [C_2mim][MetSO_4] greatly affected vanillin production. As shown in Fig.2, the optimal [C_2mim][MetSO_4] addition was 40 µL. The biotransformation of isoeugenol to vanillin was increased in ionic liquids possessing strongly coordinating anions as HSO_4 since it leads to many possible types of interactions, including hydrogen bonding, van der Waals, ionic, and dipolar interactions and increase the interaction of the enzyme and the substrate. A higher concentration of

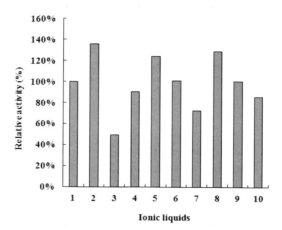

Figure 1. Effects of different kinds of ionic liquids on the biotransformation of isoeugenol to vanillin by *Bacillus fusiformis* CGMCC1347.

Note: 1: Control, without ionic liquid; 2: 1-ethyl-3-methylimidazolium methylsulfate[C_2mim][MetSO_4]; 3: Choline nitrate; 4: Choline acetate; 5: Tetramethyl ammonium acetate; 6: Tetrabutylammonium acetate; 7: 1-n-Butyl-3-methylimidazolium methylsulfate; 8: 1,3-dimethylimidazolium methylsulfate; 9: 1-Butyl-3-methylimidazolium Hexafluorophosphate; 10: 1,2 - dimethyl tetrafluoroborate.

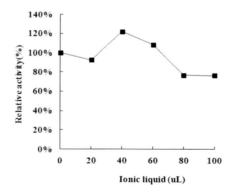

Figure 2. Effects of [C_2mim][MetSO_4] addition on the biotransformation of isoeugenol to vanillin by *Bacillus fusiformis* CGMCC1347.

IL not only causes high ionic strength in the enzymatic reaction medium that might inactivate the isoeugenol monooxygenase, but also leads to high viscosity of the reaction mixture, limiting the diffusion of isoeugenol which results in a drop in the enzymatic reaction (Wang J, 2013). Based on this study, [C_2mim][MetSO_4]was found to be more suitable than the other ILs as co-solvents in the enzymatic reaction medium and its suitable addition was 40 µL in 10 mL reaction buffer.

3.2   *Effects of isoeugenol amount and the ionic liquid/isoeugenol*

For an enzyme-catalysed reaction, there is usually a hyperbolic relationship between the rate of reaction and the concentration of substrate. At low concentration of substrate, there is a steep increase in the rate of reaction with increasing substrate concentration. As the concentration of substrate increases, the enzyme becomes saturated with substrate. As soon as the catalytic site is empty, more substrate is available to bind and undergo the reaction. The rate of formation of product now depends on the activity of the enzyme itself, and adding more substrate will not affect the rate of the reaction to any significant effect.

As shown in Fig.3, the suitable isoeugenol addition for this biotransformation was 400 µL and IL was 40 µL. Further more isoeugenol couldn't increase vanillin production.

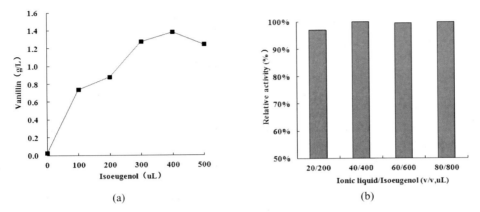

(a)   (b)

Figure 3.   Effects of isoeugenol amount on the biotransformation of isoeugenol to vanillin by *Bacillus fusiformis* CGMCC1347. (a) isoeugenol ranged from 0 to 500 µL with fixed 40 µL [C_2mim][MetSO_4]; (b) isoeugenol ranged from 20 to 800 µL with fixed 1:10 (v/v) of [C_2mim][MetSO_4]/isoeugenol.

3.3   *Effects of initial pH*

It is well known that pH plays a crucial role in enzymatic reaction. In general, variation in pH will alter the ionic state of substrate and enzymes involved in the reaction. In this system, initial pH ranged from 6 to 8.5. As a result, in this pH range, it had no obvious effect on this biotransformation (data not shown).

3.4   *Effects of reaction time*

As shown in Fig. 4, with the addition of 40 µL and 400 µL isoeugenol into the reaction liquid, the vanillin concentration increased linearly during the initial 60 h and reached a maximal level of 1.38 g/L. The vanillin concentration reached the reaction balance in the following 12 h.

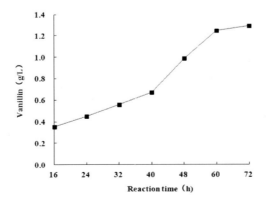

Figure 4.   Effects of reaction time on the biotransformation of isoeugenol to vanillin by *Bacillus fusiformis* CGMCC1347 with addition of IL.

4 CONCLUSION

In this paper, an ionic liquid (IL)-containing buffer system was first applied in the conversion of isoeugenol to vanillin by *Bacillus fusiformis* CGMCC1347. [C_2mim][MetSO_4] was the suitable ionic liquid tested for this biotransformation. The optimal biotransformation conditions were as following: [C_2mim][MetSO_4] 40 μL, isoeugenol 400 μL for 10 mL reaction liquid in 50-mL flask, phosphate buffer (pH 7.0) 50 mM, 37°C, 180 r/min. The Maximum vanillin concentration reached 1.38 g/L in 60 h.

ACKNOWLEDGEMENT

This work was supported by Shenzhen Dedicated Funding of Strategic Emerging Industry Development Program (JCYJ20140418091413576).

REFERENCES

Ashengroph, M., I. Nahvi and J. Amini (2013) "Application of Taguchi Design and Response Surface Methodology for Improving Conversion of Isoeugenol into Vanillin by Resting Cells of Psychrobacter sp CSW4." *Iranian Journal of Pharmaceutical Research,* 12(3), 411–421.

Ashengroph, M., I. Nahvi, H. Zarkesh-Esfahani and F. Momenbeik (2011) "Candida galli Strain PGO6: A Novel Isolated Yeast Strain Capable of Transformation of Isoeugenol into Vanillin and Vanillic Acid." *Current Microbiology,* 62(3), 990–998.

Ashengroph, M., I. Nahvi, H. Zarkesh-Esfahani and F. Momenbeik (2012) "Conversion of Isoeugenol to Vanillin by Psychrobacter sp Strain CSW4." *Applied Biochemistry and Biotechnology,* 166(1), 1–12.

Druaux, D., G. Mangeot, A. Endrizzi and J. M. Belin (1997) "Bacterial bioconversion of primary aliphatic and aromatic alcohols into acids: Effects of molecular structure and physico-chemical conditions." *Journal of Chemical Technology and Biotechnology,* 68(2), 214–218.

Li, Y. H., Z. H. Sun and P. Zheng (2004) "Determination of vanillin, eugenol and isoeugenol by RP-HPLC." *Chromatographia,* 60(11–12), 709–713.

Moniruzzaman M, N. K., Kamiyaa N, Goto M, (2010) "Recent advances of enzymatic reactions in ionic liquids." *Biochemical Engineering Journal,* 48, 295–314.

Priefert, H., S. Achterholt and A. Steinbuchel (2002) "Transformation of the Pseudonocardiaceae Amycolatopsis sp strain HR167 is highly dependent on the physiological state of the cells." *Applied Microbiology and Biotechnology,* 58(4), 454–460.

Ryu, J. Y., J. Seo, S. Park, J. H. Ahn, Y. Chong, M. J. Sadowsky and H. G. Hur (2013) "Characterization of an Isoeugenol Monooxygenase (Iem) from Pseudomonas nitroreducens Jin1 That Transforms Isoeugenol to Vanillin." *Bioscience Biotechnology and Biochemistry,* 77(2), 289–294.

Su, F., D. L. Hua, Z. B. Zhang, X. Y. Wang, H. Z. Tang, F. Tao, C. Tai, Q. L. Wu, G. Wu and P. Xu (2011) "Genome Sequence of Bacillus pumilus S-1, an Efficient Isoeugenol-Utilizing Producer for Natural Vanillin." *Journal of Bacteriology,* 193(22), 6400–6401.

Wang J, S. G., Yu L , Wu F, Guo XJ (2013) "Enhancement of the selective enzymatic biotransformation of rutinto isoquercitrin using an ionic liquid as a co-solvent." *Bioresource Technology,* 128, 156–163.

Yang, R. L., N. Li and M. H. Zong (2012) "Using ionic liquid cosolvents to improve enzymatic synthesis of arylalkyl beta-D-glucopyranosides." *Journal of Molecular Catalysis B-Enzymatic,* 74(1–2), 24–28.

Zhao, L. Q., Z. H. Sun, P. Zheng and J. Y. He (2006) "Biotransformation of isoeugenol to vanillin by Bacillus fusiformis CGMCC1347 with the addition of resin HD-8." *Process Biochemistry,* 41(7), 1673–1676.

Zhao, L. Q., Z. H. Sun, P. Zheng and L. L. Zhu (2005) "Biotransformation of isoeugenol to vanillin by a novel strain of Bacillus fusiformis." *Biotechnology Letters,* 27(19), 1505–1509.

Medicine Sciences and Bioengineering – Wang (Ed.)
© *2015 Taylor & Francis Group, London, ISBN: 978-1-138-02684-1*

New method for producing diosgenin

Xiang Li, Li-ping Wang, Chun-lan Shi & Bin Zhang
*College of Chemistry and Chemical Engineering, Shaanxi University of Science and Technology, Xi'an,
ShaanXi, China*

ABSTRACT: A new method for diosgenin is introduced. The new method can achieve the
purpose of the diosgenin clean production under low cost.

1 INTRODUCTION

Dioscorea Zingiberensis C.H Wright (DZW), generally known as "Yellow Ginger", contains 5%
of dioscin, which, under the effect of acid or enzyme, will be hydrolyzed into Diosgenin, which is
a raw material needed in synthesizing about 400 different kinds of steroid hormones. On the basis
of laboratory studies, 500 kg of DZW is used as main raw material and ultrasonic-assisted extraction method is adopted, surfactant is introduced to improve the dioscin solubility. Flocculation of
dioscin is the key to this new method for producing diosgenin (appreciated into New Method).
Five experiments were carried out and the yield rate of diosgenin, material cost, discharge of
wastewater, the COD, BOD and color of wastewater as the evaluation criteria to study the influence this new method will have on the production of diosgenin. Based on this, a comparison is
made between this method and the traditional method, and it is discovered that the new method
can produce the most diosgenin; the material cost is the lowest; the discharge of wastewater and
its COD, BOD is the least, and they all meet the national discharge standard for companies of this
type, and they also basically meet the national discharge standard for newly-established companies
that produce diosgenin, so it is a very promising clean production method.

2 MATERIALS AND METHODS

2.1 *New method for producing diosgenin*

2.2 *Control experiment*

The procedure of the control experiment is similar to one of the new method. Their differences
lie in: 1). Ethanol of 95% is used as extraction agent. 2). Replace the flocculation technology
with vacuum concentration technology, ethanol and dioscin extractum are obtained after vacuun
concentration. Then dioscin extractum become diosgenin by acidolysis, neutralization, filtration,
drying and supercritical fluid extraction, The processing conditions are same as the new method
for producing diosgenin.

3 RESULTS AND DISCUSSIONS

3.1 *The yield of diosgenin*

Do the experiments according to 2.2, and the yields of diosgenin are shown in Table 1.

Table 1. the yield rates of the three experimental methods.

Experiment NO		1	2	3	4	5	Mean value
The new method	Output of diosgein/kg	11.98	11.91	12.31	12.66	12.64	12.30
	Yield of diosgenin/%	2.396	2.382	2.462	2.532	2.528	2.471
The control method	Output of diosgein/kg	11.31	11.49	11.61	11.96	10.98	11.47
	Yield of diosgenin/%	2.262	2.298	2.322	2.392	2.196	2.294
The traditional method	Output of diosgein/kg	10.95	10.96	10.93	10.95	10.93	10.94
	Yield of diosgenin/%	2.189	2.192	2.186	2.190	2.185	2.188

Note: The output of diosgenin is obtained by 500kg DZW in their respective experimental conditions, the yield of diosgenin = the output of diosgenin × its purity /500 × 100%.

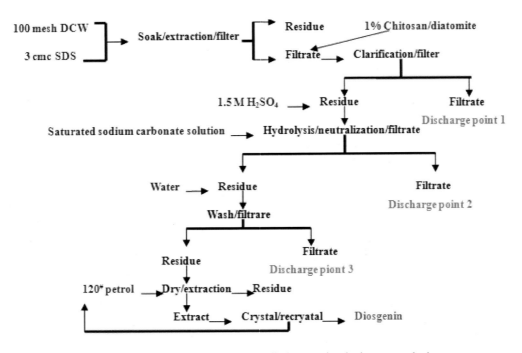

Figure 1. The technological processes and wastewater discharge points in the new method.

It can be seen from Table 1 that the new method (using 25.8×10^{-3} mol/L of Sodium dodecyl sulfate as extraction agent) has the highest yield of diosgenin, to 2.471%; the traditional method has the lowest yield of diosgenin, at 2.188%, the yield of diosgenin of the control method (using 75% of ethanol as extraction agent) fall in between, at 2.294%. So the yield of diosgenin of the new method is 0.117% higher than one of the control methods.

3.2 Raw material cost of the three methods

Do the experiments according to 2.2, and record the raw material consumption in the process of diosgenin production by each, and then work out the raw material cost with reference to the price for the raw material. The results are shown in Table 2.

It can be seen from Table 2 and Table 3 that the new method has the lowest raw material cost, about 300,000 yuan, and that is only 33.34% of the control experiment and 84.75% of the traditional method.

Table 2. The cost of raw material.

	The new method	The control method	The traditional method
Yield of diosgenin/%	2.471	2.294	2.188
The cost of raw material/yuan/ton	302,113	906,277	356,490

Table 3. Comprehensive assessment on the pollution of the two methods.

	Wstewater discharge/m³/t	COD/mg/mL	BOD mg/mL	Color index
The traditionl method	427	31076	6218	474
The new mothod	442	293	58	76
The discharge standard of the old factory	600	400	60	100
The discharge standard of the new factory	400	300	50	80

3.3 *Environmental pollution of the new method and traditional method*

The wastewater discharge and test the COD, BOD, color of the wastewaters. The results are as in Table 3.

It can be seen from Table 3, using the new method, the wastewater discharge, its COD, BOD and color, can reach the discharge standard of the old factory, and after a simple treatment they can also meet the discharge standard of the old factory.

4 CONCLUSION

Using the yield of diosgenin, raw material cost, wastewater discharge, wastewater properties as a comprehensive evaluation criteria, it can be seen that this method, under current technological conditions, is a very promising method to realize the clean production of diosgenin.

ACKNOWLEGEMENTS

This work was supported by Shaan Xi Education Department Project (2012JC06), The Dr scientific research funds (BJ13-10), Jiangxi plan projects (ZBBF60011), Jiujiang projects (131).

REFERENCES

Huang Wen, Huazhang Zhao, Jinren Ni(2008), The best utilization of D.Zingiberensis C.H. Wright by an ecofriendly process[J].Bioresource technology,99(15):7405–7411.
Yuqing Zhang, Linru Tang, Xuan An, etc(2009). Modification of cellulase and its application to extraction of diosgenin from Dioscorea zingiberensis C.H.Wright[J]. Biochemical Engineering Journal 47:80–86.
Li Xiang, Ma Jianzhong, Xia Jing (2011). Surfactant assisted ethanol extraction of Dioscin [J]. Journal of Medicinal Plants Research, 5(3) :324–331.
Li Xiang (2012). Study on the key technologies of diosgenin cleaner production and resources utilization of Dioscorea zingiberensis[D]. Shaan xi university of science and technology.
Zhang Liming, Zuo Beimei, Wu Peilong, etc(2012). Ultrasound effects on the acetylation of dioscorea starch isolated from Diosorea zingiberbensis C.H.Wright [J]. Chemical Engineering and Processing: Process Intensification, 54:29–36.

Medicine Sciences and Bioengineering – Wang (Ed.)

Sulfate-reducing bacteria anaerobic metabolism carbon source test of Huainan coal

Chun Qi, Xiao-guang Ge*, Shuo Liu & Guang-xiu Zhao
School of Resources and Environmental Engineering, Hefei University of Technology, Hefei, Anhui, China

Liu Yang & Yong-kang Ye
School of Biotechnology and Food Engineering, Hefei University of Technology, Hefei, Anhui, China

ABSTRACT: A study on relationship between Sulfate-Reducing Bacteria (SRBs) in groundwater under the coal mine and coal samples in Permian formation taken from the Huainan Panbei coal mine was done. The water samples from borehole were detected with 16SrRNA gene sequencing and systematically compared. A SRB strain of Desulfovibrio genus was detected out. A GC-MS test matched 21 macromolecule organic compounds by methanol extraction of coal samples. From SRB-carbon source adaptability comparison test, it is found that butyleret hydroxytoluen and 2-hexyl-1-Decanol were good carbon sources for SRBs' anaerobic metabolism, while Naphthalene,2,6-dimethyl was not effectively degradaed as the carbon source. The conclusions suggested carbon sources needed by sulfate reduction in groundwater in coal fields could come from surrounding coal seams themselves.

1 INTRODUCTION

Sulfate reduction occurs in different anaerobic/anoxic and organism-rich environments such as ocean bottoms, hot springs, soils, sludge, oil, gas, and coal fields, and often was accompanied with methanogenesis in the nature (Wawrik *et al*., 2012, Wentzel *et al*., 2013), and was known to produce by SRBs (sulfate reducing bacteria). We recently found strong rotten egg smells and black bacteria mats at the orifices of drainage boreholes at the coal mine's wickets in Huainan coal-field in China, which meant the presence of SRBs in groundwater in coal-bearing strata (Wawrik *et al*., 2012, An *et al*., 2013, Ge *et al*., 2011).

The aim of our work was to verify if SRBs anaerobic metabolism in groundwater in coal seams could use and how to utilize the macromolecular organic compounds in the coals.

2 MATERIALS AND METHODS

2.1 *Sample sources*

The groundwater samples were taken from a drainage borehole at 530 m depth in a Panbei coal mine in Anhui, China. The samples were smelly and contained black flocs and the temperature at 38.4°C. We scraped bacterial mats attached on the borehole collar into two 250-ml glass bottles with a sterilized spoon, and filled the bottles with the water overflowed from borehole orifice, then sealed the bottle with a Teflon-lined cap, and sent them to the laboratory on the same day, and stored under 4°C.

---

*Project (41172216) supported by the National Natural Science Foundation of China;
Corresponding author: Tel.:+86 551 62902983. E-mail: xgge@hfut.edu.cn, xgge.cn@qq.com.

Coal samples were taken from coal seam A1-3 of the Lower Permian Shanxi Formation, and were saved with sealed HDPE bags.

2.2 The enrichment, isolation and naming of SRBs

2.2.1 Medium components and method of enrichment and separation

SRB enrichment medium (Postgate, 1984): The medium contained the following constituents (in 1L volume): KH_2PO_4 0.5g, NH_4Cl 1.0 g, Na_2SO_4 4.5 g, $CaCl_2$ 0.06 g, $MgSO_4 \cdot 7H_2O$ 2.0 g, $FeSO_4 \cdot 7H_2O$ 0.5 g, yeast extract 1.0 g, L-cysteine 0.2 g, lactate 3 ml; distilled water was added into a culture flask to be seeded. The pH was adjusted to about 7.2. After oxygen was removed with nitrogen filling, most media, together with culture flask, were sterilized in autoclave under 1×10^5 Pa. But $FeSO_4 \cdot 7H_2O$ and L-cysteine were UV lamp-treated due to their poor heat resistance (Jiménez-Rodríguez et al., 2009). Configured medium was poured into a medical brine bottle of 250 ml and 1ml of bacteria sample was inoculated on the sterile table, then anaerobically cultured at 35°C.

SRBs isolation: Enriched bacterial liquid was diluted to 10 times under the protection of nitrogen, isolated and cultured using Hungate rolling-tube anaerobic technique (Hungate & Macy, 1973) . This procedure was repeated 20 times to obtain pure colonies.

A scanning electron microscope (SEM) was used to take photos and observe the SRB after 6d of cultivation. The procedure included: the bacterial liquid centrifugation, glutaraldehyde fixation, ethanol dehydration, freeze-drying, Gold plating, and microscopic imaging (Bozzola & Russell, 1999). Microscopic imaging and photo taking of final samples were carried out on the field emission scanning electron microscope (SU8020, Hitachi, Japan).

2.2.2 SRB gene phylogenetic tree

The DNA of separated bacteria was extracted by Ezup column extraction kit and polymerase chain reaction amplification (PCR) of 16S rRNA was performed using the primer AprA-1-FW/ AprA-5-RV (Etebu, 2013), then was sent to the Shanghai Shenggong Company for gene sequencing after recycled by SanPro gel extraction kit. The measured sample sequence similarity analysis was performed in the GenBank DNA sequence database using the BLAST program on the NCBI website. The sequences highly homologous with this strain were selected to establish a phylogenetic tree by the N-J method using software MEGA5.1.

2.3 GC-MS analysis of the organic components in coal samples

2.3.1 Organic components extraction from coal

8 g of coal sample was transferred to a 150 ml beaker after drying, smashing (JP-150A-8 mill) and sieving through 200 mesh, and 50 ml of methanol solvent was added to the beaker. The solid-liquid organic mixture was extracted in an ultrasonic cleaning machine (KQ218) for 1h, and extracted in a Soxhlet extractor (YMST-250Q) at 60°C for 80h; then the supernatants were centrifuged in a rotary evaporator at 120rpm till 10ml of concentrated extracts was obtained.

2.3.2 Coal analysis with gas chromatography-mass spectrometry (GC-MS)

The component profile of the coal sample extract was measured with a gas-chromatography- mass spectrometry (RUKER Scion SQ). Work conditions: DB-5 capillary column (30.0m × 250 μm × 0.25 μm), carrier gas N_2, airflow rate 1.0ml/min, inlet temperature 300°C, programmed rising column temperature: maintaining 100°C for 2min, then increasing to 300°C, at 10°C/min, keeping 10 min; MS conditions: EI source 70eV, ion source 230°C; mass scanning: 30-500amu. The measured chromatographies were retrieved with NIST compound mass spectral library database to obtain the chemical species of the corresponding compounds (Liu et al., 2003).

2.4 Observation on SRBs degrading carbon sources

2.4.1 Methods

Three typical organic compounds were selected which were abundant at the coal's GC-MS organic component profile and easily purchasing from markets. Each of them was treated as a substitute of the carbon source sodium-lactate in the SRBs enrichment medium mentioned above. Each was added into the medium at 2 g/l concentration, and a distilled water sample was also added as a control. SRBs were cultured in each medium in an anaerobic incubation flask. The four incubation flasks were put in a shock incubator cultured at 35°C. The produced gas in each flask was extracted with sampling needle, and the culture solution in each incubation flask was extracted under nitrogen protecting ones every 72 h. All of their H_2S and SO_4^{2-} contents were measured during the incubation period.

2.4.2 Measurement

a. Gas H_2S was measured with a Gas-Phase Molecular Absorption Spectrometry (AJ-2100) (Shyla & Nagendrappa, 2012). b. Anion SO_4^{2-} was measured by turbidimetry techniques.

2.5 Verification of sulfur transformation in SRBs culture process

Three pieces of glass, in size of 3 mm × 3 mm × 0.5 mm, were immersed in each culture flask beforehand. One piece glass was taken from each culture flask under nitrogen protection and was put into a plastic tube filled with nitrogen, after 0 d, 6 d and 15 d, respectively. Then they were sent to a vacuum freeze drier (DZF-6030B) to be dried more than 2 d. Then the medium components were detected with XPS (ESCALAB250, Thermo Co. USA), and the spectrum peak distribution of sulfur S2p BE was focusedly observed.

3 TEST RESULTS AND DISCUSSION

3.1 SRBs' isolation and appraisal results

1ml of original groundwater sample from the coal mine was inoculated in enriching medium, oxygen was removed with nitrogen filling. A part of culture in the bottle turned black after 3d of anaerobical incubation, and most turned black after 6d. A wetted lead acetate paper turned dark as being put at the bottle mouth, which indicates that H2S gas occurred and a large number of SRBs had reproduced. It can be observed from the scanning electron micrograph (Figure 1), that most cells are short arc and cell size (0.3 ~ 0.4 μm) × (1.5 ~ 2 μm).

3.2 SRB phylogenetic tree

A 384 bp of nucleotide sequence was obtained from the isolated strain, named as S890, after PCR amplification and 16S rRNA gene sequencing. The measured sample sequence similarity analysis was performed with the GenBank DNA sequence database using the BLAST program on the

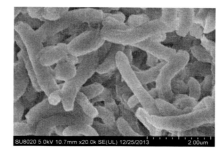

Figure 1. Scanning electron micrograph of SRB after anaerobicly cultured 5d (× 20000).

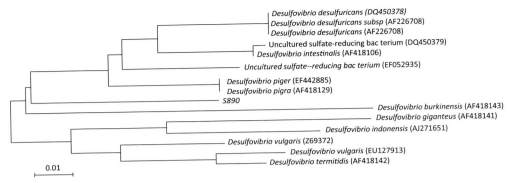

Figure 2. Phylogenetic tree based on 16S rRNA sequences of strain S890 and related species using Neighbor-Joining method.

NCBI website. 14 pieces of sequences highly homologous with the strain were selected to establish a neighbor-joining phylogenetic tree by MEGA5.1 shown in Figure 2. The sequence similarity between strain S890 and *Desulfovibrio piger* was of the highest level, meant the strain belonged to *Desulfovibrio*, a common SRB genus.

3.3 Analysis results of coal samples organic components

Total ionic chromatogram (TIC) of the methanol extracts of Huainan mine's coal sample was gained by GC-MS measurement, as shown in Figure 3. The chief period in the TIC was $t = 5–20$ min. The most prominent 24 peaks were numbered in the figure, and 21 essential organic compounds were matched by NIST library index, and their names were listed in Table 1.

All these organic compounds were senior chain hydrocarbons, cyclic hydrocarbons, aromatic hydrocarbons and their derivatives, which contain above 11 carbon atoms in carbon chains. Butyleret hydroxytoluen, 2-hexyl-1-Decanol, Naphthalene, 1,4,5,8-tetramethyl and 11,14-Octa-decadienoic acid, methyl ester, etc. were most abundant among the 21 compounds. A small amount of organosulfur compound 2-Myristynoyl pantetheine and organonitrogen compound 2-Azido-2,4,4,6,6-pentamethylheptane were also found, and coincided with the facts a little of organic sulfur and organic nitrogen depositing within the coals (Thomas, 2012).

3.4 Comparison of the carbon source adaptability to SRBs

3.4.1 Carbon source choice
Three types of organic compounds 2-hexyl-1-Decanol (HED for short), butyleret hydroxytoluen (BHT) and 2,6-Dimethylnaphthalene (DIN) were chosen as samples for the carbon source adaptability comparison test, because the former two compounds were abundant, and the third could be as the representative of four kinds of mult-methylnaphthalenes (See Table 1) .

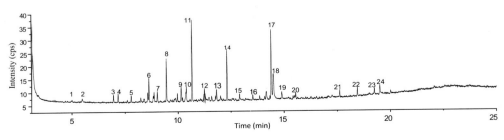

Figure 3. Methanol extracts GC-MS total ions chromatogram of Huainan coal.

Table 1. Identified compounds in methanol extracts of Panbei coal by GC-MS.

No	Formula	Compound name
1, 4	$C_{22}H_{42}O_4$	Bis(2-ethylhexyl) adipate
2	$C_{15}H_{28}O_2$	Cyclohexanecarboxylic acid,octyl este
3	$C_{11}H_{18}O_3$	3,3-Dimethyl-1,5-dioxaspiro[5.5]undecan-9-one
5, 18	$C_{18}H_{34}O_2$	Oleic acid
6	$C_{11}H_{10}$	1-methylnaphthalene
7	$C_{12}H_{12}$	2,6-Dimethylnaphthalene
8	$C_{15}H_{24}O$	butyleret hydroxytoluen
9	$C_{13}H_{14}$	Naphthalene,2,3,6-trimethyl-
10	$C_{13}H_{14}$	Naphthalene,1,4,6-trimethyl)
11, 21	$C_{16}H_{34}O$	2-hexyl-1-Decanol
12	$C_{17}H_{34}O_2$	Methyl Palmitate
13	$C_{25}H_{44}N_2O_5S$	2-Myristynoyl pantetheine
14	$C_{14}H_{16}$	Naphthalene,1,4,5,8-tetramethyl-
15	$C_{20}H_{14}O_2$	9,10-Ethanoanthracene,9,10-dihydro-11,12-diacethyl-
16	$C_{32}H_{54}O_4$	Didodecyl phthalate
17	$C_{19}H_{34}O_2$	11,14-Octadecadienoic acid,methyl ester
19	$C_{19}H_{38}O_2$	Heptadecanoic acid,16-methyl-, methyl ester
20	$C_{16}H_{14}$	Phenanthrene,2,7-dimethyl-
22	$C_{21}H_{44}$	Heptadecane,2,6,10,15-tetramethyl-
23	$C_{16}H_{32}O_2$	4-Propionyloxytridecane
24	$C_{12}H_{25}N_3$	2-Azido-2,4,4,6,6-pentamethylheptane

DIN (purity > 98%) was purchased from Sinopharm Chemical Reagent (Shanghai, China); HED (purity > 97%) from Sigma-Aldrich Chemistry (Steinheim, Germany); DIN (purity > 98%) from Kasei Kogyo (Tokyo, Japan).

3.4.2 *Test results*

The three kinds of chemicals as well as distilled water were added to the medium substrates to form four groups, namely BHT group, HED group, DIN group and control group (no carbon source).

It can be seen from Figure 4(a) that H_2S generated in BHT and HED group after 6 days of inoculation, and the top rate occurred after 18 days, and HED group was slightly larger than BHT group. The H_2S concentration in DIN group and the control group almost unchanged.

It can be seen from Figure 4(b) that the concentration of substrate SO_4^{2-} in BHT group and HED group began to decrease after 6 days of inoculation, and decreasing rate of SO_4^{2-} in BHT group and

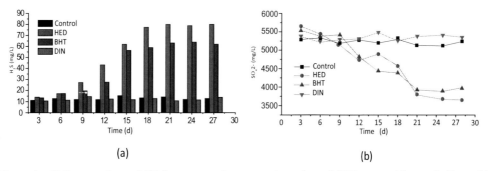

(a)   (b)

Figure 4. H_2S generation and SO_4^{2-} concentration comparison plots of SRBs anaerobic metabolism with carbon sources as BHT (butyleret hydroxytoluen) group, HED (2-hexyl-1-Decanol) group, DIN (2,6-Dimethyl naphthalene) group and Contol (No carbon) group.

HED group reached to 27.9% and 35.2%, respectively, after 27 days, while SO$_4^{2-}$ concentrations in DIN group and the control group were not obviously changed during these days. Both tests reflected that butyleret hydroxytoluen and 2-hexyl-1-Decanol could anaerobic degraded by SRBs effectively, but Naphthalene, 2,6-dimethyl could not be effectively degraded as a carbon source by SRBs.

3.5   *Sulfur valence changes based on XPS*

Preset glasses were taken out from the culture flasks of BHT group, HED group, DIN group and a control group to XPS tests after freeze-drying at the end of 0d, 6d and 15d, respectively. Their XPS spectra of e-counting vs. binding energy (B.E.) were shown in Figure 5 (a) ~ (d).

It can be found from Figure 5 that the initial states of all 4 XPS spectra shows a single peak at 168–169 eV corresponding to the sulfates S2p peaks, which indicated that SO$_4^{2-}$ were dominant before the bacteria cultured. After 6d of incubation, a peak of BHT or HED group at about 160 – 163 eV corresponding to sulfide S2p peaks appeared in addition to sulfate peak. the XPS spectra peaks of BHT or HED group declined further at 168–169 eV segment and rised further at 160 ~ 163 eV segment after 15d, which indicated that sulfate reduction caused by SRBs metabolism were very intensive, while 160–163 eV sulfide peaks of the DIN group and control group never appeared obviously, meant their sulfate reduction did not happen massively. These test results also coincided with the changing processes of ion SO$_4^{2-}$ and gas H$_2$S.

3.6   *Explanation on carbon sources degradation differences*

It could be roughly explained by "electron cloud" theory of organic chemistry, the reason why there are differences among the three carbon source degradation by SRBs anaerobic metabolism (See Figure 6).

All the three chemicals, BHT, HED and DIN, consist mainly of hydrocarbyls ('C-H' bond), but two former chemicals also possess 'hydroxy' ('H-O' bonds). As electron cloud on the hydroxy is

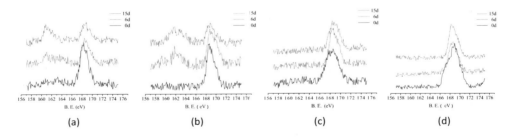

| (a) | (b) | (c) | (d) |

Figure 5.   X-ray photoelectron spectroscopy (XPS) spectra of several carbon sources during different SRBs degradation phases, (a) = BHT (butyleret hydroxytoluen) group, (b) = HED (2-hexyl-1-Decanol) group, (c) = DIN (2,6-Dime-thyl naphthalene) group, (d) = control (no carbon source) group; B.E. represents binding energy; 0d,6d,15d, represent after 0 day, 6 days and 15 days of incubation, respectively.

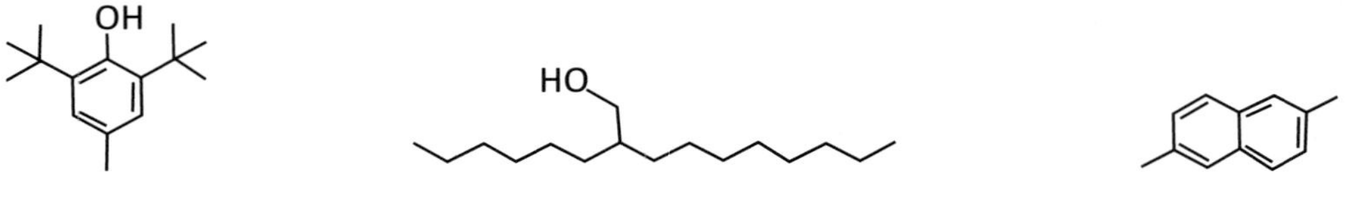

(a) butyleret hydroxytoluenl   (b)2-hexyl-1-Decanol   (c) Naphthalene,2,6-dimethyl-

Figure 6.   Chemical structure diagrams of three experimental organic carbon sources.

strongly bias oxygen atom, H-O bond is weakened, hydrogen atoms are easily dissociated by ions in the medium, such as Na^+, etc. Their resultants combine with polar water molecules in emulsifying style, can be easily utilized by SRBs in water solution. But the naphthalene ring and two methyls in third chemical are all linked by the C-H bond, and has high stability (McMurry, 2012). The poor, liberation properties make it hard to be utilized by SRBs.

The test results confirmed that carbon sources of sulfate reduction in the coal seam groundwater could directly come from the coal itself. There might be more organic compounds in coal seam being degraded by the anaerobic metabolism of other bacteria.

4 CONCLUSION

1. Enriched, isolated and purified water samples were detected with 16SrRNA gene sequencing and systematically compared. A SRB strain of *Desulfovibrio* genus was confirmed. It indicates that there are SRBs in the groundwater in this coal field and sulfate reduction is happening.
2. GC-MS test matched 21 main organic compounds after compounds methanol extraction of coal samples. These compounds were senior chain hydrocarbons, cyclic hydrocarbons, aromatic hydrocarbons and their derivatives. No medium or small organic molecules containing less than 11 carbon atoms was measured on the chromatogram.
3. From the detected organic compounds, three types of organic compounds butyleret hydroxytoluen, 2-hexyl-1-Decanol and Naphthalene,2,6-dimethyl- were chosen as samples for 27 days SRB-carbon-source adaptability comparison test. The results shows that after SRBs inoculated to each culture solution, butyleret hydroxytoluen and 2-hexyl-1-Decanol groups were H_2S generated, and their SO_4^{2-} concentrations decreased 27.9% and 35.2%, after 27 days, respectively. While Naphthalene,2,6-dimethyl group could not be effectively degraded as a carbon source by SRBs, XPS spectra comparison of precipitation during the experiment process showed the similar effects.

REFERENCES

An, D., Caffrey, S. M., Soh, J., Agrawal, A., Brown, D., Budwill, K., Dong, X.L. & Gieg, L.M. (2013) Metagenomics of Hydrocarbon Resource Environments Indicates Aerobic Taxa and Genes to be Unexpectedly Common. *Environmental science & technology*, 47(18), 10708–10717.

Bozzola, J.J. & Russell, L.D. (1999) *Electron microscopy: principles and techniques for biologists*, 2nd edition. Sudbury: Jones & Bartlett Learning. pp. 17–46.

Etebu, E. (2013). Potential Panacea to the Complexities of Polymerase Chain Reaction (PCR). *Advances in Life Science and Technology*, 13(1), 53–59.

GE, X. G., Yang, L., Peng, S. & Li, F. (2011) Isolation and identification of a SRB strain from coal mine groundwater and its characteristics. *Journal of Hefei University of Technology*, 34(3), 420–423.

Hungate, R. E. & Macy, J. (1973) The roll-tube method for cultivation of strict anaerobes. *Bulletins of the Ecological Research Committee*, 17, 123–126.

Jiménez-Rodríguez, A.M., Durán-Barrantes, M.M., Borja, R., Sánchez, E., Colmenarejo, M. F. & Raposo, F. (2009) Heavy metals removal from acid mine drainage water using biogenic hydrogen sulphide and effluent from anaerobic treatment: effect of pH. *Journal of hazardous materials*, 165(1), 759–765.

Liu, Z., Zong, Z. & Wei, X. (2003) GC/MS analysis of Datong raw and oxidized coal extract using methanol/tetrahydrofuran mixed solvent. *Journal of Fuel Chemistry and Technology*, 31(2), 177–180.

McMurry, J. E. (2012) *Organic Chemistry*, 8th edition. Helmot: Cengage Learning, pp.34-39, pp.50–62.

Shyla, B. & Nagendrappa, G. (2012) New spectrophotometric methods for the determinations of hydrogen sulfide present in the samples of lake water, industrial effluents, tender coconut, sugarcane juice and egg. *Spectrochimica Acta: Molecular and Biomolecular Spectroscopy*, 96, pp. 776–783.

Thomas, L. (2012) *Coal geology*. Chichester: John Wiley & Sons. pp. 103–106.

Wawrik, B., Mendivelso, M., Parisi, V. A., Suflita, J.M., Davidova, I.A., Marks, C.R., Van Nostrand, J.D., Liang, Y.T., Zhou, J.Z. & Huizinga, B.J. (2012) Field and laboratory studies on the bioconversion of coal to methane in the San Juan Basin. *FEMS microbiology ecology*, 81(1), 26–42.

Wentzel, A., Lewin, A., Cervantes, F. J., Vallas, s. & Kotlar, H.k. (2013) Deep Subsurface Oil Reservoirs as Poly-extreme Habitats for Microbial Life. *A Current Review. In Polyextremophiles*. Springer Netherlands, pp. 439–466.

Medicine Sciences and Bioengineering – Wang (Ed.)
© *2015 Taylor & Francis Group, London, ISBN: 978-1-138-02684-1*

Optimization of PCR-SSCP analysis conditions on the analysis of microbial communities of the strong-flavor Chinese liquor fermentation

Xin-xin Chen & Lin Yuan[1,*]
College of Life Science, Inner Mongolia University, Hohhot, Inner Mongolia, China

ABSTRACT: The microbial communities of fermented grains were complex during the strong-flavor Chinese liquor fermentation. In this study, by using Single Strand Conformation Polymorphism (SSCP), we optimized the influence factors of microbial communities, including the size of PCR production, concentration of gel, cross-linking degree and temperature of the electrophoresis. Based on SSCP profiles, the optimizing conditions are as follows. The target fragments were PCR-amplified using 16S rDNA V3 region (about 200bp) primers. The volume ratio of denaturing buffer and sample was 1:2. The best gel concentration was 14% and the weight ratio of acrylamide and bis-acrylamide was 49:1. Then electrophoresis for 18h at 4°C with 300 V constant voltage.

1 INTRODUCTION

Pits, which has a variety of micro-organism, is the foundation of strong-flavor Chinese liquor production. Especially, the quality of strong-flavor Chinese liquor production is largely affected by the microorganism. Fermented grains, including a wide range of micro-organism and a complex relationship, mainly come from the wine environment, daqu and pit mud (Lan Pu *et al.*, 2011). It is difficult to analyze fermented grains micro-organism communities by the traditional methods of strain separation, physiological and biochemical analysis.

With the development of modern molecular biology, single-strand conformation polymorphism analysis (SSCP) becomes a new molecular biology area. Generally, the single-stranded nucleotide mutation is detected by using DNA single-strand conformation polymorphism to electrophoresis in non-denaturing polyacrylamide gel. Because of its high sensitivity and simple operation, SSCP is widely used in gene polymorphism analysis and other gene mutation detection, such as cancer genes, tumor-suppressor genes, genetic disorders, autoimmune diseases and infectious diseases (Fang Gui & Zhuoran Zhang, 2005). SSCP technology has made great progress on the analysis of complex microbial community structure (Yan Wang *et al.*, 2009). Kornelia Smalla *et al.* has concluded that SSCP method is more accurate in the analysis of micro-organism community's diversity (Kornelia Smalla *et al.*, 2007).

However, none of the PCR-SSCP method has been applied to analyze all environmental samples. Each sample must consider its unique physical, chemical and biological characteristics, and optimized a special method (Lixin Baoa *et al.*, 2008). In this paper, fermented grains as samples, we studied the factors which impacted on the quality of SSCP profiles. Under optimum conditions, we improved the profile resolution and readability. Obviously, it provided a quick, strong repeatability, high sensitivity method for analysis fermented grain micro-organism community structure.

---

[1]Inner Mongolia University, No.235 West College Road, Hohhot, Inner Mongolia, P.R.C ZIP:010021
yuan0079@163.com

2 MATERIALS AND METHODS

2.1 *Samples*

All of the fermented grain samples were collected from the Hetao Liquor Industry Group in the west of China. The fermented grain samples were collected and stored in −20°C rapidly. This experiment adopted the 13th, 28th, 43th, 60th days fermented grain samples.

2.2 *DNA extraction*

Washing samples three times by adding ultrapure water, centrifuging and discarding the supernatant. DNA extraction buffer and SDS (20%) were added to the samples, vortex for 1 min. The mixture was incubated at 65°C for 20 min, centrifuged at 12000 rpm/min for 10 min, transferred the supernatant into a new tube. Adding an equal volume of chloroform / isoamyl alcohol(v/v,24:1) into the supernatant, centrifuged at 12000 rpm/min for 10 min. The supernatant was added 0.6 times the volume of supernatant precooling isopropyl alcohol, incubated at −20°C for at least 30 min. Then centrifuged at 13000 rpm/min for 10 min. 0.1 × TE buffer was added into pellets and after RNaseA digestion, stored at −20°C.

2.3 *PCR amplification*

Amplification of the partial sequence of 16S rDNA V3 region was performed with the universal primers 338F-1F (5′-ACT CCT ACG GGA GGC AGC AG-3′) and 533R-1R (5′-TTA CCG CGG CTG CTG GCA C-3′). Target fragments were about 190bp. 16S rDNA V4-5 region was performed with the universal primers 519F (5′-CAG CAG CCG CGG TAA TAC-3′)and 926R (5′-CCG TCA ATT CCT TTG AGT TT-3′). Target fragments were about 400bp. The 25 μL PCR reaction system was performed, containing 2.5 μL 10 × PCR buffer (Mg2+), 4.0 μL dNTP, 0.5 μL Taq polymerase (5 U/μL), 0.5 μL of each primer (20 μmol/L), 2.5 μL Template DNA (100ng/μL) and 18.5μL DD water. All amplification systems were determined as follows: 35 cycles, 94°C for 30 s, 57°C for 30 s and 72°C for 20 s, and a final elongation at 72°C for 5 min. The PCR products were separated with 2% agarose gel.

2.4 *PCR-SSCP analysis*

Mixing loading buffer and PCR product, and the mixture was denatured by boiling 10 min, then removing it on ice over 10 min. The denatured samples were added in non-denaturing polyacrylamide gel electrophoresis in 1 × TBE buffer.

After electrophoresis, washing the gel with DD water for twice. Silver stained 15 min, washed 3–5 times. Then put it into precooling color reagent. After the gel color became black, we replaced liquid of color reagent, until bands appeared. Substituted stop buffer for color reagent to stop the color reaction. Finally, added DD water, store.

2.5 *Optimization of PCR-SSCP analysis conditions*

In SSCP analysis, denaturing buffer and sample volume ratio, the length of DNA fragments had a great influence on the clarity and sensitivity of SSCP profiles. We studied on the ratio of three different denaturing buffer and the sample (Table 1), two kinds of DNA fragments length and polyacrylamide gel conditions (Table 2), six different combinations of polyacrylamide gel concentration (Table 3), and the influence of temperature on SSCP profile quality. Although 16% gel could separate a certain number of microbial groups, the microbial community diversity had not shown. Due to the large concentration of gel, many bands could not be separated. Therefore, 16% gel was not considered for the test (Aijie Wang *et al.*, 2008).

Table 1. Optimization of the ratio of denaturing buffer and samples.

Test	Denaturing buffer	Samples
1	5μL	5μL
2	7.5μL	5μL
3	10μL	5μL

Table 2. The length of DNA fragment and polyacrylamide gel conditions.

Test	Length of DNA fragment	Concentration of polyacrylamide gel
1	190bp	10%
2	400bp	10%

Table 3. The optimization of gel conditions.

Test	Gel concentration	Degree of cross-linking
1	10%	29:1
2	10%	49:1
3	12%	29:1
4	12%	49:1
5	14%	29:1
6	14%	49:1

3 RESULTS AND ANALYSIS

3.1 *Effect of the ratio of denaturing buffer and the samples on SSCP*

Some of the references indicated that high concentrations of denaturing buffer easily lead to Single-stranded template DNA chain, which cannot be formed inside hydrogen bonds and stable three-dimensional structure, thereby affecting the SSCP profiles. The volume ratio of the denaturing buffer and the samples were 1:1, 1:1.5, and 1:2, respectively. Then made the DNA denaturation for SSCP (Fig. 1). Thus, when denaturing buffer and samples in the proportion of 1:2, SSCP profile band neat and high definition, it was beneficial for subsequent sequencing analysis.

3.2 *Effect of the length of 16s rDNA amplification fragments on SSCP profile*

With the V3 and V4-5 region primer amplification of PCR product, after degeneration, electrophoresis in the gel concentration of 10% polyacrylamide gel, we got the SSCP profiles (Figure 2). Lane 1–4 were V3 primers amplification product, lane 5-8 were V4-5 region primers amplification product. Lane 1–4 with a rich band and separating effect was good, the migration rate of lane 5–8 samples was relatively slow, and the bands were little and poor readability. So the smaller segments of nucleic acid, the higher SSCP detection sensitivity.

3.3 *Effect of gel conditions on SSCP*

3.3.1 *Effect of gel concentration*

Different proportion polyacrylamide gel affected the mass fraction of water in the gel, which directly led a change in DNA sample migration rate. The results (Fig. 3) show that under the same conditions of cross-linking degree, 14% polyacrylamide gel SSCP profiles, which could separate more bands, and the bands were more clear, diversity and readability, was the most suitable. It could well reflect the fermented grains of microbial diversity and dominance.

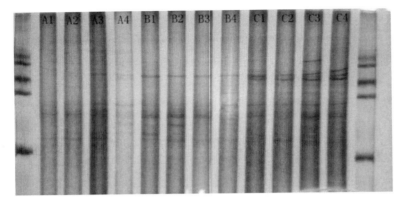

Figure 1.　The optimization of the ratio of denaturing buffer and sample.

Note: the A, B, C corresponded test 1,2,3 in table 1

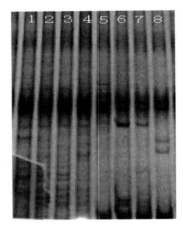

Figure 2.　different fragment size product SSCP profiles.

Note: the lane 1–4 and 5–8 respectively corresponding to test 1 and 2 in table 2

3.3.2　Cross-linking degree optimization

SSCP analysis using non-denaturing polyacrylamide gel, gel pore size was determined by the chain length and the degree of cross-linking. Chain length depends on the concentration of polymerization of acrylamide. Acrylamide and N, N '- methylene double the proportion of acrylamide (Acr: Bis) determined the amount of cross-linking degree. When Acr:Bis = 49:1, electrophoresis fastest and we could obtain better separation of bands and higher resolution. It indicates that a high degree of cross-linking could promote the separation of some SSCP bands (Taiyun We et al., 2002). Richness of bands, therefore, this condition of profile had large distribution range. (Figures 3,4).When Acr:Bis = 29:1, bands were with poor clarity. That is likely due to unstablity of the conformation of single-stranded DNA under this cross-linking degree.

In order to further improve the resolution of the gel effect, we chose 200 bp DNA fragments, and discussed the influence of the quality of SSCP profiles under 29:1 and 49:1 of the ratio of Acr and Bis, respectively. As shown in Figure 3, with the sixth group of the experimental conditions, the SSCP profile was the optimal method. That is, Acr:Bis = 49:1 is the best cross-linking degree, which could be used in the fermented grains of microbial community structure analysis.

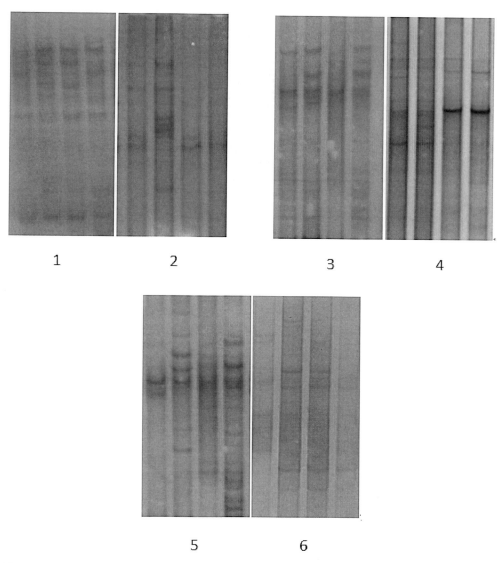

Figure 3.　SSCP profiles under different condition of gel.

Note: the picture 1-6 corresponding test 1-6 in table 3

3.3.3　*Influence of temperature on gel*

It is generally believed that maintaining a constant gel temperature is one of the most critical condition in SSCP analysis. The temperature could directly affect the detection of differences in nucleotide by affecting the formation of single-stranded DNA conformation and the stability of the internal forces. Generally, operation of the PCR-SSCP method is performed at 4°C. It is difficult to control temperature conditions, because of the phenomenon that temperature rises when electrophoresis occurs. This test takes a lower voltage, circulating water cooling, and air cooling measures to ensure a constant temperature during electrophoresis. The results show that by using 300 V and 18 h, the SSCP profiles under the condition of 4°C (Figure 4B) was bright yellow, bands

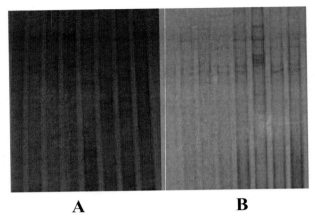

A   B

Figure 4.   The comparison of SSCP profiles at room temperature (A) and 4°C(B).

were clear and easy to observe. While SSCP profiles formed at room temperature electrophoresis conditions (Figure 4A), gel was black and could not be easily observed. When the temperature is unstable, the electrophoretic bands proned to bending. Therefore, SSCP profiles obtained at 4°C had a higher resolution and readability.

4 CONCLUSION

Due to the complexity of fermented grain community structure, the SSCP method requires more higher when using PCR-SSCP method to analyse microbial community structure in fermented grains. By SSCP conditional optimization analysis, we indicated that under the condition of bacterial 16S rDNA V3 region (about 200bp) PCR amplification fragments, denaturing buffer and sample volume ratio weight 1:2, boiling degeneration for 10 min, ice bath over 10min, the gel concentration was 14%, acrylamide and bis-acrylamide weight ratio of 49:1 and electrophoresis for 18h at 4°C with 300 V constant voltage, silver staining, we could obtain a more ideal SSCP profiles. In conclusion, in recent years, PCR-SSCP study gradually was taken seriously. However, this method is still seldom applied to study the aspect of liquor-making microorganism. We explore this method, with the hope that it can be used as a reference in the future application of research liquor-making microorganism.

ACKNOWLEDGEMENTS

I would like to express my gratitude to all those who helped me during the writing of this Paper, especially Lin Yuan teacher selfless help. The corresponding author of this paper is Lin Yuan (Inner Mongolia University, No.235 West College Road, Hohhot, Inner Mongolia, P.R.C ZIP:010021 E-mail: yuan0079@163.com).

REFERENCES

Aijie Wang, Hongjing Kan, Zhengguo Yu. (2008) Optimization and testing of SSCP method of microbial community structure of activated sludge.Microbiology, 35(7),1164–1169.

Kornelia Smalla, Miruna Oros-Sichler, Annett Milling, et al. (2007) Bacterial diversity of soils assessed by DGGE, T-RFLP and SSCP fingerprints of PCR-amplified 16S rRNA gene fragments: Do the different methods provide similar results.Journal of Microbiological Methods, 69,470–479.

Lan Pu, Lu Li, Cishan Xie.(2011) The variation tendency of Zaopei microbes in strong-flavor Chinese Liquor pits . Liquor-Making Science & Technology, 2011(1),17–19.

Lixin Bao, Jianzheng Li, Yan Zhao. (2008) Optimization of PCR-SSCP of anaerobic sludge microbial communities.Science & Technology Review, 26(2),28–32.

Taiyun Wei, Hanxin Lin, Lianhui Xie. (2002) Optimization of PCR-SSCP analysis conditions.Journal of Fujian Agriculture and Forestry University (Natural Science Edition),31(1),32–52.

Wenxue Zhang, Zongwei Qiao, Xiangliang Lv. (2004) Research progress of strong-flavor Chinese Liquor pits microorganisms. Liquor-making, 31(2),31–35.

Yan Wang, Xiquan Shen, Zufang Wu. (2009) The application of PCR - SSCP method in analysis of microbial community polymorphism. Biotechnology,19(3),84–87.

Author index

An, L.-P., 341
Ang, S.S., 373

Bai, G., 805
Bai, Y., 587
Bao, M.-Z., 305
Bian, L., 203
Bradshaw, T., 13

Cai, F.-Y., 577
Cao, D., 671
Cao, D.-F., 125
Cao, X.-M., 759
Cao, Y.-C., 221
Cao, Y.-N., 367
Che, Z.-M., 671
Chen, C., 705
Chen, G., 181
Chen, H., 85, 353
Chen, J.-G., 149, 253, 501, 619
Chen, L.-M., 533
Chen, N., 759
Chen, P., 3, 7, 45, 167, 173, 227
Chen, R.-X., 811
Chen, T., 137
Chen, W.-B., 811
Chen, X.-X., 829
Chen, X.-Z., 231
Chen, Y.-L., 811
Cheng, F., 277
Cheng, X.-F., 403
Cheng, X.-L., 221
Chi, Q., 193
Chiang, J.K., 469
Chu, C.-C., 469
Chu, L., 317
Cui, G.-H., 587
Cui, S.-Y., 93
Cui, X.-Y., 461
Cui, Y., 187

Dai, B.-G., 525
Debnath, S., 13
Deng, H., 733, 805
Deng, J.-J., 475
Deng, Y.-L., 199, 559, 565, 749
Ding, C., 449

Ding, Y.-F., 93
Dong, S.-F., 587
Dong, Y.-H., 421
Dou, J., 733, 805
Du, L., 181
Du, P.-G., 341, 663
Du, X., 79
Du, X.-X., 513, 623

Fan, J.-R., 79
Fan, X.-T., 149, 501
Fan, Y.-B., 89
Fan, Z., 317
Fan, Z.-L., 713
Fang, J.-M., 811

Gan, Q.-Z., 571
Gao, D.-S., 237
Gao, D.-Y., 317
Gao, G., 607
Gao, L.-H., 737
Gao, S.-M., 137
Gao, W., 701
Gao, X.-J., 687
Gao, Z., 449
Ge, M.-H., 181
Ge, N., 481
Ge, X.-G., 821
Gong, D.-C., 277
Gong, H.-W., 79, 85
Gong, J.-H., 543
Gong, R., 265
Gu, J.-J., 701
Gu, Y.-F., 203
Guan, Q.-X., 323, 331, 357
Guan, X.-Y., 505
Guo, C.-J., 613
Guo, D.-L., 793
Guo, G., 93
Guo, L., 51, 299
Guo, L.-J., 289
Guo, Q., 265
Guo, S.-D., 667
Guo, X., 713
Guo, X.-S., 357
Guo, Y.-R., 733, 805
Guo, Z.-Y., 207

Han, J., 421
Han, J.-S., 677
Han, L.-Q., 587
Han, T., 727
Han, W.-F., 671
Han, X., 341
Han, Y.-D., 167, 227
Hao, Y.-H., 461
Hazra, B., 13
He, B.-W., 391
He, H.-B., 277
He, H.-K., 641
He, J., 177
He, J.-C., 415
He, J.-T., 187, 409, 529
He, Y.-Q., 19
Hong, J., 181
Hou, C.-J., 305
Hou, Q.-X., 283, 595
Hou, W.-Y., 125
Hou, X.-M., 69
Hu, C., 495
Hu, D.-D., 293
Hu, H.-B., 657, 723
Hu, H.-S., 657
Hu, S.-L., 683
Hu, X., 317
Hua, R.-M., 311
Huang, F.-J., 443
Huang, G.-Q., 125
Huang, X., 115, 181
Huang, X.-W., 539
Huo, D.-Q., 305

Ji, Y.-B., 759
Jia, H., 149, 253, 501
Jia, L.-L., 277
Jia, X.-R., 385
Jiang, D.-Y., 465
Jiang, H., 385
Jiang, L., 79, 311, 671
Jiang, L.-L., 51
Jiang, M., 63
Jiang, S., 341
Jiang, T.-Z., 143, 697
Jiang, W., 403
Jiang, W.-H., 521, 591

Jiang, X.-Z., 259
Jiang, Y., 125
Jiang, Y.-G., 155
Jie, L.-X., 727
Jin, G.-L., 277
Jin, X.-D., 461
Jin, Z., 397
Jing, S., 521, 619

Kang, X.-J., 475
Khoo, T.J., 13
Kong, F.-L., 133
Ku, H.-L., 121

Lee, C.-L., 121
Lei, J.-C., 305
Lei, M., 105
Lei, R.-X., 551, 783
Li, A.-J., 641
Li, A.-N., 683
Li, B., 719
Li, F., 577
Li, H., 149, 253, 501, 619
Li, J., 733
Li, J.-J., 533
Li, J.-Y., 79
Li, K., 227, 421
Li, K.-Q., 641
Li, L., 249
Li, L.-F., 347
Li, M.-J., 461
Li, N., 465
Li, P.-F., 51
Li, Q.-S., 69
Li, R., 63
Li, S., 653
Li, S.-M., 481
Li, T.-B., 93
Li, W.-L., 587
Li, X., 525
Li, X.-L., 211, 525
Li, X.-Z., 775
Li, Y., 125, 283, 317, 495, 595
Li, Y.-B., 215, 571
Li, Y.-J., 305
Li, Y.-M., 75
Li, Y.-Q., 93
Li, Y.-Y., 421, 805
Li, Z.-C., 705
Li, Z.-S., 187
Li, Z.-Z., 203
Liang, C.-T., 99
Liang, F., 45, 173
Liang, J.-Q., 415
Liang, J.-S., 763
Liang, S.-W., 99, 323, 357, 705
Liang, T.-G., 69

Liang, X.-S., 203
Liang, Y.-B., 759
Lin, F.-K., 559
Lin, H.-B., 671
Lin, J.-X., 323
Lin, L., 25
Lin, S.-Y., 693
Liu, B., 705
Liu, C.-J., 221
Liu, D.-L., 713
Liu, H., 283, 595, 727, 799
Liu, H.-M., 543
Liu, H.-Q., 347
Liu, J., 243, 581
Liu, J.-M., 737
Liu, J.-N., 551, 783
Liu, K.-G., 89
Liu, L., 733
Liu, Q.-C., 57
Liu, Q.-L., 283, 595
Liu, S., 821
Liu, S.-N., 109
Liu, W.-C., 85
Liu, X.-J., 505
Liu, Y., 143, 687, 701
Liu, Y.-C., 551, 783
Liu, Y.-H., 627
Liu, Y.-X., 109
Liu, Z.-H., 89, 743
Lu, A.-P., 63
Lu, J.-H., 85
Lu, J.-Y., 603
Lu, L., 323, 331, 357
Lu, Y., 13
Lu, Z.-T., 455
Lu, Z.-W., 427
Lui, H.-Y., 529
Lun, Y.-Z., 193
Luo, G.-C., 603
Luo, X.-G., 305
Lv, A., 391
Lv, H.-Q., 231
Lv, L., 317
Lv, X.-F., 749
Lv, Y.-X., 161

Ma, C., 243, 713
Ma, D.-P., 783
Ma, J., 129, 133
Ma, J.-G., 435
Ma, L., 475
Ma, X.-M., 283
Mang, J., 187, 409, 529
Manoharan, A., 373
Mei, C.-L., 409
Meng, H., 39
Meng, L., 539, 577

Meng, Y., 671
Miao, M., 155
Miao, M.-S., 51, 299
Miao, Y., 367
Miao, Z.-M., 653
Ming, Z.-J., 155
Mu, X.-M., 133

Nian, H.-J., 533
Niu, H.-Q., 265
Niu, L.-L., 539, 577

Ou, Y., 753
Ouyang, J.-M., 215, 571

Pan, F., 449
Pan, Y.-H., 45, 167, 173
Peng, J., 177
Peng, L., 559, 565
Pu, S.-P., 177

Qazzaz, M., 13
Qi, A.-R., 481
Qi, C., 821
Qian, M., 539
Qin, F.-Q., 495
Qin, H.-L., 277
Qin, J.Y.-X., 237
Qin, X.-J., 69
Qing, H., 199, 559, 565, 749
Qiu, W.-B., 693
Qiu, X.-D., 623
Qiu, Y.-H., 155
Qiu, Y.-W., 687
Qu, H.-Y., 79

Rao, Y.-T., 599
Ren, Y.-W., 3, 7
Rong, S.-Z., 461
Rong, Y.-Q., 99
Rong, Y.-Y., 323, 331
Ruan, H.-L., 603

Shao, Y.-K., 187, 409, 529
Shen, K.-W., 475
Shen, Y.-L., 737
Shi, H.-H., 63
Shi, L., 737
Shi, W.-L., 367
Shi, W.-M., 347
Soliman, S.S.M., 775
Song, C.-P., 211
Song, D.-X., 759
Song, H.-W., 713
Song, J., 713
Song, Y.-L., 137
Srichan, T., 13

Sui, C.-H., 587
Sun, G., 109
Sun, H.-X., 253, 501
Sun, J., 753
Sun, J.-H., 149, 253, 501, 517
Sun, W., 591
Sun, W.-J., 75, 149, 501, 513, 521, 619, 623
Sun, Y., 99, 125
Sun, Y.-F., 221
Sun, Z., 397

Tan, X., 57
Tan, Y., 249
Tang, Y., 379
Tang, Y.-J., 653
Tian, J., 31
Tian, L.-M., 265
Tian, S., 51
Tian, X.-F., 317
Tian, Y.-X., 323
Tong, D., 391

Ullah, K., 559, 565

Voravuthikunchai, S.P., 13

Wan, S.-J., 385
Wang, A.-X., 687
Wang, C., 89
Wang, C.-M., 149, 253, 501, 513
Wang, D.-K., 125
Wang, D.-X., 249
Wang, F., 353, 357
Wang, F.-L., 199
Wang, G.-H., 341, 517
Wang, H.-Q., 663
Wang, H.-W., 277
Wang, H.-Z., 737
Wang, J.-F., 811
Wang, J.-H., 207, 211, 449, 701
Wang, J.-J., 697, 737
Wang, J.-L., 93
Wang, J.-Q., 187, 409, 529
Wang, J.-Z., 449
Wang, L., 125, 397
Wang, L.-R., 63
Wang, M.-L., 283, 595
Wang, N.-L., 89
Wang, P., 421, 533
Wang, Q., 293
Wang, Q.-K., 177
Wang, R., 525
Wang, R.-M., 653
Wang, S., 607, 713
Wang, S.-M., 99, 323, 331, 353, 357, 705

Wang, S.-P., 181
Wang, T.-C., 627
Wang, W., 775
Wang, W.-H., 763
Wang, W.-J., 481
Wang, W.-P., 155
Wang, W.-Q., 293
Wang, X.-D., 31
Wang, X.-H., 199, 749
Wang, X.-Y., 489
Wang, Y., 133, 475
Wang, Y.-B., 353
Wang, Y.-J., 435
Wang, Y.-M., 409
Wang, Y.-T., 409
Wang, Z., 677
Wang, Z.-H., 129
Wang, Z.-Q., 3
Wei, G.-D., 743
Wei, J.-Y., 713
Wei, Q.-G., 427
Wei, X.-X., 551
Wei, Z., 89
Wen, C.-P., 231
Wen, X.-L., 215
Wen, X.-S., 743
Wen, Y., 79, 85
Wiart, C., 13
Wu, C.-W., 331
Wu, H.-C., 3, 7
Wu, H.-Y., 565
Wu, L.-H., 347, 677
Wu, Q., 125
Wu, Q.-H., 461
Wu, X., 93
Wu, X.-C., 581
Wu, X.-X., 475
Wu, Y., 657, 723
Wu, Z.-Z., 443

Xi, W., 277
Xia, F.-J., 647
Xia, G.-H., 265
Xia, Y., 633
Xiao, Y., 161, 539
Xie, B.-J., 559, 565
Xie, D.-M., 627
Xie, F., 283
Xie, Y.-H., 727, 799
Xie, Z.-J., 231
Xie, Z.-X., 627
Xin, Z.-Y., 587
Xing, R.-Q., 713
Xing, X.-F., 277
Xing, Y.-G., 671
Xing, Y.-S., 633
Xu, B., 277

Xu, B.-F., 57
Xu, B.-Q., 89
Xu, C.-R., 759
Xu, G.-Y., 517, 587
Xu, H., 465
Xu, J., 763
Xu, Q.-L., 671
Xu, X.-Y., 551
Xu, Z.-H., 409
Xu, Z.-T., 767
Xu, Z.-X., 187, 529
Xv, G.-Y., 341

Yan, C., 237
Yan, J.-F., 79, 85
Yan, L., 187
Yan, S., 75
Yan, X.-Y., 137
Yang, D., 481
Yang, D.-Y., 89
Yang, F., 331, 599
Yang, H., 403
Yang, H.-M., 367
Yang, L., 775, 821
Yang, L.-L., 259
Yang, M., 305
Yang, S.-D., 481
Yang, W., 455
Yang, W.-A., 495
Yang, W.-D., 719
Yang, X.-P., 243, 581
Yang, Z.-Y., 783
Yao, D.-Z., 633
Yao, J., 391
Yao, J.-H., 317
Yao, X.-J., 551
Ye, J., 753
Ye, R., 379
Ye, X., 237
Ye, Y.-K., 821
Yin, Y.-K., 461
Yin, Y.-L., 775
You, X., 85
Yu, C.-S., 143
Yu, Y., 713
Yu, Y.-B., 687
Yu, Z.-G., 193
Yuan, L., 829
Yuan, S.-L., 525

Zeng, B., 311
Zeng, F., 199
Zhang, C., 259
Zhang, C.-X., 749
Zhang, C.-Y., 253, 501
Zhang, D., 39
Zhang, D.-F., 671

Zhang, H., 115, 293, 767
Zhang, H.-H., 203
Zhang, H.-L., 25
Zhang, H.-M., 641
Zhang, H-X., 799
Zhang, H.-X., 525, 727
Zhang, J., 435, 455
Zhang, J.-C., 799
Zhang, J.-H., 543
Zhang, J.-J., 533
Zhang, L., 533
Zhang, L.-H., 181
Zhang, L.-Y., 265, 367
Zhang, M.-C., 341
Zhang, M.-H., 455, 687
Zhang, P., 627
Zhang, P.-D., 243, 581
Zhang, S.-Z., 293
Zhang, W.-X., 203
Zhang, X.-G., 155
Zhang, X.-W., 783
Zhang, X.-Y., 793

Zhang, Y., 155
Zhang, Y.-L., 713
Zhang, Y.-Q., 143, 743
Zhang, Z.-G., 385
Zhang, Z.-Y., 3, 7
Zhang, Z.-Z., 641
Zhao, D., 115, 759
Zhao, F., 89
Zhao, G.-X., 821
Zhao, H.-S., 767
Zhao, J., 167
Zhao, J.-H., 125, 435
Zhao, J.-Y., 93, 723
Zhao, L., 323, 331, 357, 753
Zhao, L.-Q., 385, 811
Zhao, S.-W., 623
Zhao, W., 115
Zhao, W.-X., 587
Zhao, W.-Y., 623
Zhao, X., 701
Zhao, X.-C., 753
Zhao, Y., 249

Zhen, Z., 687
Zheng, G., 63, 481
Zheng, H.-R., 539, 577
Zheng, X., 115
Zheng, X.-D., 551, 657, 723, 783
Zhong, L., 211
Zhong, R.-G., 283
Zhong, W.-J., 719
Zhou, J.-H., 489
Zhou, J.-Z., 603
Zhou, Q.-W., 641
Zhou, Q.-X., 161
Zhou, S.-D., 701
Zhou, S.-H., 265
Zhou, T., 775
Zhou, Y., 249
Zhou, Y.-H., 385
Zhou, Z., 465
Zhu, H.-H., 775
Zou, X., 427
Zuo, J., 105